W9-BYT-100

PATHOLOGY OF TUMOURS
IN LABORATORY ANIMALS

Volume III – Tumours of the Hamster

THE INTERNATIONAL AGENCY FOR RESEARCH ON CANCER

The International Agency for Research on Cancer (IARC) was established in 1965 by the World Health Assembly, as an independently financed organization within the framework of the World Health Organization. The headquarters of the Agency are at Lyon, France.

The Agency conducts a programme of research concentrating particularly on the epidemiology of cancer and the study of potential carcinogens in the human environment. Its field studies are supplemented by biological and chemical research carried out in the Agency's laboratories in Lyon, and, through collaborative research agreements, in national research institutions in many countries. The Agency also conducts a programme for the education and training of personnel for cancer research.

The publications of the Agency are intended to contribute to the dissemination of authoritative information on different aspects of cancer research. A complete list is printed at the back of this book.

INTERNATIONAL LIFE SCIENCES INSTITUTE

The International Life Sciences Institute (ILSI) was established in 1978 to stimulate and support scientific research and educational programmes related to nutrition, toxicology, and food safety. ILSI promotes the resolution of health and safety issues by encouraging cooperation in these programmes among scientists in universities, industry, and government agencies. ILSI is grateful for the opportunity to collaborate with the International Agency for Research on Cancer in the publication of this volume, which will make an important contribution towards improved interpretations of animal studies.

WORLD HEALTH ORGANIZATION

INTERNATIONAL AGENCY FOR RESEARCH ON CANCER
INTERNATIONAL LIFE SCIENCES INSTITUTE

Pathology of Tumours in Laboratory Animals

Volume III – Tumours of the Hamster

Second Edition

Edited by

V.S. TURUSOV AND U. MOHR

IARC Scientific Publications No. 126

INTERNATIONAL AGENCY FOR RESEARCH ON CANCER
LYON, FRANCE
1996

Published by the International Agency for Research on Cancer,
150 cours Albert Thomas, F-69372 Lyon cedex 08, France

Distributed by Oxford University Press, Walton Street, Oxford, UK OX2 6DP (Fax: +44 1865 267782) and in
the USA by Oxford University Press, 2001 Evans Road, Carey, NC 27513, USA (Fax: +1 919 677 1303).
All IARC publications can also be ordered directly from IARC*Press*
(Fax: +33 72 73 83 02; E-mail: press@iarc.fr).

IARC Library Cataloguing in Publication Data

Pathology of tumours in laboratory animals – – 2nd ed./
    editors, V.S. Turusov, U. Mohr
    Contents: v. 2. Tumours of the hamster

(IARC Scientific Publications; 126)

1. Hamsters   2. Neoplasms – pathology   3. Rodent diseases – pathology
I. Turusov, V.S. II. Mohr, U. III. Series

ISBN 92 832 2126 5   (NLM Classification: QZ 206)
ISSN 0300–5085

Printed in the United Kingdom

CONTENTS

FOREWORD

Alongside its activities in descriptive and analytical epidemiology and in evaluation of carcinogenicity of chemical and other risk factors, IARC has always carried out a programme of laboratory research. An important component of this work has been the use of animal models in studies of carcinogenesis, and one outcome was the publication, between 1973 and 1982, of the series of volumes on Pathology of Tumours in Laboratory Animals. These volumes have been extensively in demand and are referred to widely.

The hamster is not as widely used in carcinogenicity testing as the mouse and the rat. Nevertheless, it remains a very useful model for studies in many fields of experimental carcinogenesis and provides valuable information for comparative pathology and virology. New findings have been incorporated wherever possible and relevant, so as to ensure that this series, of which this is the third and last volume, reflects the latest developments in this area of research.

IARC is particularly grateful to Dr Vladimir Turusov, who initiated and guided the first edition through to publication, and to Dr Ulrich Mohr for their great efforts in compilation and checking of the large amount of material included in this new edition. The Agency is also pleased to be associated on this occasion with the International Life Sciences Institute, which has jointly sponsored the publication with IARC.

Paul Kleihues, M.D.
Director, IARC

INTRODUCTION

The series Pathology of Tumours in Laboratory Animals was initiated by the International Agency for Research on Cancer almost 30 years ago, and the three volumes (tumours of the rat, part 1 and part 2, tumours of the mouse and tumours of the hamster) appeared in 1973, 1976, 1979 and 1982 respectively.

In 1987 the Agency started preparing a new edition of the series. The first volume of the second edition, tumours of the rat, appeared in 1990 and the second on tumours of the mouse in 1994.

The present volume differs considerably from the first edition that appeared in 1982. The chapter in the first edition that covered all the organs of the alimentary tract has been replaced with separate chapters each describing the tumours of the major parts of this system: the oral cavity with the oesophagus and forestomach, the glandular stomach, and the intestines. New chapters are included on tumours of the nasal cavity and tumours of the gallbladder. On the other hand, tumours of the pituitary gland, thyroid gland, the parathyroid gland and the adrenal gland, subjects of separate chapters in the first edition, are now brought together in one chapter covering the tumours of the endocrine system. Likewise, tumours of the integumentary scent gland, previously an independent chapter, are now included with tumours of the skin. Considerable changes have also been made in the authorship of the volume. New authors are responsible for eleven of the chapters, and have joined with the original authors in several others. These changes mean that this is effectively a new book, by no means simply an update of the first edition.

The structure of each chapter in the first edition (normal structure of the organ in question, classification, morphology and biology of tumours, spontaneous tumours, methods of induction, comparative aspects, references and illustrations) has been largely retained. The contributors were asked to describe – or at least to mention – all tumours that have been reported to occur in the organ concerned. Although the terminology proposed by WHO for human tumours has been used wherever possible, a list of the most widely used synonyms is included, as many different terms have been applied for almost every tumour, particularly across different species.

This volume has been prepared in the hope of providing service and help to experimental pathologists working with the hamster. The editors would be grateful for any criticisms, missing references or pathological or photographic material that can be taken into consideration in any future editions.

Editors: V.S. Turusov
U. Mohr

CONTRIBUTORS

Dr P. Bannasch
Institute for Experimental Pathobiology
German Cancer Research Center
Im Neuenheimer Feld
6900 Heidelberg
Germany

Dr S. W. Barthold
Yale University School of Medicine
Section of Comparative Medicine
333 Cedar Street
P.O. Box 3333
New Haven, CT 06510
USA

Dr L.D. Berman
Mallory Institute of Pathology
784 Massachusetts Avenue
Boston, MA 02118
USA

Dr A. Cardesa
Department of Anatomic Pathology
Hospital Clinic
University of Barcelona Medical School
Villarroel 170
08036 Barcelona
Spain

Dr F. Cruz-Sanchez
Department of Anatomic Pathology
Hospital Clinic
University of Barcelona Medical School
Villarroel 170
08036 Barcelona
Spain

Dr D.L. Dungworth
Department of Veterinary Pathology
University of California
Davis, CA 95616
USA

Dr H. Ernst
Fraunhofer-Institut für Toxikologie und
  Aerosolforschung
3000 Hannover 61
 Germany

Dr M. Emura
Institut für Experimentelle Pathologie
Medizinische Hochschule Hannover
3000 Hannover 61
Germany

Dr P.L. Fernandez
Department of Pathology,
Hospital Clinic
University of Barcelona Medical School
Villarroel 170
08036 Barcelona
Spain

Dr S. Fukushima
First Department of Pathology
Osaka City University Medical School
1-4-54 Asahi-machi,
Abeno-ku
Osaka 545
Japan

Dr F.N. Ghadially
Department of Laboratory Medicine
Ottawa Civic Hospital
1053 Carling Avenue
Ottawa
Canada K1Y 4E9

Dr R. Ghadially
Department of Dermatology
University of California at San Francisco
Veterans Administration Medical Center
San Francisco, CA
USA

Dr B. Gorin (deceased)

Dr A. Hagiwara
Department of Pathology
Nagoya City University Medical School
1 Kawasumi
Mizuho-cho
Mizuho-ku
Nagoya 467
Japan

Dr K. Hakoi
Department of Pathology
Nagoya City University Medical School
1 Kawasumi
Mizuho-cho
Mizuho-ku
Nagoya 467
Japan

Dr G.B. Hubbard
Department of Laboratory Animal Medicine
Southwest Foundation for Biomedical Research
P.O. Box 28147
San Antonio, TX 78228-0147
USA

Dr K. Kamino
Institut für Experimentelle Pathologie
Medizinische Hochschule Hannover
3000 Hannover 61
Germany

Dr T. Kato
Department of Pathology
Nagoya City University Medical School
1 Kawasumi
Mizuho-cho
Mizuho-ku
Nagoya 467
Japan

Dr A. D. Kelman
Departments of Pathology and Microbiology,
Boston University School of Medicine,
Boston, MA,
USA

Dr D.J. Kim
Chemotherapy Division
National Cancer Center Research Institute
5-1-1 Tsukiji, Chuo-ku,
Tokyo 104
Japan

Dr Y. Kurata
First Department of Pathology
Nagoya City University Medical School
1 Kawasumi
Mizuho-cho
Mizuho-ku
Nagoya 467
Japan

Professor U. Mohr
Institut für Experimentelle Pathologie
Medizinische Hochschule Hannover
D-3000 Hannover 61
Germany

Dr M. A. Moore
Department of Pathology
Nagoya City University Medical School
1 Kawasumi
Mizuho-cho
Mizuho-ku
Nagoya 467
Japan

Dr F.K. Mostofi
Department of Veterinary Pathology
Armed Forces Institute of Pathology
6825 16th Street NW
Washington, DC 20306-6000
USA

Dr H. Okamiya
Department of Pathology
National Institute of Hygienic Sciences
Kamiyoga 1-18-1
Setagaya-ku
Tokyo 158
Japan

Dr J.M. Pletcher
Department of Veterinary Pathology
Armed Forces Institute of Pathology
6825 16th Street NW
Washington, DC 20306-6000
USA

Dr P.M. Pour
Eppley Institute for Research in Cancer and Allied
  Disease
Department of Microbiology
University of Nebraska Medical Center
600 South 42nd Street,
Omaha, NR 68198-6805
USA

Dr J.L. Ribas
Department of Genitourinary Pathology
Armed Forces Institute of Pathology
Washington, DC, 20306-6000
USA

Dr R. E. Schmidt
Zoo/Exotic Pathology Service
2825 Kovr Drive
West Sacramento, CA 95605
USA

Dr H. M. Schüller
Experimental Oncology Laboratory
Department of Pathology
College of Veterinary Medicine
University of Tennessee
P.O. Box 1071
Knoxville, TN 37901–1071
USA

Dr M.-A. Shibata
First Department of Pathology
Nagoya City University Medical School
1 Kawasumi
Mizuho-cho
Mizuho-ku
Nagoya 467
Japan

Dr M. Takahashi
Department of Pathology
National Institute of Hygienic Sciences
Kamiyoga 1-18-1
Setagaya-ku
Tokyo 158
Japan

Dr W. Thamavit
Department of Pathology
Faculty of Science
Mahido University
Rama VI
Bangkok 10400
Thailand

Dr T. Tomioka
Eppley Institute for Research in Cancer and Allied
    Disease
Department of Pathology
University of Nebraska Medical Center
Omaha, Nebraska 68105
USA

Dr H. Tsuda
Chemotherapy Division
National Cancer Center Research Institute
5-1-1 Tsukiji, Chuo-ku
Tokyo 104
Japan

Dr V.S. Turusov
Cancer Research Centre of the Academy of
    Medical Sciences
Kashirskoye Shosse, 24
115478 Moscow
Russia

Dr G. M. ZuRhein
Department of Pathology and Laboratory of
    Medicine
University of Wisconsin Medical Center
1300 University Avenue
Madison, Wisconsin 53706
USA

REVIEWERS

M. Aufderheide   Medizinische Hochschule Hannover, Institut für
Experimentelle Pathologie, Hanover, Germany

P. Bannasch   Abteilung für Cytopathologie, Deutsches Krebs-
forschungszentrum, Heidelberg, Germany

C.C. Capen   Department of Veterinary Biosciences, Ohio State
University, Columbus, OH, USA

W.W. Carlton   Department of Veterinary Pathobiology, Purdue University,
School of Veterinary Medicine, West Lafayette, IN, USA

D.L. Dungworth   Department of Veterinary Pathology, University of
California, Davis, CA, USA

H. Ernst   Fraunhofer-Institut für Toxikologie und Aerosolforschung,
Hanover, Germany

G.C. Hard   American Health Foundation, Valhalla, NY, USA

C.F. Hollander   Laboratoires Merck Sharp & Dohme-Chibret, Riom, France

G.J. Krinke   Ciba-Geigy AG, Basle, Germany

E. Kunze   Pathologisches Institut der Universität Göttingen,
Göttingen, Germany

F J.C Roe   Roe Partners Pathtox Services, London, UK

C. Zurcher   IVVO – TNO, Leiden, The Netherlands

Tumours of the skin

F.N. GHADIALLY AND R. GHADIALLY

Since the first historic production of tumours of the rabbit skin by Yamagiva & Ishikawa (1918), cancer research workers have extended the study of cutaneous carcinogenesis to a number of other animal species. Cutaneous carcinogenesis has many attractions, perhaps the most important being the fact that the skin provides an opportunity for easy, continuous and accurate observation of its lesions as does no other organ, and that tumours can be raised here not only by a large variety of chemicals but also by various physical and biological agents.

Of the animal species recently added to the list of those used for cutaneous carcinogenesis, the hamster stands out as undoubtedly the most important. At least three points set the hamster apart from other species: (1) it has a costovertebral spot in which tumours can be raised by hormonal means (Kirkman & Dodge, 1982); (2) it has small pigmented spots in the skin (comprising networks of melanocytes around some of the hair follicles), from which melanotic tumours can be readily produced; and (3) it has a cheek pouch, which can be exteriorized and used as a glabrous area for carcinogenesis, so that one may compare tumours arising from hairy and non-hairy epithelia.

In common with the skin of many laboratory rodents, hamster skin also yields a crop of epithelial and mesenchymal tumours of various types. These include keratoacanthomas, papillomas, squamous cell carcinomas, sebaceous adenomas, basal cell tumours, dermatofibromas and dermatofibrosarcomas. The commonest of the epithelial tumours produced in the skin by chemical carcinogenesis bears a close morphological and behavioural resemblance to the keratoacanthoma of man. Studies of these tumours in rabbit (Whitely, 1957; Ghadially, 1958b), mouse, hamster (Ghadially, 1959), rat (Ghadially, 1961), hedgehog (Ghadially, 1960a), chicken (Rigdon, 1959), duck (Rigdon, 1956a,b) and man (Ghadially, 1961, 1971, 1975; Ghadially *et al.*, 1963) have shown that these tumours arise from the hair follicles.

The skin with its appendages is a complex dynamic organ, which produces a bewildering variety of tumours. If the histogenesis and behaviour of these tumours is to be understood, one must first recall certain relevant points regarding the biology and morphology of the hair follicles, the small pigmented spots and the costovertebral spots. We shall therefore commence by examining the morphology and function of these structures.

NORMAL STRUCTURE

Hair follicles and cycles of growth

It is now well known that hair growth is discontinuous and occurs in cyclic waves of active growth (hair-growth cycle) followed by periods of quiescence (Montagna, 1956; Montagna & Ellis, 1958). In some animals, such as the hamster, rabbit, rat and mouse, there is a grossly evident hair-growth cycle, seen as bilaterally symmetrical bands of actively growing hair follicles, but in others, such as the guinea-pig and man, no such hair-growth cycle occurs (Whitely & Ghadially, 1954; Ghadially 1957, 1958a). Nevertheless each hair follicle shows an independent cycle of growth and quiescence (hair-follicular cycle). The difference noted between these two groups of animals is due to the fact that in the latter, actively growing and quiescent hair follicles occur side by side in any small area of skin (mosaic pattern), while in the former each variety of follicle is grouped together in large zones (wave pattern).

Thus, except for this difference, there is a fundamental similarity between all of these animals, including man, in that each hair follicle shows cyclic periods of activity (anagen) and rest (telogen). The duration of these periods of rest and activity depends upon the type of hair. Thus, the fine coat hair on the body of hamsters and other laboratory animals usually has a brief anagen and a long telogen, while the coarse vibrissae hair and the hair in the costovertebral spot of the hamster have a long period of anagen and only a brief telogen phase (Ghadially & Barker, 1960; Ghadially, 1958a).

The morphological changes that occur during the hair follicular cycle are best illustrated in whole mounts of hamster skin (Figures 1–3). It will be observed that hair follicles are distributed as regularly spaced groups of follicles in the skin (Figure 1). The hair follicle in telogen (Figure 2) is essentially an epithelial sac containing the hair shaft. At the bottom of the epithelial sac lies the hair germ and the rounded dermal papilla.

The part of the follicle above the hair germ is formed during early life and persists more or less throughout life, so that it may be called the permanent, static, upper or superficial part of the hair follicle. When the active or growth phase (anagen) begins, the cells in the hair germ divide

rapidly to form a sac-like structure that surrounds the dermal papilla to form the hair bulb. The hair follicle now grows and extends downwards to form a large club-shaped structure (Figure 3) many times longer than the resting follicle. A new hair shaft is formed which pushes out or grows alongside the old one. After anagen comes the regression phase (catagen) when the newly formed deeper part of follicle is destroyed and the hair follicle and hair shaft move upwards so that the resting stage (telogen) is reached once more and the follicular cycle completed.

The part of the hair follicle derived from the hair germ may be described as the deeper, lower or transient part of the hair follicle, for it is built up and destroyed in each hair follicular cycle. It is important to distinguish between the deeper transient part of the follicle and the static superficial part, for two morphologically distinct tumours, type-1 and type-2 keratoacanthomas, arise from these sites (Ghadially, 1961). It is also worth noting that the sebaceous glands drain into the superficial part of the follicle, and that the junction between the superficial and deep part lies a little below the attachment of the erector pili muscle.

Small pigmented spots

The term small pigmented spot was coined by us (Ghadially & Barker, 1960) to describe pigmented spots in hamster skin which consist of networks of melanocytes and melanophages surrounding groups of pilosebaceous units (Figures 4 and 5). The term 'small' was used by us to distinguish these pigmented spots, which need a microscope for their demonstration, from the two 'large' grossly visible pigmented spots on the flank of the hamster first described by Kupperman and known as the costovertebral spots, flank organs, or the organs of Kupperman (Figures 6–9).

The discovery of the small pigmented spots stemmed from the following question: why are melanotic tumours so commonly and consistently produced in hamster skin painted with carcinogens, while in innumerable other animals, such as mice, rabbits and rats, that have been painted melanotic tumours occur extremely rarely or not at all?

It seemed to us that there could well be an anatomical difference between the skin of the hamster and that of other animals. Further, the fact that no such difference had been noted previously suggested that naked eye inspection of the skin or routine haematoxylin and eosin stained sections from randomly collected samples of skin would be unlikely to reveal any such difference, if it existed. Thus the idea of examining the entire skin covering the trunk as a whole skin mount was born. In such a preparation the small pigmented spots are easily visualized (for the technique of preparing whole mounts, see Ghadially & Barker, 1960) and their number and distribution readily appreciated.

It must be noted that the melanin-containing cells of the small pigmented spot occur only around a few of the innumerable groups of hair follicles in hamster skin and, as such these spots are rarely encountered in routine histological sections from unselected portions of skin. Even when a small pigmented spot is included in the section, only a few melanocytes are visualized and not the whole network, so that the true morphology and size of this structure is not appreciated. The actual number of small pigmented spots in the skin is very variable. Thus we have found that more spots occur with increasing age and also at any given age, females have more spots than males (Ghadially & Illman, 1966). In keeping with this is the observation that there is a marked increase in the size and number of small pigmented spots in hamsters treated with estrogen (Illman & Ghadially, 1966b). The number of spots that can be detected is also related to the hair-growth cycle. Thus the spots are readily found around hair follicles in telogen but not in

anagen except in very old animals, where a few small pigmented spots can be found around hair follicles in early anagen.

Coat colour also influences the small pigmented spots (Illman & Ghadially, 1960). The original Syrian hamster, as described by Waterhouse (1839) and Ahavoni (1932), is an agouti animal which is often referred to as the golden or brown hamster. Two well-known spontaneous mutations are the white and cream varieties. The white is not a true albino as it has black pigment in the eyes, scrotal skin and ear tips. Only an occasional small pigmented spot is found in the cream variety, but none are seen in the white hamster. However, there is ample evidence that in the white hamster networks of amelanotic melanocytes exist in this situation, and that the failure to detect the spots is due to an absence of pigment and not of melanocytes.

Ghadially and Illman (1963, 1966) also found small pigmented spots in two other species of hamsters. In the skin of the Chinese hamster (*Cricetulus criceus*), which is less than half the size of the Syrian hamster, only an occasional small pigmented spot similar to those in Syrian hamsters is seen, but many diffuse melanocytic networks are seen in the dermis. The European hamster (*Cricetus cricetus*) is 2–3 times larger than the Syrian hamster. Its skin contains numerous small pigmented spots similar to those seen in the Syrian hamster. Quevedo *et al.* (1968) have found small pigmented spots in the skin of the Mongolian gerbil.

The costovertebral spot

The costovertebral spot, flank organ or organ of Kupperman (1944) is a paired organ easily seen with the naked eye on the flank of the hamster after the hair has been removed (Figure 6). It is a black, slightly raised spot about 0.5 cm in diameter, composed of giant sebaceous glands discharging into large hair follicles (Figures 7 and 8). The follicles produce coarse hair which seems to grow continuously (long anagen, brief telogen). Melanocytic networks abound around the necks of these hair follicles. The remarkable size and extent of these is best visualized in whole mounts of skin (Figure 9). In hamsters under 10 days old, the spot appears as a white non-pigmented area which stands out from the surrounding skin (Ghadially & Barker, 1960). As regards function, it has been suggested that the secretion from the costovertebral spot of the male hamster serves to mark territory but that of the female has no such function. The marking is probably effected by a porphyrin-containing secretion from the glands in the costovertebral spot (Illman & Ghadially, 1966a), which in the summer months show a marked red fluorescence in the male animal.

MORPHOLOGY AND BIOLOGY OF TUMOURS

As already noted, the skin of the hamster is unusual in that it yields numerous melanotic tumours during cutaneous carcinogenesis. There is, however, nothing unusual about the epithelial tumours that one can produce in the skin of this animal or which arise spontaneously. Indeed, here one cannot but wonder at the amazing similarity in morphology and behaviour between the tumours raised in this and other animals and certain naturally occurring tumours of human skin. If maximum benefit is to be derived from our studies on cutaneous carcinogenesis in the hamster we must examine the epithelial tumours raised in this animal within this broader framework, and this is what we shall attempt to do.

Comparative experimental and histological studies of cutaneous tumours of man and chemical-carcinogen-induced tumours in a variety of animals including the hamster (Ghadially, 1961) have led to the following conclusions: (1) in spite of morphological differences between the skin of various species of animals, the types of benign epithelial tumours produced are remarkably similar; (2) certain basic tumour patterns can be identified, and it can be shown that each is related to a particular site of origin; (3) a benign tumour which one may call a true or primary papilloma arises from glabrous skin and other glabrous epithelia; (4) a distinctive bud-shaped tumour called type-1 keratoacanthoma arises from the superficial part of the hair follicle. Occasional exfoliation of this tumour produces a secondary papilloma; (5) a deeply placed rounded berry-shaped tumour called type-2 keratoacanthoma arises from the hair germ or deeper part of the hair follicle; (6) occasionally tumours with basal cell differentiation are also seen arising from hair follicles or surface epidermis; (7) a benign tumour called sebaceous adenoma arises from the sebaceous glands in rare instances; (8) at times the carcinogen seems to penetrate deeper and produces fibromas or sarcomas in the dermis; and (9) besides the above-mentioned lesions hamster skin also yields many melanotic tumours which arise from the perifollicular networks of melanocytes. Some of the concepts summarized above are illustrated by means of symbolic figures in the accompanying diagram. In the description which follows, the stages of development of the various tumours will be illustrated with the aid of this diagram and the corresponding histological sections of experimentally produced tumours in animals and naturally occurring tumours in man.

Since we are here concerned mainly with tumours of hamster skin, I have included a large number of examples of tumours raised in this animal by 7,12-dimethylbenz[a]anthracene (DMBA), but in order to emphasize the remarkable similarity of the lesions in various species, I have also included a few similar tumours which occur in man and which can be produced in other experimental animals.

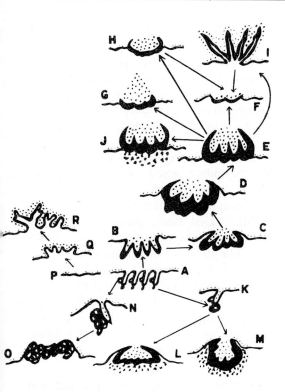

Diagram illustrating the origin and evolution of epithelial tumours. The dotted areas represent keratin; the black areas represent epithelial elements.

Only by such a broad look at the comparative pathology of these tumours can one hope to understand their histogenesis, development and behaviour.

Histological types of tumour

Epithelial tumours

    Papilloma

    Keratoacanthoma

    Squamous cell carcinoma

    Basal cell tumour

    Sebaceous adenoma

Melanotic tumours

Connective tissue tumours

    Dermatofibroma

    Dermatofibrosarcoma

Epithelial tumours

Papilloma

As is well known, this term is used to describe benign epithelial tumours composed essentially of papillary or finger-like processes. Such tumours may occur in hairy or glabrous skin, but the mode of origin in these two sites is different. The true or primary papilloma is the classical tumour of glabrous skin and many other epithelia (e.g., urinary bladder, and epithelium of various ducts). Such primary papillomas have been produced by testosterone in the skin of goldfish (Ghadially & Whitely, 1952), by 3-methylcholanthrene (MC) in the web of the ducks foot (Rigdon, 1956b) and by (DMBA) on the squamous epithelium of the exteriorized hamster cheek pouch (Ghadially & Illman, 1961) (Figures 10–18).

The hairy skin of hamsters and other animals painted with carcinogens rarely if ever yields primary papillomas. Indeed, there is very little surface epithelium between the hair follicles from which such tumours can originate. As will be shown later (p. 8), the papillomas of the hairy skin are produced by exfoliation of a type-1 keratoacanthoma. We therefore refer to these as secondary papillomas. It is now well known that chemical carcinogens enter the skin via the hair follicles and that they are retained there for a considerable period, while carcinogen lying on the surface is soon lost (Berenblum *et al.*, 1958; Suntzeff *et al.*, 1955). Under such circumstances it seems inevitable that, in a race between the hair follicle and the superficial epidermis to produce a tumour, the hair follicle is likely to win. The experimental and clinical evidence for the hair follicular origin of many cutaneous tumours is now overwhelming and has already been discussed in detail in previous papers so will not be dealt with here (Ghadially, 1961; Ghadially *et al.*, 1963a).

However, tumours of carcinogen-painted skin have so often been confused and considered identical to those arising from glabrous epithelia that it is worth looking into this briefly. Twort & Twort (1936) attempted to produce tumours from glabrous skin by forcing mice to tread on carcinogenic oil, but tumours developed quickly on the hairy face råther than on the glabrous skin of the foot pads. The absence of a reasonable stretch of glabrous (both hair- and hair-follicle-free) skin in animals commonly employed for carcinogenesis studies has for long thwarted experiments of this kind.

The hamster, however, has provided a partial solution to this problem, for when its cheek pouch is exteriorized (Figures 10–12) and used to replace an area from which the normal skin has been excised, we obtain an area of squamous epithelium free of hair follicles which shares the same external environment as skin and soon becomes keratinized and comes to resemble skin. If such an area is painted with carcinogens, true papillomas (Figures 13 and 14) are produced which are quite distinct and different from the kerato-acanthomas of hair follicular origin which arise from the hair follicles in surrounding skin.

In this experiment also the greater susceptibility to carcinogenesis of hair follicles and hence of hairy skin is clearly demonstrated, for tumours invariably arise much faster and in greater numbers on adjacent skin than on the exteriorized pouch epithelium, however carefully the carcinogen is applied to the cheek pouch. This observation and that of Twort & Twort (1936) are in keeping with human experience, for in tar workers also, tumours occur on the hairy skin on the dorsum of the hand and forearm råther than on the palm which comes in more direct contact with the tumour-producing agent.

The manner in which papillomas arise from the glabrous epithelium of the cheek pouch (is illustrated in the diagram on page 5 (P, Q, R) and Figures 15–18. The basic principles of this process have been known to pathologists (Willis, 1967) for a long time. Briefly, it appears that cellular proliferation engendered by the neo-plastic process produces an elongation and thickening of the epithelium, which is then thrown into a series of folds so as to accommodate itself in a given space. Increasingly complex folding ultimately produces a projecting, branched, sessile or pedunculated mass, which may or may not be well keratinized (Figures 13 and 14). Malignant transformation to squamous cell carcinoma also sometimes occurs. The transition from a benign to a malignant type of epithelium is quite abrupt (Figures 17 and 18), a point in keeping with our experience of human papillomas and adenomas which became malignant.

The fact that true metastasizing squamous cell carcinoma can be produced from the hair-free epithelium of the cheek pouch clearly shows that hair follicles are not a prerequisite for the production of squamous cell carcinoma. It would, however, be illogical to extend this to mean, as some have done in the past, that carcinomas of painted animal skin do not arise from the hair follicles, for all the evidence clearly shows this to be the case.

Keratoacanthoma

This is one of the commonest benign cutaneous tumours of man and experimental animals (including the hamster) painted with carcinogens (Ghadially, 1971). It is believed to arise from the hair follicles. Its main interest lies in the fact that, although its rapid growth and histological appearance may suggest a carcinoma, it frequently regresses spontaneously. In man this tumour has often been mistakenly diagnosed as squamous cell carcinoma and, at times, unnecessarily drastic surgical procedures, such as amputation of a limb, have been performed to treat this condition (Ghadially, 1958b, 1971; Ghadially, *et al.*, 19963a; Belisario, 1959; Lennox, 1960; Vickers & Ghadially, 1961; Webb & Ghadially, 1966). During the active growth phase, this tumour so closely resembles a squamous cell carcinoma that it has been used to illustrate 'typical squamous cell carcinoma' in textbooks, and indeed many student classes in histopathology have been taught the microscopic morphology of squamous cell carcinoma from sections of keratoacanthoma (Lennox, 1960; Ghadially, 1971). Such errors in diagnosis have also grossly exaggerated the recorded cure rates of squamous cell carcinoma in man, and there is ample evidence in the illustrations of many papers that in animal experiments also keratoacanthomas have been falsely reported as squamous cell carcinomas. We, too, have been guilty of the last offence for Figure 12 in an early paper of ours (Whitely & Ghadially, 1951) is almost certainly not a true squamous cell carcinoma!

Two varieties of keratoacanthoma have been identified: type 1 and type 2 (Ghadially, 1961). The former is a bud-shaped tumour which arises from the superficial part of hair follicles (Figures 19–28), the latter a more deeply placed berry-shaped or dome-shaped lesion which arises from the hair germ or deeper part of the hair follicle (Figures 29–37). Although during the early stages these lesions are morphologically distinct, in the later stages of evolution it may be difficult or impossible to distinguish them.

Type-1 keratoacanthoma. Figure 19 illustrates the naked eye appearance of type-1 keratoacanthoma on the nose of a woman and Figure 22 a remarkably similar-looking tumour which arose on the chin of a hamster whose flank had been painted with DMBA. Figures 20, 21 and 23 illustrate the histology of the mature type-1 keratoacanthoma from man, hamster and rabbit. The tumour has convex sides and a central or apical

keratinous mass. Microscopically, it shows irregular papillary processes, which represent walls of modified hair follicles separated by cores of vascular stroma. The genesis and evolution of the type-1 keratoacanthoma is illustrated in the diagram on p. 5 and Figures 19–28. In the diagram, A depicts a portion of skin with a group of hair follicles in telogen. The bud-shaped (type-1) keratoacanthoma arises as a result of a thickening and elongation of the walls of the superficial parts of adjacent hair follicles (B, C and Figure 24). The hair shafts are soon destroyed and the neoplastic epithelium produces keratinous material which accumulates in the central region of the tumour. The mature lesion (D and Figures 20 and 21) has now formed.

During the active growth phase, proliferative activity (as evidenced by numerous mitoses) dominates over differentiation (as evidenced by the amount of keratin formed). This is followed by a static phase when few or no mitoses are seen and few new epithelial cells are formed. Regression is achieved by continuing differentiation of existing epithelial cells into keratin, assisted perhaps by the reaction which occurs at the base of the tumour. The composition of the cellular exudate in the stroma and base is, however, variable. It may be composed almost entirely of lymphocytes and plasma cells, although at times many polymorphonuclear leukocytes are also seen.

As a result of such changes the lesion is progressively forced upwards and/or shrinks upwards and comes to the surface of the skin (E in the diagram on p. 5 and Figure 23). Next, the keratinous plug detaches and either is shed as one compact mass or comes off piecemeal, forming a saucer- or cup-shaped lesion (E, F, G, H in the diagram and Figures 25, 27 and 28), which ultimately disappears, leaving behind a small puckered scar. However, not all lesions regress in this manner. Thus the keratinous mass may build up to form a horn (G). The lesion may ulcerate and/or exfoliate to form a secondary papillomatous mass (I in the diagram and Figure 26). Whatever direction of development the tumour takes, the chances are that it will ultimately regress. However, sometimes, particularly when a horn is formed, these tumours behave in an indolent fashion, showing neither obvious growth nor regression for a considerable period of time.

A feature of great interest and also of considerable practical importance in diagnostic histology is the development of what may be termed pseudocarcinomatous infiltration (J in the diagram and Figure 23). Here we find columns and islands of epithelial cells breaking away from the main body of the tumour and producing a rather regular, limited infiltration of the stroma, mimicking an early well differentiated carcinoma. The distinction between this and true carcinoma will be discussed later.

Type-2 keratoacanthoma. Figures 29–31 illustrate the gross appearance of the type-2 keratoacanthoma in man, hamster and rabbit. When the tumour grows in lax tissue, such as hamster axilla (Figure 30), it is berry-shaped and only a small part of the tumour is seen on the surface. When it rests on a hard surface, such as the cheekbone (Figure 29) or the cartilage of the rabbit ear (Figure 31), it becomes dome-shaped. This rounded lesion has a smooth appearance as it is covered by stretched skin, but this in time ulcerates to release the central keratinous plug which forms in the tumour (Figures 32–37). The origin of this tumour from the hair germ or deeper part of the follicle has been clearly established and illustrated in a variety of animals (Ghadially, 1961). It would appear that cellular proliferation in this region produces the cystic lesion (K, L, M in the diagram on p. 5 and Figures 32–37) we call type-2 keratoacanthoma.

The stages of development are essentially similar to those of type-1 keratoacanthoma. During the growth phase, the tumour shows many mitoses and is predominantly cellular. During regression, the tumour cells differentiate out to form much keratin so that the tumour now shows a large central keratinous plug and a thin cup-shaped zone of epithelium. As a rule the type-2 tumour regresses rapidly, leaving behind a small scar. Pseudo-carcinomatous infiltration is more commonly encountered in type-1 than in type-2 keratoacanthoma.

The significance of the self-regressing behaviour of the keratoacanthomas (types 1 and 2) has been the subject of much speculation. The explanation proposed by us (Whitely, 1957; Ghadially, 1958b, 1961) and supported and elaborated by others (Lennox, 1960; Prutkin & Gerstner, 1966; Fleischmajer *et al.*, 1968; Ramselaar & van der Meer, 1976, 1979; Ramselaar *et al.*, 1980; Flannery & Muller, 1979) may be summarized as follows. It is well known that tumours may retain not only some of the appearances but also the properties and functions of the tissue from which they originate. The type-2 keratoacanthoma shows rapid growth and regression that is frequently complete in a few weeks. This matches well the behaviour of the hair germ and deeper part of the follicle from which the tumour arises. One may therefore suggest that the hair germ, altered by the action of a carcinogen, produces a keratoacanthoma instead of a normal follicle and that the tumour so produced recapitulates in its behaviour the cyclic life history of the deeper part of the hair follicle. In this connection, it is interesting to note that the lesion does not extend much deeper than the level attained by hair follicles in anagen.

The type-1 keratoacanthoma as a rule also regresses, but this is a more tardy process, particularly when it develops into a horn or exfoliates to form a secondary papilloma. Some may become quite indolent and lose the power of spontaneous regression. The superficial part of the hair follicle and epidermis proper do not show the explosive growth pattern of the hair germ, but they do show many cyclic rhythms or activities, which may be diurnal, associated with hormonal changes and the hair growth cycle (Chase *et al.,* 1953; Green & Ghadially, 1951; Ghadially & Green 1957). However, the extent of the morphological alterations produced is quite modest. Thus one may argue that, from tissues showing only modest cyclic changes, there arise tumours (type-1 keratoacanthoma and papilloma) that show a slow or erratic pattern of regression, while the dramatic cyclic activity of the hair germ is matched by the explosive growth and rapid regression of the type-2 keratoacanthoma.

Giant keratoacanthoma. Most keratoacanthomas of man and experimental animals are under 2.5 cm in size. However, much larger lesions called massive or giant keratoacanthoma measuring up to 12 cm in diameter have been recorded in man (Schwartz, 1979) and similar lesions can also be raised in the skin of laboratory animals. On analysis, one finds that these large tumorous masses are in fact composed of multiple confluent keratoacanthomas which have arisen in close proximity to each other. We, and others, have observed and recorded the spontaneous regression of such lesions in man and rabbit (Vickers & Ghadially, 1961; Webb & Ghadially, 1966; Belisario, 1959; Emerson *et al.,* 1971). The situation in the hamster and the mouse has not been studied in such detail, but it is my impression that progressive growth to true squamous cell carcinoma is of somewhat more frequent occurrence in these animals.

The question is often asked whether a keratoacanthoma of man can become malignant. Opinion varies on this point, but one can argue that, since any benign tumour may at times become malignant, the keratoacanthoma is hardly likely to be an exception. An unequivocal answer to this question is difficult for, when a tumour diagnosed as a keratoacanthoma spreads and metastasizes, doubt is automatically raised regarding the accuracy of the initial diagnosis. There is, however, little doubt that the squamous cell carcinoma of painted animal skin arises ultimately from a keratoacanthoma, usually of the type-1 variety.

Ultrastructure of keratoacanthomas. Electron microscopic studies of keratoacanthomas show that the tumour cells contain abundant intracytoplasmic filaments (tonofilaments), some rough endoplasmic reticulum and slightly enlarged nuclei with altered nucleoli. Abundant desmosomes are seen between tumour cells. The nuclear changes and the changes in desmosomes and rough endoplasmic reticulum are worthy of further comment.

During the growth phase of keratoacanthoma, the nucleolus is enlarged and marginated (i.e., it comes to lie close to the nuclear envelope) and at times multiple nucleoli are seen in a nucleus (Ghadially, 1988). Such nucleolar changes are seen in many malignant tumours also, but they are not the hallmark of malignancy (Oberling & Bernhard, 1961). In fact, such changes are no more than an indicator of a state of heightened protein synthesis, necessary to keep pace with new cell production. Thus, for example, when intense protein synthetic activity occurs in the regenerating liver of the rat after partial hepatectomy, 50% of the nucleoli become marginated (Swift, 1959), and Stowell (1949) has shown that nucleoli larger than those occurring in malignant hepatoma can be found in the regenerating rat liver after hepatectomy.

Desmosomes have been seen in many epithelia, but are best developed in squamous epithelia. In keratoacanthoma, desmosomes are plentiful (Fisher *et al.,* 1972) or even markedly increased in numbers (Takati *et al.,* 1971). An increase in numbers of desmosomes is also seen in human warts (Chapman *et al.*, 1963), but there is a loss of structural cohesion and a marked reduction of desmosomes in squamous cell carcinoma.

Of similar interest is the observation that the rough endoplasmic reticulum is better developed in the cells of keratoacanthomas than in those of the normal hair follicles from which these tumours arise (Prutkin, 1967), for generally speaking the rough endoplasmic reticulum in a malignant tumour is poorly developed as compared to its cell of origin (Ghadially, 1985, 1988).

Squamous cell carcinoma

As already pointed out, pseudo-carcinomatous infiltration is frequently associated with keratoacanthoma, and both in man and experimental animal this has often been mistaken for true carcinoma. In the absence of tumour deposit in distant organs or regional lymph nodes, a firm diagnosis of carcinoma may be difficult to uphold. Indeed, it would appear that here more than in any other instance our histological concepts of malignancy are severely tested and at times appear inadequate. As noted earlier, certain ultrastructural differences have been found between keratoacanthoma and squamous cell carcinoma, but their practical value in differential diagnosis remains to be determined.

The problem of distinguishing true carcinoma from the pseudo-carcinomatous infiltration arising at the margins of keratoacanthomas is illustrated by Figures 38–40. Of particular interest is Figure 40, where the resemblance to carcinoma is most marked, and indeed this lesion was at first diagnosed by others as a true carcinoma. This patient developed many small keratoacanthomas on his skin which grew and regressed (Vickers & Ghadially, 1961). He then developed a giant keratoacanthoma, 4.5 cm in diameter. Figure 40 shows the appearance of a

biopsy of this lesion, which regressed spontaneously in two months.

The manner in which the pseudo-carcinomatous infiltration of keratoacanthoma disappears is depicted in Figures 41–44, obtained from rabbit and hamster tumours. In some instances an appearance is created (Figures 41 and 42) as if the tumour cells were being strangled by the accompanying cellular infiltrate and fibrosis. In others, the infiltrating tumour cells seem to disappear largely by differentiating into masses of keratin (Figures 43 and 44).

Figure 45 shows the infiltrating edge of a DMBA-induced squamous cell carcinoma of hamster skin which produced secondary deposits in a lymph node, while Figure 46 shows lymph-node deposits from a DMBA-induced carcinoma of the skin of the hedgehog. The cellular pleomorphism and poor organization are clearly evident (Figures 45 and 46) but are lacking in the pseudo-carcinomatous infiltration of keratoacanthomas shown in Figures 38–44.

Although the distinction between true squamous cell carcinoma and keratoacanthoma may at times be difficult or impossible to make, in most instances it is easy to distinguish them if an adequate specimen is available for study. The points to look for may be summarized as follows. Keratoacanthomas are rounded or compact tumours composed of singularly well-differentiated squamous epithelium which shows little pleomorphism or anaplasia, and has a strong tendency to form masses of keratin. Squamous cell carcinomas even when well-differentiated show more pleomorphism, and keratin production is, comparatively speaking, quite scanty. The pseudo-carcinomatous infiltration of the keratoacanthoma as a rule presents a smooth, regular, well-demarcated front, in contrast to the irregular extensions of a true carcinoma. Such infiltration is of limited extent (depth) and as a rule does not extend beyond the level of the hair follicles and cutaneous glands in the region. A high-power view of the infiltrative zone of a keratoacanthoma during its growth phase may be virtually indistinguishable from a similar view of true carcinoma, but in later stages the presence of cellular infiltrate and marked stromal fibrosis assists the diagnosis of keratoacanthoma. Further, at this stage, the epithelial cells themselves show no proliferative activity and in fact are found to be in various stages of degeneration, necrosis and dissolution.

The occurrence of mitoses in these tumours must be interpreted with caution. As one would expect in young lesions in the growth phase, numerous mitotic figures are found but this must not allow one to be persuaded that the lesion is a carcinoma. Closer examination will reveal that these are only bipolar mitoses of normal appearance, and not the bizarre multipolar ones characteristic of true squamous cell carcinoma. In older lesions which are in the static or regressive phase it is difficult to find a single mitotic figure.

An interesting difference between squamous cell carcinoma and benign lesions of human skin is that the former fluoresce red under ultraviolet radiation, while the latter rarely do so. Opinion has varied regarding the value of this 'live coal' fluorescence in the diagnosis of these lesions. Some have found this phenomenon specific enough to be useful in the diagnosis of squamous cell carcinoma, while others have cast doubts regarding both the specificity and usefulness of this phenomenon (Belisario, 1959).

A study (Ghadially, 1960b) involving a large number of experimentally produced skin tumours in the hamster, rabbit, mouse and hedgehog has shown that ulcerated squamous cell carcinomas invariably show a brilliant red fluorescence, while only a rare benign epithelial tumour shows a weak red fluorescence. It is now clear that the red fluorescence is due to the presence of protoporphyrin, which lies on the surface but not in the substance of the carcinoma (Ghadially & Neish, 1960). It would appear that the porphyrin is produced by the growth of certain organisms, such as *Staphylococcus pyogenes* and *Escherichia coli,* on the ulcerated surface of the carcinoma. Such organisms, when grown on blood agar to which δ-aminolaevulinic acid is added, produce colonies which also show an intense red fluorescence (Ghadially *et al.,* 1963b). This suggests that the red fluorescence of squamous cell carcinoma is due to the action of bacteria on a protoporphyrin precursor derived from the tumour and/or its host.

Basal cell tumour

Tumours composed of cells resembling basal cells of the epidermis and its appendages occur in man, and also in animals painted with carcinogens. Such tumours show many morphological variations. The best known of these is the rodent ulcer or basal cell carcinoma of man.

In the minds of many, the etiology of basal cell carcinoma is firmly linked with solar radiation. It is not too well known that basal cell tumours also occur in the skin of man exposed to carcinogenic hazards and animal skin painted with carcinogens. Little is known about the factors which determine whether a tumour of basal or squamous differentiation will arise in painted skin. It is possible that the carcinogen used may be a factor, for rat skin painted with 2-anthramine (2-aminoanthracene) produces quite a crop of basal cell tumours (Lennox, 1955). The same carcinogen has been reported to produce squamous cell tumours and adnexal tumours in the hamster, but the exact nature of the latter was not mentioned (Shubik *et al.,* 1960). Basal cell tumours have been produced in hamster skin following application of benzo-[*a*]pyrene (BP) dissolved in carbo-wax and water (Schinz & Fritz-Niggli, 1954).

From my experience of painting a variety of species of animals with DMBA, I am more impressed with the species differences. In the rabbit and mouse, basal cell tumours are very rarely produced, but a few are almost always encountered when rats or hamsters are painted with DMBA. It is also my impression that when the carcinogenic stimulus is weak (low dose and/or fewer applications) and tumour production tardy, basal cell carcinomas are likely to be produced. However, further work is needed to test the validity or otherwise of such impressions. The hamster seems to be ideally suited for such studies for in my experience this animal more than any other is highly prone to basal cell tumour production. All the basal cell tumours illustrated here (Figures 47–52) were produced in hamster skin by DMBA (Ghadially, unpublished data).

Figure 47 shows a basal cell tumour where the tumour architecture and small size of basal cell are well contrasted with the squamous differentiation of an adjacent keratoacanthoma, a part of which is also included in the picture for comparison. Basal cell tumours of man often contain a variety of other cells besides basal cells, such as clear cells, sebaceous cells and cells showing squamous differentiation. This is also the case in some of the hamster tumours (Figure 48).

The hamster tumour shown in Figure 49 is reminiscent of the so-called 'cystic rodent ulcer' of man, for here we have a lesion the wall of which (Figure 50) contains basal cells showing palisading and also cells of sebaceous differentiation adjacent to the cavity of the cyst. In Figure 51 we have an ulcerated tumour apparently arising from the surface of hamster skin which may be considered the equivalent of the rodent ulcer or multiple superficial small basal cell carcinomas known to occur in human skin. The hamster tumour in Figure 52 contains basal cells surrounding numerous small and large hair follicles, some of which are probably produced by the tumour. This tumour could therefore be considered the equivalent of the trichoepithelioma of man.

Sebaceous adenoma

This is a rare tumour of human skin and it is also rarely seen during cutaneous carcinogenesis. The two tumours illustrated here are the only ones that we have raised in the many hamsters painted with DMBA. Their origin in the sebaceous glands is clearly demonstrated in the early lesion depicted in Figure 53. Further growth of the tumour displaces and destroys adjacent structures, so that the site of origin is no longer evident. The tumour then appears as a lobulated structure composed of irregular islands of neoplastic sebaceous tissue (Figure 54).

Melanotic tumours

Perhaps the most fascinating aspect of cutaneous carcinogenesis in the hamster is the ease with which melanotic tumours can be raised in the skin of this animal. Prior to the first production of such tumours by Della Porta *et al.* (1965a,b) one had come to regard the melanocyte as a cell resistant to attack by chemical carcinogens. True, a few melanotic tumours had been seen in mice and other animals painted with carcinogens, but the extreme rarity of such reports among the countless studies on cutaneous carcinogenesis seemed only to add weight to this idea.

As pointed out earlier, it was this discrepancy of response between the skin of the hamster and other animals to chemical carcinogens which led to the search for and discovery of the small pigmented spots and their perifollicular network of melanocytes from which the melanotic tumours arise (Ghadially & Barker, 1960). It seems now that the susceptibility of the hamster and the resistance of other species to melanotic tumour production can be explained by simple mechanistic concepts, such as the anatomical position of the melanocytes and the entry of carcinogen via the hair follicles, rather than by any intrinsic immunity or susceptibility of the melanocyte to chemical carcinogenic stimulation.

Melanotic tumours have been produced by painting hamster skin with DMBA, MC, dibenz[*a*]anthracene, 4-nitroquinoline 1-oxide, β-propiolactone and urethane. The last-named carcinogen is also effective when injected into or fed to the animal.

Nomenclature. A melanoma is a tumour of melanocytes. This term does not imply that the tumour is either benign or malignant and as such it could be justifiably employed to cover melanocytic tumours of all behavioural patterns. However, in clinical medicine the term melanoma is commonly used to indicate the malignant tumour of melanocytes. In order to avoid confusion, the term melanoma is best avoided and one should refer to the tumour as either benign melanoma or malignant melanoma.

Examples of malignant melanoma include the malignant melanoma of the skin of man and the Fortner melanoma of the skin of hamsters. Both stem from the melanocytes at the dermo-epidermal junction. The compound naevus or the junction naevus of man is an example of a benign melanoma, but this term is rarely if ever used. Similarly, junction naevi (benign melanoma) are seen in hamsters that develop spontaneous melanomas like the Fortner melanoma. In both man and hamster, malignant melanomas at times arise from these naevi.

The tumours produced in carcinogen-painted hamster skin are referred to either by the non-committal term (i.e., could be benign or malignant) 'melanotic tumours' or as 'blue naevi', because in analogy with the human state such tumours arise from deeply placed dermal melanocytes or according to some from neural elements (e.g., from Schwann cells of cutaneous nerves). Blue naevi in both man and hamster are almost always but not invariably benign.

Two varieties of cutaneous blue naevi are recognized in man: the ordinary blue naevus (also called 'common blue naevus') and the cellular blue naevus. The latter is larger, tends to be hypomelanotic and, as its name implies, is more cellular. A similar distinction can also be made in the hamster blue naevi, where the larger tumours are much more cellular and generally hypomelanotic.

In carcinogen-painted hamster skin, there is the added difficulty of deciding at what stage one is to regard a given lesion as a neoplasm rather than a hyperplastic proliferation of cells. In painted hamster skin, some of the melanotic lesions produced are quite small and such lesions (less than 1 mm in diameter) sometimes regress with cessation of painting. Arbitrary criteria are therefore used by most workers. It is now customary to call slightly raised lesions, 2 mm or more in diameter, melanotic 'tumours' or'blue naevi', while smaller lesions are often referred to as pigmented lesions.

Since in this text we deal primarily and extensively with carcinogen-induced melanotic tumours which are now frequently referred to as blue naevi, it is essential to explain the reason for this. Most of the human blue naevi are blue or bluish-grey, but some are dark brown. Most hamster naevi do not have a bluish hue, they are in fact quite black. Despite this, such lesions are called 'blue naevi' as explained below.

When a collection of cells containing melanin occurs in a superficial plane in the skin (as in the common human naevus at the dermo-epidermal junction), they produce a brown or black lesion, but if such cells occur deep in the dermis, the lesion has a bluish tint. The blue colouration is an optical effect produced by deeply sited melanin viewed through the overlying epidermis and superficial dermis. While small blue naevi composed of pigmented cells lying deep in the dermis are blue, the larger lesions where the cells lie under a stretched or attenuated epidermis are not. This is why some human blue naevi have a brown appearance. The hamster skin is so thin (epidermis is only about 2 to 3 cells thick) that virtually all these tumours appear black. Here, the bluish or greyish hue of some tumours stems chiefly from a relative paucity of melanin in the tumour. Thus the colour of the lesion is of secondary importance, and the term blue naevus is today employed for any blue, brown or black lesion composed of extra-epithelial pigment cells, be they in the skin, prostate, lymph node, endocervix or middle ear (Jao *et al.*, 1971; Rios & Wright, 1976; Levene, 1980; Goldman, 1981). The fact that the blue naevi of hamsters are carcinogen-induced tumours (very rarely metastasize) and not naevi in the strict sense of the word (i.e., birth mark or a developmental defect) has also not deterred students of this subject from calling these tumours 'blue naevi', simply because these are tumours derived from pigment cells situated in the dermis. Finally, it is worth noting that the cells in blue naevi (human and hamster) are often referred to as naevus cells. This at least has the merit of circumventing the arguments as to whether these cells are neoplastic melanocytes or Schwann cells.

In summary, the term 'melanoma' or 'malignant melanoma' refers to the malignant cutaneous melanoma of man and its equivalent the Fortner melanoma and some other spontaneously occurring melanomas in hamsters, while the term blue naevus refers to the human tumours of this name and the equivalent carcinogen-induced cutaneous melanotic tumour or blue naevus of hamster skin.

Morphology. In this section we deal with the melanotic tumours or blue naevi produced by chemical carcinogens in the common Syrian hamster, which has a brown or agouti coat. Tumours produced in other varieties and species of hamster will be dealt with later.

The melanotic tumours that arise in the skin are almost invariably multiple, and vary in size from approximately 2 mm to 1 cm in diameter; only rarely are larger tumours produced. The small pigmented spots from which melanotic tumours arise are widely distributed in hamster skin, but the bulk of them lie in the dorsolateral skin posterior to the costovertebral spots. It is in this region that melanotic tumours are most frequently produced, although of course this will also depend upon which region of the skin is painted. Another common site of tumour incidence is the skin of the ears, chin and face. This is no doubt due to the cleaning activities of the animals, which transfer the carcinogen to these sites from the painted area of skin. The small pigmented spots are more numerous in females than in males and, as one might expect, more tumours are produced in females than in males when similar doses of carcinogens are applied (Illman & Ghadially, 1960; Ghadially & Illman, 1966).

The light microscopic appearance of these tumours is related to their size. The early lesions present as a sheath of pigmented melanocytes growing around a pilosebaceous unit (Figure 55). Appearances such as these clearly indicate the origin of these tumours from the perifollicular networks of the small pigmented spots. Large tumours (Figures 56–59) present as a heavily pigmented rounded mass lying in the dermis. These tumours are so heavily pigmented that cytological details can only be observed in bleached sections (Figure 57). In the smaller tumours the main cell type is spindle-shaped, while in the larger tumours many of the cells are polyhedral and have indistinct cell boundaries. Larger tumours tend to be somewhat less pigmented than smaller ones. Whatever the size of the tumour, it is almost invariably separated from the superficial epidermis by some dermal connective tissue. Junctional activity of the type seen in the junctional naevus and malignant melanoma of man and in similar spontaneous hamster melanotic tumours is not encountered. Thus, as mentioned before, the carcinogen-induced melanotic tumours of the hamster more resemble the blue naevus of man rather than human junctional naevus or malignant melanoma. (For further discussion on this point, see pp. 15–16).

Infiltration of deeper structures and secondary deposits to distant organs are only rarely seen, yet many of the larger-sized melanotic tumours are not difficult to transplant.

Effect of coat colour. We noted earlier that, besides the golden or brown Syrian hamster, we also have a cream and a white variety in which the number and type of small pigmented spots are somewhat different. In whole mounts of skin, the common agouti hamster is seen to be well endowed with small pigmented spots containing well melanized melanocytes. The skin of the cream variety contains only an occasional such spot, and none are seen in the white hamster. This is due to the fact that the perifollicular networks of melanocytes in the white hamster are amelanotic (the situation regarding the cream variety is not as clear) and not that such networks are absent. These amelanotic networks can be occasionally identified in histological section. An excellent illustration of this may be seen in the paper by Rappaport *et al.,* (1961). Further proof of the existence of amelanotic melanocytic networks has been obtained by painting the skin of the white hamster with 1% croton oil in acetone (Quevedo *et al.,* 1961b). The amelanotic melanocytes are then stimulated to produce melanin, and small pigmented spots similar to those in the agouti animal are seen. It is interesting to note that croton oil does not induce proliferation of melanocytes and

melanotic tumour formation even if it is applied for a prolonged period.

However, if the skin of the various colour varieties is painted with similar doses of carcinogen, interesting differences in tumour production are noted (Illman & Ghadially, 1960; Rappaport *et al.,* 1961; Quevedo *et al.,* 1961b). Thus fewer but larger melanotic tumours are produced in the skin of the white, as compared to the brown hamster, but none are observed in the cream animal. The yield of epithelial tumours is also low and tardy in the cream hamster.

The melanotic tumours produced in the white variety may be melanotic, hypomelanotic or amelanotic, the naked eye appearance varying from black through various shades of grey to pink. However, even the best melanized tumour does not show the quantity and concentration of pigment found in the tumours raised in the common agouti animal. Except for differences in pigment content, the histological and cytological features of the melanotic tumours produced in the white and brown variety are similar (Figures 60–62). Behaviourally, however, the amelanotic tumours appear to be somewhat more aggressive in that they grow faster and are both larger and more readily transplantable.

The resistance of the cream variety to melanotic tumour production after painting with carcinogen may be due either to a paucity of small pigmented spots or to genetic or strain resistance to the action of the carcinogen. Data available on carcinogenesis in this variety are too scanty to allow an accurate analysis of the situation.

Other species. Besides the Syrian hamster, small pigmented spots and associated perifollicular networks of melanocytes have been found in the Chinese hamster (*Cricetulus criseus*), the European hamster (*Cricetus cricetus*), and the Mongolian gerbil (*Meriones unguiculatus*).

In the Chinese hamster (Ghadially & Illman, 1963), only a few small pigmented spots of morphology similar to that of the Syrian hamster occur. However, besides this there are large diffuse dermal networks of melanocytes in this animal; these extend over an oval or elongated area, come in contact with many groups of hair follicles, and produce large lenticular melanotic tumours when the skin is painted with carcinogen. The pigmented spots in the European hamster are similar to those in the Syrian hamster, but this animal has not yet been painted with carcinogens (Ghadially & Illman, 1960). Melanotic tumours have been raised from the small pigmented spots in the gerbil by Quevedo *et al.* (1968).

Resistance of costovertebral spots. Many investigators have found that the costovertebral spot is most resistant to tumour production by chemical carcinogens. Even when the spot was carefully painted so as to focus the attack on it as far as possible, we found that numerous melanotic tumours arose from the perifollicular networks of melanocytes in the skin outside the spot rather than in the large networks in the spot itself. Berenblum *et al.* (1958) have pointed out that hair follicles in telogen retain carcinogen longer than hair follicles in anagen and that this may be due to the flushing action of the sebaceous glands, which are much larger during anagen. Perhaps the large sebaceous glands in the spot act in a similar fashion and rid themselves rapidly of carcinogens.

Even so, it is not completely impossible to raise melanotic tumours within the costovertebral spot and we have succeeded in doing this on one occasion. Microscopically, the morphology of the tumour was similar to that of the melanotic tumours from the small pigmented spots, in that it was composed mainly of well melanized spindle-shaped cells. The atrophic remnants of the sebaceous glands of the costovertebral spot lay compressed beneath the tumour, clearly indicating that the tumour had arisen from the

melanocytic networks which lie mainly around the neck of the hair follicles above and around the superficial parts of the sebaceous glands.

Histogenesis. Throughout this chapter the importance of the hair follicle in cutaneous carcinogenesis has been emphasized, as also the evidence supporting the origin of the melanotic tumours from perifollicular networks of the small pigmented spots. This theory first proposed by us (Ghadially & Barker, 1960) has now been confirmed and upheld by many other workers (Chernozemsky, 1966; Parish & Searle, 1966; Quevedo *et al.,* 1961b; Mishima & Oboler, 1965; Walters *et al.,* 1967; Della Porta, 1966).

However, cutaneous melanocytes are found in sites other than the perifollicular networks and one has to consider the possibility that an occasional melanotic tumour may arise from such melanocytes also. Thus, in common with many animals including man and various laboratory rodents, hamster skin contains melanocytes situated in the bulbs of hair follicles. A few amelanotic melanocytes also occur at the dermo-epidermal junction (Mishima & Oboler, 1965), and it has been suggested that the spontaneous melanomas of the hamster probably arise from these cells. There is, however, no evidence whatsoever suggesting that carcinogen-induced melanotic tumours of hamster skin arise from either the melanocytes in the hair bulb or at the dermo-epidermal junction. Hair follicles are as a rule richly supplied with neural elements. Such elements, and particularly Schwann cells, are abundant in the region of the melanocytic networks and it has been suggested (Nakai & Rappaport, 1963) that the melanotic tumours may be of endoneural or Schwann cell origin.

A similar suggestion has also been put forward by Straile (1964) who believes that there are two distinct possibilities regarding the histogenesis of the melanotic tumours, namely that: (1) the perifollicular melanocytes proliferate, and invade and envelope the neural elements; or (2) the neural elements of the richly innervated hair follicles proliferate to produce the tumour.

One can see no fundamental difficulty in accepting the neural hypothesis. Since both melanocytes and Schwann cells are derived from the neural crest, it is conceivable that these two closely related cells are intermutable. Indeed, one may recall that in man the origin of pigmented nerve sheath tumours has been explained by a similar thesis. Yet the evidence (in the case of the hamster) on which this hypothesis is based is no more than that neural elements are present in this region and that Schwann cells are abundant in the early perifollicular melanotic tumours in painted hamster skin. One might argue that this is only to be expected since this is a region well endowed with neural elements, and that as such these elements are bound to become incorporated in any tumour originating in this region. It seems to me that, since melanocytes are also abundant at this site, there is neither need nor justification for evolving an alternative hypothesis. The supporters of the neural hypothesis or other hypotheses, such as the origin of these tumours from bulbar melanocytes, do not even attempt to explain why the hamster is so susceptible to melanotic tumour production while other common laboratory animals are not. Surely all these species have melanocytes in the hair bulbs, and abundant perifollicular neural structures! Then why do they, too, not produce abundant melanotic tumours like the hamster?

It seems to me that no alternative hypothesis proposed so far explains all the observed phenomena and that there is now overwhelming evidence in support of the idea that the melanotic tumours of painted hamster skin arise from the perifollicular melanocytic networks of the small pigmented spot. This evidence may be summarized as follows: (1) only animals with small pigmented spots, like the various species and varieties of hamsters and gerbils, yield abundant melanotic tumours when painted with carcinogens; (2) the distribution of melanotic tumours produced matches well with the distribution of the small pigmented spots in hamster skin; (3) females normally have many more pigmented spots than males and they also yield many more melanotic tumours on skin painting; (4) the paucity of pigmented spots in the cream hamster correlates well with the failure to produce melanotic tumours in this variety. (There may, however, be an alternative explanation; see p. 15; (5) the state of melanization of the tumour correlates well with the degree of melanization of the pigmented spots, for amelanotic and hypomelanotic tumours arise in the white variety, while heavily melanized tumours occur in the brown hamster; (6) in the Chinese hamster the large elongated and lenticular melanotic tumours match well with the similar shaped more diffuse dermal networks in its skin; (7) histological studies have repeatedly shown that the early tumour consists of a ring or mantle of melanocytes around the hair follicle, clearly arising from the networks of the spot; (8) as expected, absence of junctional activity with superficial epidermis is a constant feature; (9) the costovertebral spot is resistant to carcinogenic action, but when a melanotic tumour is raised, it clearly originates from the perifollicular networks, and rides above the sebaceous glands which are displaced downwards; and (10) ultrastructural study (Ghadially *et al.*, 1986) of human blue naevi and carcinogen-induced hamster blue naevi has shown that both the hamster and the human tumours are composed almost entirely of cells acceptable as melanocytes and melanophages. This is discussed further in a later section dealing with the ultrastructure of these tumours.

Mechanisms of melanotic tumour production. It is well established by fluorescence microscopy that carcinogens enter the skin via the pilosebaceous apparatus (Simpson & Cramer, 1943; Berenblum *et al.*, 1958) and indeed, as we have seen, a majority of tumours arise from these structures and not the surface epidermis. Further, it has been shown in the mouse that a carcinogen such as MC is retained 2–3 times as long in the quiescent (telogen) as in the active (anagen) follicle (Berenblum *et al.*, 1958). One of the earliest and most dramatic effects of carcinogenic action in the mouse and hamster skin is the destruction and disappearance of sebaceous glands of hair follicles in telogen (Suntzeff *et al.*, 1955; Ghadially & Barker, 1960).

Bearing these points in mind, we can explain the mechanism of origin of the melanotic tumours as follows. The carcinogen enters the hamster skin via the hair follicles and sebaceous glands. Since the perifollicular network of melanocytes is in places closely applied to the sebaceous glands, direct transfer of carcinogen from sebaceous glands to melanocytes probably occurs. The destruction of the sebaceous glands brought about by the carcinogen must further aid the transfer of carcinogen from the sebaceous glands to melanocytes. The melanocytes, thus repeatedly stimulated by numerous applications of carcinogen, ultimately produce a melanotic tumour.

It seems to us that there can be little doubt that in the hamster the peculiar anatomical arrangement of the melanocytes around the sebaceous gland and hair follicle neck places these cells in a most vulnerable position for attack by carcinogens, and that herein lies the explanation of the observation that the hamster is more liable to develop melanotic tumours than the rabbit and the mouse, in which similar melanocytic networks do not occur.

Trauma and melanoma. It has long been held that malignant melanoma of man can arise as a result of trauma to a mole (naevus or benign melanoma) or even normal skin, but some workers do not accept this thesis (for a critique and references, see Ghadially *et al.*, 1960; Ghadially, 1966). They believe that as yet there is no authenticated case of a mole having become malignant as a result of trauma and that the local appearance of a malignant melanoma after incomplete removal of a supposed benign naevus indicates that the lesion was already malignant before removal (Belissario, 1959).

This controversy led to a study of the effect of trauma on melanotic tumours. Ghadially *et al.* (1960) traumatized some 80 carcinogen-induced melanotic tumours in the hamster by various means such as cutting, pricking, squeezing, shaving and suturing, yet not a single tumour metastasized or showed a rapid increase in size. Indeed, quite a few regressed or even disappeared.

Deeply infiltrating and destructive malignant melanomas can be produced in certain viviparous fishes by hybridization (e.g., *Xiphophorus maculatus* x *X. helleri*). Trauma to the skin of such fishes does not precipitate melanoma production or increase their incidence (Ghadially, 1966).

Similar studies using a transplantable Fortner melanoma have been carried out in which the tumours were subjected to incisional and excisional biopsies (Paslin, 1973). No significant adverse effect, such as accelerated growth or a greater incidence of metastasis, was seen after incisional biopsies, while excisional biopsy resulted in significantly fewer metastases than incisional biopsies or no biopsies. However, Riggins and Ketcham (1965) have reported that incisional biopsy of the Cloudman S91 melanoma in mice does produce a small but significant increase in the incidence of metastasis.

Experiments such as the ones reported in this section are interesting but the results are difficult to extrapolate to man. However, the collective evidence seems to suggest that trauma to benign melanotic lesions and biopsies of malignant melanomas may not be quite as dangerous as one might suspect.

Ultrastructure of melanomas and blue naevi. Ultrastructural studies have shown that human and hamster melanomas and blue naevi, whether benign or malignant, are composed of neoplastic melanocytes which contain melanosomes in various stages of development and non-neoplastic melanophages (which are in fact histiocytes) which contain compound melanosomes, which are single membrane-bound lysosomal bodies containing many melanosomes derived by phagocytosis of melanosomes produced by the tumour cells. It is extremely uncommon for non-neoplastic Schwann cells to produce melanosomes, but there does occur a tumour called the melanotic schwannoma (for details see Ghadially, 1985, 1988), in which neoplastic Schwann cells produce numerous melanosomes. This tumour also contains non-neoplastic melanophages. The equivalent of this human tumour has not been reported to occur in hamsters. Therefore no further reference will be made to this tumour.

It is now well established that melanin synthesis occurs in a specialized organelle in the melanocyte called the melanosome (Seiji *et al.*, 1961). It is now clear that this organelle contains tyrosinase, an enzyme which is involved in the oxidation of the colourless amino acid tyrosine to the pigmented polymers we call the melanins (eumelanins are brownish-black, phaeomelanins are yellowish-red). Dopa (3,4-dihydroxyphenylalanine) is an intermediate compound formed during the first stage of this oxidative reaction. Thus when either dopa or tyrosine is presented to cells containing tyrosinase, they show increased pigmentation. This is the basis of the dopa reaction (Bloch, 1927) and the tyrosinase reaction (Fitzpatrick *et al.*, 1950); both reveal the presence of the only enzyme known to be involved in melanin synthesis, namely tyrosinase.

The classification of melanosomes developed by Fitzpatrick *et al.* (1971) recognizes four stages of melanosome development. The first or earliest contains no melanin. The last stage is the fully mature melanin granule, where the internal structure of the melanosome is totally masked or destroyed by melanin deposition. The earlier stages possess an active tyrosinase system, the last stage does not. The ontogeny of melanosomes has been the subject of excellent reviews (Toda *et al.*, 1968; Fitzpatrick *et al.*, 1971). It is now generally held that tyrosinase is synthesized by the ribosomes of the rough endoplasmic reticulum and transported via this organelle to the Golgi complex, where it is parcelled off into small vesicles (melanosome stage I). The vesicles then enlarge and elongate to form an oval organelle melanosome stage II (also called premelanosome), in which a characteristic striated or coiled filamentous structure develops. Deposition of melanin on the structure heralds the next stage (melanosome stage III, also called premelanosome or partially melanized melanosome), and the completion of this process produces a uniformly electron-dense granule without discernible internal structure (melanosome stage IV, mature melanosome or melanin granule).

Most ultrastructural studies of the hamster melanoma have used transplantable tumour lines derived from the Fortner melanomas or similar spontaneously occurring melanomas which developed in other laboratories. Both melanotic and amelanotic primary tumours have been used for transplantation, and also melanotic and amelanotic variants derived by selectively transplanting well pigmented and poorly pigmented portions of a single tumour. It would appear that the degree of pigmentation is a property of the tumour itself and is not significantly altered by the colour of the host, but tumours have been found to grow more slowly in albino hamsters (Hesselbach, 1959).

All human amelanotic melanoma studies so far have found stage II or III melanosomes to be present (Ghadially, 1985), but rodent melanomas (including those of the hamster) often lack organelles that can be confidently identified as stage II or III melanosomes (Bomirski *et al.*, 1973; Pandov *et al.*, 1976). Needless to say, amelanotic melanomas lack well melanized melanosomes and melanin granules, i.e., stage IV melanosomes, but these are found in abundance in the melanotic versions of the tumour (Epstein & Fukuyama, 1970). The number of melanosomes varies greatly from tumour to tumour and within the cells of the same tumour, and there is also a variation in size and morphology of the melanosomes. Quite bizarre variations in size have been noted in carcinogen-induced melanotic tumour cells in white hamsters (Rappaport *et al.*, 1963).

In our (Ghadially *et al.*, 1986) comparative study of 12 human blue naevi and 18 carcinogen-induced hamster blue naevi (also called melanotic tumours), we found that the naevus cells in the ordinary blue naevi and in the hamster small blue naevi presented fusiform or oval profiles. Profiles of this shape were at times seen in the human cellular blue naevi and in the larger more cellular hamster blue naevi, but more often than not the profiles of these closely packed cells were rounded or of an irregular shape.

Some of the melanotic tumours (Figures 63 and 64) of man and hamster contained so many melanosomes that it was difficult to detect various cell organelles and often the cells seemed to contain little besides melanosomes and a few mitochondria. The hypermelanotic tumours (Figures 65 and 66) of man and hamster contained far fewer melanosomes, which were usually also much smaller. In quite substantial portions of these tumours one could find only a rare melanosome or no melanosomes, but there were a few better pigmented areas where quite a few melanosomes were present.

The melanosomes in the naevus cells were largely solitary, but occasionally small aggregates of melanosomes, mimicking compound melanosomes, or true compound melanosomes limited by a membrane were present (Figures 63 and 65).

In the melanotic blue naevi, most of the melanosomes were stage IV melanosomes (Figure 67) and only a few stage III melanosomes and fewer stage II melanosomes were detected. In the hypomelanotic tumours, stage III melanosomes showing patchy melanization predominated. However, several stage IV melanosomes and some stage II melanosomes with characteristic striated (100 nm periodicity) internal structures were also present (Figure 68).

Several types of solitary melanosomes were seen in the naevus cells. Granular melanosomes (Figure 68) as well as rounded and elongated melanosomes were found in tumours from both species. However, the granular melanosomes were much more common in the human material, while the rounded and elongated melanosomes were more common in the hamster. Further such melanosomes in hamster tumours at times contained rounded structures which have been variously referred to as 'electron-lucent bodies', 'holes' or 'vesicles' (Ghadially *et al.*, 1986). Giant melanosomes with a diameter (up to about 2.3 μm) markedly greater than the usual melanosomes were at times seen in the naevus cells of hamster tumours, but they were not detected in the naevus cells of human blue naevi.

Organelles such as rough endoplasmic reticulum and Golgi complex were quite sparse in the naevus cells of human and hamster tumours but at times several cell processes arising from these cells were detected. These processes varied from short and plump to long and slender. The plump processes often contained some melanosomes. Some of the cell processes were acceptable as microvilli. Unlike the cell processes seen in schwannomas (Ghadially, 1985), the cell processes in the blue naevi did not intertwine, inter-digitate or wrap around structures (like collagen fibrils in the matrix) to form pseudomesaxons. Invaginations of the cell membrane to form mesaxons were also not detected. Thus the cell processes found in these tumours clearly support the idea that the cells are neoplastic melanocytes and not Schwann cells.

Despite a diligent search, neither a basal lamina surrounding a group of cells nor an external lamina surrounding solitary cells was detected in human ordinary blue naevi or their equivalent– the hamster small blue naevi. On very rare occasions, however, small ill-defined patches or minute segments of basal lamina-like material could be discerned.

This situation also prevailed in about half the human cellular blue naevi and their equivalent – the hamster larger blue naevi. In the remainder, a small minority of the cells in each tumour showed clear evidence of basal lamina or external lamina formation in that sizeable seg-ments of a slender basal lamina or external lamina was detected. However, in one human tumour and one hamster tumour (Figure 67) quite a thick (at times continuous) external lamina was seen adjacent to a few cells. It must be stressed that even in these tumours only a few cells in some areas showed evidence of lamina production.

As is well known Schwann cells have an external lamina but melanocytes do not therefore, the failure to find this feature in most tumours and in most areas of the remainder shows that the overwhelming majority of cells are acceptable as melanocytes. One may therefore surmise that blue naevi (human and hamster) are tumours of dermal melanocytes (probably derived from migrant neural crest cells which failed to reach the epidermis) and that the occasional production of external lamina found in these tumours is an infrequent aberration engendered by the neoplastic state, which reflects the close kinship between the melanocyte and Schwann cell. The occurrence of basal and external laminae in cellular blue naevi and the hamster larger blue naevi, but their virtual absence in ordinary blue naevi and small hamster blue naevi, supports such an idea and suggests that lamina formation is a late event which tends to develop only when a blue naevus has attained a certain level of size and cellularity.

As mentioned earlier (p. 17), much has been made of 'neural elements' (i.e., nerves) in these tumours and it has been suggested that blue naevi arise from Schwann cells in these nerves. We too saw several cutaneous nerves in sections of human and hamster blue naevi, but they appeared to be 'trapped' or 'accidentally included' nerves, uninvolved in the neo-plastic process. No melanosomes were detected in the scores of nerves encoun-tered, but in one instance a cell in a nerve contained compound melanosomes. No external lamina was seen around this cell, hence it is unlikely to be a Schwann cell which had endocytosed melanosomes. We are inclined to regard it as a melanophage (macrophage) which had invaded the nerve after endocytosing melanosomes in the tumour. If blue naevi were tumours of Schwann cells, we would have found melanosomes in various stages of development in Schwann cells (as in melanotic schwannoma) but this was certainly not the case. The extra-cellular matrix of the tumours was unremarkable. It contained collagen fibres and occa-sionally also elastic fibres. In contrast to the situation in schwannomas, Luse bodies (fibrous long-spacing collagen) were not found in any tumour.

Virus-like particles resembling the type-C virus particles of Bernhard and Granboulan (1962) have been seen in transplanted hamster melanomas (Balda *et al.*, 1973). Epstein and Fukuyama (1970) found such virus-like particles within the cisternae of the rough endoplasmic reticulum of a transplantable melanoma and we have seen a similar distribution of virus particles in Ehrlich ascites tumour cells (Ghadially, 1988). The significance of the presence of virus particles in hamster melanomas is not known but there is little reason to believe that this is the causative agent, for viruses are now known to be associated with many transplantable mouse carcinomas and sarcomas.

Connective tissue tumours

Dermatofibroma and dermatofibrosarcoma

In experimental animals painted with carcinogens, one occasionally finds a tumour that has arisen from dermal fibroblasts. Depending upon histological appearance, behaviour and transplantability, such tumours may be designated either as dermatofibromas or dermatofibrosarcomas. Histologically, these tumours are similar to tumours produced in subcutaneous tissue by injections of carcinogens. The well-differentiated members of this group contain spindle cells which resemble fibroblasts, and a matrix containing collagen fibres. In the more aggressive ones, the cells are pleomorphic and the matrix is scanty.

The manner in which cutaneously applied carcinogens reach the dermis is debatable. The most plausible explanation is that they arrive there via the cracks or ulcers so often produced in painted skin. It is also possible that rupture of sebaceous glands may release carcinogens in this area. Among the various laboratory species, the rat and the hamster are very susceptible to dermatofibrosarcoma production, while the rabbit is highly resistant. This matches well with the fact that

sarcomas are readily produced by subcutaneous injections of a variety of carcinogens in the former two species but not in the latter.

SPONTANEOUS TUMOURS

Spontaneous tumours of the skin (Kirkman & Algard, 1968) are of rather rare occurrence in the hamster, perhaps the only exception being melanomas, which are not uncommon in certain strains.

Of the epithelial tumours, basal cell carcinomas have been more frequently reported than squamous cell carcinomas. As is well known, in both man and experimental animals, basal cell carcinomas very rarely metastasize. It is therefore interesting to note that a metastasizing basal cell carcinoma which arose on the nostril of a hamster has been described. A spontaneous keratoacanthoma has been noted to occur in the hamster and also a sweat-gland cystadenocarcinoma or possibly hidradenoma.

Melanotic tumours showing a high degree of aggressiveness, as evidenced by frequent secondary deposits in lymph nodes and distant organs, occur spontaneously in the Syrian hamster (Fortner, 1957; Fortner & Allen, 1958, 1959). These malignant melanomas are markedly different from the chemical-carcinogen-induced melanotic tumours, both in morphology and behaviour. Personal experience and a review of the literature suggest that this spontaneous tumour arises in only certain hamster colonies. For instance, in the thousands of animals bred and reared in our laboratory we have never seen a single example. In susceptible animals junctional naevi occur, and the malignant melanomas are reported to arise from such naevi. This situation is, of course, very similar to that in man, but quite different from the experimental induction of melanotic tumours of hamster skin.

The incidence of these tumours was found to be about 2% (Fortner & Allen,

1959), males being affected much more frequently than females. This also contrasts with the experimentally produced melanotic tumours, where females are more susceptible.

The site distribution is also markedly different, there being no predilection for areas where small pigmented spots abound. Mitotic activity and cellular pleomorphism are characteristic of these malignant tumours, which may be melanotic or amelanotic. The capacity of the amelanotic variety to grow and metastasize exceeds that of the melanotic version, a point evident in both the primary tumour and its transplants. This situation, at least, is similar to that seen in experimentally induced melanotic tumours but not to that seen in man, where both pigmented and non-pigmented melanomas have a devastating capacity to metastasize.

Thus it would appear that the spontaneous tumours and their precursor lesions are the equivalent of the malignant melanoma and junctional naevi of man, while the experimentally produced tumour is probably the equivalent of the blue naevus, which only rarely undergoes malignant transformation. It is interesting to note that, at least in some blue naevi of man (Lund & Kraus, 1962), pilosebaceous follicles occur and the situation is then somewhat reminiscent of the small pigmented spots of hamster skin and the melanotic tumours arising from them.

INDUCTION OF TUMOURS

Tumours can be produced in the skin of experimental animals by a variety of physical, chemical and biological agents. In the hamster, most of the work has been done with chemical carcinogens. Information regarding, for instance, the effect of ionizing radiations or viral agents is scanty. Melanotic tumours, including malignant melanomas, have been noted after irradiation with X-rays, but it is not certain whether they were produced as a result of this treatment (Oberman & Riviere, 1966). Repeated exposure to ultraviolet radiation has failed to produce melanomas, but papillomas, keratoacanthomas and squamous cell carcinoma have been reported to occur (Stenback, 1975).

Some studies suggest that tumours can be produced in hamster skin by viral agents. Graffi *et al.* (1968a,b) have reported the occurrence of epithelial tumours of hair follicular origin in hamsters which were injected when new-born with hamster embryo tissue cultivated *in vitro*. Virus particles morphologically similar to agents of the papovavirus group were found in the tumour cells. Fortner (1965) reported the occurrence of malignant cutaneous and haematological abnormalities in young hamsters injected subcutaneously with material initially obtained from an animal that had spontaneously developed malignant melanoma. The nature of the cutaneous tumours was uncertain, as also the viral etiology.

Shope rabbit papillomavirus was found by Nagaeva (1966) to be incapable of producing tumours in adult guinea-pigs, hamsters, rats and mice, but when virus-containing material was inoculated into newborn animals of these species, only the Syrian hamsters responded with papillomatosis of the ears, nose, mouth, feet and tail.

Many chemical carcinogens can produce tumours in the skin of hamsters. The extensive earlier literature on this subject has been most ably reviewed by Homburger *et al.* (1968, 1969), so I shall only briefly record certain interesting aspects, giving occasional references.

The first tumours raised in hamster skin were basal cell carcinomas, produced by the repeated application of benzo[a]-pyrene (BP) (Schintz & Fritz-Niggli, 1954). Since then, tumours have been produced in hamster skin by the topical application of BP, DMBA, dibenz[a,h]anthracene,benz-[a]anthracene, 3-methylcholanthrene

(MC), 2-aminoanthracene, 4-nitroquinoline-*N*-oxide, β–propiolactone (Parish & Searle, 1966) and urethane. The last-named carcinogen is also effective when injected into or fed to the animal. Hamster skin is about as susceptible to tumour production by DMBA as mouse or rabbit skin. Rats are slightly more resistant and guinea-pigs very markedly so.

The widely accepted two-stage theory of carcinogenesis, based on studies of cutaneous carcinogenesis in mouse and rabbit skin, is not demonstrable in hamster skin. Ghadially *et al.* (1960) found that trauma does not act as a co-carcinogenic stimulus (it is poor or ineffective in the mouse also) and it has also been shown by others that croton oil and Tween-60 do not have a promoting action. This however applies only to cutaneous carcinogenesis, for in the cheek pouch the co-carcinogenic activity of croton oil and Tween-60 is demonstrable.

The costovertebral spot is very resistant to chemical carcinogenesis, but is highly susceptible to malignant transformation by hormonal imbalance. Subcutaneous implantation of estrogen/androgen mixtures produces tumours which are of great importance for fundamental studies on hormonal carcinogenesis and the hormone dependence of tumours. Our knowledge of these tumours stems almost entirely from the work of Kirkman, Algard and their colleagues (Kirkman & Dodge, 1982).

REFERENCES

Ahavoni, B. (1932) Die Muriden von Palästina und Syrien. *Z. Säugetierk.*, 7, 166–240

Balda, B.R., Birkmayer, G.D. & Braun-Falco, O. (1973) Particle-associated RNA-directed polymerase and 70S RNA in the hamster melanoma A Mel 3. *Arch. Derm. Forsch.*, 248, 229–236

Belisario, J.C. (1959) *Cancer of the Skin*, London, Butterworths, pp. 82–93

Berenblum, I., Haran-Ghera, N. & Trainin, N. (1958) An experimental analysis of hair cycle effect in mouse skin carcinogenesis. *Br. J. Cancer*, 12, 402–413

Bernhard, W. & Granboulan, N. (1962) Morphology of oncogenic and non-oncogenic mouse viruses. In: Wolstenholme, G.E.W. & O'Connor, M.C., eds, *Ciba Foundation Symposium on Tumour Virus of Murine Origin*, London, Churchill, pp. 6–49

Bloch, B. (1927) Das Pigment. In: *Handbuch der Haut- und Geschlechtskrankheiten*, Vol. 1, Berlin, Springer-Verlag, pp. 434–541

Bomirski, A., Zawrocka-Wrzolkowa, T. & Pautsch, F. (1973) Electron microscopic studies on transplantable melanotic and amelanotic melanomas in hamsters. *Arch. Derm. Forsch.*, 246, 284–298

Chapman, G.B., Drusin, L.M. & Todd, J.E. (1963) Fine structure of the human wart. *Am. J. Pathol.*, 42, 619–642

Chase, H.B., Montagna, W. & Malone, J.D. (1953) Changes in the skin in relation to the hair growth cycle. *Anat. Rec.*, 116, 75–81

Chernozemsky, I. (1966) Changes in the skin of Syrian hamster after a single application of 9,10-dimethyl-1,2-benzanthracene. In: Della Porta, G. & Muhlbock, O., eds, *Structure and Control of the Melanocyte*, Berlin, Heidelberg, New York, Springer-Verlag, pp. 274–280

Della Porta, G. (1966) Discussion. In: Della Porta, G. & Muhlbock, O., eds, *Structure and Control of the Melanocyte*, Berlin, Heidelberg, New York, Springer-Verlag, pp. 283–285

Della Porta, G., Rappaport, H., Saffiotti, U. & Shubik (1956a) Induction of melanotic lesions during skin carcinogenesis in hamsters. *Arch. Pathol.*, 61, 305–313

Della Porta, G., Rappaport, H., Saffiotti, U., Spencer, K. & Shubik, P. (1956b) The induction of cutaneous melanotic tumours in hamsters. *Proc. Am. Ass. Cancer Res.*, 2, 102

Emerson, C.W., Hillman, J.W., McSwain, B. & Wood, F. (1971) Keratoacanthoma vs. squamous cell carcinoma. *J. Bone Jt Surg.*, 53-A, 143–146

Epstein, W.L. & Fukuyama, K. (1970) Light and electron microscopic studies of a transplantable melanoma associated with virus-like particles. *Cancer Res.*, 30, 1241–1247

Fischer, E.R., McCoy II, M.M. & Wechsler, H.L. (1972) Analysis of histopathologic and electron microscopic determinants of keratoacanthoma and squamous cell carcinoma. *Cancer*, 28, 1387–1397

Fitzpatrick, T.B., Becker, S.W., Jr, Lerner, A.B. & Montgomery, H. (1950) Tyrosinase in human skin; demonstration of its presence and its role in human melanin formation. *Science*, 112, 223–225

Fitzpatrick, T.B., Quevedo, W.C., Jr, Szabo, G. & Seiji, M. (1971) Biology of the melanin pigmentary system. In: Fitzpatrick, T.B., Arndt, K.A., Clark, W.H., Eisen, A.Z., Van Scott, E.J. & Vaughan, J.H., eds, *Dermatology in General Medicine*, New York, Maidenhead, McGraw-Hill, pp. 117–146

Flannery, G.R. & Muller, H.K. (1979) Immune response to human keratoacanthoma. *Br. J. Derm.*, 101, 625–632

Fleischmajer, R., Lara, J.V. & Charoenvej, P. (1968) Intradermal 3-methylcholanthrene in rabbits and mice. *Dermatologica*, 136, 85–94

Fortner, J.G. (1957) Spontaneous tumors, including gastrointestinal neoplasms and malignant melanomas, in the Syrian hamster. *Cancer*, 10, 1153–1156

Fortner, J.G. (1965) The production of skin lesions and lymphocytic leukemia in the Syrian (golden) hamster. *Br. J. Cancer*, 19, 620–626

Fortner, J.G. & Allen, A.C. (1958) Hitherto unreported malignant melanomas in the Syrian hamster: an experimental counterpart of the human malignant melanoma. *Cancer Res.*, 18, 98–104

Fortner, J.G. & Allen, A.C. (1959) Comparative oncology of melanomas in hamsters and man. In: Gordon, M., ed., *Pigment Cell Biology*, New York, Academic Press, pp. 85–98

Ghadially, F.N. (1957) The effect of transposing skin flaps on the hair growth cycle in the rabbit. *J. Pathol. Bact.*, 74, 321–325

Ghadially, F.N. (1958a) Effect of trauma on growth of hair. *Nature*, 181, 993

Ghadially, F.N. (1958b) A comparative morphological study of keratoacanthoma of man and similar experimentally produced lesions in rabbit. *J. Pathol. Bact.*, 75, 441–453

Ghadially, F.N. (1959) The experimental production of keratoacanthomas in the hamster and the mouse. *J. Pathol. Bact.*, 77, 277–282

Ghadially, F.N. (1960a) Carcinogenesis in the skin of the hedgehog. *Br. J. Cancer*, 14, 212–215

Ghadially, F.N. (1960b) Red fluorescence of experimentallly induced and human tumours. *J. Pathol. Bact.*, 80, 345-351

Ghadially, F.N. (1961) The role of the hair follicle in the origin and evolution of some cutaneous neoplasms of man and experimental animals. *Cancer*, 14, 801–816

Ghadially, F.N. (1966) Trauma and melanoma production. *Nature*, 211, 1199

Ghadially, F.N. (1971) Keratoacanthoma. In: Fitzpatrick, T.B., Arndt, K.A., Clark, W.H., Eisen, A.Z., Van Scott, E.J. & Vaughan, J.H., eds, *Dermatology in General Medicine*, New York, Maidenhead, McGraw-Hill, pp. 425–436

Ghadially, F.N. (1985) *Diagnostic Electron Microscopy of Tumours*, 2nd edition, London, Butterworths

Ghadially, F.N. (1988) *Ultrastructural Pathology of the Cell and Matrix*, 3rd edition, London, Butterworths

Ghadially, F.N. & Barker, J.F. (1960) The histogenesis of experimentally induced melanotic tumours in the Syrian hamster (*Cricetus auratus*). *J. Pathol. Bact.*, 79, 263–271

Ghadially, F.N. & Green, H.N. (1957) Effect of adrenal hormones and adrenalectomy on mitotic activity. *Br. J. Exp. Pathol.*, 38, 100–110

Ghadially, F.N. & Illman, O. (1961) Carcinogenesis in the explanted cheek pouch of the Syrian hamster (*Cricetus auratus*). *J. Pathol. Bact.*, 81, 45–48

Ghadially, F.N. & Illman, O. (1963) The histogenesis of experimentally produced melanotic tumours in the Chinese hamster (*Cricetulus criseus*). *Br. J. Cancer*, 17, 727–730

Ghadially, F.N. & Illman, O. (1966) Small pigmented spots in hamsters. In: Della Porta, G. & Muhlbock, O., eds, *Structure and Control of the Melanocyte*, Berlin, Heidelberg, New York, Springer-Verlag, pp. 259–268

Ghadially, F.N. & Neish, W.J.P. (1960) Porphyrin fluorescence of experimentally produced squamous cell carcinoma. *Nature*, 188, 1124

Ghadially, F.N. & Whitely, H.J. (1952) Hormonally induced epithelial hyperplasia in the goldfish (*Carrasius auratus*). *Br. J. Cancer*, 6, 246–248

Ghadially, F.N., Illman, O. & Barker, J.F. (1960) The effect of trauma on the melanotic tumours of the hamster. *Br. J. Cancer*, 14, 647–650

Ghadially, F.N., Barton, B.W. & Kerridge, D.F. (1963a) The aetiology of keratoacanthoma. *Cancer*, 16, 603–611

Ghadially, F.N., Neish, W.J.P. & Dawkins, H.C. (1963b) Mechanisms involved in the production of red fluorescence of human and experimental tumours. *J. Pathol. Bact.*, 85, 77–92

Ghadially, F.N., Ghadially, R. & Lalonde, J.-M.A. (1986) A comparative ultrastructural study of cutaneous blue naevi of humans and hamsters. *J. Submicrosc. Cytol.*, 18, 417–432

Goldman, R.L. (1981) Blue naevus of the lymph node capsule: report of a unique case. *Histopathology*, 5, 445–450

Graffi, A., Schramm, T., Bender, E., Graffi, I., Horn, K.H. & Bierwolf, D. (1968a) Cell-free transmissible leukoses in Syrian hamsters, probably of viral aetiology. *Br. J. Cancer*, 22, 577–581

Graffi, A., Schramm, T., Graffi, I., Bierwolf, D. & Bender, E. (1968b) Virus-associated skin tumours of the Syrian hamster: preliminary note. *J. Natl Cancer Inst.*, 40, 867–873

Green, H.N. & Ghadially, F.N. (1951) Relation of shock, carbohydrate utilization, and cortisone to mitotic activity in the epidermis of the adult male mouse. *Br. Med. J.*, 1, 496–498

Hesselbach, M.L. (1959) Control of melanization of X-91 tumours by selective transfer and biochemical studies of the tumours produced. In: Gordon, M., ed., *Pigment Cell Biology*, New York, Academic Press, pp. 189–210

Homburger, F. (1968) The Syrian golden hamster in chemical carcinogenesis research. *Prog. Exp. Tumor Res.*, 10, 163–237

Homburger, F. (1969) Chemical carcinogenesis in the Syrian golden hamster, a review. *Cancer*, 23, 313–338

Illman, O. & Ghadially, F.N. (1960) Coat colour and experimental melanotic tumour production in the hamster. *Br. J. Cancer*, 14, 483–488

Illman, O. & Ghadially, F.N. (1966a) Red fluorescence in costovertebral spots of hamsters. *Nature*, 210, 843

Illman, O. & Ghadially, F.N. (1966b) Effect of oestrogen on the small pigmented spots in hamsters. *Nature*, 211, 1303–1304

Jao, W., Fretzin, F., Christ, M.L. & Prinz, L.M. (1971) Blue nevus of the prostate gland. *Arch. Pathol.*, 91, 187–191

Kirkman, H. & Algard, F.T. (1968) Spontaneous and nonviral-induced neoplasms. In: Hoffman, R.A., Robinson, P.F. & Magalhaes, H., eds, *The Golden Hamster*, Ames, Iowa State University Press, pp. 227–240

Kirkman, H. & Dodge, A.H. (1982) Tumours of the integumentary scent gland. In: Turusov, V.S., ed., *Pathology of Tumours in Laboratory Animals*, Vol. III, *Tumours of the Hamster*, Lyon, IARC, pp. 199-219

Kupperman, H. (1944) Hormone control of a dimorphic pigmentation area in the golden hamster (*Cricetus auratus*). *Anat. Rec.*, 88, 442

Lennox, B. (1955) The production of a variety of skin tumours in rats with 2-anthramine, and a comparison with the effects in mice. *Br. J. Cancer*, 9, 631–639

Lennox, B. (1960) Histopathology of tumours: some topics of recent interest. *Recent Adv. Pathol.*, 7, 1–34

Levene, A. (1980) On the natural history and comparative pathology of the blue naevus. *Ann. R. Coll. Surg. Engl.*, 62, 327–334

Lund, H.Z. & Kraus, J.M. (1962) Melanotic tumours of the skin. In: *Atlas of Tumour Pathology*, Washington, DC, Armed Forces Institute of Pathology, pp. 1–134

Mishima, Y. & Oboler, A.A. (1965) Differential chemical carcinogenesis in three distinct melanocyte systems of Syrian (golden) hamsters. *J. Invest. Derm.*, 44, 157–169

Montagna, W. (1956) *The Structure and Function of Skin*, New York, Academic Press

Montagna, W. & Ellis, R.A., eds (1958) *The Biology of Hair Growth*, New York, Academic Press

Nagaeva, L.I. (1966) Development of tumours in Syrian hamsters during their infection by Shope rabbit papilloma virus [in Russian]. *Vopr. Virus*, 11, 194–197

Nakai, T. & Rappaport, H. (1963) Carcinogen-induced melanotic tumours in animals. *Natl Cancer Inst. Monogr.*, 10, 297–322

Oberling, C. & Bernhard, W. (1961) The morphology of the cancer cell. In: Brachet, J. & Mirsky, A.E., eds, *The Cell*, Vol. 5, New York, Academic Press, pp. 405–496

Oberman, B. & Riviere, M.R. (1966) Experimental melanoma in hamsters. In: Della Porta, G. & Muhlbock, O., eds, *Structure and Control of the Melanocyte*, Berlin, Heidelberg, New York, Springer-Verlag, pp. 268–272

Pandov, H.I., Pandov, L.P. & Franks, L.M. (1976) Tumour growth and melanogenesis in hamster tumours *in vivo* and *in vitro:* growth, cytochemistry and ultrastructure of tissue culture cell lines. *Eur. J. Pathol.*, 11, 27–37

Parish, D.J. & Searle, C.E. (1966) The carcinogenicity of beta-propiolactone and 4-nitroquinoline N-oxide for the skin of the golden hamster. *Br. J. Cancer*, 20, 206–209

Paslin, D.A. (1973) The effects of biopsy on the incidence of metastases in hamsters bearing malignant melanoma. *J. Invest. Derm.*, 61, 33–38

Prutkin, L. (1967) An ultrastructural study of the experimental keratoacanthoma. *J. Invest. Derm.*, 48, 326–336

Prutkin, L. & Gerstner, R. (1966) A histochemical study of keratoacanthoma experimentally produced. *Dermatologica*, 132, 16–26

Quevedo, W.C., Jr, Cairns, J.M. & Smith, J.A. (1961a) The effects of croton oil and 7,12-dimethylbenz[a]anthracene (DMBA) on melanocytes in hamsters. *Am. Zool.*, 1, 381

Quevedo, W.C., Jr, Cairns, J.M., Smith, J.A., Bock, F.G. & Burns, R.J. (1961b) Induction of melanotic tumours in the white (partial albino) Syrian hamster. *Nature*, 189, 936–937

Quevedo, W.C., Jr, Bienicki, T.C., Fausto, N. & Magalini, S.I. (1968) Induction of pigmentary changes in the skin of the Mongolian gerbil by chemical carcinogens. *Experientia*, 24, 585–586

Ramselaar, C.G. & van der Meer, J.B. (1976) The spontaneous regression of keratoacanthoma in man. *Acta Derm. (Stockh.)*, 56, 245–251

Ramselaar, C.G. & van der Meer, J.B. (1979) Non-immunological regression of dimethylbenz[a]anthracene-induced experimental keratoacanthomams in the rabbit. *Dermatologica*, 158, 142–151

Ramselaar, C.G., Ruitenberg, E.J. & Kruisinga, W. (1980) Regression of induced keratoacanthomas in anagen (hair growth phase) skin grafts in mice. *Cancer Res.*, 40, 1668–1673

Rappaport, H., Pietra, G. & Shubik, P. (1961) The induction of melanotic tumours resembling cellular blue naevi in the Syrian white hamster by cutaneous application of 7,12-dimethylbenz[a]anthracene. *Cancer Res.*, 21, 661–666

Rappaport, H., Nakai, T. & Swift, H. (1963) The fine structure of normal and neoplastic melanocytes in the Syrian hamster with particular reference to carcinogen-induced malanotic tumors. *J. Cell Biol.*, 16, 171–186

Rigdon, R.H. (1956a) Trauma and cancer; experimental study in white Pekin duck. *Arch. Pathol.*, 61, 443–449

Rigdon, R.H. (1956b) Tumours induced in skin without follicles: experimental study in duck. *Cancer Res.*, 16, 804–807

Rigdon, R.H. (1959) Keratoacanthoma, experimentally induced with methylcholanthrene in chicken. *Arch. Derm.*, 79, 139–147

Riggins, R.S. & Ketcham, A.S. (1965) Effect of incisional biopsy on the development of experimental tumor metastases. *J. Surg. Res.*, 5, 200–206

Rios, C.N. & Wright, J.R. (1976) Melanosis of the prostate gland: report of a case with neoplastic epithelium involvement. *J. Urol.*, 115, 616–617

Schinz, H.R. & Fritz-Niggli, H. (1954) Benzpyren-Karzinom beim Goldhamster. *Strahlentherapie*, 94, 554–560

Schwartz, R.A. (1979) Multiple persistent keratoacanthomas. *Oncology*, 36, 281–285

Seiji, M., Fitzpatrick, T.B. & Birback, M.S.C. (1961) The melanosome: a distinctive subcellular particle of mammalian melanocytes and the site of melanogenesis. *J. Invest. Derm.*, 36, 243–252

Shubik, P., Pietra, G. & Della Porta, G. (1960) Studies of skin carcinogenesis in the Syrian golden hamster. *Cancer Res.*, 20, 100–105

Simpson, W.L. & Cramer, W. (1943) Fluorescence studies of carcinogens in skin. 1. Histological localization of 20-methylcholanthrene in mouse skin after single application. *Cancer Res.*, 3, 362–369

Stenback, F. (1975) Species-specific neoplastic progression by ultraviolet light on the skin of rats, guinea-pigs, hamsters and mice. *Oncology*, 31, 209–225

Stowell, R.E. (1949) Alterations in the nucleic acids during hepatoma formation in rats fed p-dimethylaminoazobenzene. *Cancer*, 2, 121–131

Straile, W.E. (1964) Carcinogen-induced melanotic tumors of the tylotrich (hair) follicle.
Nature, 202, 403–404

Suntzeff, V., Cowdry, E.V. & Croninger, A.B.
(1955) Microscopic visualization of
degeneration of sebaceous glands caused by
carcinogens. *Cancer Res.*, 15, 637–640

Swift, H. (1959) Studies on nucleolar function.
In: Zirkle, R.E., ed., *Symposium on Molecular
Biology*, Chicago, University of Chicago
Press, pp. 266–303

Takaki, Y., Masutani, M. & Kawada, A. (1971)
Electron microscopic study of keratoacanthoma. *Acta Derm.-Venereol. (Stockh.)*,
51, 21–26

Toda, K., Hori, Y. & Fitzpatrick, T.B. (1968)
Isolation of the intermediate "vesicles"
during ontogeny of melanosomes in
embryonic chick retinal pigment epithelium. *Fed. Proc.*, 27, 722

Twort, J.M. & Twort, C.C. (1936) Variable
sensitivity of different sites of skin of mice
to carcinogenic agents. *J. Pathol. Bact.*, 42,
303–316

Vickers, C.F.H. & Ghadially, F.N. (1961) Kerato-
acanthomata associated with psoriasis. *Br. J.
Derm.*, 73, 120–124

Walters, M.A., Roe, F.J.C. & Levene, A. (1967)
The induction of tumours and other lesions
in hamsters by a single subcutaneous injection of 9,10-dimethyl-1,2-benzanthracene
or urethane on the first day of life. *Br. J.
Cancer*, 21, 184–189

Waterhouse, C.R. (1839) Description of a new
species of hamster (*Cricetus auratus*). *Proc.
Zool. Soc. Lond.*, 7, 57–58

Webb, A.J. & Ghadially, F.N. (1966) Massive or
giant keratoacanthoma. *J. Pathol. Bact.*, 91,
505–509

Whitely, H.J. (1957) Effect of hair growth cycle
on experimental skin carcinogenesis in the
rabbit. *Br. J. Cancer*, 11, 196–205

Whitely, H.J. & Ghadially, F.N. (1951) The
naturally occurring effect of zones of hair
growth on experimental carcinogenesis in
the rabbit. *Br. J. Cancer*, 5, 353–357

Whitely, H.J. & Ghadially, F.N. (1954) Hair
replacement in the domestic rabbit. *J.
Anat.*, 88, 13–18

Willis, R.A. (1967) *Pathology of Tumours*,
London, Butterworths, p. 120

Yamagiwa, K. & Ichikawa, K. (1918) Experimental study of pathogenesis of carcinoma.
J. Cancer Res., 3, 1–29

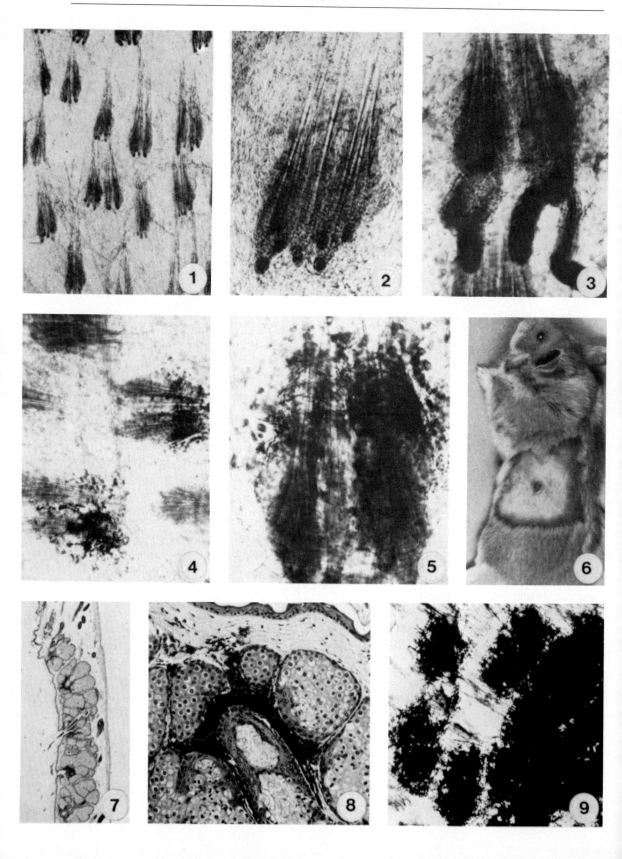

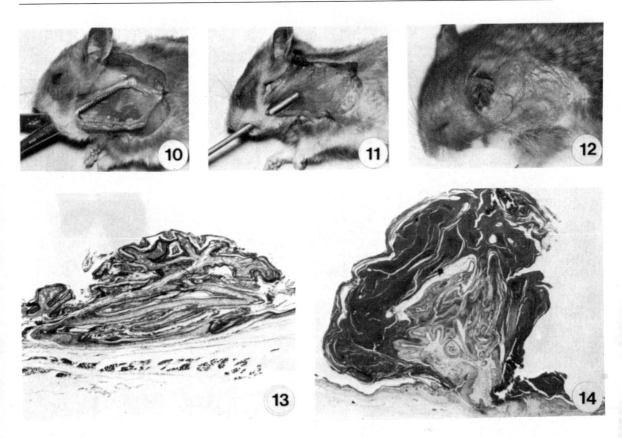

Figure 1. Whole mount of hamster skin, showing groups of hair follicles in telogen. H & E; × 65

Figure 2. High-power view of Figure 1, showing hair follicles in telogen. Note hair shafts, superficial part of follicle and the rounded dermal papilla. H & E; × 270

Figure 3. Hamster hair follicles in early anagen. Note that the superficial part of the follicles resembles that shown in Figure 2. Arising from the bottom are dark club-shaped structures which represent the deeper part of the follicle formed from the hair germ. H & E; × 270

Figure 4. Whole mount of hamster skin, showing two small pigmented spots and groups of numerous hair follicles. H & E; × 65

Figure 5. High-power view of one of the small pigmented spots illustrated in Figure 4, showing network of dendritic melanocytes surrounding pilosebaceous units in the region of the neck and sebaceous glands. H & E; × 170

Figure 6. Adult male hamster with hair clipped on the flank to show a normal pigmented costovertebral spot

Figure 7. Normal costovertebral spot. Note large sebaceous glands and hair follicles in anagen. The melanocytic networks around the necks of some of the pilosebaceous units can just be discerned. H & E; × 14

Figure 8. High-power view of costovertebral spot illustrated in Figure 7, showing a melanocytic network and large sebaceous glands. H & E; × 130

Figure 9. Whole mount of hamster skin showing melanocytic networks of the costovertebral spot. Unstained; × 22

Figure 10. Exteriorization of cheek pouch. An ellipse of skin has been excised, revealing the cheek pouch with forceps within. An incision opening the cheek pouch has been made after it has been anchored by a suture to the skin.

Figure 11. Exteriorization of cheek pouch. Further stage of operation, showing early stage of suturing of cheek pouch to skin margin. Probe demonstrates communication between mouth and cheek pouch.

Figure 12. Final result of operation. Glabrous epithelium of cheek pouch area once occupied by hairy skin.

Figure 13. Papilloma raised on exteriorized cheek pouch by DMBA. H & E; × 13

Figure 14. Keratotic papilloma raised on exteriorized cheek pouch by DMBA. H & E; × 13

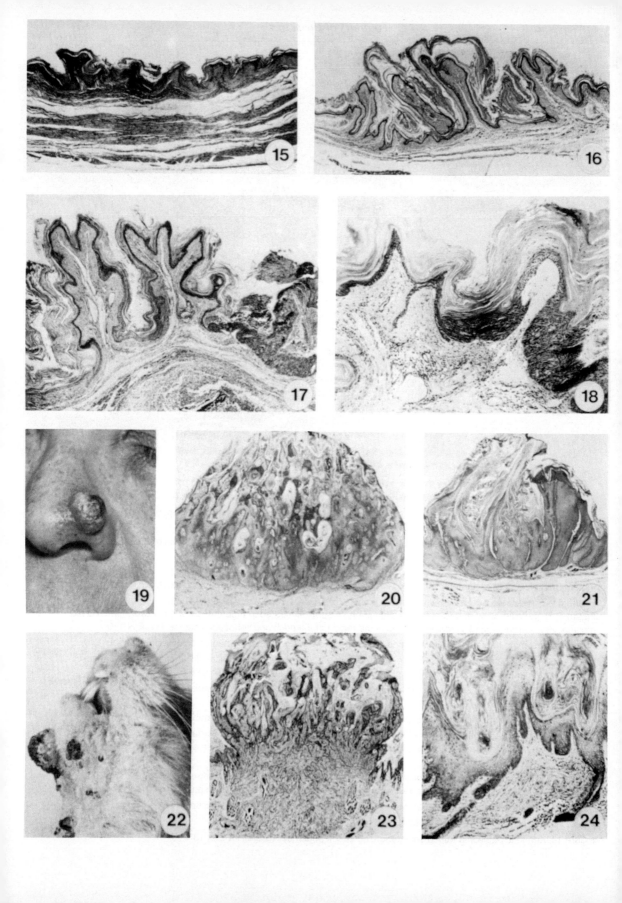

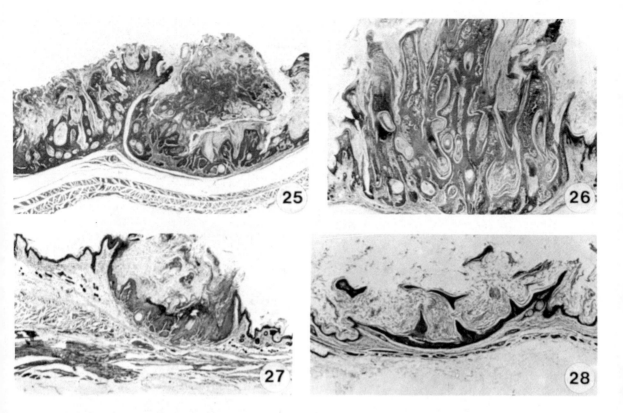

Figure 15. Early stage of development of a papilloma from cheek-pouch epithelium. H & E; × 17

Figure 16. A more advanced stage of papilloma formation on cheek pouch. H & E; × 13

Figure 17. Portion of a fully formed papilloma. Epithelium on right-hand side of the picture shows in situ malignant transformation. H & E; × 30

Figure 18. Abrupt transition from benign to malignant epithelium is seen on the surface of a papilloma raised on the exteriorized cheek pouch by DMBA. H & E; × 60

Figure 19. Type-1 keratoacanthoma on the nose of a woman. This bud-shaped lesion is similar to the hamster tumour illustrated in Figure 22.

Figure 20. Mature type-1 keratoacanthoma in man. H & E; × 9

Figure 21. Type-1 keratoacanthoma produced on hamster skin by DMBA. H & E; × 9

Figure 22. Type-1 keratoacanthoma in hamster; bud-shaped lesion on chin with apical keratinous plug. Compare with Figure 19

Figure 23. DMBA-induced type-1 keratoacanthoma in rabbit, showing well marked pseudo-carcinomatous infiltration. H & E; × 9

Figure 24. An early stage of development of type-1 keratoacanthoma in hamster. Note that the hyperplastic changes affect only the superficial part of the hair follicles; the deeper parts appear unaltered. H & E; × 70

Figure 25. Two confluent type-1 keratoacanthomas in hamster. The one on the left is exfoliating to produce a secondary papilloma while the one on the right has formed a pyramidal keratinous mass which is becoming detached. Further stage of evolution would lead to lesions similar to those shown in Figures 27 and 28. H & E; × 10

Figure 26. An early stage of exfoliation of type-1 keratoacanthoma in hamster probably leading to the formation of a secondary papilloma. H & E; × 10

Figure 27. Regressing keratoacanthoma in hamster. Note cup-shaped base and large keratinous mass. H & E; × 11

Figure 28. Keratoacanthoma in hamster just before complete regression. H & E; × 57

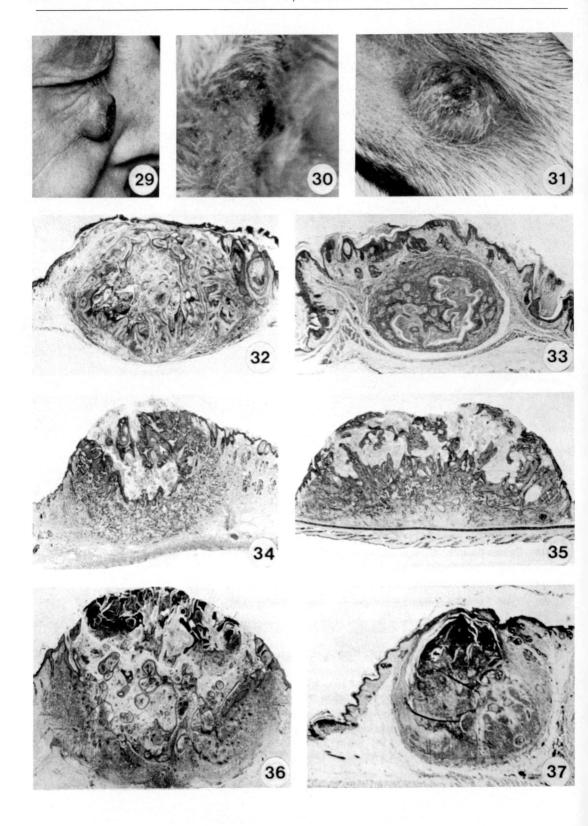

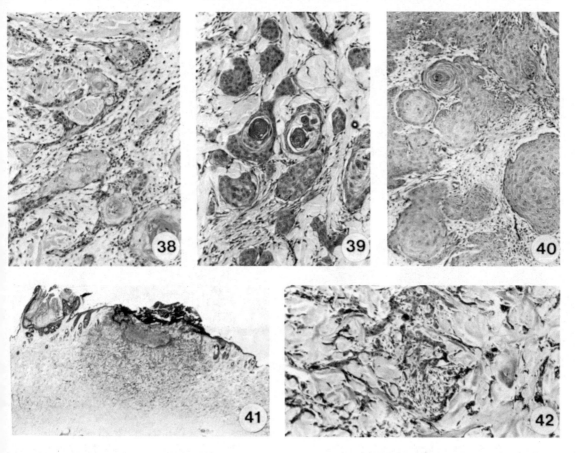

Figure 29. Type-2 keratoacanthoma in man. This lesion is covered by stretched skin which has ulcerated (dark area) and exposed the keratinous mass

Figure 30. Type-2 keratoacanthoma in hamster. A deeply placed berry-shaped lesion arising in axillary skin, ulceration of stretched skin revealing keratinous mass (dark area). Compare with Figure 29

Figure 31. Type-2 keratoacanthoma in rabbit. Smooth dome-shaped lesion on inner ear. Vessels are seen in stretched skin, as also a dark area representing the underlying keratinous plug.

Figure 32. Type-2 keratoacanthoma in mouse. Compare with Figures 33 and 37. H & E; × 11

Figure 33. Type-2 keratoacanthoma in hamster similar to lesions in Figures 32 and 37. H & E; × 10

Figure 34. Type-2 keratoacanthoma in rabbit. Lesion produced on the flank with DMBA by Dr H.J. Whitely. This lesion shows surface ulceration of the cystic tumour with discharging keratinous mass. Note the well-marked pseudocarcinomatous infiltration. H & E; × 7

Figure 35. Type-2 keratoacanthoma in rabbit. Same tumour as in Figure 31. Growth against the cartilaginous plate of the ear has flattened the base of the lesion. H & E; × 9

Figure 36. Type-2 keratoacanthoma in hamster. Much of the lesion has differentiated out to form keratin. When this is shed, a cup-shaped lesion difficult to distinguish from a regressing type-1 lesion is produced. H & E; × 7

Figure 37. Type-2 keratoacanthoma in hamster. Mature lesion about to produce surface ulceration and discharge its keratinous plug. H & E; × 9

Figure 38. Margin of keratoacanthoma in man, mimicking a well differentiated squamous cell carcinoma. Note infiltration of stroma by lymphocytes. H & E; × 96

Figure 39. Margin of a keratoacanthoma in rabbit, mimicking a well differentiated squamous cell carcinoma. Note stromal fibrosis and the singularly well differentiated islands of infiltrating epithelium. H & E; × 96

Figure 40. Biopsy specimen from a giant keratoacanthoma in man which regressed. The histological picture mimicks a squamous cell carcinoma. Note lymphocytic infiltration of stroma, and absence of cellular and nuclear pleomorphism. H & E; × 165

Figure 41. Regressing type-1 (left) and type-2 (centre) lesions in rabbit. H & E; × 8

Figure 42. High-power view of margin of type-2 lesion illustrated in Figure 41. Note dense fibrous tissue and inflammatory cells apparently destroying columns of infiltrating epithelial cells. H & E; × 96

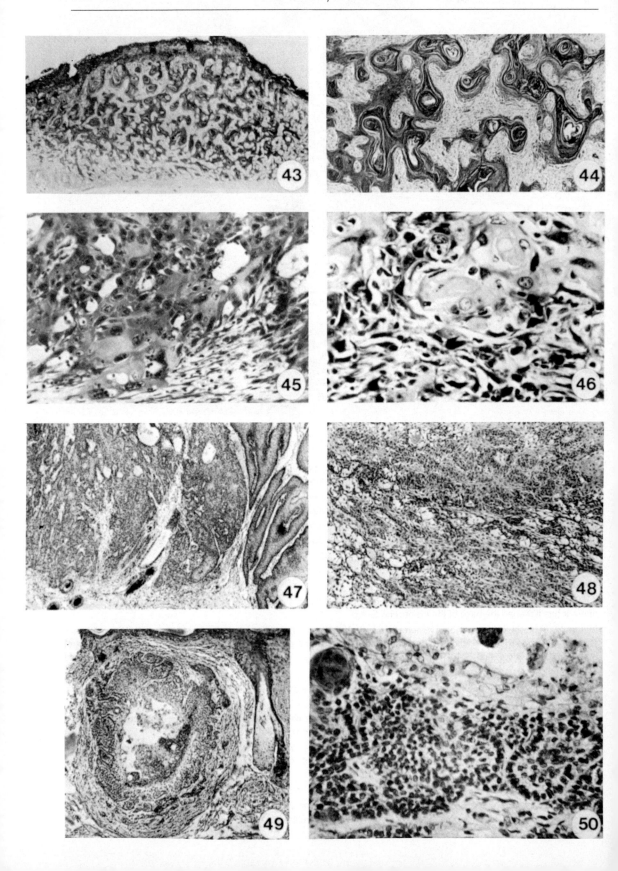

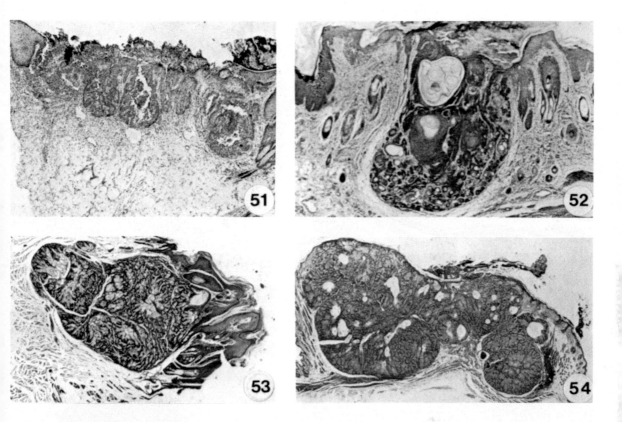

Figure 43. Non-equatorial section through a regressing keratoacanthoma in hamster, showing marked keratinization of infiltrating epithelium. H & E; × 9

Figure 44. High-power view of Figure 43. Note how the infiltrating epithelium is differentiating out to form large concentric keratinous masses. H & E; × 29

Figure 45. Infiltrating edge of DMBA-induced squamous cell carcinoma in hamster; it produced lymph-node deposits. H & E; × 165

Figure 46. Lymph-node deposits from a cutaneous squamous cell carcinoma produced in hedgehog by DMBA painting. H & E; × 260

Figure 47. The difference in architecture and cellular morphology between a basal cell tumour (left) and a keratoacanthoma with typical squamous differentiation (in hamster) is illustrated in this photomicrograph. H & E; × 31

Figure 48. Basal cell tumour in hamster. Besides basal cells, this tumour also contains clear cells (bottom left-hand corner) and squamous cells (top right-hand corner). H & E; × 52

Figure 49. Cystic basal cell tumour in hamster. H & E; × 60

Figure 50. High-power view of Figure 49. Adjacent to cyst cavity (top right) are cells showing sebaceous differentiation. Further out in the wall of the cyst are palisade basal cells. H & E; × 290

Figure 51. Ulcerated superficial basal cell tumour in hamster. H & E; × 28

Figure 52. A hamster tumour resembling the trichoepithelioma of man. H & E; × 17

Figure 53. Sebaceous adenoma in hamster. (Surface of skin is to right of picture). The lobulated adenoma is seen arising from a gland adjacent to a hyperplastic hair follicle. H & E; × 13

Figure 54. Further stage of evolution of sebaceous adenoma. H & E; × 10

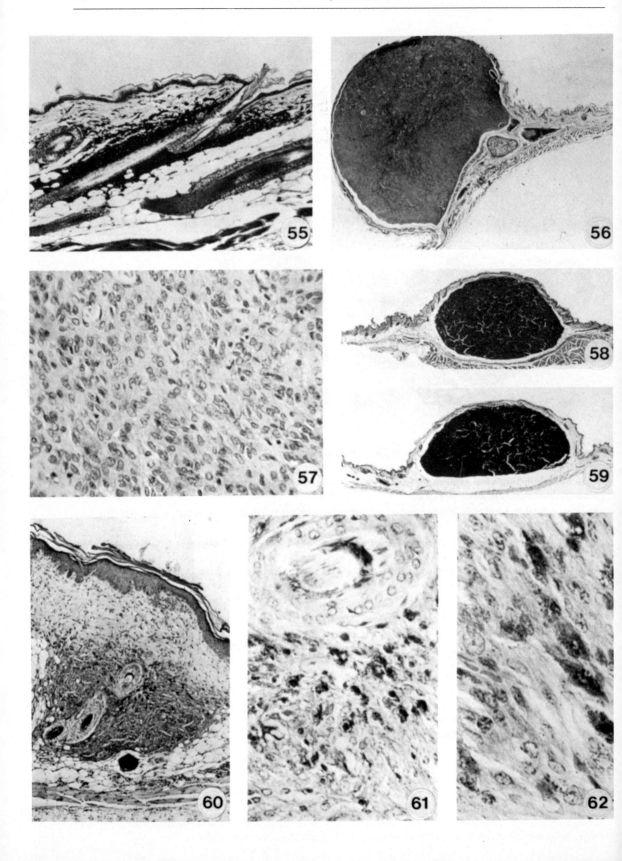

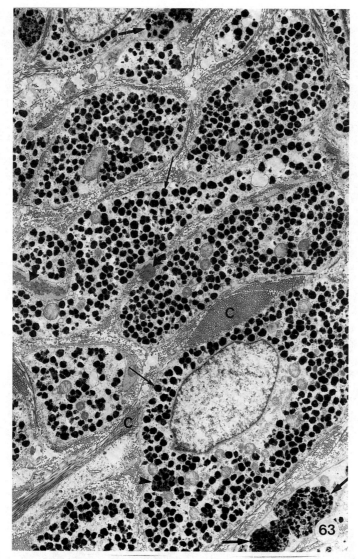

Figure 55. An early lesion in DMBA-painted hamster skin illustrating a melanotic tumour arising from the perifollicular network of melanocytes of a small pigmented spot. The young tumour is seen as a sheath enveloping a pilosebaceous unit. H & E; × 87

Figure 56. Melanotic tumour in hamster, arising at the root of the ear. H & E; × 10

Figure 57. High-power view of tumour illustrated in Figure 56. Bleached. H & E; × 296

Figures 58 and 59. Typical intensely pigmented melanotic tumours produced in the agouti animal by DMBA painting. H & E; × 10

Figure 60. An early lesion illustrating a hypomelanotic tumour arising from a melanotic network in a white hamster. Compare with Figure 55. H & E; × 87

Figure 61. High-power view of tumour illustrated in Figure 60. The tumour cells are in close contact with a hair follicle seen at the top of the picture. H & E; × 520

Figure 62. High-power view of another hypomelanotic tumour produced in the white hamster. The bulk of the tumour cells contained no melanin. Only a few densely pigmented cells were seen scattered throughout the tumour. H & E; × 870

Figure 63. Human melanotic cellular blue naevus. Several naevus cells containing solitary melanosomes (thin arrows) and melanophages containing compound melanosomes (thick arrows) are seen. A small compound melanosome (arrowhead) is present in a naevus cell also. Note the collagen fibres (C) and elastic fibres (curved arrowheads) in the matrix. Note also the absence of an external lamina. × 3600 (From Ghadially *et al.*, 1986)

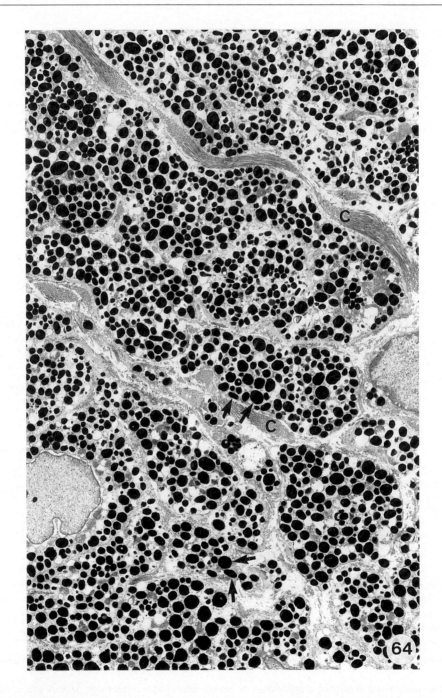

Figure 64. Hamster melanotic blue naevus. The naevus cells contain numerous rounded and elongated solitary (arrows) melanosomes. Note the collagenous matrix (c) and the absence of an external lamina. × 2800 (From Ghadially *et al.,* 1986)

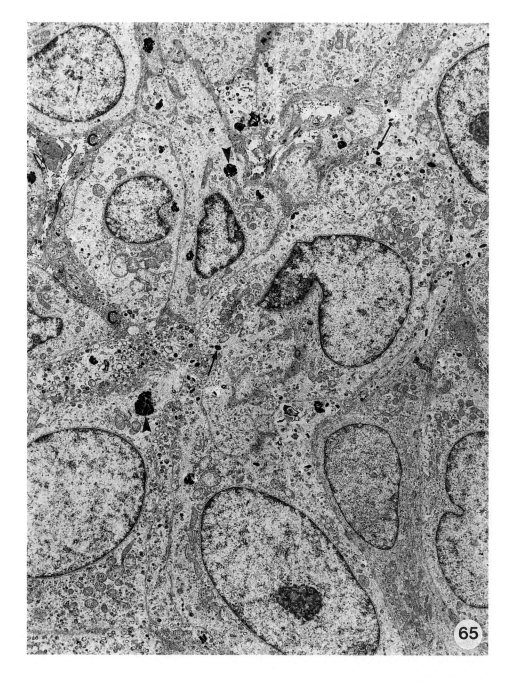

Figure 65. Human hypomelanotic cellular blue naevus. Depicted here is the better melanized portion of the tumour, where many of the naevus cells contain several small solitary melanosomes (arrows) and some compound melanosomes (arrowheads). In the major part of the tumour, no melanosomes or only one or two melanosomes per cell were found. Note the sparse matrix containing some collagen fibrils (C). No external lamina is evident. × 2300

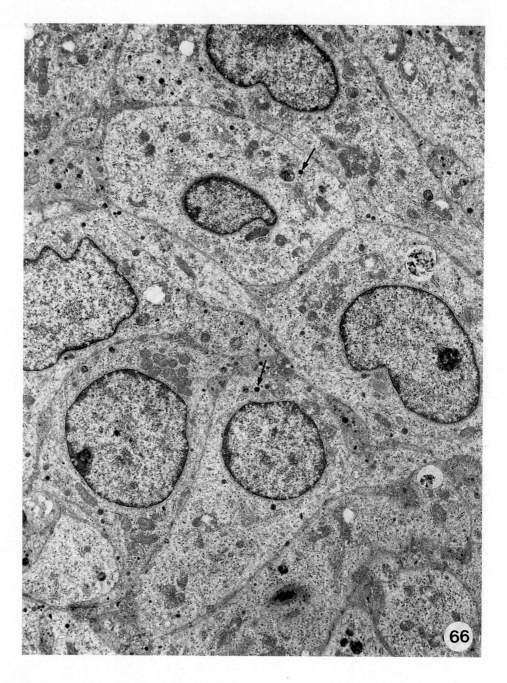

Figure 66. Hamster hypomelanotic blue naevus. The closely packed naevus cells contain a few small rounded melanosomes (arrows). No external lamina is seen here nor was one detected at higher magnification. × 2500 (From Ghadially, 1985)

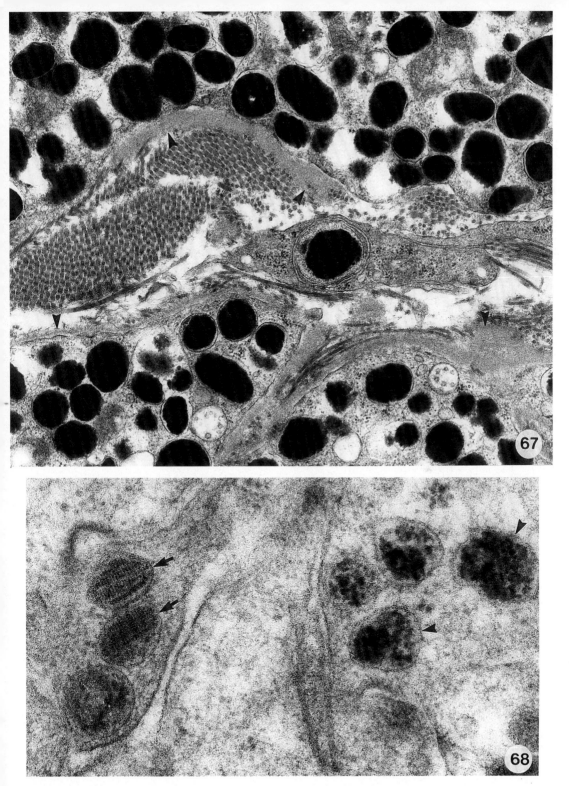

Figure 67. Hamster melanotic blue naevus. Interrupted external lamina or external lamina-like material (arrowheads) of varying thickness is seen adjacent to tumour cells. The cells contain stage IV melanosomes. × 16 200 (From Ghadially *et al.*, 1986)

Figure 68. Hamster hypomelanotic blue naevus. Two oval stage II or III melanosomes (arrows) with characteristic striated internal structure are seen in the cell on the left. The cell on the right contains granular melanosomes (arrowheads). × 115 000 (From Ghadially, 1985)

Tumours of the mammary gland

P.L. Fernandez, A. Cardesa and K. Kamino

There are very few reports on the experimental induction of tumours of the mammary gland in the hamster. Nevertheless, consideration of the hamster model would seem to be of interest, in view of the fact that the oral administration of 3-methylcholanthrene (MC) to this species resulted in the induction of mammary gland carcinomas after short periods of time (Della Porta, 1961). In certain aspects, this is a more striking occurrence than in the rat (Huggins *et al.*, 1959), since spontaneous mammary tumours are exceedingly rare in the hamster, and since in this animal prolonged stimulation with synthetic estrogens did not result in the development of tumours of the breast (Kirkman, 1959).

NORMAL STRUCTURE AND HISTOLOGY

As in the rat and mouse, the mammary glands of the hamster are arranged in the form of two Vs with their points located in the axillary and inguinal regions. Usually, in the hamster, the nipples are not regularly spaced. As a rule, the hamster has seven pairs of nipples, but there may also be six nipples on one side and eight on the other. Microscopically, the mammary gland of the adult hamster female undergoes a sequence of changing patterns which, in general, according to Michel and Steiner (1969), may be described as follows. The parenchymal structure of the breast in non-pregnant, sexually mature hamsters is composed of a few mammary complexes. They consist primarily of a ductal system, lined on the inside mainly by concentrically disposed, cuboidal epithelial cells, with rounded, chromatin-rich nuclei. Externally, the ducts are surrounded by soft connective tissue and by fat tissue. From the fourth day of pregnancy, a progressive enlargement of the mammary complexes becomes evident. As a result of growth and differentiation of the terminal ducts, acini are developed; this completes the formation of the glandular lobules (Figures 1A and 1B). At the 12th day of pregnancy the acini of some lobules already show that secretion has begun. At this stage, the ducts and the acini have a cuboidal epithelium in which myoepithelial cells are also present. At the 15th day, the small mammary ducts are filled with milk. Three hours after delivery the mammary gland is fully functioning, showing all the phases of secretion of an apocrine gland. Three days after weaning, the acini and the ducts already show marked signs of stagnation with intense accumulation of secretions. The epithelial covering of the acini is no longer recognizable. At the same time a marked increase in the amount of connective tissue on the lobules takes place. Eight days after weaning, the involutional changes of the breast tissue are so far advanced that there is no recognizable difference from the non-pregnant, sexually mature female hamster.

HISTOLOGICAL TYPES OF TUMOUR

Benign
   Fibroadenoma
   Adenoma
   Cystadenoma

Malignant
   Papillary carcinoma
   Cribriform carcinoma
   Follicular carcinoma
   Carcinosarcoma

Fibroadenoma

Fibroadenoma is a tumour composed of ductal adenomatous structures surrounded by abundant benign fibromatous stroma. We are aware of three recorded cases of mammary fibroadenoma in hamsters (Toth *et al.*, 1961; Homburger, 1983; Ernst *et al.*, 1989).

Adenoma

This benign tumour consists of a proliferation of usually medium-sized closely packed glands with round nuclei and scanty atypia. Apocrine features can be also found (Figure 2A, B).

Cystadenoma

A case of spontaneous mammary cystadenoma has been reported by Ernst *et al.* (1989).

Carcinoma

The majority of the reported tumours primarily originating from the mammary gland were carcinomas. According to Della Porta (1961), such carcinomas were often multiple, with as many as six occurring in one animal (Figure 3). Grossly, their diameter ranged from 0.4 to 3 cm at death. They had solid portions alternating with necrotic areas, and cystic formations often filled with blood-stained fluid (Figure 4A). Histologically, the tumours were invariably adenocarcinomas, showing either irregular glandular structures with papillary projections or a follicular or cribriform pattern (Figure 4B, C). Some tumours were seen to grow intraductally, occupying the lumen of the larger mammary ducts, which are located underneath the skin, sometimes with a rather exuberant papillary pattern. In two out of ten females with mammary carcinoma, the tumour metastasized to both local and distant lymph nodes. The lymph-node metastasis of one of the tumours showed cystic changes and abundant papillary projections, even though the primary tumour was follicular in pattern. Transplants of tumours from two different donors were both successful; both tumours grew in untreated hamsters of both sexes. An interesting additional observation in this study was that the mammary glands not affected by the tumours showed dilatation and hyperplasia of the ducts and evidence of secretion (Figure 5).

Carcinosarcoma

Two instances of mammary carcinosarcomas in hamster females were reported by Bain *et al.* (1959). This type of tumour is usually solid, and has a double epithelial and mesenchymal malignant component. It can display a nodular arrangement and extensive necrotic areas (Figure 6A). Malignant neoplastic glands coexist with a very cellular stroma (Figure 6B) in which atypia and mitoses are also observed. The neoplastic cells sometimes show remarkable atypia as well as intense proliferative activity with numerous abnormal mitoses (Figure 6C, D).

SPONTANEOUS TUMOURS

Spontaneous malignant tumours of the breast are very rare in hamsters. According to Kirkman (1959), in more than 30 different types of tumour oserved in his colony of Syrian hamsters, no mammary tumours were observed. In other large-scale studies of spontaneous tumours in Syrian (*Mesocricetus auratus*) and European hamster (*Cricetus cricetus* L.), no malignant tumours of the mammary gland have been recorded (Fortner, 1957, 1961; Pour *et al.*, 1976; Homburger 1983; Fabry, 1985; Ernst *et al.*, 1989). We are aware of one solitary cystic adenocarcinoma of the mammary gland in a hamster observed by Habermann (see Eddy *et al.*, 1958). Dunham and Herrold (1962) reported two breast adenocarcinomas in females among 375 variously manipulated hamsters of both sexes, which they considered as spontaneous. Fortner *et al.* (1961) described a spontaneously occurring transplantable mammary tumour, from which, in the primary host, metastases were not found; in the 91st transplant generation, however, metastasis occurred in the axillary and inguinal lymph nodes. The original tumour showed a 4 × 2.5 cm, dark red–brown cut surface. The consistency was soft and it was subcutaneously attached to a prominent mamma on the right side. The histology was that of an adenocarcinoma arising in the large mammary ducts and invading adjacent stroma. Necrosis and haemorrhage were extensive. The tumour cells were large, polygonal, with nuclei of varying size. There was an abundant vascular stroma which contained many fibroblasts, neutrophils, lymphocytes, plasma cells and occasionally mast cells. With successive passage of this mammary tumour to hamsters, the number of mitoses increased from 1 per high-power field to 3 and 5. The nuclei also contained more nucleoli and the cytoplasm became more basophilic. The hormone sensitivity of the tumour was not known in detail. The tumour appeared to grow faster in males, and did not respond well to cortisone acetate, estradiol or testosterol propionate (Schabel *et al.*, 1961).

Malignant spontaneous breast tumours seem to be more frequent in other species such as the Russian hamster (*Phodopus sungorus*), in which adenocarcinomas have been reported (Cooper *et al.*, 1991; Lawrie & Megahy, 1991).

A few spontaneous benign tumours have been reported in Syrian and European hamsters, including fibroadenomas and cystadenomas (Homburger, 1983; Ernst *et al.*, 1989).

INDUCTION OF TUMOURS

Studies by Della Porta (1961) on tumour induction in hamsters by oral administration of MC showed that this method generated mammary carcinoma after short latency periods. Of the 70 MC-treated hamster females, 10 had a total of 26 mammary carcinomas. As many as six tumours were found in one animal. No mammary tumours were seen in males. The age of the animals at the beginning of the experiment seemed to play an interesting role in tumour induction. In 20 hamster females whose treatment with MC was started at five weeks of age, mammary carcinomas developed in seven animals, whereas among the same number of females receiving the same treatment but started at 12 weeks of age, only one animal had mammary carcinoma. In another group of 30 females in which the treatment was started at 15 weeks of age, only two animals developed carcinoma.

The mode of action of MC on the breast tissue of hamsters is not well understood, but it is suggested that a hormonal influence may be involved, because most of the hamsters with mammary cancer also had both proliferation of the endometrial stroma and ovarian thecomas. Nevertheless, no mammary tumours have been reported after administration of diethylstilbestrol alone, even though many hamsters have been treated in his way in order to induce renal tumours (Kirkman, 1959). However, Bain *et al.* (1959) reported the occurrence of two mammary carcinosarcomas in females in which MC was implanted in the gallbladder, and estradiol subcutaneously. The part that the pituitary gland may play in the induction of mammary tumours in the hamster is not known. Isologous pituitary grafts in the kidney of golden hamsters resulted in stimulation of the production of sufficient prolactin to affect the mammary gland and to cause diffuse acinar hyperplasia, often accompanied by milk secretion, ductal hyperplasia, and ectasia of the breast of female hamsters, but no mammary tumours were observed (Della Porta, 1962).

Two mammary adenocarcinomas and one mammary fibroadenoma were recorded after administration to hamsters of 0.2–0.4 % urethane in the drinking-water for about 10 months (Toth *et al.*, 1961). Rivière *et al.* (1964) observed that, in one-month-old female golden hamsters whose dorsal region was painted twice a week with urethane in acetone solution, or which received urethane in their drinking-water, mammary tumours developed after 12–18 months in 4 out of 20 painted animals, and in 2 out of 20 orally treated animals. Histologically, the tumours were papillary carcinomas. In another experiment, after injection of urethane into adult hamsters (Toth, 1971), one adenocarcinoma of the breast was also found. Homburger *et al.* (1971) showed that susceptibility to mammary tumour induction by MC in females varied among different hamster lines. In addition, Homburger *et al.* (1972) showed that susceptibility to mammary tumours was higher in the inbred hamsters in their colony than in non-inbred hamsters.

The mammary gland of the hamster has been recently reported as target organ for vinyl chloride carcinogenesis (Gold *et al.*, 1991).

COMPARATIVE ASPECTS

From the morphological standpoint, carcinomas of the mammary gland in female hamsters, like normal lobular structures, have a certain resemblance to their counterparts in women. In the hamster, they are mainly ductal in origin, and in women the great majority also arise from mammary ducts. The papillary and cribriform patterns of growth, which are frequent in hamsters, are also common in women. The follicular or acinar pattern observed in hamsters shows certain similarities to the characteristic follicular pattern of the so-called juvenile carcinoma of the breast seen in children and young women (Norris & Taylor, 1970).

With the regard to the risk of exposure of women to the carcinogens that have been shown to act on female hamster breast tissue, it should be noted that MC or structurally related carcinogenic steroids may be endogenously produced (Clayson, 1962). The gut, with the help of the intestinal flora, using bile acids or cholesterol as the starting point, is the organ where these reactions most commonly take place (Reddy *et al.*, 1978). Although it has been shown that such reactions are important mainly as a fundamental stage in the promotion of colon cancer, it should be remembered that, in the hamster model for mammary cancer using MC, breast tumours and colonic tumours occurred concomitantly.

The other carcinogen with organotropism for the mammary gland of hamsters, urethane, has been found in beverages (Löfroth & Gjevall, 1971) and, according to Schmähl (1970), has been used as a solvent in the processing of progesterone.

ACKNOWLEDGEMENTS

The authors are indebted to Dr Giuseppe Della Porta for providing photographic material for this chapter and to Mrs T. Roch for secretarial work.

REFERENCES

Bain, G.O., Allen, P.B.R., Silbermann, O. & Kowalewski, K. (1959) Induction in hamsters of biliary carcinomas by intra-cholecystic methylcholanthrene pellets. *Cancer Res.*, 19, 93–96

Clayson, D.B. (1962) *Chemical Carcinogenesis*, London, Churchill, p. 340

Cooper, J.E., Knowler, C. & Pearson A.J. (1991) Tumours in Russian hamsters (*Phodopus sungorus*). *Vet. Rec.*, 128, 335–336

Della Porta, G. (1961) Induction of intestinal, mammary, and ovarian tumors in hamsters with oral administration of 20-methyl-cholanthrene. *Cancer Res.*, 21, 575–579

Della Porta, G. (1962) Isologous pituitary implants in the kidney of golden hamsters. *Tumori*, 49, 139–146

Dunham, L.J. & Herrold, K.M. (1962) Failure to produce tumors in the hamster cheek pouch by exposure to ingredients of betel quid. Histopathologic changes in the pouch and other organs by exposure to known carcinogens. *J. Natl Cancer Inst.*, 29, 1047–1067

Eddy, B.E., Stewart, S.E., Young, R. & Mider, G.B. (1958) Neoplasms in hamsters induced by mouse tumor agent passed in tissue culture. *J. Natl Cancer Inst.*, 20, 747–761

Ernst, H., Kunstyr, I., Rittinghausen I. & Mohr, U. (1989) Spontaneous tumors of the European hamster (*Cricetus cricetus* L.). *Z. Versuchstierkd.*, 32, 87–96

Fabry, A. (1985) The incidence of neoplasms in Syrian hamsters with particular emphasis on intestinal neoplasia. *Arch. Toxicol.* (suppl.), 8, 124–127

Fortner, J.G. (1957) Spontaneous tumors, including gastrointestinal neoplasms and malignant melanomas, in the Syrian hamster. *Cancer*, 10, 1153–1156

Fortner, J.G. (1961) The influence of castration on spontaneous tumorigenesis in the Syrian (golden) hamster. *Cancer Res.*, 21, 1491–1498

Fortner, J.G., Mahy, A.G. & Cotran, R.S. (1961) Transplantable tumors of the Syrian (golden) hamster. II. Tumors of the hematopoietic tissues, genitourinary organs, mammary glands and sarcomas. Cancer chemotherapy screening data X. *Cancer Res.*, 21, 199–234

Gold, L.S., Slone, T.H., Manley N.B. & Bernstein, L. (1991) Target organs in chronic bioassays of 533 chemical carcinogens. *Environ. Health Perspect.*, 93, 233–246

Homburger, F. (1983) Background data on tumor incidence in control animals (Syrian hamster). *Prog. Exp. Tumor Res.*, 26, 259–265.

Homburger, F., Kerr, C.S. & Hsueh, S.S. (1971) Influence of genetic factors on the induction of mammary and intestinal adenocarcinomas in inbred Syrian golden hamsters. *Nature* , 234, 28–29.

Homburger, F., Hsueh, S.S., Kerr, C.S. & Russfield, A.B. (1972) Inherited susceptibility of inbred strains of Syrian hamsters to induction of subcutaneous sarcomas and mammary and gastrointestinal carcinomas by subcutaneous and gastric administration of polynuclear hydrocarbons. *Cancer Res.*, 32, 360–366

Huggins, C., Briziarelli, G. & Sutton, H., Jr (1959) Rapid induction of mammary carcinoma in the rat and the influence of hormones on the tumors. *J. Exp. Med.*, 109, 25–41

Kirkman, H. (1959) Estrogen-induced tumors of the kidney in the Syrian hamster. *Nat. Cancer Inst. Monogr.*, 1, 1–57

Lawrie, A.M., Megahy, I.W. (1991) Tumours in Russian hamsters. *Vet. Rec.*, 128, 411–412

Löfroth, G. & Gjevall, T. (1971) Diethylpyrocarbonate: formation of urethan in treated beverages. *Science*, 1974, 1248–1250

Michel, G. & Steiner, A. (1969) Zum Bau der Milchdrüse des syrischen Goldhamsters (*Mesocricetus auratus* W.). *Z. Versuchstierk.*, 11, 320–331

Norris, H.J. & Taylor, H.B. (1970) Carcinoma of the breast in women less than thirty years old. *Cancer*, 26, 953–959

Pour, P., Mohr, U., Althoff, J., Cardesa, A. & Kmoch, N. (1976) Spontaneous tumors and common diseases in two colonies of Syrian hamsters. IV. Vascular and lymphatic systems and lesions of other sites. *J. Natl Cancer Inst.*, 56, 963–974

Reddy, B.S., Weisburger, J.H. & Wynder E.L. (1978) Colon cancer: bile salts as tumor promoters. In: Slaga, T.J., Sivak, A. & Boutwell, R.K., eds, *Carcinogenesis*, Vol. 2, *Mechanisms of Tumor Promotion and Cocarcinogenesis*, New York, Raven Press, pp. 453–464

Rivière, M.R., Perrier, M. T., Chouroulinkov, I. & Guérin, M. (1964) Tumeurs mammaires développées chez le hamster femelle après application cutanée ou ingestion d'uréthane. *C. R. Séanc. Soc. Biol.*, 158, 440-443

Schabel, F.M., Jr, Skipper, H.E., Fortner, J.G., Thompson, J.R., Laster, W.R., Jr, Moore, J.H., Kelley, C.A. & Farnell, D.R. (1961) Experimental evaluation of potential anticancer agents. II. Studies on the growth characteristics, metastases, and drug response of hamster neoplasms of diverse "sites of origin". Cancer chemotherapy screening data X. *Cancer Res.*, 21, 235–339

Schmähl, D. (1970) *Entstehung, Wachstum und Chemotherapie maligner Tumoren*, Aulendorf, Editio Cantor, pp. 145–146

Toth, B. (1971) Tumor induction by repeated injections of urethan in newborn and adult hamsters: Age influence. II. *J. Natl Cancer Inst.*, 46, 81–93

Toth, B., Tomatis, L. & Shubik, P. (1961) Multipotential carcinogenesis with urethan in the Syrian golden hamster. *Cancer Res.*, 21, 1537–1541

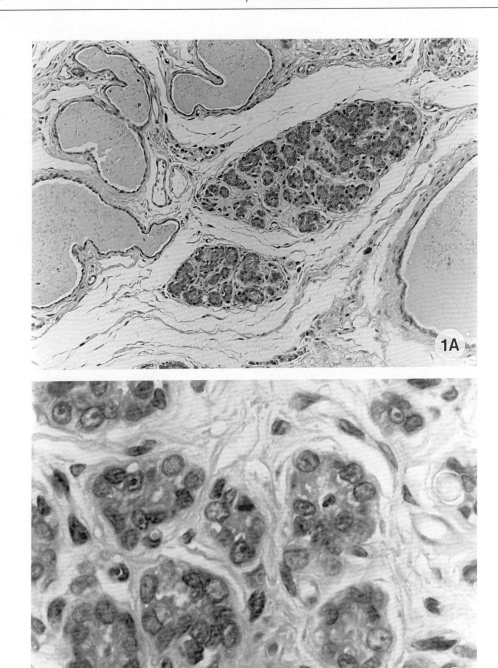

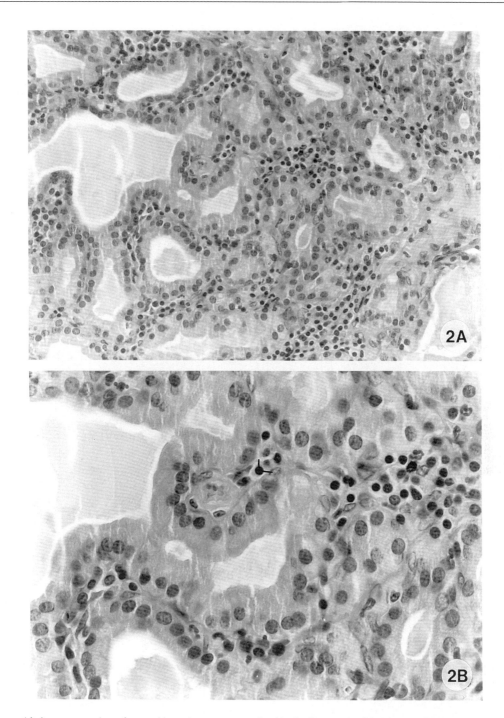

Figure 1A. Low-power view of normal hamster mammary gland in the first week of pregnancy. Mammary complexes are composed of terminal ducts and acini surrounded by connective tissue. Large dilated ducts are also seen. H&E; × 100

B. Acini are lined by cuboidal epithelial cells. Myoepithelial cells are not yet evident. H&E; × 600.

Figure 2A. Adenoma is composed of medium-sized glands, some of them irregular, with a rather monomorphic cellularity. Inflammatory infiltrate is seen in the stroma. H&E; × 200

B. Higher magnification of adenoma showing round nuclei with scarce or no atypia and apocrine features with granular eosinophilic cytoplasm. H&E; × 400

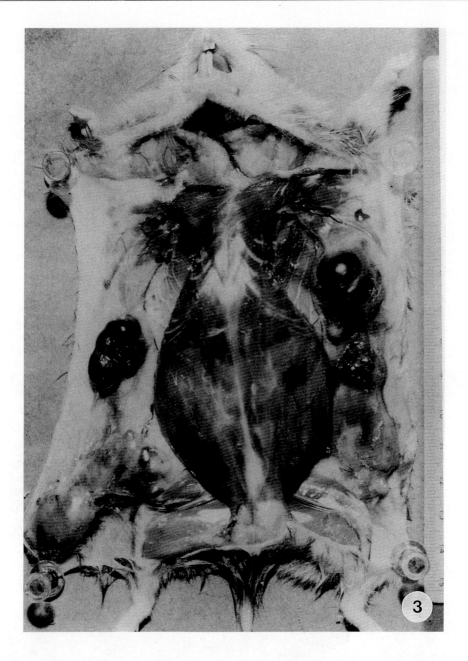

Figure 3. Several mammary carcinomas, the largest measuring up to 2.5 cm in greatest dimension, arising along the right and left milk lines of a female hamster.

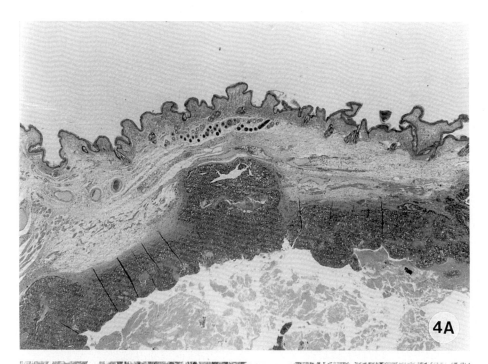

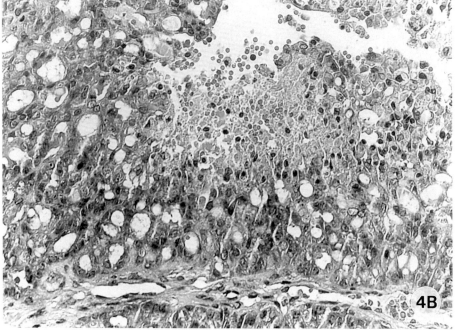

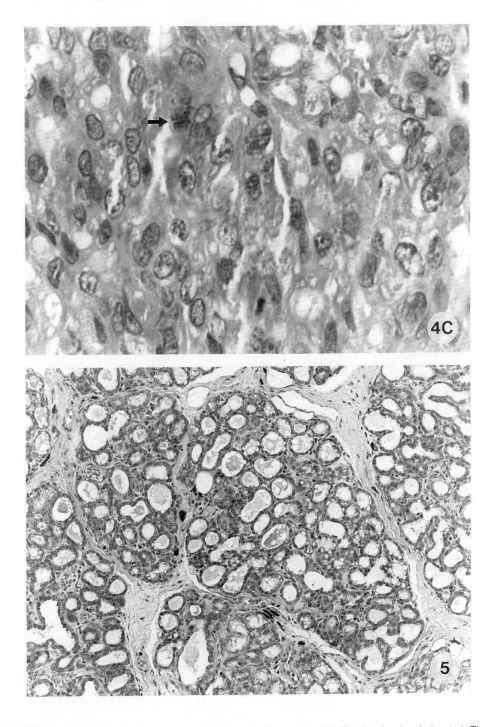

Figure 4A. Large cystic adenocarcinoma underneath the skin. The tumour is infiltrating the dermis (centre). The cyst was filled with necrotic and haemorrhagic fluid. H&E; ×10

B. The same tumour, showing solid areas with central necrosis and a cribriform pattern. H&E; ×200

Figure 4C. A higher-power view shows nuclear atypia with prominent nucleoli and mitotic figures (arrow). H&E; ×600

Figure 5. Lobular architecture is preserved in this hyperplastic mammary gland, with numerous dilated acini and signs of secretion on the right. H&E; ×100

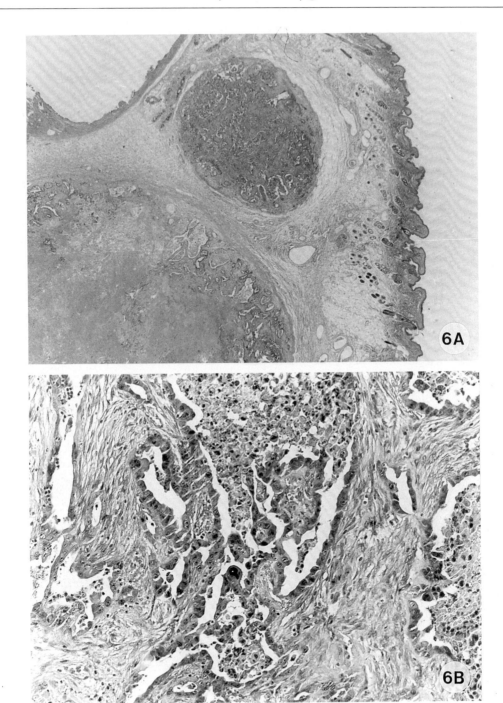

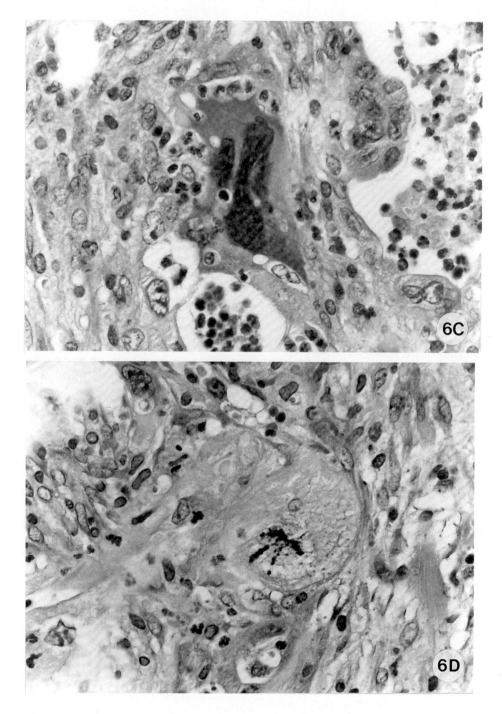

Figure 6A. Carcinosarcoma composed of several neoplastic nodules and cysts. Extensive necrotic areas are seen at the left lower corner. H&E; ×20

B. The tumour is composed of irregular neoplastic glands and a very cellular fibrous stroma. Glands are filled with cell debris and inflammatory cells. H&E; ×100

C. Scattered epithelial cells show intense atypia. H&E; ×400

D. Mitoses were abundant in this tumour, sometimes with monstrous forms. H&E; ×400

Tumours of the oral cavity, buccal pouch, oesophagus, forestomach and salivary glands

M. Takahashi and H. Okamiya

The fact that hamsters have buccal pouches has determined their wide use for investigations of oral carcinogenesis, while simultaneous dermal application allows comparison in the same animals between epithelia with and without a pilosebaceous apparatus.

The carcinogen-induced squamous cell carcinoma of the hamster buccal pouch is a well documented tumour, demonstrating biological progression through clearly defined preneoplastic and neoplastic stages, which is often compared with cancers arising from human cervical and oral mucosal tissues.

NORMAL STRUCTURE

Oral cavity and buccal pouch

The free margins of the lips form a three-cornered flap which blocks the mouth opening when the mouth is closed. The hard palate is 15.0–16.5 mm long and runs from the caudal edge of the incisor teeth to the caudal end of the last molars. The oral cavity is lined with keratinized, stratified squamous epithelium. Cornification may be slight, incomplete or even absent.

There are two well developed buccal pouches which are located on the lateral side of the neck and head beneath the cheek skin. The pouches are internal muscular sacs opening on each side of the vestibulum oris and extending dorso-caudally to the shoulder. The pouch wall is, histologically, composed of four layers: stratified squamous epithelium on the surface, dense fibrous connective tissue, longitudinal striated muscle fibres, and loose areolar or submuscular connective tissues where the pouch joins the underlying structures (Bivin *et al.,* 1987).

Oesophagus

The oesophagus runs mainly mid-sagittally along the dorsal aspect of the trachea. Its length is about 5 cm, the last centimetre being caudal to the diaphragm. The oesophageal wall is composed of four coats: mucosa, sub-mucosa, muscularis, and adventitia or serosa. The mucosa consists of keratinized stratified epithelium in longitudinal folds and lamina propria, with neither glands nor muscularis mucosa. The muscularis consists throughout of inner circular and outer longitudinal skeletal muscle sheets. The adventitia comprises loose fibro-elastic connective tissue that extends to the adjacent organs. In the intra-abdominal region of the oesophagus, the adventitia is replaced by the serosa — a thin layer of loose fibro-elastic connective tissue covered by mesothelium.

Forestomach

The stomach of the hamster is compartmentalized, consisting of a non-glandular forestomach separated from the glandular stomach by a distinct border called the limiting ridge. The separation is a constriction with a sphincter-like muscular structure which may regulate movement of ingested material between the sections of the stomach. The oesophagus enters the stomach through the wall of the lesser curvature at the junction between the two compartments.

The forestomach is lined by stratified squamous epithelium characteristic both histologically and ultrastructurally of the rumen, but contains no papillae.

Salivary glands

The major salivary glands include submaxillary, parotid and sublingual varieties. The submaxillary gland is associated with a retrolingual gland. In addition, smaller salivary glands with serous and mucous acini are situated randomly in the buccal areas but always at the orifices of the buccal pouches. Histologically, salivary glands are composed of tubuloacinar structures.

Submaxillary glands contain a granular tubular segment which functions as part of the intralobular duct system. The acini are morphologically and histochemically intermediate between mucous and serous acini. The parenchyma of the hamster submaxillary gland is similar to that of the rat and mouse (Flon & Gerstner, 1968). Narrow intercalated ducts connect the acini to the branches of the granular convoluted tubules. These tubules are continuous with the striated duct segments of the excretory system.

The parotid gland is located below the ear and is structurally similar to those in other mammals. One central, one ventral, and two dorsal ducts emerge from each parotid salivary gland. These ducts run first along the lateral margin of, and then across, the masseter muscle. The gland is entirely covered by the buccal pouch and ends near the maxillary edge of the entrance to the buccal pouch. The parotid gland contains serous acini and ducts with granule formation.

The sublingual gland is closely adherent to the lateral surface of the submaxillary gland at the narrow cephalid pole. The gland is composed of mucous acini, serous demilunes, and numerous myoepithelial cells.

MORPHOLOGY AND BIOLOGY OF TUMOURS

Histological types of tumour

Oral cavity, buccal pouch, oesophagus and forestomach

Epithelial tumours
    Squamous cell papilloma
    Squamous cell carcinoma
       Well differentiated
       Poorly differentiated

Non-epithelial tumours
    Fibrosarcoma
    Mixofibroma
    Spindle cell sarcoma

Salivary glands

Epithelial tumours
    Adenoma
    Adenocarcinoma

Non-epithelial tumours
    Fibrosarcoma
    Malignant mesenchymoma

Oral cavity, buccal pouch, oesophagus and forestomach

Squamous cell papilloma

Squamous cell papillomas are white or grey, grossly papillomatous lesions which may be single or multiple, small or large and confluent, pedunculated or sessile, warty or cauliflower-like outgrowths from normal, slightly altered or diffusely thickened mucosa. Tumours beyond a certain size in the forestomach or oesophagus may cause obstruction, but even very large papillomas, where hyperkeratotic tumour masses occupy almost the entire lumen, show neither serosal invasion nor metastases.

Squamous cell papillomas (Figures 2–5) are usually exophytic growths of mucosal epithelium consisting of arborized finger-like projections from the surface. In most instances, they are fibroepithelial neoplasms on a connective tissue stalk characterized by delicate or bulky processes covered by hyperkeratotic stratified squamous epithelium with a well arranged basal layer demonstrating numerous mitoses. The pale nuclei within the epithelial layers vary considerably in size. Nucleoli are markedly enlarged and basophilic. Parakeratosis and dyskeratosis, as well as areas of acanthosis or slightly atypical dysplastic cells, may sometimes be observed. Enlarged vessels and sometimes lymphocytic infiltration are present in the stromal stalks.

Papillomas may be difficult to distinguish from epithelial hyperplasia (Figures 1, 13, 14, 16–20), especially when small. Tumours in which the squamous epithelium is arranged in branched finger-like processes supported by a fibrovascular core and without invasive growth are defined as benign.

Squamous cell carcinoma

Squamous cell carcinomas are characterized by downward projecting sheets, nests or anastomosing cords of squamous tumour cells that invade the underlying structures. These malignant tumours may either develop from benign, papillary tumours as described above or evolve directly from atypical epithelium. In both cases, the malignant nature of any individual tumour can usually be confirmed only by histological examination.

Masses of cells may originate in hyperplastic mucosal areas and extend beneath slightly altered or normal-looking epithelia, invading the underlying tissues and causing thickening, induration and destruction of the muscular wall or adhesion to adjacent tissues. Tumour surfaces are sometimes ulcerated and necrotic, and cut tumour masses may

sometimes demonstrate prominent intramural growth with necrosis and haemorrhage. Carcinomas may also be accompanied by acanthotic and hyperkeratotic mucosa or papillomas in the adjacent mucosa.

Two main types of tumour may be distinguished based on the degree of cellular differentiation: well differentiated (Figures 6–10, 15, 21–24) and poorly differentiated (Figures 11, 12). Epithelia demonstrating characteristics of both types may occasionally be observed within a single tumour.

Well differentiated squamous cell carcinomas are characterized by a distinct tendency for differentiation towards normal squamous epithelium. Areas of keratinization and formation of horn pearls may be observed with cells showing relatively few abnormalities. Buds and nests of neoplastic epithelial cells sometimes show fairly uniform basal cell layers but no sign of keratinization. Neoplastic cells may occasionally be pleomorphic and hyperchromatic; signs of hyperplasia and loss of the normal nucleus to cytoplasm relationship as well as frequent mitotic figures may be observed.

Poorly differentiated squamous cell carcinomas lack signs of squamous cell differentiation such as keratinization or horn pearl formation, and demonstrate cellular and nuclear atypia. Dissociated epithelial cells, vacuolization of the cytoplasm, prominent nucleoli and hyperchromatism of nuclei are often present. Tumour cells are arranged as solid sheets separated by thin stromal elements or as strands or groups of cells intermingled with connective tissue.

Non-epithelial tumours

Fibrosarcomas can be induced in the buccal pouch (Siegel & Shklar, 1969) and they are malignant circumscribed or infiltrating tumours containing reticulin and collagen produced by predominantly spindle-shaped cells showing no evidence of other forms of cellular differentiation. The histological picture consists mainly of interlacing, densely cellular fascicles of more or less uniform spindle cells. Mitotic figures are a constant feature of fibrosarcomas.

The authors found one case of myxofibroma in the buccal pouch of a hamster treated with *N*-nitroso-*N*-propyl-urethane. Histologically, the tumour was composed of myxoid and fibromatous tissue. Surrounding and mixed in the myxoid tissue, which was characterized by a loose texture with round, spindle or stellate cells and a few very fine reticulin fibres, there was a well circumscribed dense growth of matured and richly collagenous fibrous tissue.

Thorotrast administration to the submucosal tissue of the buccal pouch was found to induce spindle-cell sarcomas at the sites of treatment (Mori *et al.*, 1966). Spindle-cell sarcomas are composed of interlacing bundles of spindle-shaped cells and it is not possible to make a definite diagnosis owing to the immaturity of the tumour cells.

Salivary gland

Adenoma

The tubular adenoma may arise from the intercalated or excretory duct and consists of expansible nodules of well formed tubular structures separated by fibrous stroma.

The adenoma consists of enlarged, well differentiated acini which cause compression of the normal lobules.

Adenocarcinoma

Adenocarcinomas occur as a spectrum from the well differentiated acinar or ductular pattern to the undifferentiated carcinoma.

Non-epithelial tumours

The histological characteristics of fibrosarcoma are described in other chapters.

Malignant mesenchymoma may contain more than two immature mesenchymal components (smooth or striated muscle, cartilage, vascular tissue, osteoid, adipose, etc.).

SPONTANEOUS TUMOURS

Spontaneous neoplasms of the oral cavity, buccal pouch, oesophagus and salivary glands are infrequent in the hamster.

In the oral cavity, papillomatosis of suspected viral origin and spontaneous connective tissue tumours have been reported. Other tumours of the oral cavity include squamous cell papillomas as well as a squamous cell carcinoma and several odontomas of the molar teeth (Pour *et al.*, 1979).

There have been no reports of spontaneous epithelial neoplasms developing in the hamster buccal pouch, but this site has been used experimentally to produce lesions similar to those seen in the skin.

In the oesophagus the only reported primary tumour was a squamous cell papilloma. Secondary infiltration by a malignant lymphoma has also been described (Schmidt *et al.*, 1983).

Squamous papillomas, morphologically similar to those arising in the oesophagus, have been observed in the forestomach. The incidences of spontaneous squamous cell papillomas of the forestomach were 4.1% in females and 6.1% in males; squamous cell carcinomas developed in 0.5% of males (Dontenwill *et al.*, 1973). In hamsters the occurrence of benign lesions is much higher than in rats and mice, but no sex differences have been found (Fukushima & Ito, 1985).

There are a number of reports of occasional spontaneous adenomas (Eddy *et al.*, 1958) and adenocarcinomas (Della Porta, 1961; Kirkman, 1962; Toth & Boreisha, 1969) arising in the hamster salivary glands. One malignant mesenchymoma was described by Toth (1971) in the parotid gland of a female. Most secondary tumours affecting the salivary glands were malignant lymphomas, the neoplastic lymphocytes forming sheets that destroyed normal parenchyma. In some cases, the entire gland was replaced by tumour (Schmidt *et al.*, 1983).

INDUCTION OF TUMOURS

Inducing agents

Oral cavity, buccal pouch, oesophagus and forestomach

There have been a number of studies on the experimental production of tumours in the buccal mucosa, gingiva, palate and tongue of various animal species including hamsters (Al-Ani & Shklar, 1966; Salley & Kreshover, 1959; Eveson & MacDonald, 1981).

Salley (1954) was the first to notice the susceptibility of the buccal pouch of Syrian hamsters to 7,12-dimethylbenz[a]-anthracene (DMBA). Experiments using this animal model (Salley, 1957) revealed that four distinct lesions arise during the early stages of carcinogenesis, namely inflammation, degeneration, regeneration and hyperplasia. The hamster buccal pouch is now regarded as the most suitable model for the study of initiation and promotion in experimental oral carcinogenesis (Odukoya & Shklar, 1984).

DMBA or 3-methylcholanthrene (MC) in pellets of beeswax also produced cheek-pouch carcinomas in the experiments of Dunham and Herrold (1962).

Many substances are known to induce forestomach tumours in rats, mice and hamsters. Most compounds exert their effect when administered orally, either by diet, drinking-water or gavage. In the first edition of this book, *N*-nitroso-*N*-methyl-urea, benzo[a]pyrene, MC, 2-acetylamino-fluorene, *N*-hydroxy-aminofluorene and urethane were listed as forestomach carcinogens in Syrian golden hamsters

(Emminger & Mohr, 1982). *N*-Nitroso-*N*-methylurethane induced epidermoid carcinomas of the forestomach as well as of the oesophagus (Herrold, 1966). When 3-nitroso-1,1-diethyl-3-methylurea was subcutaneously injected into Syrian golden hamsters once weekly for 52 weeks, the animals developed mainly papillomas and squamous cell carcinomas of the forestomach and nasal cavity and haem-angioendotheliomas of the spleen (Ketkar *et al.*, 1984). One of the target organs of nitrosomethylalkylamines for tumour induction is the forestomach (Lijinsky & Kovatch, 1988).

Recently, the synthetic antioxidant butylated hydroxyanisole (BHA) at 1 or 2% addition to the diet was reported to be tumorigenic to the forestomach in Syrian golden hamsters as well as in rats (Ito *et al.*, 1983).

Salivary glands

The subject of submaxillary carcino-genesis, comprehensively reviewed by Cataldo and Shklar (1964), has received considerable attention, especially among dental researchers, since Steiner (1942) produced squamous cell carcinomas, adenocarcinomas and mixed tumours by the implantation of pellets of MC, DMBA and benzo[a]pyrene into mice, rats, guinea-pigs and rabbits.

The hamster submaxillary gland appears to respond to various topically applied carcinogens by formation of fibrosarcomas, as noted by Chaudhry *et al.* (1961b, 1966) and Levij and Polliack (1968) who used DMBA. Cataldo and Shklar (1964) implanted pellets of DMBA, without solvent, into the surgically exposed submaxillary gland of hamsters and observed fibrosarcomas developing after only three weeks of treatment. Occasionally, formations resembling so-called mixed tumours were seen but no true mixed malignant tumour occurred.

Modifying factors

Oral cavity, buccal pouch, oesophagus and forestomach

Kendrick (1964) applied DMBA in ethanol–toluene or in mineral oil at first three times a week and then less often. The first squamous cell tumours appeared at the 23rd week of the study in animals receiving DMBA in ethanol–toluene and at the 26th week of study in animals receiving DMBA in mineral oil. The latter tumours grew more slowly and tended to regress.

Tabah *et al.* (1957) applied DMBA in a saturated solution in chloroform which was allowed to evaporate. Squamous cell papillomas and carcinomas developed in 10% of the animals.

Morris (1961) studied a number of modifying factors of DMBA carcino-genesis. The optimal concentration of DMBA for high tumour yield with short latent period was found to be 0.5%, lower concentrations producing tumours more slowly and higher concentrations (such as 1.5%) being toxic. Thrice weekly appli-cation was more effective than twice weekly application. However, a smaller total dose was required to produce tumours in all animals when the carcino-gen was given twice a week than when it was applied three times a week. There were no sex differences but age proved impor-tant, hamsters aged 18 months being more resistant than younger ones up to nine weeks of age. Morris *et al.* (1961) and Mori *et al.* (1962) conducted extensive studies on the biochemistry of DMBA-induced buccal pouch tumours.

With the establishment of a two-stage carcinogenesis model in the hamster buccal pouch, it was possible to test the efficacy of a number of putative pro-moting agents implicated in human oral carcinogenesis. Thus, Elzay (1966) was able to demonstrate that alcohol acted locally as a promoting agent. Renstrup *et al.* (1961, 1962) studied the effects of chronic irritation on DMBA buccal pouch carcinogenesis using irritant wires mounted on the teeth. Although tumour incidences after 18 to 24 weeks were the same in the non-irritated as in the irritated pouches, the first tumours appeared four weeks after beginning the treatment in animals with steel wires and 10 weeks after start in hamsters without wires. This indicated that chronic irritation exerted a strong cocarcinogenic effect. Possible carcinogenicity or promotion potential of croton oil was studied by Silberman and Shklar (1963) using 0.5% DMBA as an initiator. In hamsters aged 2 to 3 months, 1% croton oil retarded the appearance of tumours. Conversely, in hamsters more than one year of age, cocarcinogenic activity was noted. Shklar (1966) also found that systemic administration of cortisone hastened DMBA carcinogenesis in the buccal pouch.

Dachi (1961, 1962) reported that chronic application of 0.5% DMBA in mineral oil until appearance of tumours required similar administration times, regardless of whether or not Tween 60 was also applied. However, when DMBA was applied only 15 times, the latent period before tumour development with Tween 60 painting was shorter (45 to 47 days) than without painting (73 to 91 days). Shklar *et al.* (1966) noted that DMBA-induced tumours appeared more rapidly and grew more invasively when metho-trexate was injected subcutaneously.

Rowe and Gorlin (1959) found that vitamin A deficiency promoted formation of epithelial tumours induced by DMBA. Furthermore, local injections of beta-carotene and canthaxanthin led to regression of DMBA-induced epidermoid carcinomas of hamster buccal pouch, the former agent being the more effective while 13-*cis*-retinoic acid had no effect in the same system (Schwartz & Shklar, 1988).

One of the major questions regarding the hamster buccal pouch as a model for intra-oral carcinogenesis is whether it is truly intra-oral. Kolas (1955) argued that since the pouch is not subject to the same environmental influences as the rest of the mouth it could not be regarded as being representative of the oral cavity proper. Furthermore, it would appear that the buccal pouch is an immunologically privileged site, as evidenced by its acceptance of both normal and neoplastic heterografts (Billingham *et al.*, 1960; Williams *et al.*, 1971).

Salivary glands

A dose–effect relationship for salivary gland tumour induction by DMBA in liquid petroleum has been established (Chaudhry & Gorlin, 1959; Chaudry *et al.*, 1959, 1961a,b). Vitamin A deficiency was found to accelerate tumour formation initiated by DMBA (Rowe & Gorlin, 1959).

Sabes *et al.* (1961, 1963) studied the effects of injections of cortisone into the submaxillary gland before injection of DMBA. The results, however, were contradictory because only occasional inhibition was found. The authors believed that their data indicated a periodicity of tumour formation, depending on 24-hour cycles. Chaudhry and Schmutz (1966) failed to find any effect of prednisolone or cortisone upon tumour formation induced by DMBA.

Epithelial changes following treatment with carcinogens (preneoplastic lesions)

Lesions produced by topical application of 0.5% DMBA to buccal pouch epithelium could be classified as hyperplasia, dysplasia or carcinoma using strict histological criteria. Electron microscopic findings indicated a progressive loss of lamina densa material of the basal membrane during carcinogenesis, accompanied by extrusion of pseudopodia from the basal cells through the gaps. These pseudopodia were frequently related to peripheral cytoplasmic microfilaments. The loss of lamina densa has been discussed in relation to the specificity of the response and to the development of features indicative of motility in transforming cells (White & Gohari, 1981).

COMPARATIVE ASPECTS

The buccal pouch is unique to the hamster and therefore no comparison with other species is possible.

Experimental induction of papillomas of the oesophagus has been reported in rats (Pozharisski, 1990) and mice (Horie *et al.*, 1965), similar features being demonstrated in all cases. In man, papilloma of the oesophagus is observed only rarely (Ming, 1973). The induction of squamous cell carcinomas of the oesophagus at high yield has been reported, primarily in the rat, but also with lower frequency in hamsters, mice and other species (Iizuka *et al.* 1982). Squamous cell carcinoma is the most frequent malignant neoplasm of the oesophagus in man, but differences from the typical rodent lesion are apparent. Although they have been described, verrucous or true papillary carcinomas of the human oesophagus are rare. Non-papillary squamous carcinomas of the fungating, ulcerative and infiltrating types, on the other hand, represent the overwhelming majority found in man (Ming, 1973).

Spontaneously occurring squamous cell carcinomas as well as papillomas of the forestomach occur more frequently in Syrian golden hamsters than in rats or mice. Epithelial hyperplasia is also common in untreated hamsters. Although a large number of agents can cause forestomach tumours in this species, the majority of the cases have been described in rats. One explanation may be that the rat is very often the species of choice in carcinogenicity studies. A forestomach is not present in primates (including man); it is thought to be the counterpart of the forestomach of ruminants. Irritants are known to produce a marked epithelial hyperplasia in this region of the stomach and it is quite likely that prolonged irritation will lead to the appearance of papillomas and carcinomas. In any event, it is difficult to see the relevance to man of tumours induced in an organ which does not exist in humans. Although findings of this sort cannot be dismissed and should be supplemented by further studies of the carcinogenicity of the compound in question, no judgement on the potential carcinogenic hazard to man is possible on the basis of the induction of this type of tumour in rodents. However, the hamster may offer an advantageous animal model for the study of the biology and mechanisms underlying the pathogenesis of stomach tumors.

ACKNOWLEDGEMENTS

The author gratefully acknowledges the assistance of Dr M.A. Moore in the preparation of this manuscript.

REFERENCES

Al-Ani, S. & Shklar, G. (1966) Effects of a chemical carcinogen applied to hamster gingiva. *J. Periodontol.*, 37, 36–42

Billingham, R.E., Ferrigan, L.W. & Silver, W.K. (1960) Cheek pouch of the Syrian hamster and tissue transplantation immunity. *Science*, 132, 1488

Bivin, W.S., Olsen, G.H. & Murray, K.A. (1987) Morphophysiology, III. Digestive system, In: Van Hoosier, G.L. & McPherson, C.W., eds, *Laboratory Hamsters*, Orlando, FL, Academic Press, pp. 12–19

Cataldo, E. & Shklar, G. (1964) Chemical carcinogenesis in the hamster sub-maxillary gland. *J. Dental Res.*, 43, 568–579

Chaudhry, A.P. & Gorlin, R.J. (1959) Experimental carcinogenesis in submaxillary glands of hamsters. *J. Dental Res.*, 38, 713–714

Chaudhry, A.P., Singer, L. & Gorlin, R.J. (1959) Effects of vitamin A deficiency on experimental carcinogenesis in sub-maxillary glands of hamsters. *J. Dental Res.*, 38, 714

Chaudhry, A.P., Reynolds, D.H., Gorlin, R.J. & Vickers, R.A. (1961a) Experimental carcinogenesis in submandibular glands of hamsters. *J. Dental Res.*, 40, 426–432

Chaudhry, A.P., Singer, L., Gorlin, R.J. & Vickers, R.A. (1961b) Effects of vitamin A deficiency on experimental carcinogenesis in submandibular glands of hamsters. *J. Dental Res.*, 40, 327–330

Chaudhry, A.P. & Schmutz, J.A., Jr (1966) Effects of prednisolone and thalidomide on induced submandibular gland tumors in hamsters. *Cancer Res.*, 26, 1881–1886

Dachi, S.F. (1961) Effects of Tween 60 upon experimental oral carcinogenesis in the hamster. *J. Dental Res.*, 40, 648–649

Dachi, S.F. (1962) Effects of polyoxyethylene sorbitan monostearate (Tween 60) upon experimental oral carcinogenesis in the hamsters. *J. Dental Res.*, 41, 476–483

Della Porta, G. (1961) Induction of intestinal, mammary, and ovarian tumors in hamsters with oral administration of 20-methylcholanthrene. *Cancer Res.*, 21, 575–579

Dontenwill, W., Chevalier, H.J., Harke, H.P., Lafrenz, U. & Reckzeh, G. (1973) Spontaneous tumors in Syrian golden hamsters. *Z. Krebsforsch.*, 80, 127–158

Dunham, L.J. & Herrold, K.M. (1962) Failure to produce tumors in the hamster cheek pouch by exposure to ingredients of betel quid. Histopathologic changes in the pouch and other organs by exposure to known carcinogens. *J. Natl Cancer Inst.*, 29, 1047–1067

Eddy, B.E., Stewart, S.E., Young, R. & Mider, G.B. (1958) Neoplasms in hamsters induced by mouse tumor agent passed in tissue culture. *J. Natl Cancer Inst.*, 29, 1047–1067

Elzay, R.P. (1966) Local effect of alcohol in combination with DMBA on hamster cheek pouch. *J. Dental Res.*, 45, 1788

Emminger, A. & Mohr, U. (1982) Tumors of the oral cavity, cheek pouch, salivary glands, oesophagus, stomach and intestines. In: Turusov, V.S., ed., *Pathology of Tumours in Laboratory Animals*, Vol. III, *Tumours of the Hamsters* (IARC Scientific Publications No. 34), Lyon, IARC, pp. 45–68

Eveson, J.W. & MacDonald, D.G. (1981) Hamster tongue carcinogenesis. I. Characteristics of the experimental model. *J. Oral Pathol.*, 10, 322

Flon, H. & Gerstner, R. (1968) Salivary glands of the hamster. I. Submandibular gland: a histochemical study after preservation with various fixatives. *Acta Histochem.*, 31, 234–253

Fukushima, S. & Ito, N. (1985) Squamous cell carcinoma, forestomach, rat. In: Jones, T.C., Mohr, U. & Hunt, R.D., eds, *Digestive System* (Monographs on Pathology of Laboratory Animals), Berlin, Heidelberg, New York, Springer-Verlag, pp. 292–295

Herrold, K.M. (1966) Epidermoid carcinomas of esophagus and forestomach induced in Syrian hamsters by *N*-nitroso-*N*-methylurethan. *J. Natl Cancer Inst.*, 37, 389–394

Horie, A., Hohchi, S. & Kuratsune, M. (1965) Carcinogenesis in the esophagus. II. Experimental production of esophageal cancer by administration of ethanolic solution of carcinogens. *Gann*, 56, 429–441

Iizuka, T., Kato, H., Ichimura, S. & Kawachi, T. (1982) Experimental esophageal carcinoma in rats, rabbits, dogs and other species. In: Pfeiffer, C.J., ed., *Cancer of the Esophagus*, Vol. II, Boca Raton, FL, CRC Press, Chap. 12

Ito, N., Fukushima, S., Imaida, K., Sakata, T. & Masui, T. (1983) Induction of papilloma in the forestomach of hamsters by butylated hydroxyanisole. *Gann*, 74, 456–461

Kendrick, F.J. (1964) Some effects of a chemical carcinogen and a cigarette smoke condensate upon hamster cheek pouch mucosa. *Health Sci.*, 24, 3698–3699

Ketkar, M.B., Mohr, U. & Lijinsky, W. (1984) The carcinogenic effect of 1,1-diethyl-3-methyl-3-nitrosourea in Syrian golden hamsters. *Cancer Lett.*, 23, 177–182

Kirkman, H. (1962) A preliminary report concerning tumors observed in Syrian hamsters. *Stanford Med. Bull.*, 20, 163

Kolas, S. (1955) Investigation of normal human saliva for possible anticarcinogenic action and chemical carcinogenesis in mucous membranes. *Oral Surg.*, 8, 1192

Levij, I.S. & Polliack, A. (1968) Potentiating effect of vitamin A on 9,10-dimethyl-1,2-benzanthracene carcinogenesis in the hamster cheek pouch. *Cancer*, 22, 300–306

Lijinsky, W. & Kovatch, R.M. (1988) Comparative carcinogenesis by nitrosomethylalkylamines in Syrian golden hamsters. *Cancer Res.*, 48, 6648–6652

Ming, S.C. (1973) Tumors of the esophagus and stomach. In: *Atlas of Tumor Pathology*, 2nd ser., fasc. 7. Washington, DC, Armed Forces Institute of Pathology, p. 11

Mori, M., Miyaji, T., Murata, I. & Nagasuna, H. (1962) Histochemical observations on enzymatic processes of experimental carcinogenesis in hamster cheek pouch. *Cancer Res.*, 22, 1323–1326

Mori, T., Sakai, T., Okamoto, T., Tamura, N., Nozue, Y., Ishida, T. & Umeda, M. (1966) Preliminary report on a spindle-cell sarcoma in the Syrian hamster produced by thorotrast. *Gann*, 57, 431–433

Morris, A.L. (1961) Factors influencing experimental carcinogenesis in the hamster cheek pouch. *J. Dental Res.*, 40, 3–15

Morris, A.L., Scott, D.B.M. & Reiskin, A.B. (1961) Carcinogenesis in the hamster cheek pouch. I. Correlation of histopathology with soluble sulfhydryl groups. *Cancer Res.*, 21, 1352–1359

Odukoya, O. & Shklar, G. (1984) Initiation and promotion in experimental oral carcinogenesis. *Oral Surg.*, 58, 315–320

Pour, P., Althoff, J., Salmasi, S. & Stepan, K. (1979) Spontaneous tumors and common diseases in three types of hamsters. *J. Natl Cancer Inst.*, 63, 797–811

Pozharisski, K.M. (1990) Tumours of the oesophagus, In: Turusov, V.S. & Mohr, U., eds, *Pathology of Tumours in Laboratory Animals*, Vol. I, *Tumours of the Rat*, 2nd edition (IARC Scientific Publications No. 99), Lyon, IARC, pp. 109–128

Renstrup, G., Smulow, J.B. & Glickman, I. (1961) Carcinogenesis and mechanical irritation in the cheek pouch of hamster. *J. Dental Res.*, 40, 649

Renstrup, G., Smulow, J.B. & Glickman, I. (1962) Effect of chronic mechanical irritation on chemically induced carcinogenesis in the hamster cheek pouch. *J. Am. Dental Assoc.*, 64, 770–777

Rowe, N.H. & Gorlin, R.J. (1959) The effect of vitamin A deficiency upon experimental oral carcinogenesis. *J. Dental Res.*, 38, 72–83

Sabes, W.R., Chaudhry, A.P. & Gorlin, R.J. (1961) Effects of cortisone on experimental carcinogenesis in the hamster submandibular gland. *J. Dental Res.*, 40, 646–647

Sabes, W.R., Chaudhry, A.P. & Gorlin, R.J. (1963) Effects of cortisone on chemical carcinogenesis in hamster pouch and submandibular salivary gland. *J. Dental Res.*, 42, 1118–1130

Salley, J.J. (1954) Experimental carcinogenesis in the cheek pouch of the Syrian hamster. *J. Dental Res.*, 33, 253–262

Salley, J.J. (1957) Histologic changes in the hamster cheek pouch during early hydrocarbon carcinogenesis. *J. Dental Res.*, 36, 48–55

Salley, J.J. & Kreshover, S.J. (1959) The effect of topical application of carcinogens on the palatal mucosa of the hamster. *Oral Surg.*, 12, 501–508

Schmidt, R.E., Eason, R.L., Hubbard, G.B., Young, J.T. & Eisenbrandt, D.L. (1983) Alimentary system. In: Schmidt, R.E. & Eason, R.L., eds, *Pathology of Aging Syrian Hamsters*, Boca Raton, FL, CRC Press, pp. 45–66

Schwartz, J. & Shklar, G. (1988) Regression of experimental oral carcinomas by local injection of beta-carotene and cantha-xanthin. *Nutr. Cancer*, 11, 35–40

Scott, D.B.McN., Morris, A.L., Reiskin, A.B. & Pakoskey, A.M. (1960) Changes in hexo-kinase and dehydrogenases for glucose-6-phosphate and 6-phospho-gluconate during carcinogenesis in the hamster cheek pouch. *Fed. Proc.*, 19, 397

Scott, D.B.McN., Morris, A.L., Reiskin, A.B. & Pakoskey, A.M. (1962) Carcinogenesis in the hamster cheek pouch. II. Changes in enzymes of glucose-6-phosphate oxidation. *Cancer Res.*, 22, 857–866

Shklar, G. (1966) Cortisone and hamster buccal pouch carcinogenesis. *Cancer Res.*, 26, 2461–2463

Shklar, G., Cataldo, E. & Fitzgerald, A.L. (1966) The effect of methotrexate on chemical carcinogenesis of hamster buccal pouch. *Cancer Res.*, 26, 2218–2224

Siegel, W.V. & Shklar, G. (1969) The effect of dimethylsulfoxide and topical triamcino-lone on chemical carcinogenesis of hamster buccal pouch. *Oral Surg.*, 27, 772–779

Silberman, S.T. & Shklar, G. (1963) The effect of a carcinogen (DMBA) applied to the hamster's buccal pouch in combination with croton oil. *Oral Surg.*, 16, 1344–1355

Steiner, P.E. (1942) Comparative pathology of induced tumors of the salivary glands. *Arch. Pathol.*, 34, 613–624

Tabah, E.J., Gorecki, Z., Ritchie, A.C. & Skoryna, S.C. (1957) Effects of saturated solutions of tobacco tars and of 9,10-dimethyl-1,2-benzanthracene on the hamster's cheek pouch. *Proc. Am. Ass. Cancer Res.*, 2, 254

Toth, B. (1971) Tumor induction by repeated injections of urethan in newborn and adult hamsters: age influence. II. *J. Natl Cancer Inst.*, 46, 81–93

Toth, B. & Boreisha, I. (1969) Tumorigenesis with isonicotinic acid hydrazide and urethan in the Syrian golden hamster. *Eur. J. Cancer*, 5, 165–171

White, F.H. & Gohari, K. (1981) A quantitative study of lamina densa alterations in hamster cheek pouch carcinogenesis. *J. Pathol.*, 135, 277–294

Williams, D.E., Evans, D.M.D. & Blamey, R.W. (1971) The primary implantation of human tumours to the hamster cheek pouch. *Br. J. Cancer*, 25, 533–537

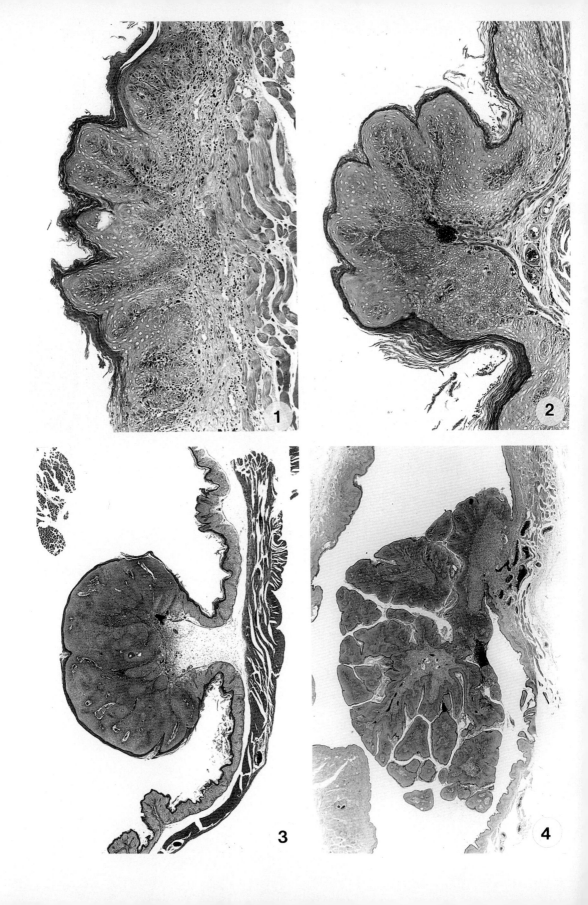

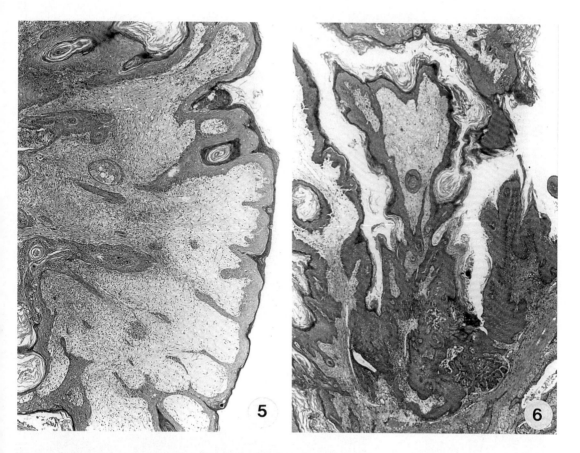

Figure 1. Epithelial hyperplasia and hyperkeratosis of the buccal pouch. H & E; × 50

Figure 2. Squamous cell papilloma of the buccal pouch. H & E; × 50

Figure 3. Squamous cell papilloma of the buccal pouch. Polypoid outgrowth on a narrow stalk with a stromal core of loose connective tissue. H & E; × 20

Figure 4. Squamous cell papilloma of the buccal pouch. Exophytic growths of mucosal epithelium consisting of arborized finger-like projections from the surface. H & E; × 15

Figure 5. Squamous cell papilloma of the buccal pouch with remarkable myxomatous stroma.
H & E; × 30

Figure 6. Well differentiated squamous cell carcinoma of the buccal pouch. H & E; × 30

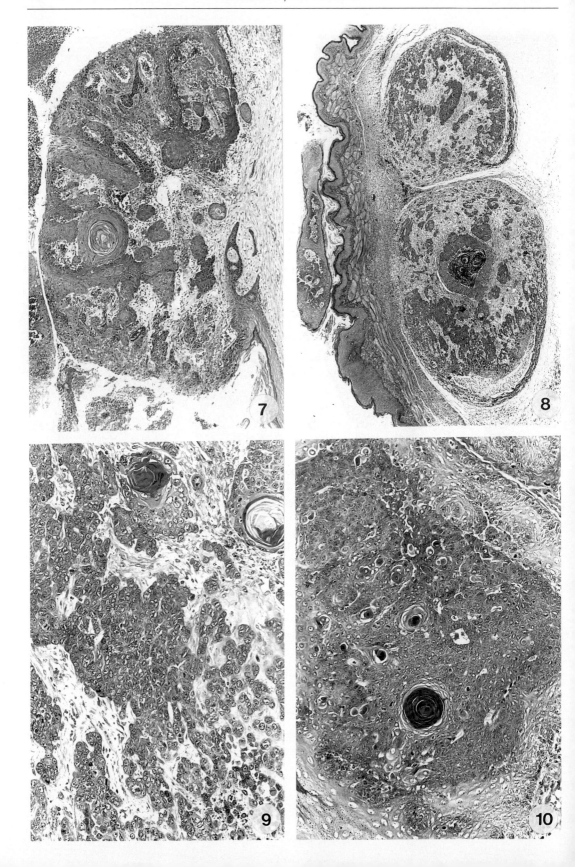

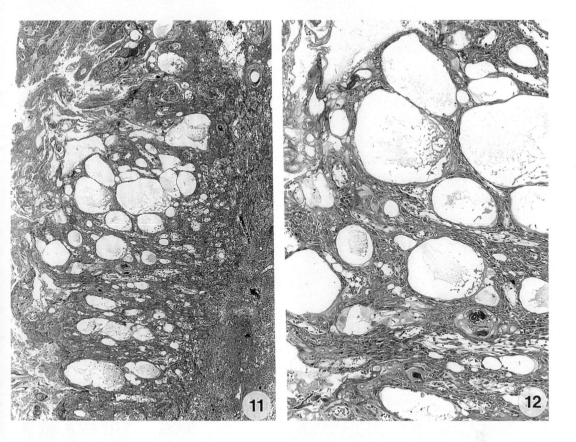

Figure 7. Well differentiated squamous cell carcinoma of the buccal pouch. H & E; × 30

Figure 8. Well differentiated squamous cell carcinoma of the buccal pouch. Tumour formation can be seen at outside of the buccal pouch. H & E; × 30

Figure 9. Higher magnification of Figure 8. Tumour cells have invaded the underlying connective tissues. × 140

Figure 10. Well differentiated squamous cell carcinoma of the buccal pouch. Keratinized epithelial pearls are formed. H & E; × 120

Figure 11. Poorly differentiated squamous cell carcinoma of the buccal pouch with conspicuous cyst formation. H & E; × 30

Figure 12. Higher magnification of Figure 11. The cysts are lined by squamous epithelial cells. × 75

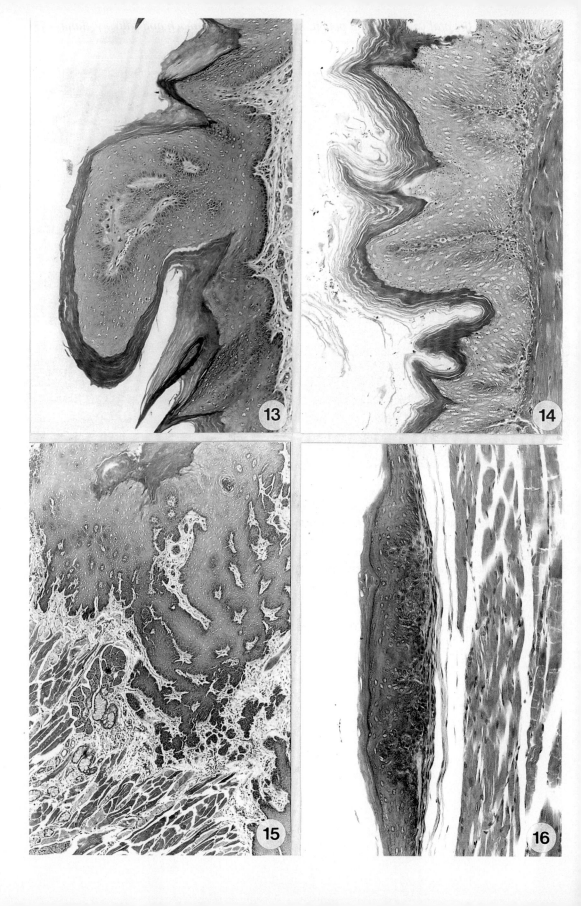

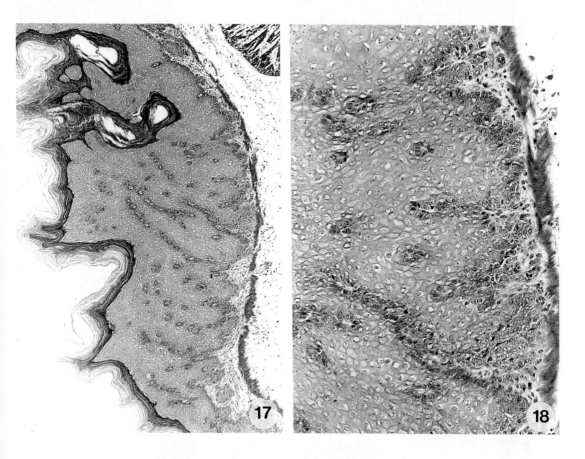

Figure 13. Epithelial hyperplasia of the tongue with well differentiated squamous epithelium. H & E; × 100

Figure 14. Epithelial hyperplasia and hyperkeratosis of the tongue. H & E; × 120

Figure 15. Well differentiated squamous cell carcinoma of the tongue. Marked downward growth of the epithelial cells is evident. H & E; × 30

Figure 16. Epithelial hyperplasia of the oesophagus. H & E; × 120

Figure 17. Epithelial hyperplasia and hyperkeratosis of the forestomach. H & E; × 40

Figure 18. Higher magnification of Figure 17. Note well differentiated epithelium without atypism. × 150

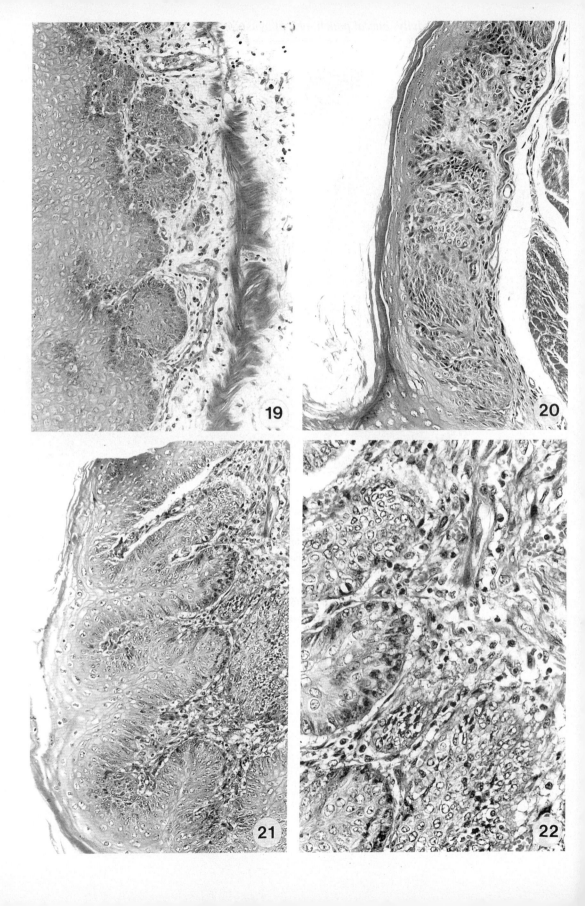

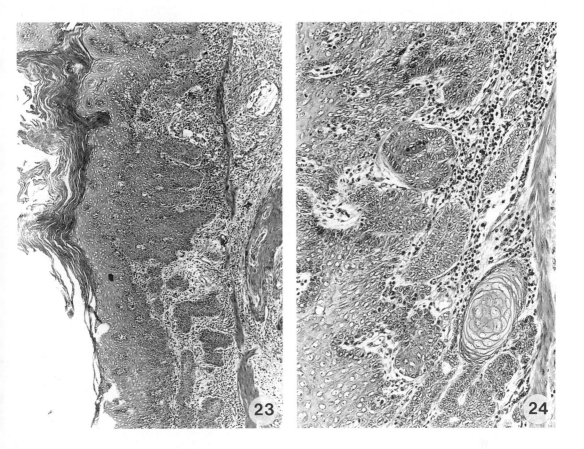

Figure 19. Epithelial hyperplasia of the forestomach. Slight downward growth of the basal cells is seen. H & E; ×150

Figure 20. Atypical hyperplasia of the forestomach. Atypical cells can be seen at basal cell portion.
H & E; ×150

Figure 21. Well differentiated squamous cell carcinoma of the forestomach with parakeratosis.
 H & E; × 150

Figure 22. Higher magnification of Figure 21. Focal invasive growth can be seen. × 300

Figure 23. Well differentiated squamous cell carcinoma of the forestomach. Cords and funiculi of neoplastic epithelial cells are observed infiltrating into the submucosal tissue. H & E; × 40

Figure 24. Well differentiated squamous cell carcinoma of the forestomach. The neoplastic cells invade the muscularis mucosa. H & E; ×140

Tumours of the liver

M.A. MOORE, W. THAMAVIT AND P. BANNASCH

The liver of the hamster, and particularly the Syrian hamster, demonstrates a wide range of morphological and biochemical alterations in response to chemical and physical insult. Some are clearly the result of acute toxicity of chemical agents or in some cases physical damage, while others are unequivocally members of the classes of tumours and their pre-stages which can arise in this organ. There are morphological entities, however, which are less easy to categorize, such as proliferative changes involving hepatocytes and ductular cells which require particular diagnostic care. The present review attempts to clarify the relationships between morphological changes encountered in histopathological investigation of the hamster liver, as well as focusing attention on comparability with lesions arising in other rodents and man.

NORMAL STRUCTURE

The hamster liver is composed of three major (left lateral, middle, right lateral) and two minor caudal lobes. Attached to the underside of the middle, split lobe lies the gallbladder and major bile duct, which is in communication with the common pancreatic duct flowing into the duodenum.

Histologically, the parenchyma is typically divided into acinar structures similar to those observed in other species, without any dividing septae. The major intrahepatic duct gives rise to intermediate and first-order bile ductules, the latter forming portal triads with the hepatic venules and arterioles. The bile duct/ductule epithelium is lined throughout by cuboidal cells with single, central nuclei of irregular outline, organized on a basement membrane. Goblet cells are not normally observed. The larger, oblong hepatocytes are arranged as bilayer sheets stretching from the zone 1 periportal areas to the zone 3 centrilobular venules (after Rappaport, 1976). Those in zone 3 are slightly larger with more cytoplasm. Nuclei are rounded with one or more nucleoli.

MORPHOLOGY AND BIOLOGY OF TUMOURS

Histological types of tumour

Epithelial tumours

Epithelial neoplasms and associated lesions arising in the hamster liver are divided into two broad categories depending on the cell of origin: hepatocellular (parenchymal) or cholangiocellular (bile duct/ductule), the latter including the gallbladder as an extrahepatic extension.

Hepatocellular lesions

Toxic or reactive lesions. Toxicity in the hamster liver is manifested by single cell or coagulative necrosis and is often associated with scattered alteration of individual hepatocytes demonstrating pronounced increase in size of the cytoplasm and nuclear atypia. As in the rat, such megalocytosis does not appear to be preneoplastic (Taper & Bannasch, 1979), although it is commonly observed after application of high doses of hepatocarcinogens, especially in zones 1 and 2. Chronic hepatic injury may result in cirrhotic changes with pseudo-lobular regenerative appearance, hepatocytes displaying considerable pleomorphism in size and shape and the lobular boundaries becoming pronounced due to proliferation of bile-duct cells between adjacent portal triads.

Preneoplastic hepatocellular lesions. After treatment with nitrosamines or other carcinogens, focally altered hepatocyte populations rapidly become evident. In the early stages these usually demonstrate increased basophilia, possibly related to carcinogen toxicity. Later, larger foci are found to be composed of clear cells (see Figure 1) (rich in glycogen, as demonstrated by staining with periodic acid–Schiff reagent (PAS)–diastase; Moore *et al.*, 1985), mixtures of clear, acidophilic and basophilic cells, cells storing lipid in excess, or basophilic cells (Figures 2–5). Although detailed histochemical or immunohistochemical studies of these populations have not been performed, hamster foci are known to demonstrate, like their counterparts in the rat liver, alterations in enzyme phenotype. These have been shown in some cases to include increase in the glutathione *S*-transferase placental form (GST-P) (Figure 6) (Moore *et al.*, 1985, 1987b, 1988) and decrease in capacity for iron loading (Stenbäck *et al.*, 1986). However, they are negative for gamma-glutamyltranspeptidase (GGT) and also do not normally demonstrate increased glucose-6-phosphate dehydrogenase (G6PD) activity, two commonly used markers of rat liver lesions. While decreased glucose-6-phosphatase and adenosine triphosphatase may be apparent (Figure 7), none of the alterations so far investigated would appear to lend itself to more accurate diagnosis than relying on morphology alone, since expression is very variable. However, morphological and enzyme phenotypic similarities between altered foci and larger nodules and hepatocellular carcinomas argue strongly for a direct histogenetic role in neoplasia.

Hepatocellular adenoma (synonyms: benign liver cell tumour; benign hepatoma; neoplastic nodule; hyperplastic hepatic nodule). These benign lesions, presenting as single nodules, characteristically demonstrate compres-sion of the surrounding parenchyma, varying in size from approximately 5 mm to 2–3 cm in diameter (Figure 8). Development of hepatocellular adenomas is usually associated with fibrotic or cirrhotic changes resulting in a pseudo-lobular appearance, although single lesions can arise in livers of otherwise normal architecture. Sometimes protruding above the liver surface, they are smooth and firm in surface, brown-yellow in colour, well demarcated and rounded.

Microscopically, conspicuous differences in nodular size or cytological character and lack of portal triads and/or central veins are diagnostic features. Adenomas comprise the same cell types observed in foci, most often being of mixed cell or basophilic character. In the latter case they may be difficult to distinguish from normal parenchyma on morphological grounds alone. Care must therefore be given to distinguishing whether portal triads and central veins can be identified within the lesions, in which case diagnosis of normal tissue within pathologically altered liver is considered to be correct (Greenblatt, 1982). Cytological features tend to be homogeneous throughout individual lesions.

In contrast to normal hepatocytes, those within adenomas usually form solid aggregates or irregular sheets or plates varying greatly in cell thickness. Although the sinusoids may be compressed, all stages through irregularly widened sinusoids to peliosis hepatis may be apparent. Occasionally, areas of changes resembling spongiosis hepatis may be observed within adenomas (cf. Bannasch *et al.*, 1981; Tatematsu *et al.*, 1980). Whether this is a neoplastic or pre-neoplastic lesion arising from peri-sinusoidal cells, as indicated in the rat liver (Bannasch *et al.*, 1981), remains unclear.

Hepatocellular carcinoma (synonyms: malignant hepatoma; liver cell carcinoma; adenocarcinoma). These are malignant tumours composed of cells resembling hepatocytes. Major diagnostic criteria for distinction from adenomas are the presence of distant metastasis, un-equivocal evidence of local invasion at some distance from the tumour mass, intravascular spread within the liver and isogenic or homologous transplantability. Nuclear and cytological abnormalities are very common in hamster hepatocytes under various conditions and are therefore not a reliable sole basis for distinguishing between benign and malignant hepato-cellular lesions. However, if they are found in association with microinvasion of the surrounding parenchyma and/or haemor-rhage and necrosis, diagnosis of a carci-noma may be warranted (Greenblatt, 1982).

Grossly, hepatocellular carcinomas are multinodular in appearance, varying in size from a few millimetres to centimetres in diameter, often occupying one or more liver lobes. They may be solitary lesions but are more commonly observed in livers demonstrating a range of cystic and nodular changes, sometimes together with cholangiocellular tumours. Metastases are most frequently found on the under surface of the diaphragm, anterior abdominal wall, upper abdominal lymph nodes and in the lungs (Greenblatt, 1982). The adrenal glands, kidneys, uterus and spleen may also be occasionally involved. Compared to human hepatocellular tumours, those in the hamster appear to metastasize relatively rarely (30% as opposed to 60%; Greenblatt, 1982). Finger-like projections of tumour tissue into the surrounding parenchyma are typical, distinctly rounded borders being generally associated with benign lesions.

Histologically, the majority of hamster hepatocellular carcinomas are well differentiated and of solid (Figure 9) or trabecular (Figure 10) morphology. Ana-plastic variants are very rare, as are mixed tumours also demonstrating bile-duct-like elements. Although some lesions may contain PAS-positive clear cells, more usual is a homogeneously basophilic population arranged in irregular cell plates and masses many cell layers thick. Nuclei are often enlarged and markedly irregular in shape, suggesting polyploidy (Figure 11). A coarse chromatin pattern and prominent nucleoli are usual but may also be evident in adenomas and smaller foci.

Cholangiocellular lesions

Toxic and reactive lesions. Proliferation of bile duct epithelium is a common response in the hamster to a variety of insults, physical, toxic and/or carcino-genic (Figure 12). Care must be taken to distinguish between diffuse lesions which may occur throughout large areas or indeed the whole liver and focal changes which belong to the pre-neoplastic category. In the former case, development of the lesion commences around the portal triads but rapidly spreads out in a stellate fashion so that adjacent portal areas become joined. Pseudolobules may result. In older animals and those infected with the liver fluke parasite *Opisthorchis viverrini*, proliferating ductular cells are often observed to be accompanied by lymphocytic infiltration and later to be embedded in amyloid deposits (S. Sriurairatna *et al.*, personal commu-nication). In the latter case, very large areas of the parenchyma may become replaced (Figures 13–17). In addition, lesions of the large ducts, which are otherwise rare, are caused by the physical presence of the flukes and their sucker action. Included are breakdown in the integrity of the epithelium, periductal fibrosis and inflammation. Granuloma formation is a common accompanying lesion (Bhamarapravati *et al.*, 1978).

Cystic structures (synonym: cystic cholangioma). In the case of focal proliferations, multilocular cystic structures lined by flattened epithelium often result (Figure 18), these sometimes assuming lobular proportions, when the term cystadenoma may be applied (Figures 19 and 20). However, they appear to have no direct histogenetic relationship to cystadenocarcinoma or other malignant tumour development. To the authors' knowledge, no malignant populations have been observed to arise within cystadenomas of the hamster liver, even under the conditions of their very extensive development after multiple doses of *N*-nitrosobis(2-hydroxypropyl)-amine. Mitotic figures and evidence of bromodeoxyuridine (BrdU) incorporation are rare.

Early bile duct proliferation may be accompanied by inflammatory infiltration. Fibrosis is apparent but not extensive, especially in the cystic lesions. Mucous secretion in simple bile duct hyperplasia or cyst formation is very limited and goblet cells are not apparent.

Atypical bile duct proliferation. Various morphological types of proliferating ductal/ductular cells, ranging from normal cuboidal through enlarged, basophilic to the flattened cyst type, may be observed. While studies of biochemical phenotype have been very limited, in one investigation, some basophilic cells, but not the other types, showed an increase in GST-P (Moore *et al.*, 1988). Since other lesions considered to participate in hamster bile duct neoplasia are also positive for this 'marker' enzyme, this is suggestive of a histogenetic link leading to proposal of the epithet 'atypical'.

Cholangiofibrosis. Focally altered populations of bile duct cells demonstrating increased mucous secretion, often accompanied by goblet cell metaplasia, are termed cholangiofibroses (Figure 21). They are further characterized by more extensive fibrosis than areas of simple bile duct proliferation or cysts and cellular atypia similar to those seen in malignant adenocarcinomas. Areas of cholangiofibrosis are regarded as being preneoplastic in nature, but on reaching acinar proportions may be difficult to distinguish from cholangiofibromas or cholangiocellular carcinomas, no encapsulation being evident. Massive increase in fibrosis and formation of desmoplastic stroma makes differential diagnosis particularly difficult.

Cholangiofibroma. Expansively growing cholangiocellular lesions of larger than liver acinus dimensions may be termed cholangiofibromas when extensive fibrosis is evident (Bannasch & Massner, 1976). Histologically they are otherwise indistinguishable from areas of fibrosis (Figure 22) and indeed correspond to the 'nodules of cholangiofibrosis' of Terao and Nakano (1974).

Histochemical and immunohistochemical investigations have demonstrated a number of alterations in enzyme phenotype within areas of cholangiofibrosis and cholangiofibromas Increases in GST-P and G6PD but not GGT appear typical, as are high rates of BrdU incorporation (Figures 23 and 24).

Cholangiocellular carcinoma (synonyms: bile duct carcinoma; biliary adenocarcinoma; cystadenocarcinoma). This is defined as a malignant tumour arising from the intrahepatic ductular epithelium. Grossly, tumours appear as solid, grey–white masses without sharp demarcation from the surrounding parenchyma. Metastases may be evident on the diaphragm surface, in the abdominal lymph nodes and commonly in the lungs (Greenblatt, 1982).

Carcinomas arising from the intrahepatic duct/ductular epithelium in the Syrian hamster present as two broad types, some individual lesions, however, being capable of demonstrating areas of both morphological categories. One form is moderately to poorly differentiated adenocarcinoma (Figures 25 and 26), the other is cystadenocarcinoma (Figures 27 and 28). Diagnosis of well differentiated cholangiocellular adenocarcinomas may be difficult without morphological evidence of progressive infiltration or metastatic spread. Microscopically, the component epithelial cells are pleomorphic, ranging from columnar to cuboidal in shape, forming distorted ductal structures. Goblet cells may be present in well and moderately differentiated adenocarcinomas. Prominent mucin production by epithelial elements is typical of the cystadenocarcinoma category. Large pools of alcian blue and/or PAS-positive material may also be observed in the stroma.

Gallbladder lesions

Gallbladder adenoma. Atypical (dysplastic) proliferations and papillary projections, on fibrous stalks, into the gallbladder lumen can be induced by carcinogen administration. Both are characterized by enlarged epithelial cells of columnar morphology, usually demonstrating increased mucin production and occasional goblet cell metaplasia (Figure 29).

Gallbladder carcinoma. Carcinomas occupying the entire gallbladder with local invasion of the mucosa are occasional findings along with benign lesions (Figures 30 and 31). Metastasis to the liver, regional lymph nodes, kidney and adrenal has been reported (Greenblatt, 1982), but diagnosis is usually dependent on the presence of atypia and clear evidence of

invasion, especially into the parenchyma. Care must be taken in differentiation from inflammatory papillary hyperplasia.

Mesenchymal lesions

Peliosis hepatis (synonyms: angiomatous cysts, acute haemorrhagic cystic degeneration). Acute or chronic treatment with carcinogens and other agents causing hepatocellular necrosis can induce peliosis hepatis, a multifocal widening of the blood spaces between hepatocyte cords (Figure 32), sometimes with endothelial proliferation, when distinction from a haemangioma may be difficult.

Haemangioma and angiosarcoma (synonyms: haemangiosarcoma; haemangioendothelioma; reticuloendothelial sarcoma). Well differentiated capillary and cavernous forms of haemangiomas and malignant angiosarcomas are common in the hamster liver after chronic carcinogen administration. Grossly, lesions may be multiple or single, varying in size from just visible with the naked eye to almost lobular proportions, when death due to peritoneal haemorrhaging often occurs. Metastases are common (>30%) with angiosarcomas, particularly to the lungs.

Microscopically, foci of endothelial proliferation appear as precursor lesions. Tumour cells are elongated and spindle-shaped with oval nuclei, growing along and into the sinusoids, with eventual production of cyst-like structures supported by stromal elements (Figures 33 and 34).

SPONTANEOUS TUMOURS

Although foci of altered hepatocytes and cystic bile ducts may be common in older animals, both hepatocellular and cholangiocellular carcinomas occur only rarely in untreated Syrian hamsters (for review of early literature see Dontenwill *et al.*, 1973). Typical findings have been rather less than 1% incidences of combined epithelial lesions (Dontenwill *et al.*, 1973; Fortner, 1957; Yabe *et al.*, 1972), although in one colony with a high prevalence of bile duct proliferation and cirrhosis, up to 6% of animals with such general lesions also demonstrated neoplastic development, cholangiocellular tumours being most common (Chesterman & Pomerance, 1965). Since random breeding procedures are normally used, variation in spontaneous tumorigenesis might well be the result of genetic heterogeneity, although in the case cited, high levels of infection with *Hymenolepis* cestode parasites may have played a causal role. A recent comparison of two colonies, however, revealed considerable differences, no epithelial tumours being found in 301 Eppley hamsters, whereas in the Hannover colony, incidences of over 3% were noted for both 'hepatomas' and cholangiomas in males and cholangiomas and cholangiocarcinomas were respectively observed in 6.8 and 2.5% of females (Pour *et al.*, 1976).

Gallbladder tumours are very rare in untreated hamsters, although 1% incidences of polyps were found in the Hannover colony reviewed by Pour and his co-workers (1976). While haemangiomas and haemangioendotheliomas have also been described to develop spontaneously in hamsters, incidences are normally lower than 1% (Dontenwill *et al.*, 1973; Pour *et al.*, 1976).

INDUCTION OF TUMOURS

Liver tumours can be induced in Syrian golden hamsters with a wide variety of chemical carcinogens including members of the azo-dye, acetylamine, polycyclic hydrocarbon and nitrosamine groups. Both hepatocellular and cholangiocellular lesions as well as vascular tumours on occasion develop in response to application of nitrosodimethylamine (Herrold, 1967; Lijinsky *et al.*, 1987; Tomatis & Cefis, 1967; Tomatis *et al.*, 1964), nitrosodiethylamine (Herrold, 1964; Herrold & Durham, 1963; Lijinsky *et al.*, 1987), nitrosohydroxypropylamines and other derivatives (Kokkinakis *et al.*,

1989; Lijinsky *et al.*, 1984; Pour *et al.*, 1975) or the nitrosamine precursors nitrite and aminopyrine (Bergman & Wahlin, 1981), azoalkanes (Lijinsky *et al.*, 1987), 2-acetylaminofluorene (Maljugina, 1958; Della Porta *et al.*, 1959) or *o*-aminoazotoluene (Tomatis *et al.*, 1961). Carbon tetrachloride induces only hepatocellular carcinomas, although this is associated with marked biliary hyperplasia (Della Porta *et al.*, 1961). Treatment with hexachlorobenzene is also associated with dose-dependent production of hepatic nodules and malignant endothelial lesions (Cabral *et al.*, 1977). In addition, urethane (Toth *et al.*, 1961) similarly causes development of hepatocellular and haemangiocellular tumours, whereas administration of synthetic estrogens to castrated male Syrian hamsters fed alpha-naphthoflavones induces multinodular carcinomas in 80–100% of cases (Li & Li, 1984). Streptozotocin, at diabetogenic doses, has been demonstrated to induce hepatic adenomas in both Chinese and Syrian hamsters (Bell *et al.*, 1984; Berman *et al.*, 1973), a low incidence of cholangiocellular lesions also being observed after long-term treatment in the former strain.

Biliary carcinomas can also be induced by intracholecystic methylcholanthrene pellets (Bain *et al.*, 1959) and high doses of aflatoxin B1 (Moore *et al.*, 1982). Feeding of nitrosodimethylamine after introduction of cholesterol pellets is associated with production of gallbladder carcinomas (Kowalewski & Todd, 1971). Intraperitoneal injection of nitrosobis-(2-hydroxypropyl)amine (Pour *et al.*, 1975), and 3,2-dimethyl-4-aminobiphenyl (Hasegawa *et al.*, 1992) also can cause development of polyp-like adenomas and adenocarcinomas in the hamster gallbladder.

Nitrosamines (see above) and dimethylhydrazine (Moore *et al.*, 1987a; Toth, 1972) are efficient inducers of haemangiomas and haemangiosarcomas, especially when given repeatedly. This can lead to extensive loss of animals by internal haemorrhage. Characteristic cystic angiomatous tumours can also be readily generated by injection of polyomavirus into newborn hamsters (Defendi & Lehman, 1964; Stanton, 1965). The lesions develop very rapidly (within weeks) and metastasize to the lungs).

A number of compounds or treatment regimens have been demonstrated capable of modifying carcinogen-initiated liver lesion induction or development in the hamster, as in the rat (Moore & Kitagawa, 1986). For example, phenobarbital (Makino et al., 1986, but not Stenbäck et al., 1986) and clofibrate (Mizumoto et al., 1988a) both promote hepatocellular adenoma and carcinoma development after initiation with N-nitrosobis(2-hydroxypropyl)amine. No tumour development was observed with clofibrate alone, however, and no effect on cholangiocellular or gallbladder lesions was evident. On the other hand, deoxycholic but not lithocholic acid at 0.5% enhanced induction of gallbladder polyps as well as cholangiocarcinomas, but exerted no effect on hepatocellular lesions (Makino et al., 1986), in contrast to findings in the rat (Tsuda et al., 1984). Testosterone has been found to inhibit, and follicle-stimulating hormone to stimulate, production of cystic liver by acetylaminofluorene without, however, any influence on malignant lesions (Dontenwill & Mohr, 1961).

As with the rat liver, agents may exert inhibitory as well as enhancing effects during both initiation and subsequent so called 'promotion stages'. Thus prior treatment with the hormone dehydroepiandrosterone or the synthetic phenolic antioxidant butylated hydroxyanisole inhibited induction of hepatic and ductular preneoplastic lesions by N-nitrosobis(2-hydroxypropyl)amine (Moore et al., 1988). The numbers of foci of altered hepatocytes (GST-P-positive) were also reduced by post-initiation administration of butylated hydroxyanisole or another antioxidant, vitamin E, while carbazole acted as a promoter under the same conditions (Moore et al., 1987a,b).

After N-nitrosobis(2-hydroxypropyl)-amine initiation, successive cycles of choline-deficient diet together with ethionine then methionine combined with the same carcinogen gave a 52% yield of cholangiocellular carcinoma in 10 weeks as well as hepatic nodules. The conclusion was of selective growth within initiated populations after the transfer from the toxic ethionine to the proliferation-stimulating methionine (Mizumoto et al., 1988b).

Proliferation occurring within the bile duct epithelium apparently also exerts strong enhancing effects by itself. Thus increased cell turnover in cholangioles after incomplete bile duct obstruction was found to significantly enhance development of cholangiocellular carcinomas after nitrosamine initiation (Kinami et al., 1990). Although heavy infestation with *Opisthorchis viverrini* parasites in Syrian golden hamsters is associated with a range of proliferative and inflammatory changes, particularly involving the ducts, under normal circumstances these do not include tumours. Indeed, repeated infection of both males and females with 50, 25 or 13 metacercariae, as many as 10 times, did not result in any tumour development after one year (Thamavit et al., personal communication). However, when acting in concert with carcinogen exposure (for example, nitrosodimethylamine or nitrite and aminopyrine precursors), parasite infestation exerts distinct promoting effects on cholangiocellular carcinoma development (Thamavit et al., 1978, 1987a). This influence is independent of whether the parasite is applied before or after carcinogen treatment (Flavell & Lucas, 1982, 1983). Furthermore, application of parasites in combination with carcinogenic regimens capable of inducing hepatocellular carcinomas also results in marked enhancement of hepatic adenoma yields (Thamavit *et al.*, 1987b, 1988a,b). In both ductal and parenchymal compartments, the effect appears to be primarily dependent on proliferation acting in the post-initiation phase.

COMPARATIVE ASPECTS

Neoplastic and preneoplastic lesions arising in epithelial, whether ductal or parenchymal, or endothelial compartments of the hamster liver are very similar to those seen in other rodents and also man. Thus the types of hepatocellular foci observed are directly comparable with the clear, mixed and basophilic lesions described for the rat (Bannasch, 1976; Bannasch *et al.*, 1984) and human (Karhunen & Penttilä, 1987). Histogenetic relationships between the various types in the hamster remain to be clarified but a sequence leading from smaller glycogen-storing populations to basophilic nodules and carcinomas would appear likely (see Bannasch *et al.*, 1984). While the fact of altered enzyme phenotype appears to be shared by rat, mouse and also human foci and nodules (Thung & Gerber, 1981; Fischer *et al.*, 1986), there are clear inter-species differences. For example, while GST-P is increased in at least a proportion of lesions in both hamsters and rats (Moore *et al.*, 1985; Tatematsu *et al.*, 1985), G6PD and GGT are conspicuously lacking in the hamster, in clear contrast to the rat (Moore & Kitagawa, 1986). G6PD is often elevated in mouse foci but not GGT (Vesselinovitch *et al.*, 1985). Whether further investigation of hamster lesions will reveal any coordinated shift in phenotype like that indicated for rat foci and nodules (Hacker *et al.*, 1982; Bannasch *et al.*, 1984) remains open, as does the question of whether selective growth advantage under Solt–Farber-type conditions (Solt *et al.*, 1977) is a common characteristic independent of species. Similarities between species with regard to inducibility and capacity for modulation of development clearly exist, as noted

above. However, in contrast to the rat, the hamster is relatively insensitive to hepatic carcinogenesis by most aminoazo-dyes, thioacetamide, ethionine and aflatoxin (Terracini & Della Porta, 1961) and the plasticizer di(2-ethylhexyl)phthalate does not appear to cause liver tumour development in the Syrian hamster (Schmezer *et al.*, 1988), in contrast to the case with F344 rats and B6C3F1 mice (Kluwe *et al.*, 1982).

As argued earlier for the rat, the term 'hepatocellular adenoma' as used in the National Toxicology Program nomenclature for benign nodular hepatocellular lesions in rats (Maronpot *et al.*, 1986) is superior to the other synonyms which have appeared in the literature, since it is in line with terminology in man. Application of the term 'hyperplastic liver nodule' appears inappropriate, since by definition, hyperplasia is an increase in tissue-specific cell numbers in the presence of extracellular growth factors which ceases on removal of the stimulus. For this reason Bannasch and co-workers have proposed the use of stop-type experiments in which exposure to the carcinogen is limited and only persisting lesions are observed (Bannasch *et al.*, 1984). The term neoplastic nodule has also been applied to adenomas (see workshop report of Squire & Levitt, 1975).

The proposed sequence leading from early bile duct proliferation through cholangiofibrosis and cholangioma/cholangiofibroma development to cholangiocellular carcinomas in the rat (Bannasch & Massner, 1976, 1977; Bannasch & Reiss, 1971) would appear to be also relevant to the hamster case (Moore *et al.*, 1986; Reuber, 1968). However, the cystic cholangiomas which can arise from areas of cholangiofibrosis in the rat (Bannasch & Reiss, 1971) are not evident in the hamster. Increased mucin production and goblet metaplasia have been similarly described for human cholangiocellular carcinomas and gallbladder tumours

(Chan *et al.*, 1976; Kozuka *et al.*, 1984; Yamagiwa & Tomiyama, 1986), this transient feature having been emphasized earlier for rat cholangiocellular (Bannasch & Massner, 1976; Terao & Nakano, 1974) and hamster intrahepatic and gallbladder neoplasia of ductal type.

Comparison of response to a variety of carcinogens reveals the hamster bile duct epithelium to be far more sensitive to tumour induction than that of the rat. The process can be significantly enhanced by proliferative stimuli such as that provided by liver fluke infestation, similar findings having been reported for man (Hou, 1956; Kurathong *et al.*, 1985). This fact, the presence of a gallbladder and the reliability of the hamster liver–*N*-nitroso-bis(2-hydroxypropyl)amine model underlies its use for investigation of factors relevant to biliary cirrhosis-associated neoplasia (cf. the reports of Falchuk *et al.*, 1976, and Melia *et al.*, 1984, in man).

ACKNOWLEDGEMENTS

The authors would like to express their thanks to the late Professor K. Sato of Hirosaki University for generous provision of antibody to GST-P.

REFERENCES

Bain, G.O., Allen, P.R.B., Silbermann, O. & Kowalewski, K. (1959) Induction in hamsters of biliary carcinoma by intracholecystic methylcholanthrene pellets. *Cancer Res.*, 19, 93–95

Bannasch, P. (1976) Cytology and cytogenesis of neoplastic (hyperplastic) hepatic nodules. *Cancer Res.*, 36, 2555–2562

Bannasch, P. & Massner, B. (1976) Histogenese und Cytogenese von Cholangiofibromen und Cholangiocarcinomen bei Nitrosomorpholinvergifteten Ratten. *Z. Krebsforsch.*, 87, 239-255

Bannasch, P. & Massner, B. (1977) Die Feinstruktur des Nitrosomorpholin-induzierten Cholangiofibroms der Ratte. *Virchows Arch. [Cell Pathol.]*, 24, 295–315

Bannasch, P. & Reiss, W. (1971) Histogenese und Cytogenese cholangiocellularer Tumoren bei Nitrosomorpholin-vergifteten Ratten. Zugleich ein Betrag zur Morphogenese der Cystenleber. *Z. Krebsforch.*, 76, 193–215

Bannasch, P., Bloch, M. & Zerban, H. (1981) Spongiosis hepatis. Specific changes of the perisinusoidal cells induced in rats by *N*-nitrosomorpholine. *Lab. Invest.*, 44, 252–264

Bannasch, P. & Hacker, H.J., Klimek, F. & Mayer, D. (1984) Hepatocellular glycogenosis and related pattern of enzymatic changes during hepatocarcinogenesis. *Adv. Enzyme Regul.*, 22, 97–121

Bell, R.H., Jr, Hye, R.J. & Miyai, K. (1984) Streptozotocin-induced liver tumors in the Syrian hamster. *Carcinogenesis*, 5, 1235–1238

Bergman, F. & Wahlin, T. (1981) Tumour induction in Syrian hamsters fed a combination of aminopyrine and nitrite. *Acta Pathol. Microbiol. Scand.*, Sect. A, 89, 241–245

Berman, L.D., Hayes, J.A. & Sibay, T.M. (1973) Effect of streptozotocin on the Chinese hamster (Cricetulus griseus). *J. Natl Cancer Inst.*, 51, 1287–1294

Bhamarapravati, N., Thamavit, W. & Vajrasthira, S. (1978) Liver changes in hamsters infected with a liver fluke of man, *Opisthorchis viverrini*. *Am. J. Trop. Med. Hyg.*, 27, 787–794

Cabral, J.R.P., Shubik, P., Mollner, T. & Raitano, F. (1977) Carcinogenic activity of hexachlorobenzene in hamsters. *Nature*, 269, 510–511

Chan, S.T., Chan, C.W. & Ng, W.L. (1976) Mucin histochemistry of human cholangiocarcinoma. *J. Pathol.*, 118, 165–170

Chesterman, F.C. & Pomerance, A. (1965) Cirrhosis and liver tumours in a closed colony of golden hamsters. *Br. J. Cancer*, 19, 802–811

Defendi, V. & Lehman, J.M. (1964) The nature of hemorrhagic lesions induced by polyoma virus in hamsters. *Cancer Res.*, 24, 329–343

Della Porta, G., Shubik, P. & Scortecci, V. (1959) The action of *N*-2-fluorenyl-acetamide in the Syrian golden hamster. *J. Natl Cancer Inst.*, 22, 463–487

Della Porta, G., Terracini, B. & Shubik, P. (1961) Induction with carbon tetrachloride of liver cell carcinomas in hamsters. *J. Natl Cancer Inst.*, 26, 855–863

Dontenwill, W. & Mohr, U. (1961) Proliferationsfoerdende und -hemmende Wirkung der Geschlechtshormone bei Behandlung von Goldhamstern mit Carcinogenen. *Z. Krebsforsch.*, 64, 381–389

Dontenwill, W., Chevalier, H.J., Harke, H.P., Lafrenz, U. & Reckzeh, G. (1973) Spontantumoren des syrischen Goldhamsters. *Z. Krebsforsch.*, 80, 127–158

Falchuk, K.R., Lesser, P.B., Galdabini, J.J. & Isselbacher, K.J. (1976) Cholangiocarcinoma as related to chronic intrahepatic cholangitis and hepatolithiasis. *Am. J. Gastroenterol.*, 66, 57–61

Fisscher, G., Hartmann, H., Droese, M. Schauer, A. and Boch, K..W. (1986) Histochemical and immunohistochemical detection of putative preneoplastic foci in women after long-term use of oral contraceptives. *Virchows Arch. (Cell Pathol.)*, 50, 321-337

Flavell, D.J. & Lucas, S.B. (1982) Potentiation by the human liver fluke *Opisthorchis viverrini* of the carcinogenic action of *N*-nitrosodimethylamine upon the biliary epithelium of the hamster. *Br. J. Cancer,* 46, 985–989

Flavell, D.J. & Lucas, S.B. (1983) Promotion of *N*-nitrosodimethylamine-initiated bile duct carcinogenesis in the hamster by the human liver fluke, *Opisthorchis viverrini*. *Carcinogenesis*, 4, 927–930

Fortner, J.G. (1957) Spontaneous tumors, including gastrointestinal neoplasms and malignant melanomas in the Syrian hamster. *Cancer*, 10, 1153–1156

Greenblatt, M. (1982) Tumours of the liver. In: Turusov, V.S., ed., *Pathology of Tumours in Laboratory Animals*, Vol. III, *Tumours of the Hamster* (IARC Scientific Publications No. 34), Lyon, IARC, pp. 69–102

Hacker, H.J., Moore, M.A., Mayer, D. & Bannasch, P. (1982) Correlative histochemistry of some enzymes of carbohydrate metabolism in preneoplastic and neoplastic lesions in rat liver. *Carcinogenesis*, 3, 1265–1272

Hasegawa, R., Ogawa, K., Takaba, K., Shirai, T. & Ito, N. (1972) 3,2'-Dimethyl-4-aminobiphenyl-induced gallbladder carcinogenesis and effects of ethinyl estradiol in hamsters. *Jpn J. Cancer Res.*, 83, 1286–1292

Herrold, K.M. (1964) Effect of route of administration on the carcinogenic action of diethylnitrosamine (*N*-nitrosodiethylamine). *Br. J. Cancer*, 18, 763–767

Herrold, K.M. (1967) Histogenesis of malignant liver tumours induced by dimethylnitrosamine. An experimental study in Syrian hamsters. *J. Natl Cancer Inst.*, 39, 1099–1104

Herrold, K.M. & Dunham, L.J. (1963) Induction of tumors in the Syrian hamster with diethylnitrosamine (*N*-nitrosodiethylamine). *Cancer Res.*, 23, 773–777

Hou, P.C. (1956) The relationship between primary liver cancer and infestation with *Clonorchis sinensis*. *J. Pathol. Bact.*, 72, 239–246

Karhunen, P.-J. & Penttilä, A. (1987) Preneoplastic lesions of human liver. *Hepatogastroenterol.*, 34, 10–15

Kinami, Y., Ashida, Y., Seto, K., Takashima, S. & Kita, I. (1990) Influence of incomplete bile duct obstruction on the occurrence of cholangiocarcinoma induced by diisopropanolnitrosamine in hamsters. *Oncology*, 47, 170–176

Kluwe, W.M., Haseman, J.K., Douglas, J.F. & Huff, J.E. (1982) The carcinogenicity of dietary di(2-ethylhexyl)phthalate (DEHP) in Fischer 344 rats and B6C3F1 mice. *Toxicol. Appl. Pharmacol.*, 72, 46–60

Kokkinakis, D.M. & Scarpelli, D.G. (1989) Carcinogenicity of *N*-nitroso(2-hydroxypropyl)(2-oxopropyl)amine, *N*-nitroso-bis-(2-hydroxypropyl)amine and cis-*N*-nitroso-2,6,dimethylmorpholine administered continuously in the Syrian hamster, and the effect of dietary protein on *N*-nitroso(2-hydroxypropyl)(2-oxopropyl)amine carcinogenesis. *Carcinogenesis*, 10, 699–704

Kowalewski, K. & Todd, E.F. (1971) Carcinoma of the gallbladder induced in hamsters by insertion of cholesterol pellets and feeding dimethylnitrosamine (35293). *Proc. Soc. Exp. Biol. (N.Y.)*, 136, 482–486

Kozuka, S., Kurtashina, M., Tsubone, M., Hachisuka, K. & Yasui, A. (1984) Significance of intestinal metaplasia for the evolution of cancer of the biliary tract. *Cancer*, 54, 2277–2285

Kurathong, S., Lerdvirasirikul, P., Wougpaitoon, V., Pramoolsinsap, C., Kanjanapitak, A., Varawithaya, W., Phupradit, P., Bunyaratvej, S., Upatham, S. & Brockelman, W.Y. (1985) *Opisthorchis viverrini* infection and cholangiocarcinoma: a prospective case-control study. *Gastroenterology*, 89, 151–156

Li, J.-J. & Li, S.A. (1984) High incidence of hepatocellular carcinomas after synthetic estrogen administration in Syrian golden hamsters fed α-naphthoflavone: a new tumor model. *J. Natl Cancer Inst.*, 73, 543–547

Lijinsky, W., Saavedra, J.E., Knutsen, G.L. & Kovatch, R.M. (1984) Comparison of the carcinogenic effectiveness of *N*-nitroso-bis(2-hydroxypropyl)amine, *N*-nitroso-bis(2-oxopropyl)amine, *N*-nitroso(2-hydroxypropyl)(2-oxopropyl)amine and *N*-nitroso-2,6-dimethylmorpholine in Syrian hamsters. *J. Natl Cancer Inst.*, 72, 685–688

Lijinsky, W., Kovatch, R.M. & Riggs, C.W. (1987) Carcinogenesis by nitrosodialkylamines and azoxyalkanes given by gavage to rats and hamsters. *Cancer Res.*, 47, 3968–3972

Maljugina, L.L. (1958) Tumours produced in hamsters by 2-acetylaminofluorene [in Russian]. *Vopr. Oncol.*, 4, 279–283

Makino, T., Obara, T., Ura, H., Kinugasa, T., Kobayashi, H., Takahashi, S. & Konishi, Y. (1986) Effects of phenobarbital and secondary bile acids on liver, gallbladder, and pancreas carcinogenesis initiated by *N*-nitroso(2-hydroxypropyl)amine in hamsters. *J. Natl Cancer Inst.*, 76, 967–975

Maronpot, R.R., Montgomery, C.A., Jr, Boorman, G.A. & McConnell, E.E. (1986) National Toxicology Program nomenclature for hepatoproliferative lesions in rats. *Toxicol. Pathol.*, 14, 263–273

Melia, W.M., Johnson, P.J., Neuberger, J., Zaman, S., Portmann, B.C. & Williams, R. (1984) Hepatocellular carcinoma in primary biliary cirrhosis: detection by alpha-fetoprotein estimation. *Gastroenterology*, 87, 660–663

Mizumoto, K., Kitazawa, S., Eguchi, T., Nakajima, A., Tsutsumi, M., Ito, S., Danda, A. & Konishi, Y. (1988a) Modulation of *N*-nitroso-bis(2-hydroxypropyl)amine-induced carcinogenesis by clofibrate in hamsters. *Carcinogenesis*, 9, 1421–1425

Mizumoto, K., Tsutsumi, M., Denda, A. & Konishi, Y. (1988b) Rapid production of pancreatic carcinoma by initiation with *N*-nitroso-bis(2-oxopropyl)amine and repeated augmentation pressure in hamsters. *J. Natl Cancer Inst.*, 80, 1564–1567

Moore, M.A. & Kitagawa, T. (1986) Hepatocarcinogenesis in the rat: the effect of promotors and carcinogens in vivo and in vitro. *Int. Rev. Cytol.*, 101, 125–173

Moore, M.R., Pitot, H.C., Miller, E.C. & Miller, J.A. (1982) Cholangiocellular carcinomas induced in Syrian golden hamsters administered aflatoxin B1 in large doses. *J. Natl Cancer Inst.*, 68, 271–278

Moore, M.A., Satoh, K., Kitahara, A., Sato, K. & Ito, N. (1985) A protein cross-reacting immunohistochemically with rat glutathione S-transferase placental form as a marker for preneoplasia in Syrian hamster pancreatic- and hepatocarcinogenesis. *Jpn. J. Cancer Res. (Gann)*, 76, 1–4

Moore, M.A., Fukushima, S., Ichihara, A., Sato, K. & Ito, N. (1986) Intestinal metaplasia and altered enzyme expression in propyl-nitrosamine-induced Syrian hamster cholangiocellular and gallbladder lesions. *Virchows Arch., B, Cell Pathol.*, 51, 29–38

Moore, M.A., Thamavit, W. & Ito, N. (1987a) Comparison of lesions induced in the Syrian golden hamster by diethylnitrosamine, dimethylhydrazine, and dibutylnitrosamine: influence of subsequent butylated hydroxyanisole treatment. *J. Natl Cancer Inst.*, 78, 295–301

Moore, M.A., Tsuda, H., Thamavit, W., Masui, T. & Ito, N. (1987b) Differential modification of development of preneoplastic lesions in the Syrian golden hamster initiated with a single dose of 2,2'-dioxo-*N*-nitrosodipropylamine: influence of subsequent butylated hydroxyanisole, alpha-tocopherol, or carbazole. *J. Natl Cancer Inst.*, 78, 289–293

Moore, M.A., Thamavit, W., Hiasa, Y. & Ito, N. (1988) Early lesions induced by DHPN in Syrian golden hamsters: influence of concomitant *Opisthorchis* infestation, dehydroepiandrosterone or butylated hydroxyanisole administration. *Carcinogenesis, 9,* 1185–1189

Pour, P., Krueger, F.W., Althoff, J., Cardesa, A. & Mohr, U. (1975) Effect of betaoxidised nitrosamines in Syrian golden hamsters. III. 2,2-dihydroxy-di-*n*-propylnitrosamine. *J. Natl Cancer Inst.,* 54, 141–145

Pour, P., Mohr, U., Althoff, J., Cardesa, A. & Kmoch, N. (1976) Spontaneous tumors and common diseases in two colonies of Syrian hamsters. II. Respiratory tract and digestive system. *J. Natl Cancer Inst.,* 56, 937–948

Rappaport, A.M. (1976) The microcirculatory concept of normal and pathological hepatic structure. *Beitr. Pathol.,* 157, 215–243

Reuber, M.D. (1968) Histogenesis of cholangiofibrosis and well-differentiated cholangiocarcinoma in Syrian hamsters given 2-acetamidofluorene or 2-diacetamidofluorene. *Gann,* 59, 239–246

Schmezer, P., Pool, B.L., Klein, R.G., Komitowski, D. & Schmael, D. (1988) Various short-term assays and two long-term studies with the plasticizer di(2-ethylhexyl)phthalate in the Syrian golden hamster. *Carcinogenesis, 9,* 37–43

Solt, D.B., Medline, A. & Farber, E. (1977) Rapid emergence of carcinogen-induced hyperplastic lesions in a new model for the sequential analysis of liver carcinogenesis. *Am. J. Pathol.,* 88, 595–618

Squire, R.A. & Levitt, M.H. (1975) Report of a workshop on classification of specific hepatocellular lesions in rats. *Cancer Res.,* 35, 3214–3223

Stanton, M.F. (1965) Transplantability, morphology, and behaviour of polyoma virus-induced hepatic haemangiomas of hamsters. *J. Natl Cancer Inst.,* 35, 201–213

Stenbäck, F., Mori, H., Furuya, K. & Williams, G.M. (1986) Pathogenesis of dimethylnitrosamine-induced hepatocellular cancer in hamster liver and lack of enhancement by phenobarbital. *J. Natl Cancer Inst.,* 76, 327–333

Taper, H.S. & Bannasch, P. (1979) Histochemical differences between so-called megalocytosis and neoplastic or preneoplastic liver lesions induced by *N*-nitrosomorpholine. *Eur. J. Cancer,* 15, 189–196

Tatematsu, M., Takano, T., Hasegawa, R., Imaida, K., Nakanowatari, J. & Ito, N. (1980) A sequential quantitative study of the reversibility or irreversibility of liver hyperplastic nodules in rats exposed to hepatocarcinogens. *Gann,* 71, 843–855

Tatematsu, M., Mera, Y., Ito, N., Satoh, K. & Sato, K. (1985) Relative merits of immunohistochemical demonstration of placental A, B and C forms of glutathione S-transferase as markers of altered foci during liver carcinogenesis. *Carcinogenesis, 6,* 1621–1626

Terao, K. & Nakano, M. (1974) Cholangiofibrosis induced by short-term feeding of 3-methyl-4-dimethylaminobenzene to rats: an electron microscopic observation. *Gann,* 65, 249–260

Terracini, B. & Della Porta, G. (1961) Feeding with aminoazodyes, thioacetamide and ethionine. Studies in the hamster. *Arch. Pathol.,* 71, 566–575

Thamavit, W., Bhamarapravati, N., Sahaphong, S., Vajrasthira, S. & Angsubhakorn, S. (1978) Effects of dimethylnitrosamine on induction of cholangiocarcinoma in *Opisthorchis viverrini*-infected Syrian golden hamsters. *Cancer Res.,* 38, 4634–4639

Thamavit, W., Kongkanuntn, R., Tiwawech, D. & Moore, M.A. (1987a) Level of *Opisthorchis* infestation and carcinogen dose dependence of cholangiocarcinoma induction in Syrian golden hamsters. *Virchows Arch., B, Cell Pathol.,* 54, 52–58

Thamavit, W., Ngamying, M., Moore, M.A., Boonpucknavig, V. & Boonpucknavig, S. (1987b) Enhancement of DEN-induced hepatocellular nodule development by *Opisthorchis viverrini* infection in Syrian golden hamsters. *Carcinogenesis, 8,* 1351–1353

Thamavit, W., Moore, M.A., Hiasa, Y. & Ito, N. (1988a) Generation of high yields of Syrian hamster cholangiocellular carcinomas and hepatocellular nodules by combined nitrite and aminopyrine administration and *Opisthorchis viverrini* infection. *Jpn. J. Cancer Res. (Gann),* 79, 909–916

Thamavit, W., Moore, M.A., Hiasa, Y. & Ito, N. (1988b) Enhancement of DHPN-induced hepatocellular, cholangiocellular and pancreatic carcinogenesis by *Opisthorchis viverrini* infestation in Syrian golden hamsters. *Carcinogenesis*, 9, 1095–1098

Thung, S.W. & Gerber, M.A. (1981) Enzyme pattern and marker antigens in nodular 'regenerative' hyperplasia of the liver. *Cancer*, 47, 1796–1799

Tomatis, L. & Cefis, F. (1967) The effects of multiple and single administration of dimethylnitrosamine to hamsters. *Tumori*, 53, 447–452

Tomatis, L., Della Porta, G. & Shubik, P. (1961) Urinary bladder and liver cell tumors induced in hamsters with o-aminoazotoluene. *Cancer Res.*, 21, 1513–1517

Tomatis, L., Magee, P.N. & Shubik, P. (1964) Induction of liver tumors in the Syrian golden hamster by feeding dimethylnitrosamine. *J. Natl Cancer Inst.*, 33, 341–345

Toth, B. (1972) Tumorigenesis studies with 1,2-dimethylhydrazine dihydrochloride, hydrazine sulfate, and isonicotinic acid in golden hamsters. *Cancer Res.*, 32, 804–807

Toth, B., Tomatis, L. & Shubik, P. (1961) Multipotential carcinogenesis with urethane in the Syrian golden hamster. *Cancer Res.*, 21, 1537–1541

Tsuda, H., Masui, T., Imaida, K., Hasegawa, R. & Ito, N. (1984) Promotive effect of primary and secondary bile acids on the induction of γ-glutamyl transpeptidase-positive liver cell foci as a possible endogenous factor for hepatocarcinogenesis in rats. *Gann*, 75, 871–875

Vesselinovitch, S.D., Hacker, H.J. & Bannasch, P. (1985) Histochemical characterization of focal hepatic lesions induced by single diethylnitrosamine treatment in infant mice. *Cancer Res.*, 45, 2274–2280

Yabe, Y., Kataoka, N. & Koyama, H. (1972) Spontaneous tumors in hamsters: incidence, morphology, transplantation and virus studies. *Gann*, 63, 329–336

Yamagiwa, H. & Tomiyama, H. (1986) Intestinal metaplasia-dysplasia-carcinoma sequence of the gallbladder. *Acta Pathol. Jpn.*, 36, 989–997

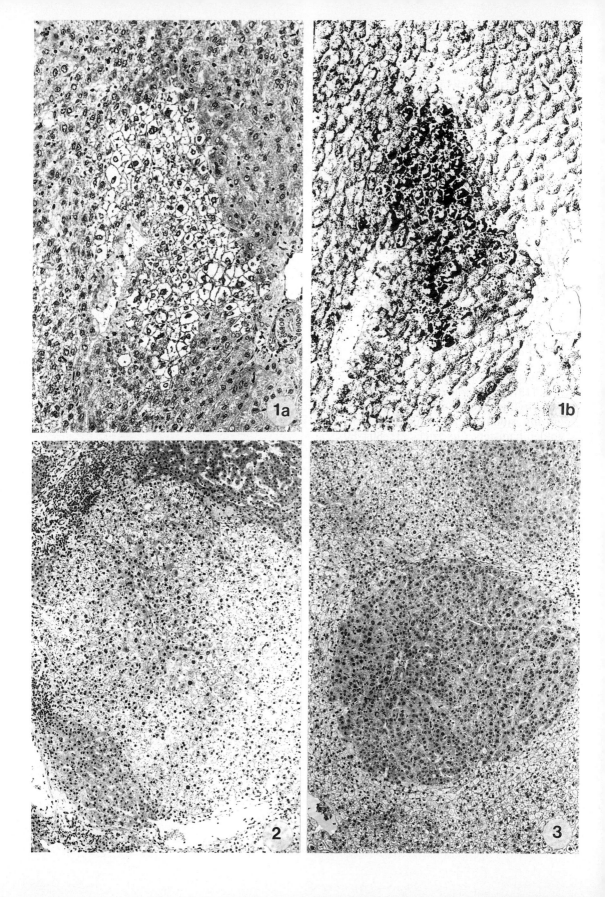

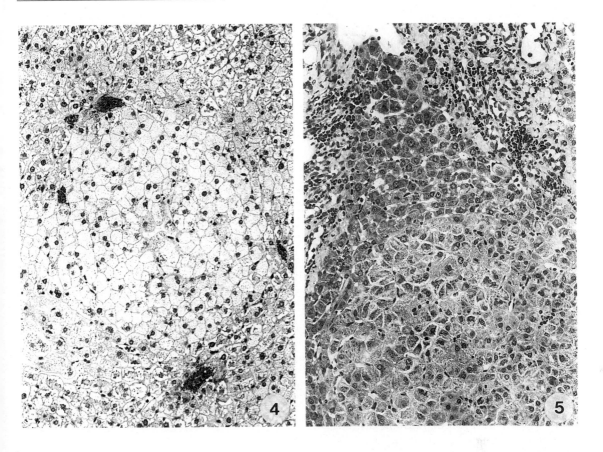

Figure 1. Clear cell focus. (a) H & E. (b) PAS. Note increase in glycogen. × 250

Figure 2. Mixed cell focus comprising clear, acidophilic and basophilic hepatocytes. H & E; × 75

Figure 3. Basophilic focus. H & E; × 100

Figure 4. Focus of fat-storing cells. H & E; ×250

Figure 5. Focus comprising acidophilic and basophilic hepatocytes in a hamster infected with *Opisthorchis viverrini*. H & E; × 250

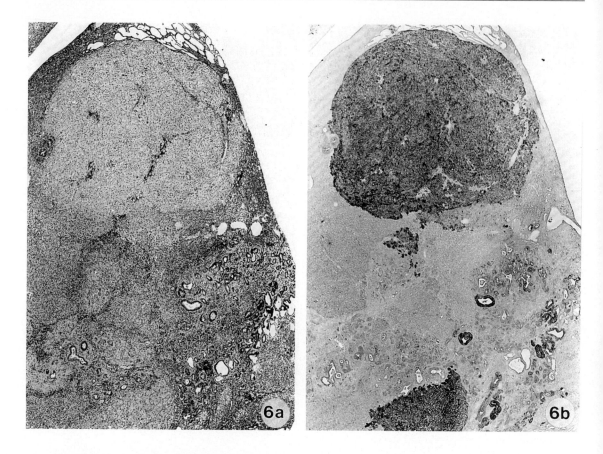

Figure 6. Low-power micrograph illustrating development of a hepatocellular adenoma, demonstrating compression of the surrounding parenchyma. (a) H & E; (b) GST-P binding (ABC immunohistochemistry); × 20

Figure 7. Semi-serial cryostat sections through *N*-nitrosobis(2-hydroxypropyl)amine-induced hepatocellular focal lesions histochemically reacted for (a) glucose-6-phosphatase; (b) succinate dehydrogenase; (c) glucose-6-phosphate dehydrogenase; (d) ATPase. × 40

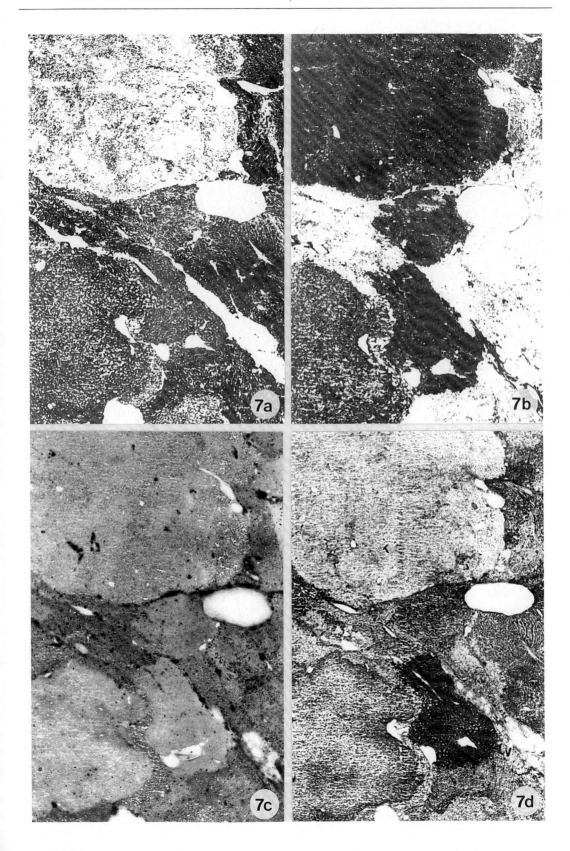

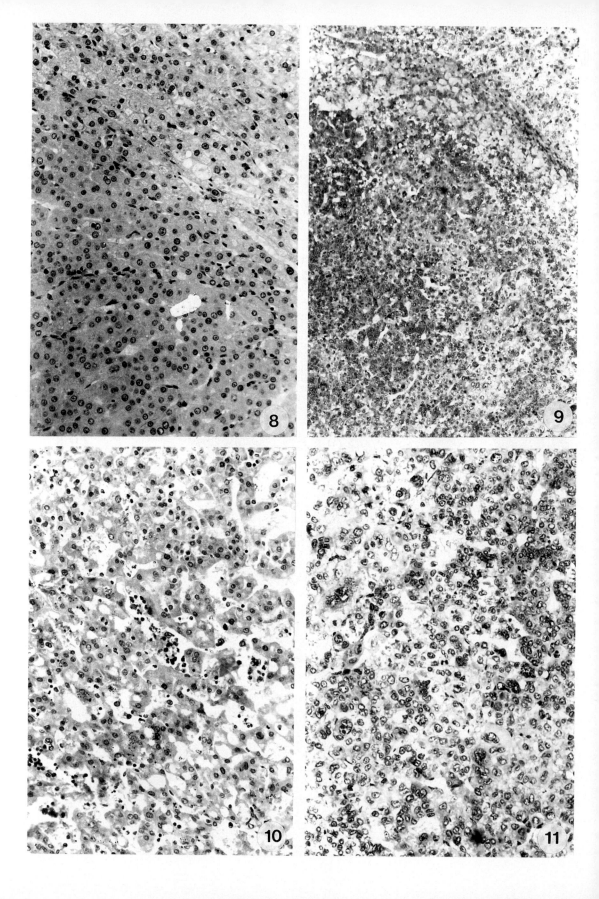

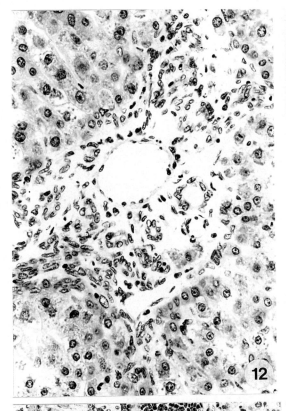

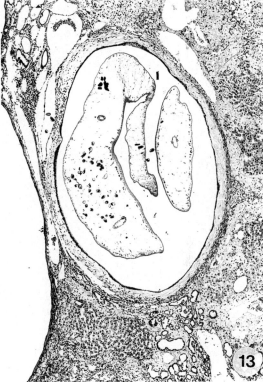

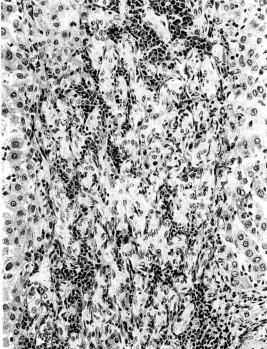

Figure 8. Edge of a hepatic adenoma. Note increased basophilia of component hepatocytes at lower left. H & E; ×250

Figure 9. Edge of solid hepatocellular carcinoma. H & E; 200

Figure 10. Area of trabecular carcinoma. H & E; ×250

Figure 11. Area of solid carcinoma illustrating cellular pleomorphism. H & E; ×250

Figure 12. Simple bile duct proliferation. H & E; ×400

Figure 13. Adult *Opisthorchis viverrini* liver flukes within a severely altered hamster liver. H & E; ×50

Figure 14. Liver fluke-associated bile duct proliferation and accompanying inflammatory infiltration. H & E; ×300

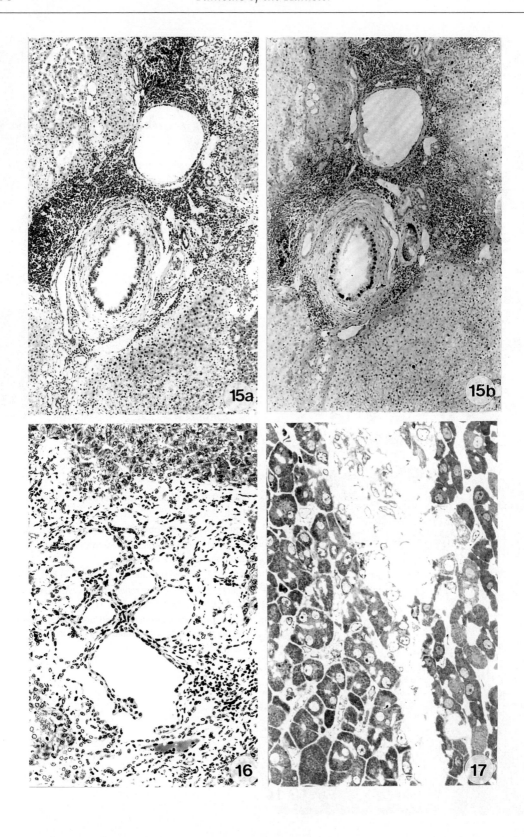

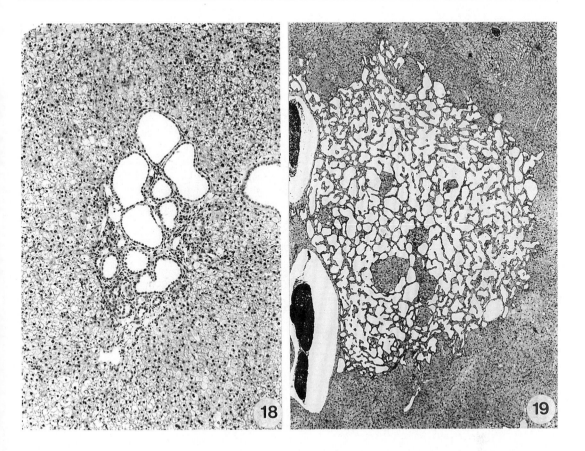

Figure 15. Serial sections through an area of periductal fibrosis and inflammation caused by infection with *Opisthorchis viverrini*. (a) H & E; (b) BrdU incorporation (ABC immunohistochemistry); ×75

Figure 16. Liver fluke-associated bile duct proliferation and amyloidosis. H & E; ×200

Figure 17. Small area of periportal amyloidosis. Semi-thin plastic embedded section. Toluidine blue; ×450

Figure 18. Cystic lesion. H & E; ×125

Figure 19. Cystadenoma. H & E; ×50

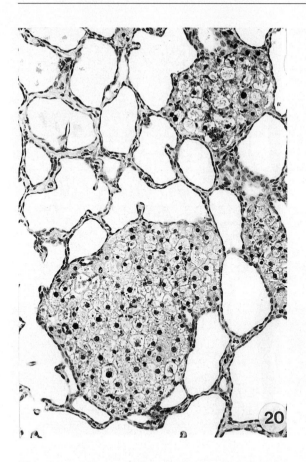

Figure 20. Detail of cystadenoma illustrating extreme flattening of the epithelium with nests of enclosed hepatocytes. H & E; ×350

Figure 21. Semi-serial sections, through an area of cholangiofibrosis. (a) H & E; (b) PAS; (c) BrdU incorporation; ×50

Figure 22. Semi-serial sections through a cholangiofibroma. (a) H & E; (b) PAS; (c) BrdU incorporation; ×50

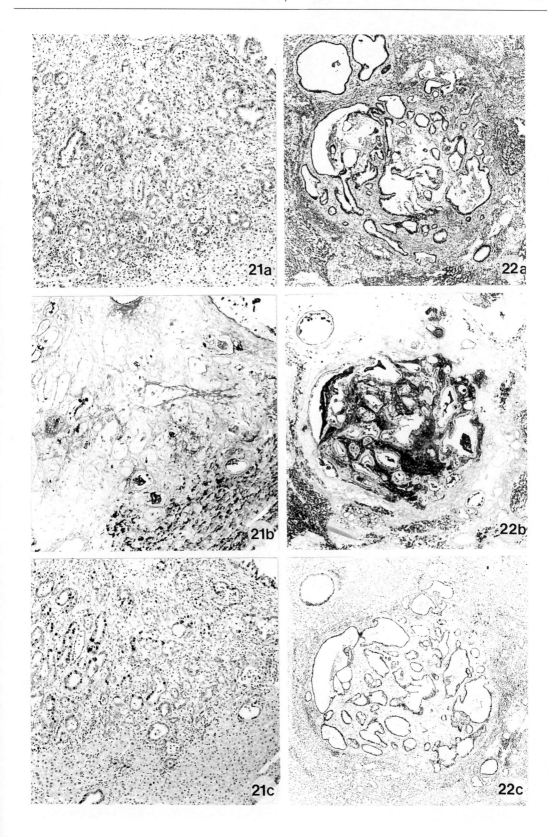

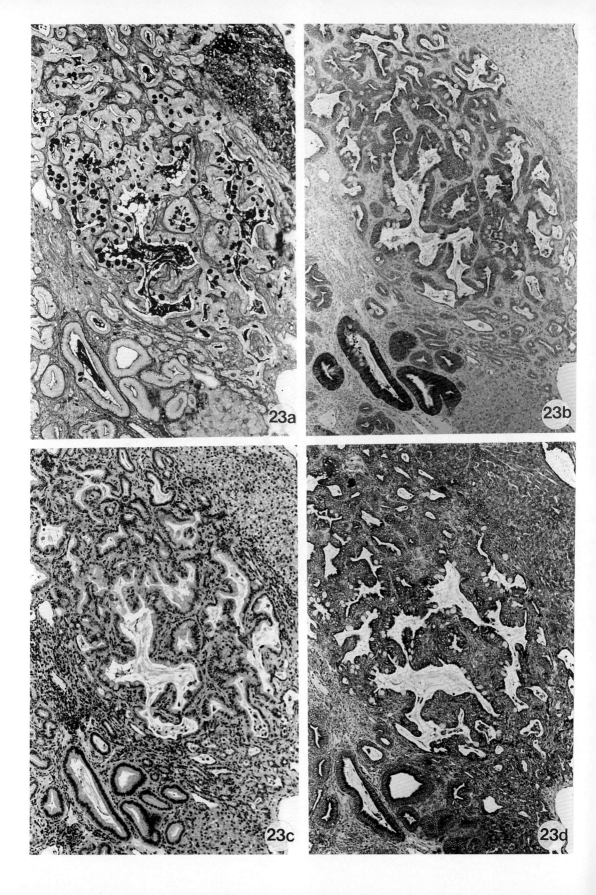

Figure 23. Semi-serial sections through an area of cholangiofibrosis ×100

(a) H & E;

(b) glutathione S-transferase P binding;

(c) Alcian blue/PAS;

(d) glucose-6-phosphate dehydrogenase binding

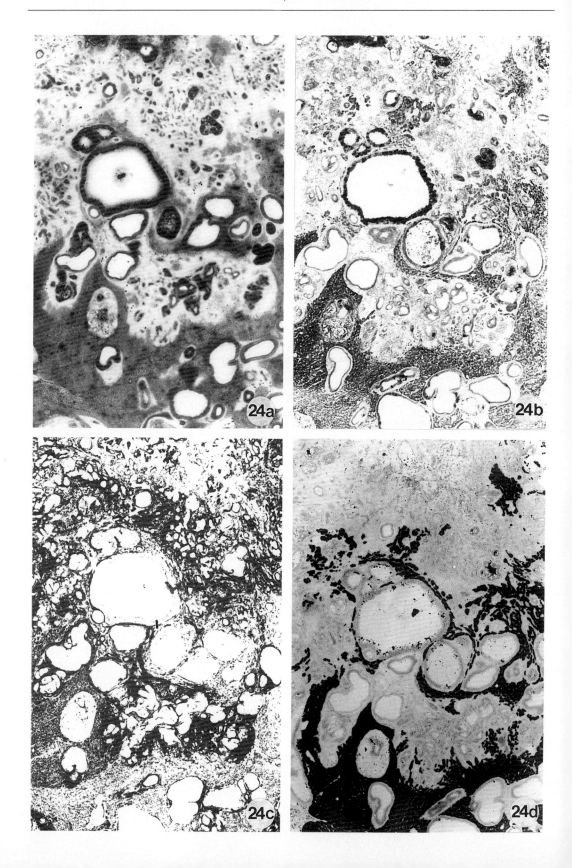

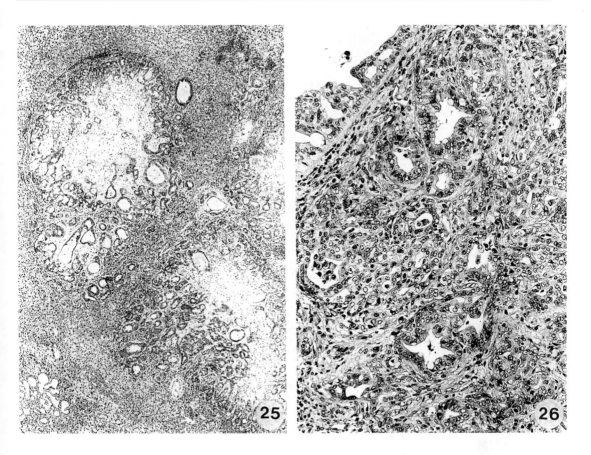

Figure 24. Semi-serial cryostat sections through an area of cholangiofibrosis reacted histochemically for (a) glucose-6-phosphatase; (b) adenosine triphosphatase; (c) succinate dehydrogenase; (d) glucose-6-phosphate dehydrogenase; ×50

Figure 25. Cholangiocellular carcinoma. H & E; × 40

Figure 26. Detail of cholangiocellular carcinoma . H & E; × 250

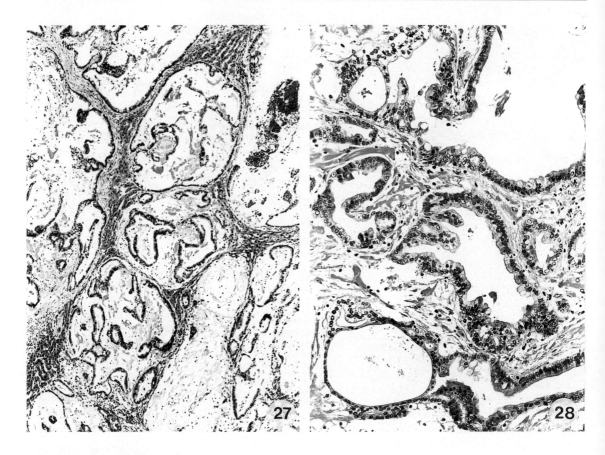

Figure 27. Cystadenocarcinoma. H & E; ×75

Figure 28. Detail of cystadenocarcinoma. H & E; ×250

Figure 29. Gallbladder polyp. Note preneoplastic goblet cell metaplasia of epithelium at top left. (a) H & E; (b) Alcian blue PAS; ×60

Figure 30. Gallbladder carcinoma. H & E; ×40

Figure 31. Detail of gallbladder carcinoma illustrating tall columnar epithelium. H & E; ×400

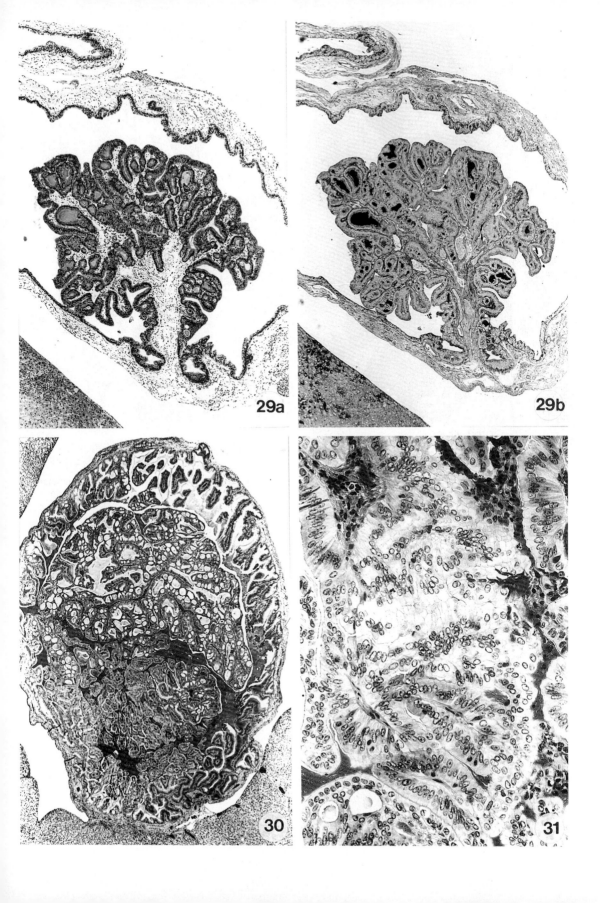

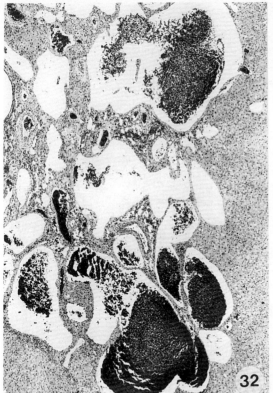

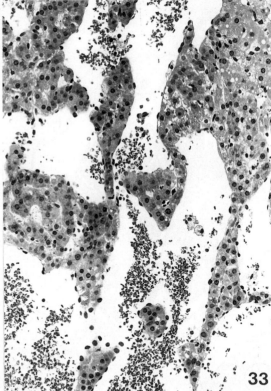

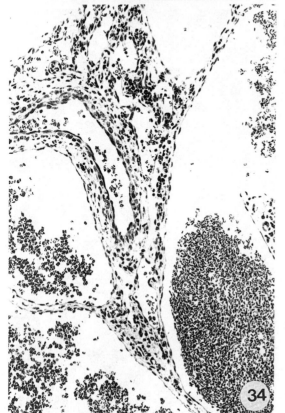

Figure 32. Peliosis hepatis. H & E; ×350

Figure 33. Haemangioma. H & E; ×40

Figure 34. Detail of haemangioma, illustrating complete endothelial lining of blood-filled cavities. H & E; ×350

Tumours of the gallbladder

V.S. Turusov and B. Gorin[1]

NORMAL STRUCTURE

The gallbladder of the hamster is located under the medial lobe of the liver. It is about 8–10 mm long, and the diameter is about 5 mm. When not distended, its mucosa forms folds covered with tall columnar epithelial cells containing dark elongated nuclei. In the distended gallbladder, the epithelial cells are cubical to low columnar (Figure 1a, b). The connective tissue under the epithelium is cellular, and in places it may be rather loose and contain few lymphoid cells and plasmacytes. Mucinous glands in the wall open onto the mucosal surface. The muscle layer is formed of smooth muscle bundles.

MORPHOLOGY AND BIOLOGY OF TUMOURS

Macroscopic appearance

Very small tumours may be detectable only if the gallbladder is opened. They appear as a white or yellowish thickening of the mucosa or nodules of varying size on the mucosa surface. Larger tumours represent the non-translucent thickening of the gallbladder wall that may be local or affect the whole organ. The lumen can be completely blocked or may remain as a narrow cavity within a tumour filled with a brownish mucoid material containing the pellet of inducing agent. In advanced cases, a nodular mass is observed firmly attached to the liver; no lumen is left and the pellet

is incorporated into the tumour tissue. The liver may be intact, but in many cases its surface becomes uneven, and the liver tissue may contain yellowish foci, mainly in the lobe to which the gallbladder is attached. This lobe may contain projections of white tumorous tissue or may be partly replaced by such tissue.

Due to the small size of many gallbladder tumours, their subdivision by naked-eye examination is hardly possible.

Histological types of tumour
Adenoma – papillary, glandular
Adenocarcinoma–exophytic or infiltrative
   highly differentiated
   poorly differentiated
   anaplastic
Other tumours

Adenoma (synonyms: papilloma, polyp)

This tumour may fill the lumen of the gallbladder totally or in part. It consists of structurally atypical papillae of varying shape, thickness and size.

The simplest lesion of this type is illustrated in Figure 2: it consists of branching thin fibrous stalks covered with normal-looking cuboidal cells. The lack of any epithelial cell atypia suggests a purely reactive nature of this lesion. This growth morphologically resembles lesions of the human gallbladder called pseudotumours (Christensen & Ishak, 1970).

More advanced tumours represent branching structures with finger-like projections covered with high columnar cells,

[1] Deceased

sometimes with hyperchromatic nuclei. Mitoses can be frequent. The papillae may be very thick and abundant, being formed of loose cellular or acellular tissue with many vessels (Figures 3 and 4). In spite of the irregularity of the general structure of such tumours, epithelium covering papillae or glands does not, in general, show any pronounced atypia, although in some areas signs of dysplasia or even carcinoma *in situ* may be seen (Figure 3d).

The distinguishing feature of these tumours is the absence of infiltrative growth into the liver, from which they are usually, although not always, separated by a thick layer of fibrous tissue or a rather loose tissue with inflammatory cells and many dilated vessels.

A papillary adenoma which has a border with the liver that is not clear-cut is illustrated in Figure 4. The connective tissue at the border with the liver contains many vessels and ductules, and may be considered as showing signs of invasive growth (Figure 4a and 4b).

The majority of adenomas are of a purely papillary structure, similar to that illustrated in Figures 2, 3 and 4. Among our material of over 20 adenomas, we found two lesions with a different structure. One consisted of several cavities separated from each other by thick connective tissue septa containing few glands and infiltrated with inflammatory cells (Figure 5). The inner surface of the cavities was uneven with a few fibrous stalks protruding into the lumen. The epithelium was tall columnar. In another case there were a few very thick and long fibrous stalks protruding into the gallbladder cavity. The epithelium of both fibrous stalks and the gallbladder was hyperplastic and unevenly thickened with signs of dysplasia (Figure 6).

Adenocarcinoma

According to the mode of growth, adenocarcinomas can be subdivided into exophytic (intravesicular) ones and those with predominantly invasive growth into the gallbladder wall and liver (infiltrative type).

In contrast to adenomas, which are mainly of a papillary structure, the majority of carcinomas are of a glandular structure. An exception is illustrated in Figure 5, where the apparently invasive growth is due to acinar elements. In human gallbladder carcinomas, a papillary pattern is also rare (Ashley, 1978). The characteristic feature of many adenocarcinomas is not the atypia of their cells or glands (they can be very well differentiated) but their invasive growth.

Exophytic (intravesicular) tumours. The gallbladder is completely replaced by tumorous tissue with no lumen left. Even histologically, the elements of the gallbladder wall may be indistinguishable and the tumour occupies a significant part of the liver lobe.

A highly differentiated adenocarcinoma (Figure 7) is formed of glands and acini of varying size but of a rather regular shape, lined with columnar, cubical or flattened epithelium. The distinguishing feature of these tumours is the lack of pronounced cell atypia in the tumour gland lining. In some areas of these tumours the epithelium lining the glands is so well differentiated that it gives an impression of reactive rather than neoplastic changes. Larger areas in the tumour may be necrotic. Stroma may be abundant, oedematous or sclerotic. Glands are sometimes transformed into thin-walled tubules with highly flattened almost indiscernible epithelium. Invasive growth into the liver and marked inflammatory reaction are typical changes.

A poorly differentiated carcinoma (Figure 8) is made up of highly atypical distorted tubuli and acini. The cells show great variation in size, and are sometimes arranged in a disorderly fashion, without forming clear-cut glandular structures.

Undifferentiated (anaplastic) carcinoma (Figure 9) does not show any distinguishable structures like tubuli or glands. The highly polymorphic and atypical cells have abundant clear cytoplasm and frequently hyperchromatic nuclei at the periphery of the cell body. Mitotic figures are rather frequent. The amount of stroma varies and in any type of carcinoma it can be very extensive and dense.

Infiltrative carcinoma is characterized by predominantly inward tumour growth, into the gallbladder wall or into the liver without exophytic tumour filling the lumen. This is illustrated in Figure 10, in which adenocarcinomatous tissue is seen in the deep parts of the gallbladder wall, while the submucosal layer is intact and the gallbladder epithelium does not show carcinomatous changes. In this case the tumour may originate from the glands in the submucosa.

Another example of a predominantly endophytic tumour is demonstrated in Figure 11; the main part of the tumour is located in the liver, completely replacing the lobe throughout its thickness (Figure 11a) while the surface epithelium shows carcinomatous changes in the form of superficial glandular-papillary growth (Figure 11b).

This type of carcinoma has also been described by Suzuki and Takahashi (1983).

Tumour spread and metastasis. Bain *et al.* (1961) observed frequent vascular invasion and direct spread to the diaphragm, bowel, pancreas and lower thoracic wall. In their material 30% of tumours metastasized to the lymph nodes, liver, peritoneum, gastric wall, diaphragm, lungs and pleura.

Other tumours

When a pellet containing 3-methylcholanthrene (MC) is placed in the gallbladder, a low incidence of connective tissue neoplasms such as fibrosarcomas and angiosarcomas may be observed (Figure 12), in addition to the epithelial tumours.

Tumour-like lesions

The lesion illustrated in Figure 2 is either a purely reactive lesion ('pseudotumour') or an early stage of a papillary adenoma. Another lesion is depicted in Figure 13. On naked-eye examination, the gallbladder looked distended, while the cut surface showed a polycystic lesion filled with a thick mucinous mass. Histologically the lesion consisted of several cystic cavities separated from each other by thin connective tissue septa with round cell infiltrates. The internal surface of these cavities was lined with mucinous epithelium, desquamated in one place and elsewhere forming small projections into the lumen. The epithelial cells had abundant vacuolated finely granular cytoplasm and peripherally located small dark nuclei. The lesion was separated from the liver by a very thin connective tissue with dilated vessels and inflammatory cells. It is not clear whether this lesion is an adenoma with mucoidization or is an example of the so-called cholecystitis glandularis proliferans. However, in the latter lesion thick fibrous bands should be present (Greenblatt, 1982), which were lacking in the above case.

Liver damage. Pronounced congestion, inflammation, necrosis (Figure 14a), proliferation of bile ducts, biliary cysts (Figure 14b) and mild cirrhotic changes are sometimes observed in liver tissue in mice with a pellet of MC implanted into the gallbladder. The severity of liver damage may not be directly correlated with the size or malignancy of the gallbladder tumour. Liver damage is more pronounced in the lobes and areas adjacent to the gallbladder. Large tumours may infiltrate the liver, which however remains otherwise intact. Relatively severe liver lesions may be observed even without any gallbladder tumour, and the degree of liver damage does not depend upon whether the cystic duct was ligated (Bain *et al.*, 1961).

INDUCTION OF TUMOURS AND MODIFYING FACTORS

In the first reported induction of gallbladder tumours in golden hamsters, a single pellet containing 6–8 mg MC was placed in the fundus of the gallbladder after incision (Bain *et al.*, 1959). The incised fundus was then ligated. The first tumour was found as early as 60 days after the operation and five months after the start of the experiment, 8 out of 14 animals sacrificed had gallbladder tumours; the experiment was terminated at eight months when 24 of the total of 39 hamsters had tumours of the gallbladder.

The cystic duct was not ligated in this experiment. It was thought that ligation of the cystic duct might be necessary to prevent excessively rapid dissolution of the pellet. The authors believed that significant intrahepatic changes (necrosis, inflammation, epithelial proliferation and atypia) might have resulted from 'back-diffusion' into the intrahepatic bile channels or gastrointestinal 'feeding' of the carcinogen so that it reached the liver in the portal venous blood. The authors referred to Fortner (1955), who observed liver necrosis and inflammation in two cats in which the cystic duct was left patent. However, in a later experiment of Bain *et al.* (1961), ligation of the cystic duct modified neither the incidence of gallbladder tumours nor the occurrence of hepatic lesions.

Suzuki and Takahashi (1983) inserted a 10 mg pellet containing 50% MC in bees-wax into the gallbladder of hamsters. The animals were killed 145–226 days after the operation and carcinoma of the gallbladder was diagnosed in 25 of 41 animals (61%).

Pellets of beeswax weighing 10 mg and containing 2 or 5 mg MC were implanted into the gallbladder by Gorin and Kruto-vskikh (1988) and Gorin *et al.* (1988). The incidences of gallbladder tumours were 39.3 and 58.3% with pellets containing 2 and 5 mg MC respectively. The tumours were found from 24 to 35 weeks after the operation. In the same experiment, the influence of the estrogen treatment on the induction of gallbladder tumours was also studied. Castrated males with a pellet containing 2 mg MC received weekly subcutaneous injections of 40 mg estradiol dipropionate for 30 weeks. The resulting tumour incidence (77.8%) was higher than in either of the groups with only an MC pellet (see above) and the tumours occurred earlier (Gorin *et al.*, 1988).

A previous attempt to elucidate the role of estrogen by Bain *et al.* (1959) showed no effect of treatment, perhaps because of the very high content of MC in the pellet.

To study the role of chronic non-specific irritation in the induction of gallbladder tumours, Kowalewski and Todd (1971) administered nitrosodiethyl-amine (NDEA) or nitrosodimethylamine (NDMA) with drinking water to hamsters with or without a cholesterol pellet implanted into the gallbladder. Among the hamsters with a cholesterol pellet and receiving NDMA, 68% (13/19) developed a gallbladder carcinoma, while no such tumour was observed in the groups receiving the nitrosamines alone or NDEA in combination with a pellet.

The above experiments indicate that the hamster is a very convenient species for induction of gallbladder tumours, yielding a high incidence with short latency. In addition, they prove the importance of nonspecific irritation and show that estrogens can have a stimu-lating role in the induction of tumours in the gallbladder.

COMPARATIVE ASPECTS

Spontaneous tumours of the gall-bladder are very rare in both domestic and laboratory animals (see also Yoshitomo & Boorman, 1993). Hoch-Ligeti *et al.* (1979) reported a high incidence of the gall-bladder adenocarcinoma in two inbred strains of guinea-pigs; this incidence was increased (in males but not in females) by whole-body gamma or X-irradiation.

Gallbladder carcinoma and gallstones have for a long time been considered linked in some way. This point of view seemed to be supported by the frequent finding of gallstones in patients with primary gallbladder carcinoma, and was the basis for numerous efforts to induce gallbladder cancer in animals, in the hope of elucidating the role of chronic non-specific irritation and chemicals or radio-active materials which might be found in the gallstones.

Lazarus-Barlow (1918) claimed to have found radium in gallstones associated with primary carcinoma of the gallbladder in humans. He inserted stones removed from human gallbladders into the gallbladders of nine rabbits: three as controls and six with radium introduced into them. Proliferative changes with atypia of columnar epithelium which appeared suggestive of carcinoma were found in all rabbits with the radium-containing stones (one of them with liver metastasis).

Various experiments have been per-formed with guinea-pigs. Kazama (1922) claimed to have produced 26 gallbladder carcinomas in 98 guinea-pigs with pebbles placed in their gallbladders, but none of the animals survived for four months. Leitch (1924) introduced soft or solid materials into guinea-pig gallbladders; gallbladder carcinomas (8 in 40 animals) were found only in animals with solid materials, and were, in the author's opinion, induced by mechanical irritation.

An attempt to induce gallbladder carcinoma by placing gallstones from non-cancerous patients into the gallbladders of 47 guinea-pigs was unsuccessful (Burrows, 1932). Equally unsuccessful were efforts to produce gallbladder tumours by placing glass beads, cholesterol pellets and MC–cholesterol pellets in the gallbladders of 32 guinea-pigs (Desforges et al., 1950). Pellets made of beeswax and containing 5% suspension of various substances (MC, calcium carbonate, ground glass, cholesterol) were implanted into the gallbladder of guinea-pigs (in one group MC plus thyroidectomy) but no carcinoma was found despite long survival (132 weeks) (Simmers & Podolak, 1963).

Petrov and Krotkina (1947) introduced various sterile solid materials into guinea-pig gallbladders. In 52 out of 100 animals, hyperplastic lesions were found and in five carcinoma (four with metastasis).

Fortner (1955) placed MC pellets in the gallbladders of dogs and cats. Five of six cats with survival of at least 23 months developed carcinoma of the gallbladder, but no gallbladder tumour was found in dogs treated in the same way.

Sternberg et al. (1960) fed dogs with a miticide, Aramite, containing as the active agents a mixture of isopropyl compounds. 9 of 19 dogs developed carcinoma of the gallbladder.

Experiments on the induction of gallbladder tumours in laboratory animals (mainly guinea-pigs) have not given easily reproducible results. Moreover, many attempts to produce gallbladder tumours failed, even with such a powerful carcinogen as MC and long periods of observation. In contrast, the experiments in hamsters have always given positive results; tumours developed with a high frequency and relatively rapidly (by laboratory standards). The tumours of the gallbladder induced experimentally in the hamster resemble human tumours both morphologically and biologically.

Human gallbladder cancers are more variable than those of the hamster (Ashley, 1978; Christensen & Ishak, 1970; Edmonson, 1967), probably simply because far more human tumours have been examined. Adenosquamous and squamous cell carcinomas are regularly observed in humans but have not yet been described in the hamster. The local spread and remote metastasis of gallbladder cancers in hamsters are also rather similar to those in man.

ACKNOWLEDGEMENT

The excellent technical assistance of Mrs Tamara G. Zabanova is highly appreciated by the authors.

REFERENCES

Ashley, D.J.B. (1978) Epithelial tumours of the gall bladder and extra-hepatic bile ducts. In: *Evans' Histological Appearances of Tumours*, 3rd edition, Edinburgh, Churchill Livingstone, pp. 603–610

Bain, G.O., Allen, P.B.R., Silbermann, O. & Kowalewski, K. (1959) Induction in hamsters of biliary carcinoma by intracholecystic methylcholanthrene pellets. *Cancer Res.*, 19, 93–96

Bain, G.O., Gort, J., Pawluk, W., Retzer, O., Husain, S. & Kowalewski, K. (1961) Further observations on methylcholanthrene induced carcinoma of gallbladder in golden hamsters. *Acta Gastro-Enterol. Belg.*, 24, 125–130

Burrows, H. (1932–33) An experimental inquiry into the association between gallstones and primary cancer of the gallbladder. *Br. J. Surg.*, 20, 607–629

Christensen, A.H. & Ishak, K.G. (1970) Benign tumors and pseudotumors of the gallbladder. *Arch. Pathol.*, 90, 423–432

Desforges, G., Desforges, J. & Robbins, S.L. (1950) Carcinoma of the gallbladder: an attempt at experimental production. *Cancer*, 3, 1088–1096

Edmondson, H.A. (1967) *Tumors of the Gallbladder and Extrahepatic Bile Ducts*, Washington, D.C., Armed Forces Institute of Pathology

Fortner, J.G. (1955) The experimental induction of primary carcinoma of the gallbladder. *Cancer*, 8, 689–700

Gorin, B.Ya. & Krutovskikh, V.A. (1988) Method of gallbladder carcinoma induction in Syrian hamsters [in Russian]. *Exp. Oncol. (Kiev)*, 10 (6), 76–77

Gorin, B.Ya., Turusov, V.S. & Parfenov, Yu.D. (1988) The influence of castration and estradiol dipropionate on methylcholanthrene-induced carcinogenesis in the gallbladder of male hamsters (in Russian). *Vopr. Oncol.*, 34 (10), 1232–1235

Greenblat, M. (1982) Tumours of the liver. In: Turusov, V.S., ed., *Pathology of Tumours in Laboratory Animals*. Vol. III, *Tumours of the Hamster* (IARC Scientific Publications No. 34), Lyon, IARC, pp. 69–102

Hoch-Ligeti, C., Congdon, C.C., Deringer, M.K. & Stewart, H.L. (1979) Adenocarcinoma of the gallbladder in guinea pigs. *J. Natl. Cancer Inst.*, 62, 381–386

Kazama, Y. (1922) Studies on the artificial production of tumors in viscera. *Jap. Med. World*, 2, 309–312

Kowalewski, K. & Todd, E.F. (1971) Carcinoma of the gallbladder induced in hamsters insertion of cholesterol pellets and feeding dimethylnitrosamine. *Proc. Soc. Exp. Biol. Med.*, 136, 482–486

Lazarus-Barlow, W.S. (1918) An attempt at the experimental production of a carcinoma by means of radium. *Proc. Roy. Soc. Med.*, 11, 1–17

Leitch, A. (1924) Gallstones and cancer of the gallbladder: an experimental study. *Br. Med. J.*, 2, 451–454

Petrov, N.N. & Krotkina, N.A. (1947) Experimental carcinoma of the gallbladder. *Ann. Surg.*, 125, 241–248

Simmers, M.H. & Podolak, E. (1963) Effect of simulated gallstones on guinea pig gallbladders. *Arch. Surg.*, 87, 583–589

Sternberg, S.S., Popper, H., Oser, B.L. & Oser, M. (1960) Gallbladder and bile duct adenocarcinomas in dogs after long term feeding of Aramite. *Cancer*, 13, 780–789

Suzuki, A. & Takahashi, T. (1983) Histogenesis of the gallbladder carcinoma induced by methylcholanthrene beeswax pellets in hamsters. *Jap. J. Surg.*, 13, 55–59

Yoshitomo, K. & Boorman, G.A. (1994) Tumours of the gallbladder. In: Turusov, V.S. & Mohr, U., eds, *Pathology of Tumours in Laboratory Animals*, Vol. 2, *Tumours of the Mouse*, 2nd edition (IARC Scientific Publications No. 111), Lyon, IARC, pp. 271–279

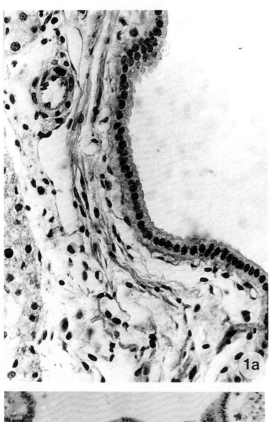

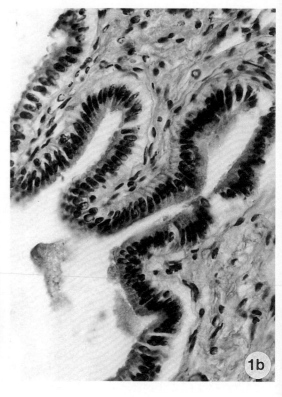

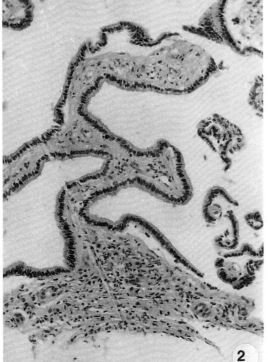

Figure 1. Normal gallbladder. H & E

(a) Gallbladder distended with formalin. Cubical to columnar epithelium. × 500

(b) Mucous membrane forms irregular folds in the non-distended gallbladder. × 600

Figure 2. Highly benign papillomatous lesion consisting of connective tissue stalks covered with a normal-looking epithelium. H & E; × 220

Figure 3. Papillary adenoma. H & E

(a) General view. Adenoma consisting of branching and anastomosing papillae of varying length and thickness. No invasive growth into the liver. × 35

(b) Detail. Rather regular arrangement and rather uniform size of cells covering papillae. Thick layer of fibrous tissue between tumour and liver. × 220

(c) Detail. Although there is a pseudostratification of epithelial cells, their pattern of arrangement is rather orderly. Rare mitosis. × 500

(d) Detail. Tumour cells look dysplastic and show a less regular arrangement than in (b) and (c). There is piling up of nuclei of various sizes, some of them normochromatic, others hyperchromatic, and mitosis is seen. Epithelial cells vary from cuboidal to very tall columnar × 600

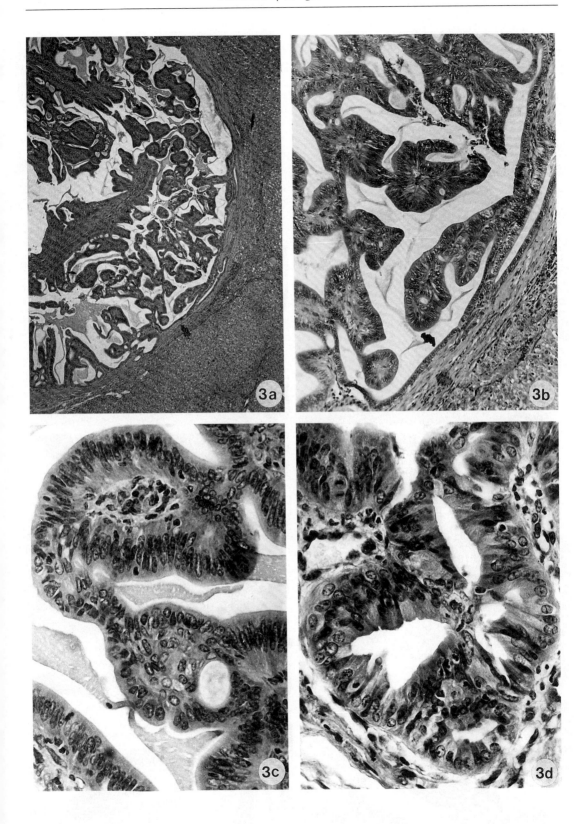

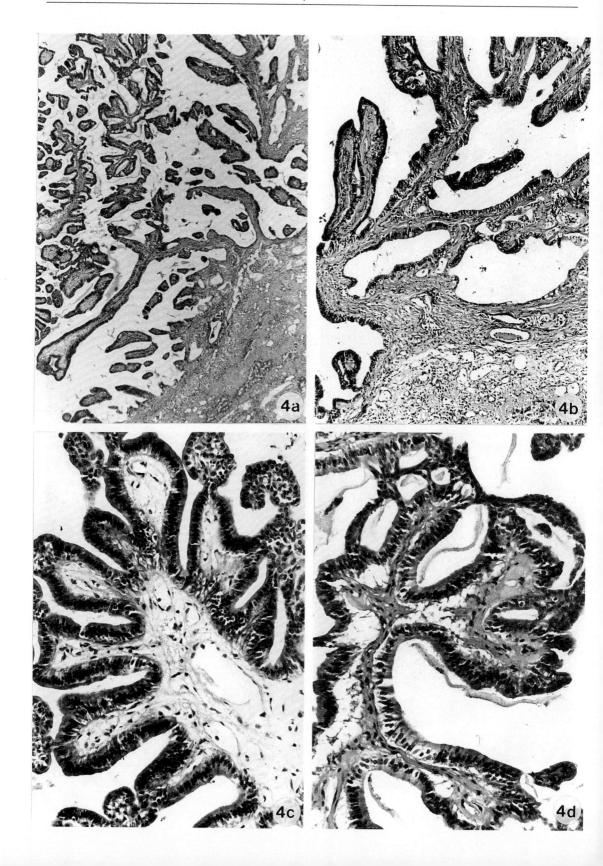

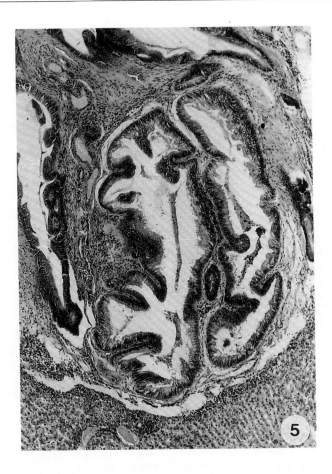

Figure 4. Intravesicular papillary tumour with signs of invasive growth. H & E

(a) General view. Numerous branching papillae. Clear-cut border with the liver is absent. × 35

(b) Detail. The epithelium lining papillae and glands is partly thickened, in other places atrophied. Connective tissue at the border with the liver contains many vessels and small ductules. This area might be considered as showing an invasive growth into the gallbladder wall. × 90

(c,d) Details. Different types of papillae and finger-like projections with loose fibrovascular stalk. Epithelium covering the papilla retains an orderly arrangement in most areas. × 220

Figure 5. Adenomatous tumour that consists of cavities lined with a tall epithelium and separated by connective tissue. A few short fibrous papillae protrude into the cavities. Epithelium is very tall columnar. H & E; × 90

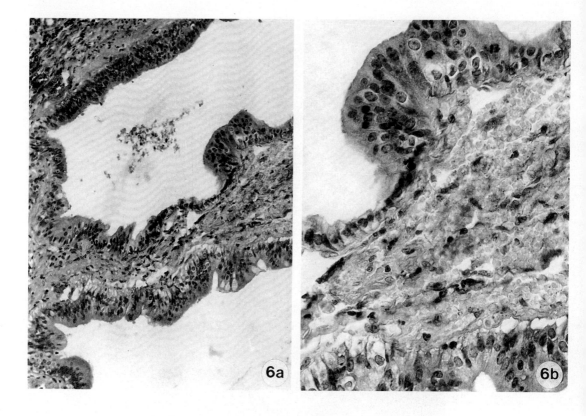

Figure 6. Part of the lesion with a thick fibrous stalk protruding into the lumen of the gallbladder

(a) Hyperplastic and unevenly thickened epithelium. H & E; × 220

(b) Detail. Moderate dysplasia of the epithelium with mitosis. H & E; × 500

Figure 7. Highly differentiated adenocarcinoma. H & E

(a) Tumour invading the liver. Massive necrosis of tumour tissue. × 35

(b) Part of the tumour at the border with the liver. Well differentiated glands and marked inflammatory reaction. × 220

(c) Tumour glands of various sizes and forms lined with normal-looking cubical epithelium and filled with mucus or cell debris. × 200

(d) This part of the tumour is formed of glands cystically dilated, with flattened atrophied epithelium, in the abundant oedematous stroma. × 220

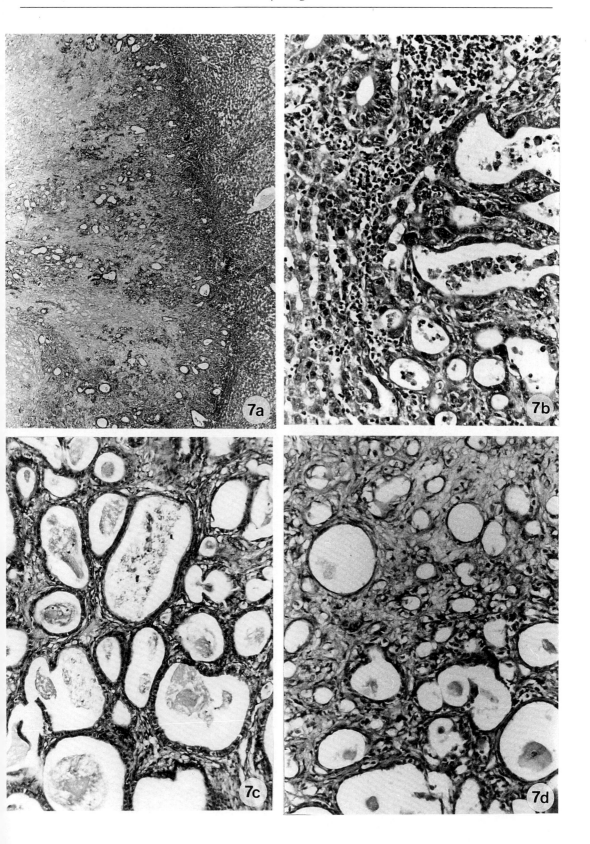

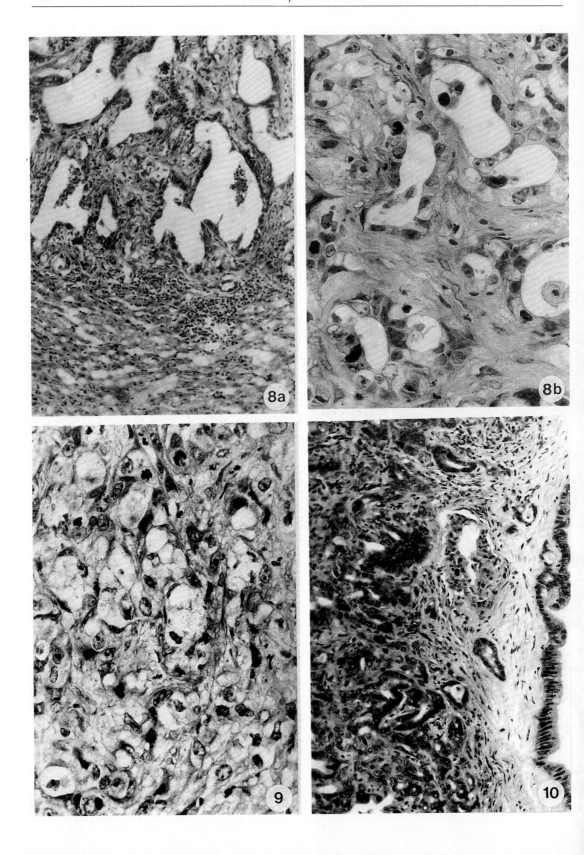

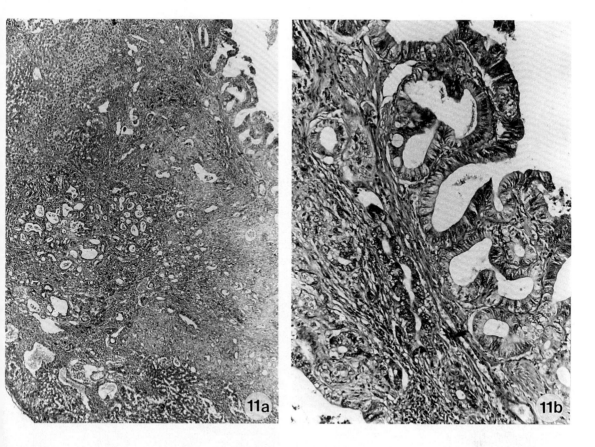

Figure 8. Poorly differentiated adenocarcinoma. H & E

(a) General view. Tumour is formed of highly atypical glandular elements. Invasive growth into the liver. × 220

(b) Glandular elements of varying size and shape; cells are highly atypical, with abundant stroma. × 500

Figure 9. Anaplastic tumour with mucoidization of highly atypical tumour cells. H & E; × 500

Figure 10. Tumour infiltrating the deep parts of the gallbladder wall; the submucosal layer is almost deprived of tumorous elements. The gallbladder epithelium in this section does not show obvious carcinomatous changes H & E; × 220

Figure 11. Predominantly endophytic tumour; (a) Highly differentiated adenocarcinoma penetrating throughout the thickness of the liver lobe. Papillomatous changes in the gallbladder epithelium (top right). H & E; × 35

(b) Detail of Figure 11a. Carcinomatous changes in the epithelium in the form of superficial glandular-papillary growth with pronounced cell and structural atypia. H & E; × 220

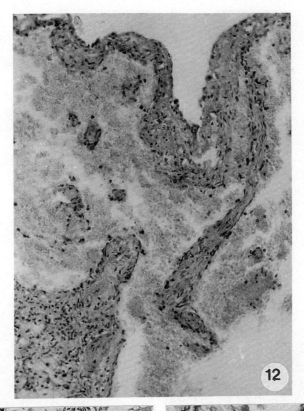

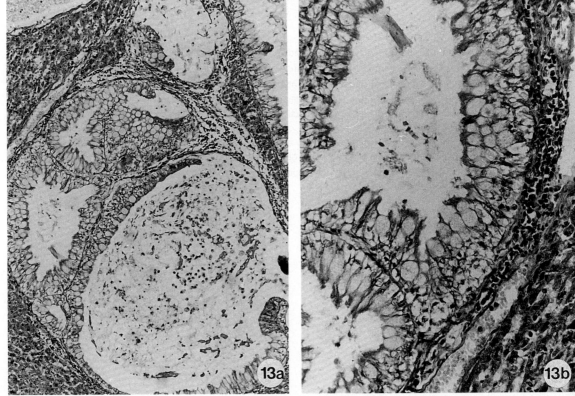

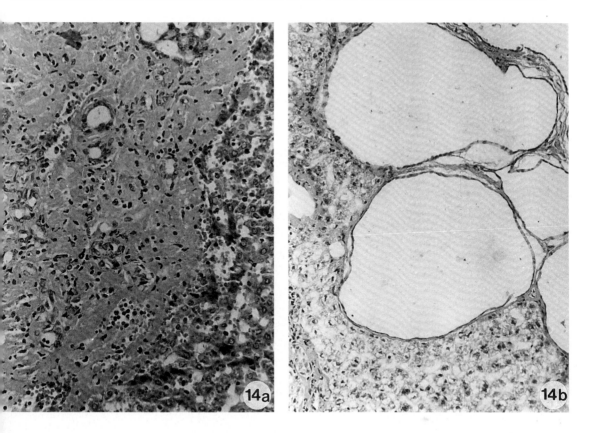

Figure 12. Angiosarcoma; macroscopically this was a small haemorrhagic nodule in the gallbladder wall. H & E; × 220

Figure 13. Mucinous lesion of the gallbladder.

(a) General view: cysts separated by thin connective tissue septa and filled with mucus and cell debris. H & E; × 90

(b) Detail. Mucinous pseudostratified epithelium, dilated vessels and inflammatory cells at the border with the liver. H & E; × 220

Figure 14. Non-tumorous liver lesions in a mouse with a methylcholanthrene pellet in the gallbladder.
H & E; × 220

(a) Necrosis of liver tissue and proliferating bile ductules at distance from the gallbladder tumour.

(b) Biliary cysts with a flattened epithelium.

Tumours of the glandular stomach

M. Takahashi and H. Okamiya

Although suitable animal models for the induction of adenocarcinoma in the glandu-lar stomachs of rats and dogs with N-methyl-N'-nitro-N-nitrosoguani-dine (MNNG) are well established, experimental production of tumours in the glandular stomach of hamsters has been only rarely reported. One reason is the complication of high sarcoma inci-dences.

NORMAL STRUCTURE

The glandular stomach in the hamster, which is separated from the forestomach by a distinct border called the limiting ridge, is divided into the fundus and pylorus and communicates with the duodenum at the pyloric ring. The surface and the glands in the fundic region are lined by four major types of columnar epithelial cells: surface mucous, mucous neck, parietal and chief cells. The pyloric mucosa is covered by foveolar epithelium with the same cellular characteristics as those of surface mucous cells in the fundic region. In addition, a fifth entero-endocrine class of cells, which are stained by methods using heavy metal salts such as chromium, silver or osmium, is present in the glands of the stomach. Fewer of these argentaffin cells are found in the fundic region of the hamster than in the rat or the rabbit (Bivin *et al.*, 1987).

MORPHOLOGY AND BIOLOGY OF TUMOURS

Histological types of tumour

Epithelial tumours
   Adenoma/adenomatous hyperplasia
   Adenocarcinoma

Non-epithelial tumours
   Fibroma
   Fibrosarcoma (spindle cell sarcoma)
   Leiomyoma
   Leiomyosarcoma

Adenoma and adenomatous hyperplasia
   Macroscopically, the adenoma is a polypoid or diverticulum-like, sharply circumscribed alteration. Adenomatous polyps are grossly observed as plaque-like or nodular lesions covered by glandular epithelium with a smooth and glossy or ulcerated surface. They often present as white or translucent nodules of various sizes, in some cases appearing as well demarcated thickenings of the mucosa accompanied by polypoid structures on the surface. The mucosal thickening is mainly due to hyperplasia of foveolar epithelial cells. Adenomatous diverticuli, in communication with the lumen, consist of various sized submucosal nodules causing thickening of the wall. They occur predominantly in the pyloric antrum.

127

Each macroscopic type of adenoma demonstrates different histological patterns (Figures 1–5). Adenomatous polyps are confined primarily to the mucosa, while in adenomatous diverticula there is prominent downward growth into the wall. Glandular cells in adenomatous polyps are mostly hyperchromatic and have cuboidal and/or columnar morphology. They are arranged to form acini and branching tubules of various sizes and shapes, independent of whether the lesion is sessile or pedunculated. At the bases of these polypoid or nodular lesions, downgrowths of neoplastic cells may form acini, branching tubules or cysts. The acini, tubules and cysts are usually lined by a single layer of neoplastic cells.

Adenomatous diverticulum lesions display more or less dilated regular glands arrayed in a honeycomb pattern. Cells are well differentiated or slightly atypical. The cyst lumens contain mucus, inflammatory exudate or necrotic debris. The tumour is frequently isolated from its surroundings by fibrous inflammatory glandular tissue which never grows beyond the stomach wall. The stroma of an adenomatous diverticulum contains fibrous connective tissue and sometimes osteoid tissue.

Adenomatous hyperplasias of the glandular stomach usually occupy only a relatively small area of the pyloric mucosa, involving a small number of pits. Cytological features are similar to those of adenomas, a well organized glandular pattern being retained with only slight cellular atypia. No infiltrative growth can be observed. Hyperplasia of foveolar epithelium and mucous cells is common in regenerative mucosa or healed ulceration and it is sometimes difficult to distinguish between hyperplastic changes and adenomas because of transitional features. However, the distribution of cell types composing the gastric mucosa may be helpful. The normal arrangement of the foveolar and mucous cells is lost in adenomas.

The role of adenomatous hyperplasia in the development of particular epithelial tumours including adenomas, is, however, difficult to define. Sometimes, the neoplastic cells seem to arise directly from normal epithelium without a preceding hyperplastic stage. It seems, therefore, that adenomatous hyperplasias, adenomas and adenocarcinomas may be independent lesions in some cases, whereas in others they represent different histogenetic stages in the neoplastic process.

Adenocarcinoma

Most cases of gastric adenocarcinoma arise in the antral region of the glandular stomach in the vicinity of the pylorus. In early stages the tumours appear as round or oval, slightly elevated solitary or multiple lesions 2–4 mm in diameter. Some cases of intramucosal carcinoma with erosion, located at the level of the mucous membrane, have also been observed.

Macroscopically, three different types can be distinguished: umbilicated or ulcerated tumours with irregular elevated margins; flowerbed-like lesions with a central area of depression; hemispherical or polypoid protruding lesions.

Histologically, carcinomas are characterized by atypically branching glands demonstrating infiltration of the submucosa as well as the muscular layer. The glands are lined by cells showing distinctive signs of malignancy, such as hyperchromasia, irregular nuclear shape, increase in nucleus:cytoplasm ratio, and frequent mitotic figures. In the advanced state, neoplastic growths may invade through all coats of the stomach, including the serosa, thus demonstrating unequivocal malignant potential.

The well differentiated type (Figures 6–8) is most frequently characterized by well preserved glandular structures with branching tubular, papillary or cystic patterns. The stroma of these tumours shows various degrees of inflammation.

Metaplastic cartilage and bone formation may also occur.

Poorly differentiated adenocarcinomas demonstrate a loss of glandular structure, the tumour cells being highly variable and polymorphic, forming irregularly arborating cords which may in some focal areas have signet ring cells. Poorly differentiated adenocarcinomas are morphologically of two different types: one with mucinous cells and the other of non-mucinous cell type.

Mucinous adenocarcinoma is a poorly differentiated tumour consisting of extensive mucous masses containing complexes of highly pleomorphic and atypical cancer cells that show no tendency to form glandular structures. Such tumours are therefore distinguishable by the excessive extracellular secretion of mucus into the surrounding tissues.

Signet-ring cell carcinoma is a mucus-secreting tumour with a tendency for intracellular accumulation of mucus which gives the cells a characteristic appearance. Single or small groups of tumour cells are observed randomly arranged between connective tissue strands.

Well differentiated adenocarcinomas rarely give rise to metastases to the lymph nodes and seldom grow into adjacent tissues and therefore care must be taken in differential diagnosis from adenomas. A reliable diagnosis of carcinoma is based on cellular and structural atypia as well as evidence of local invasion. With poorly differentiated adenocarcinomas, invasion of blood and lymph vessels and metastases into regional lymph nodes or other organs are common.

SPONTANEOUS TUMOURS

Tumours of the glandular stomach are rarely observed. Pour *et al.* (1976) reported no spontaneous development of primary neoplasms in two colonies of Syrian hamsters.

Connective tissue tumours (Figures 9–12) of the stomach such as leiomyoma, leiomyosarcoma, angiosarcoma and fibrosarcoma may occur, but are rarely reported. Schmidt *et al.* (1983) reported secondary tumours in the stomach to be all malignant lymphomas.

INDUCTION OF TUMOURS

MNNG is a potent mutagen, which has proved to be a gastric carcinogen after oral administration in the drinking water to rats, hamsters, rabbits and dogs. Adenocarcinomas and spindle cell sarcomas can be produced with high incidence in the glandular stomach of the hamster. As in rats, administration of MNNG at low concentration and for short periods induces stomach cancer (Sugimura *et al.*, 1969; Fujimura *et al.*, 1970). *N*-Ethyl-*N*'-nitro-*N*-nitrosoguanidine has also been found to be an efficient inducer of stomach cancer, particularly in rats, hamsters and dogs (Kawachi *et al.*, 1974).

COMPARATIVE ASPECTS

Gastric polyps and/or adenomas are sometimes present in certain strains of mice spontaneously and in MNNG-treated hamsters, rats and dogs but not in mice. However, a clear relationship between spontaneous lesions and carcinoma development has not been established in any of these species. In hamsters and dogs (Fujita *et al.*, 1974), the mode of induction, course of tumour development, histological type and biological behaviour of gastric adenocarcinomas are similar to those observed in the rat. The histological appearance of rodent tumours is also similar to that of human gastric cancer. In well differentiated human tumours, however, completely differentiated cells do not occur in such high numbers as in the animal tumours. Human tumours also proliferate more readily and usually metastasize with higher frequency. Metastasis to regional lymph nodes or remote organs is rare with induced cancers of the rat or hamster. The reason for this is not yet clear, but it seems that the prominent proliferation of connective tissue in and around the neoplasms observed in rats, but not in man, may be of significance.

Leiomyosarcomas in hamsters resemble those in mice and rats. In man, leiomyosarcomas are rare, comprising about 1% of stomach tumours, and generally attain large size (Ranchod & Kempson, 1977; Shiu *et al.*, 1982) with invasion of the entire stomach wall.

ACKNOWLEDGEMENTS

The author gratefully acknowledges the assistance of Dr M.A. Moore in the preparation of this manuscript.

REFERENCES

Bivin, W.S., Olsen, G.H. & Murray, K.A. (1987) Morphophysiology, III. Digestive system, In: Van Hoosier, G.L. & McPherson, C.W., eds, *Laboratory Hamsters*, Orlando, FL, Academic Press, pp. 12–19

Fujimura, S., Kogure, K., Obashi, S. & Sugimura, T. (1970) Production of tumours in glandular stomach of hamsters by N-methyl-N'-nitro-N-nitrosoguanidine. *Cancer Res.*, 30, 1444–1448

Fujita, M., Taguchi, T., Takami, M., Usugane, M., Takahashi, A. & Shiba, S. (1974) Carcinoma and related lesion in dog stomach induced by oral administration of N-methyl-N'-nitro-N-nitrosoguanidine. *Gann*, 65, 207–214

Kawachi, T., Kogure, K., Tanaka, N., Tokunaga, A., Fujimura, S., Sugimura, T., Kuwubara, N. & Takayama, S. (1974) Induction of tumors in the stomach and duodenum of hamsters by N-ethyl-N'-nitro-N-nitrosoguanidine. *Z. Krebsforsch.*, 81, 29–36

Pour, P., Mohr, U., Cardesa, A., Althoff, J. & Kmoch, N. (1976) Spontaneous tumors and common diseases in two colonies of Syrian hamsters. II. Respiratory tract and digestive system. *J. Natl Cancer Inst.*, 56, 937–948

Ranchod, M. & Kempson, R.L. (1977) Smooth muscle tumors of the gastrointestinal tract and retroperitoneum: a pathologic analysis of 100 cases. *Cancer*, 39, 255–262

Schmidt, R.E., Eason, R.L., Hubbard, G.B., Young, J.T. & Eisenbrandt, D.L. (1983) Alimentary system. In: Schmidt, R.E., ed., *Pathology of Aging Syrian Hamsters*, Boca Raton, FL, CRC Press, pp. 45–66

Shiu, M.H., Farr, G.H., Papachristou, D.N. & Hajdu, S.I. (1982) Myosarcomas of the stomach: natural history, prognostic factors and management. *Cancer*, 49, 177–187

Sugimura, T., Fujimura, S., Kogure,K., Baba, T., Saito, T., Nagao, M., Hosoi, H. & Shimosato, Y. (1969) Production of adenocarcinomas in glandular stomach of experimental animals by N-methyl-N'-nitro-N-nitroso-guanidine. *Gann Monogr. Cancer Res.*, 8, 157–196

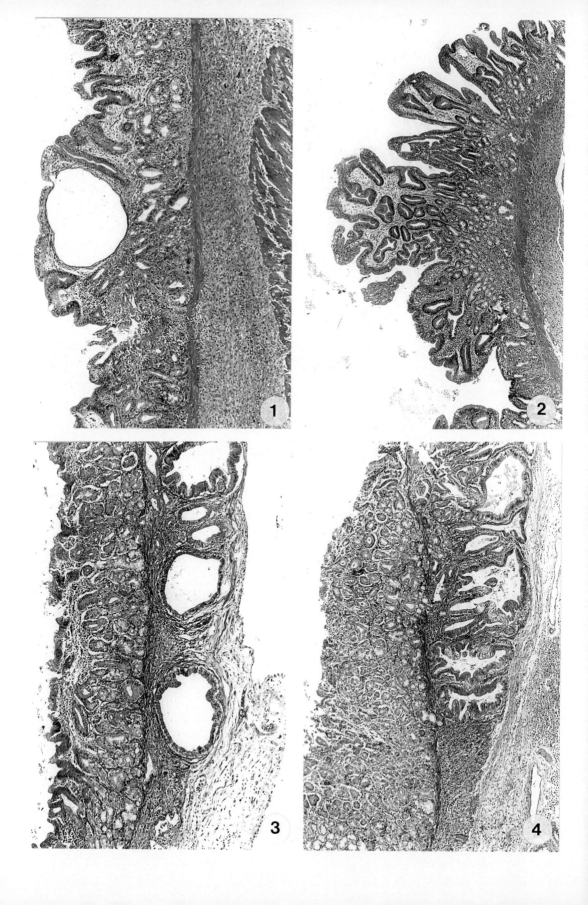

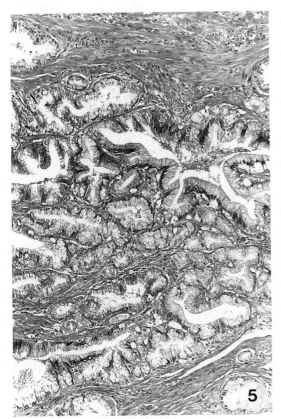
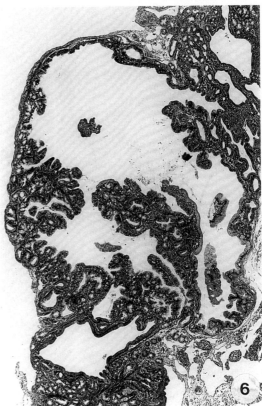

Figure 1. Adenomatous hyperplasia of the glandular stomach. Sessile growth pattern with a large cyst. H & E; × 60

Figure 2. Adenomatous hyperplasia of the glandular stomach. Exophytic growth pattern with papillary projection. H & E; × 60

Figure 3. Adenomatous diverticulum of the glandular stomach. There is prominent downgrowth into the submucosal layer. H & E; × 60

Figure 4. Adenomatous diverticulum of the glandular stomach. Cystically dilated glands are evident in the submucosal layer. H & E; × 60

Figure 5. Higher magnification of Figure 4. The lining columnar cells are tall and vacuolated without atypia; × 120

Figure 6. Well differentiated adenocarcinoma of the glandular stomach. Papillary growth into a cystic gland. H & E ; × 30

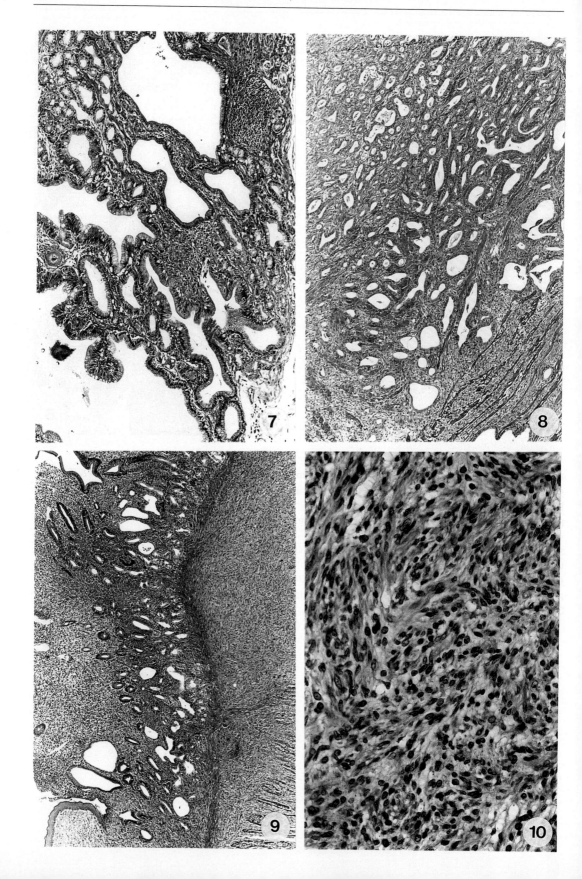

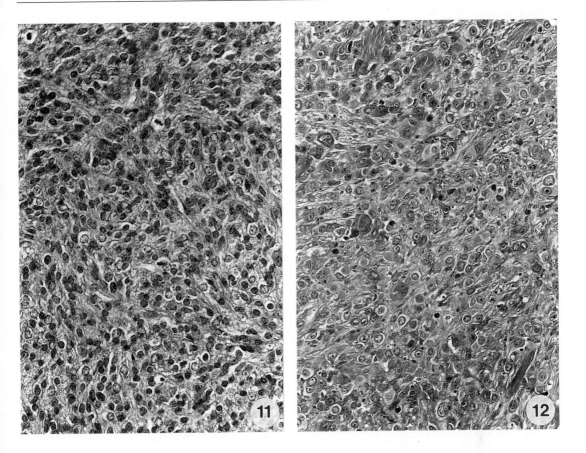

Figure 7. Higher magnification of Figure 6. The glands consist of surface epithelium and pyloric gland type cells. × 75

Figure 8. Well differentiated tubular adenocarcinoma of the glandular stomach. H & E. × 50

Figure 9. Leiomyosarcoma of the stomach. Tumour cells have invaded into the lamina propria mucosa. H & E. × 40

Figure 10. Higher magnification of Figure 9. The tumour is composed of elongated fusiform cells with eosinophilic cytoplasm. × 300

Figure 11. Undifferentiated sarcoma of the stomach, probably originating from smooth muscle cells (leiomyosarcoma). H & E ; × 300

Figure 12. Undifferentiated sarcoma. The tumour cells show marked atypia and pleomorphism. Several mitotic figures are also seen. H & E; × 150

Tumours of the intestine

M. Takahashi and H. Okamiya

Intestinal cancer can be induced in rats, mice and hamsters by indirect-acting chemical carcinogens related to either 3,2-dimethyl-4-aminobiphenyl (DMAB) or 1,2-dimethylhydrazine (DMH). Such experimental studies have aroused considerable interest because of their potential relevance to the role of environmental carcinogens and co-carcinogens in the pathogenesis of human bowel cancer. Most studies have, however, used rats and mice, and only a few reports have been published concerning hamsters (Emminger & Mohr, 1982).

NORMAL STRUCTURE

The small intestine is divided into three parts: duodenum, jejunum and ileum. The duodenum runs laterally and slightly caudally towards the right before turning to run caudally as the descending duodenal loop and making a reverse turn to the left to become the ascending duodenal loop. The jejunum is about 2.5 times the length of the duodenum and forms a number of small looplets. The ileum is short (<2 cm), continuous with the jejunum and leads into the caecum.

The caecum is slightly sacculated and divided into apical and basal portions. A groove in the external caecal wall corresponds to the location of a semilunar valve delineating the division between the two portions. There are four valves at the ileo-caecal–colic junctions. The ascending colon moves cranially along the right side of the abdominal cavity, crosses to the left side of the dorsal abdomen as the transverse colon and then turns caudally to become the descending colon before emptying through the rectum and anus.

As in other parts of the gastrointestinal tract, the wall of the intestine is made up of four layers – the mucosa, the submucosa, the muscularis and the serosa. The mucosa is covered by a simple columnar epithelium in which three types of cell can be distinguished: absorptive cells, goblet cells and endocrine cells (argentaffin cells). Absorptive cells are columnar in form and have ovoid nuclei stained in the lower part of the cells. The goblet cells are found irregularly scattered among the absorptive cells, their apical regions being distended with mucigen droplets. The basal nuclei tend to be flattened and the surrounding cytoplasm strongly basophilic. Enteroendocrine cells are single and widely scattered throughout the epithelial lining of the gastrointestinal tract. They are common in the duodenum and are sparser in the jejunum and ileum. They occur both on the villi and in the crypts. These cells are also present in limited numbers throughout the colon. In addition to the cell types already described, a further type of cell occurs in small groups only in the depths of the crypts of Lieberkuhn – the Paneth cells. These are pyramidal in form, with a round or oval nucleus situated near the base, and conspicuous secretory granules in the apical cytoplasm.

In the proximal duodenum, the submucosa is largely occupied by the Brunner's glands, whose terminal secretory portions consist of richly branched and coiled tubules arranged in lobules.

In the mucosa of the large intestine, the goblet cells are the most conspicuous element, the majority of the cells in the middle and upper portions of the crypts being of columnar absorptive type.

MORPHOLOGY AND BIOLOGY OF TUMOURS

Histological types of tumour

Epithelial tumours
    Adenoma
    Intramucosal carcinoma
    Adenocarcinoma
        Well differentiated
        Moderately differentiated
        Poorly differentiated

Non-epithelial tumours
    Leiomyoma
    Leiomyosarcoma
    Fibrosarcoma
    Haemangioendothelioma
    Spindle cell sarcoma

Intestinal lesions in the hamster are usually well differentiated tumours demonstrating glandular or cystic glandular patterns and mucus production; most arise in the colon, but they can be found in the small bowel as well.

Adenoma

Adenomas are usually papillary and of polypoid appearance with attachment to the mucosal surface by a thin fibrovascular stalk. The epithelium is thrown up into folds and is hypercellular with enlarged epithelial cells having increased basophilia. Mucus production may or may not be present. Adenomas show limitation of cellular proliferation to the area above the basement membrane.

Intramucosal carcinomas

These tumours (Figures 1 and 2) are characterized by epithelial crypts and tubules showing changes typical of well or moderately differentiated adenocarcinomas. However, step serial sectioning through individual tumours does not reveal invasion by the epithelial elements into the muscularis mucosa or beyond. The stroma of these tumours does not differ from that of invasive tumours with regard to inflammatory infiltrate.

Adenocarcinoma

Malignant lesions have more downward growth of epithelium into the stroma and out into the epithelium surrounding the polyp. Metastasis usually occurs first to regional mesenteric lymph nodes. Intestinal neoplasms have been reported as responsible for significant morbidity and mortality in hamsters (Pour *et al.*, 1976; Fortner, 1961).

Tumours with microscopically well formed glandular structures have been subclassified into well differentiated (Figures 3–10) and moderately differentiated (Figures 11 and 12) adenocarcinomas, on the basis of the degree of architectural and cytological abnormality expressed. They are characterized by epithelial crypts and tubules which differ from normal in their complex and irregular branching and dilatation. The regular pattern of grooves and crypts is replaced by an irregular system of clefts and abnormal, multiple crypt openings, which are often unevenly distributed and reduced in number. Goblet cells are reduced or absent and the absorptive cells are more numerous than normal and show layering and overlapping of nuclei. There is considerable variation in cell size and shape, with the epithelial cells being generally taller than normal but flattened or cuboidal in some areas. The cytoplasm of these cells is amphophilic and the nuclei are pleomorphic, hyperchromatic and generally larger than normal. Mitoses are scattered throughout the abnormal epithelium. With regard to histological features observed in the stroma of these tumours, most show an increase in inflammatory cells compared with the normal lamina propria but the increase is variable, both in quantity and in the ratio of polymorphonuclear to mononuclear cells. Many of these tumours show a variable degree of stromal fibrosis.

Poorly differentiated adenocarcinomas are characterized by epithelial cells lacking uniform arrangement into crypts and tubules. Small irregular cysts or tubular structures are lined by a single layer of very pleomorphic epithelial cells with hyperchromatic nuclei, variable but reduced numbers of microvilli, and either amphophilic or vacuolated cytoplasm. The basal lamina of these structures may sometimes be poorly defined or incomplete. Occasional tubules resembling those seen in well or moderately differentiated adenocarcinomas are often present at the junction of these tumours with the surrounding mucosa. The bulk of these lesions, however, consist of masses of cells arranged as cords and clumps, or as isolated cells embedded in connective tissue. Individual tumour cells show marked variation in size and shape and contain pleomorphic, hyperchromatic nuclei which are generally larger than normal. The cytoplasm of some is amphophilic and homogeneous, but in most it contains accumulations of PAS-positive material. In many cells of the latter type, mucus occupies most of the cytoplasm and the nucleus is eccentric, giving a 'signet ring' appearance. Mitotic cells are scattered throughout these tumours, but are harder to identify than in well or moderately differentiated adenocarcinomas because of the difficulty in distinguishing epithelial from stromal cells. As in well or moderately differentiated tumours, microvilli are fewer than normal. The lateral cell borders in poorly differentiated lesions are less convoluted and junction specializations are less frequent.

An additional feature observed in one third of these tumours is the presence of collections of extracellular PAS-positive material forming mucus lakes containing clumps or cords of tumour cells and closely resembling the so-called 'colloid carcinoma' seen in the human colon. The stroma of poorly differentiated tumours does not differ from that typical for cases of well or moderately differentiated adenocarcinomas.

Non-epithelial tumours

Connective tissue tumours or sarcomas may arise from the mesenchymal elements of the intestinal tract. Fibrosarcoma, leiomyosarcoma and haemangioendothelioma are the types of neoplastic lesion most frequently observed, but rhabdomyosarcomas and malignant lymphomas may also be very occasionally seen. In some cases it is not possible to make a definitive diagnosis because of a lack of clear differentiative characters of the tumour cells.

SPONTANEOUS TUMOURS

Considerable variability in incidence of tumours of the hamster digestive tract is encountered in the literature. This is the case in reports from a range of authors as well as in publications emanating from different colonies studied by the same investigator. Van Hoosier and Trentin (1979) reported numerous polyps of the intestine and squamous papillomas of the forestomach among benign lesions and noted that adenocarcinomas of the bowel were the most common malignancy observed. The caecum and colon were the usual sites for these lesions. These findings were mirrored in the Hannover colony surveyed by Pour *et al.* (1976), with a 23% incidence of gastrointestinal neoplasms; this contrasted with the observation by the same authors of a 7% incidence in the

Eppley colony. These figures also included liver and gallbladder tumours. Although adenocarcinoma of the intestine was diagnosed in 1.0% of the animals, the primary site was not always identified, the diagnosis being made on the basis of metastatic lesions. Secondary tumour growth involving the intestine was found to be due to malignant lymphomas (Schmidt *et al.*, 1983).

Fabry (1985) reported that small intestinal adenocarcinomas occurred in 0.8% of hamsters used as controls in carcinogen bioassays, indicating the incidence of intestinal tumours to be greater and more variable than that in the mouse or rat.

About 13% of reported spontaneous gastrointestinal tumours demonstrated malignant characteristics (Kirkman *et al.*, 1968). Hamsters, however, have a high incidence of proliferative enteritis, which morphologically can easily be confused with malignant neoplasia. The prevalence of true intestinal adenocarcinomas is therefore almost certainly lower than recorded in some of the earlier literature (see Strandberg, 1987).

Connective tissue tumours of the digestive system have been reported to arise at low frequencies; most of those encountered have been malignancies of one of the native connective tissue elements of the tract. Thus small numbers of leiomyosarcomas, angiosarcomas, liposarcomas and fibrosarcomas have been described, most commonly in the cheek pouches and intestines. Tumours composed of 'granular cells' in the intestinal walls of white hamsters have been described by Pour and co-workers (1973).

INDUCTION OF TUMOURS

In 1961, Della Porta noticed that experimental protocols chosen in order to obtain mammary and ovarian tumours were associated with high incidences of inflammatory changes in the intestines with hyperplastic and atypical glands in 3-methylcholanthrene-treated and control hamsters. In the treated animals, adenocarcinomas of the small and large intestines and squamous cell tumours of the forestomach were induced. Similar observations were also discussed in a review by Shubik *et al.* (1960).

Shubik *et al.* reported papillomas of the forestomach and adenomatous polyps of the colon in hamsters fed a diet containing 0.04% 2-acetylaminofluorene for 26 to 40 weeks (Della Porta *et al.*, 1959) or a 0.1% dietary *o*-amino-azotoluene supplement for 49 weeks (Tomatis *et al.*, 1961). Toth *et al.* (1961) also observed papillomas and carcinomas of the forestomach and adenomatous polyps of the caecum in hamsters ingesting 0.2 and 0.4% urethane in their drinking water for more than 40 weeks. However, as similar tumours have occasionally been observed in untreated animals, the significance of these observations remains unclear.

Lijinsky *et al.* (1987) reported on the carcinogenic effects of three nitrosamines, nitrosodimethylamine, nitrosodiethylamine and nitrosomethylethylamine, and two azoxyalkanes, azoxymethane and azoxyethane, in rats and Syrian golden hamsters. The results showed that azoxymethane induced tumours of the colon in hamsters and nitrosodiethylamine and azoxyethane were less potent carcinogens than the corresponding methyl compounds, nitrosodimethylamine and azoxymethane.

Two types of chemicals have been used to induce adenocarcinomas in the intestine of rodents as models for the human disease (Newberne & Rogers, 1985). One type is a direct-acting (complete) carcinogen which requires no metabolic activation, the two members of this group finding particular application being methylnitrosourea (MNU) and *N*-methyl-*N'*-nitro-*N*-nitrosoguanidine. MNU is the more powerful of the two. It can be given as a single dose or a small number of doses, which permits accurate studies of factors that influence tumour development before or after exposure to carcinogen. Direct-acting compounds are useful also to separate factors that influence carcinogen metabolism from factors that influence direct interactions between cellular components and active carcinogenic species.

Carcinogens of the other group require metabolic activation. Examples that are active in the hamster intestine are DMH and its metabolites, azoxymethane and methyl-azoxymethanol, administered as the acetate. Other carcinogens for which the large intestine is one of the target organs have not been widely used. Syrian golden hamsters and certain strains of inbred hamsters develop caecal and colon tumours upon oral intake or gavage of sizable amounts of 3-methylcholanthrene (Della Porta, 1961; Homburger *et al.*, 1972). Mirvish *et al.* (1981) noted that a fraction of administered polycyclic aromatic hydrocarbons was present in the colon and excreted in the faeces.

The aromatic amine carcinogen DMAB produces primarily intestinal cancer in rats (Walpole *et al.*, 1952; Spjut & Spratt, 1965), but in hamsters it causes mainly urinary bladder neoplasms, with development of only a few colon lesions (So & Wynder, 1972). Other aromatic amines that produce intestinal neoplasms in rats have also been found to induce bladder neoplasms in hamsters. For example, 3-methyl-2-naphthylamine (MeNA) is an aromatic amine which produces mammary neoplasms in female rats and intestinal neoplasms in male rats (Weisburger *et al.*, 1967; Hadidian *et al.*, 1968); both DMAB and MeNA were found to produce bladder neoplasms in hamsters following subcutaneous injection. These results suggest that the metabolism of aromatic amines (Miller & Miller, 1969; Weisburger & Weisburger, 1973) in hamsters may differ from that in rats in such a way as to result in greater urinary excretion of carcinogenic metabolites.

COMPARATIVE ASPECTS

Cancer of the colon and rectum, one of the most common visceral cancers in the world, is a major cause of human morbidity and mortality, but little is known about the etiology.

The predominant tumour location in mice is in the distal large bowel (Izumi *et al.*, 1979). DMH-induced colon adenocarcinomas in rats and hamsters are grossly and histologically similar to human colon tumours. A few adenomas have been diagnosed in rats on the basis of histological evidence of benign growth and absence of invasion through the muscularis mucosae. Progression from benign to malignant lesions has been described by Madara *et al.* (1983). Whether this occurs in the hamster remains unclear. However, rodent adenomas do not exactly mimic the human tubular or tubulovillous polyps and the evidence for progression is relatively weak, since malignant tumours are usually found earlier than or at the same time as adenomas (Maskens & Dujardin-Loits, 1981; Madara *et al.*, 1983; Takemiya *et al.*, 1982). The high doses of carcinogen used in most studies may preclude observation of the sequence of dysplasia, adenoma, and carcinoma that appears to occur in development of at least some colon tumours in man.

ACKNOWLEDGEMENTS

The author gratefully acknowledges the assistance of Dr M.A. Moore in the preparation of this manuscript.

REFERENCES

Della Porta, G., Shubik, P. & Scortecci, V. (1959) The action of N-2-fluorenyl-acetamide in Syrian golden hamster. *J. Natl Cancer Inst.*, 22, 463–487

Della Porta, G. (1961) Induction of intestinal, mammary, and ovarian tumors in hamsters with oral administration of 20-methylcholanthrene. *Cancer Res.*, 21, 575–579

Emminger, A. & Mohr, U. (1982) Tumours of the oral cavity, cheek pouch, salivary glands, oesophagus, stomach and intestines. In: Turusov, V.S., ed., *Pathology of Tumours in Laboratory Animals*, Vol. III, *Tumours of the Hamster* (IARC Scientific Publications No. 34), Lyon, IARC, pp. 45–68

Fabry, A. (1985) The incidence of neoplasms in Syrian hamsters with particular emphasis on intestinal neoplasia. *Arch. Toxicol., Suppl.* 8, 124–127

Fortner, J.G. (1961) The influence of castration on spontaneous tumorigenesis in the Syrian (golden) hamster. *Cancer Res.*, 21, 1491–1498

Hadidian, Z., Fredrickson, T.N. & Weisburger, E.K. (1968) Tests for chemical carcinogens. Report on the activity of derivatives of aromatic amines, nitrosamines, quinolines, nitroalkanes, amides, epoxides, aziridines, and purine antimetabolites. *J. Natl Cancer Inst.*, 41, 985–1036

Homburger, F., Hsueh, S.S., Kerr, C.S. & Russfield, A.B. (1972) Inherited susceptibility of inbred strains of Syrian hamsters to induction of subcutaneous sarcomas and mammary and gastro-intestinal carcinomas by subcutaneous and gastric administration of polynuclear hydrocarbons. *Cancer Res.*, 32, 360–366

Izumi, K., Otsuka, H., Furuya, K. & Akagi, A. (1979) Carcinogenicity of 1,2-dimethylhydrazine dihydrochloride in BALB/c mice. Influence of route of administration and dosage. *Virchows Arch. (Pathol. Anat.)*, 384, 263–267

Kirkman, H. & Algard, F.T. (1968) Spontaneous and nonviral-induced neoplasms. In: Hoffman, R.A., Robinson, P.F. & Magalhaes, H., eds, *The Golden Hamster. Its Biology and Use in Medical Research*. Ames, Iowa, Iowa State University Press, pp. 227–240

Lijinsky, W., Kovatch, R.M. & Riggs, C.W. (1987) Carcinogenesis by nitroso-dialkylamines and azoxyalkanes given by gavage to rats and hamsters. *Cancer Res.*, 47, 3968–3972

Madara, J.L., Harte, P., Deasy, J., Ross, D., Lahey, S. & Steel, G. Jr (1983) Evidence for an adenomacarcinoma sequence in dimethylhydrazine-induced neoplasms of rat intestinal epithelium. *Am. J. Pathol.*, 110, 230–235

Maskens, A.P. & Dujardin-Loits, R.M. (1981) Experimental adenomas and carcinomas of the large intestine behave as distinct entities: most carcinomas arise de novo in flat mucosa. *Cancer*, 47, 81–89

Miller, E.C. & Miller, J.A. (1969) Studies on the mechanism of activation of aromatic amines and amide carcinogens to ultimate carcinogenic electrophilic reactants. *Ann. NY Acad. Sci.*, 163, 731–750

Mirvish, S.S., Ghadirian, P., Wallcave, L., Raha, C., Bronczyk, S. & Sams, J.P. (1981) Effect of diet on fecal excretion and gastrointestinal tract distribution of unmetabolized benzo-(a)pyrene and 3-methylcholanthrene when these compounds are administered orally to hamsters. *Cancer Res.*, 41, 2289–2293

Newberne, P.M. & Rogers, A.E. (1985) Adenocarcinoma, colon and rectum, rat. In: Jones, T.C., Mohr, U. & Hunt, R.D., eds, *Digestive System* (Monographs on Pathology of Laboratory Animals), Berlin, Heidelberg, New York, Springer-Verlag, pp. 365–370

Pour, P., Althoff, J. & Cardesa, A. (1973) Granular cells in tumors and in nontumorous tissues. *Arch. Pathol.*, 95, 135–138

Pour, P., Mohr, U., Cardesa, A., Althoff, J. & Kmoch, N. (1976) Spontaneous tumors and common diseases in two colonies of Syrian hamsters. II. Respiratory tract and digestive system. *J. Natl Cancer Inst.*, 56, 937–948

Schmidt, R.E., Eason, R.L., Hubbard, G.B., Young, J.T. & Eisenbrandt, D.L. (1983) Alimentary system. In: Schmidt, R.E., ed., *Pathology of Aging Syrian Hamsters*, Boca Raton, FL, CRC Press, pp. 45–66

Shubik, P., Pietra, G. & Della Porta, G. (1960) Studies of skin carcinogenesis in the Syrian golden hamster. *Cancer Res.*, 20, 100–105

So, B.T. & Wynder, E.L. (1972) Induction of hamster tumors of the urinary bladder by 3,2-dimethyl-4-aminobiphenyl. *J. Natl Cancer Inst.*, 48, 1733–1738

Spjut, H.J. & Spratt, J.R., Jr (1965) Endemic and morphologic similarities existing between spontaneous colonic neoplasms in man and 3,2'-dimethyl-4-amino-biphenyl induced colonic neoplasms in rats. *Ann. Surg.*, 161, 309–324

Strandberg, J.D. (1987) Neoplastic diseases, In: Van Hoosier, G.L. Jr & McPherson, C.W., eds, *Laboratory Hamsters*, Orlando, FL, Academic Press, pp. 157–168

Takemiya, M., Miyayama, H. & Takeuchi, T. (1982) Pathogenesis of 1,2-dimethylhydrazine-induced carcinoma in rat intestine. I. The induction of mucin producing carcinomas in the rat intestine. *Acta Pathol. Jpn.*, 32, 257–264

Tomatis, L., Della Porta, G. & Shubik, P. (1961) Urinary bladder and liver cell tumors induced in hamsters with *o*-aminoazotoluene. *Cancer Res.*, 21, 1513–1517

Toth, B., Tomatis, L. & Shubik, P. (1961) Multipotential carcinogenesis with urethan in the Syrian golden hamster. *Cancer Res.*, 21, 1537–1541

Van Hoosier, G.L., Jr & Trentin, J.J. (1979) Naturally occurring tumors of the Syrian hamster. *Prog. Exp. Tumor Res.*, 23, 1–12

Weisburger, J.H., Mantel, N. & Weisburger, E.K. (1967) New carcinogenic naphthylamine and biphenyl derivatives. *Nature*, 213, 930–931

Weisburger, J.H. & Weisburger, E.K. (1973) Biochemical formation and pharmacological, toxicological and pathological properties of hydroxylamines and hydroxamic acids. *Pharmacol. Rev.*, 25, 1–66

Walpole, A.L., Williams, M.H. & Roberts, D.C. (1952) Carcinogenic action of 4-aminodiphenyl and 3,2'-dimethyl-4-amino-phenyl. *Br. J. Indust. Med.*, 9, 255–263

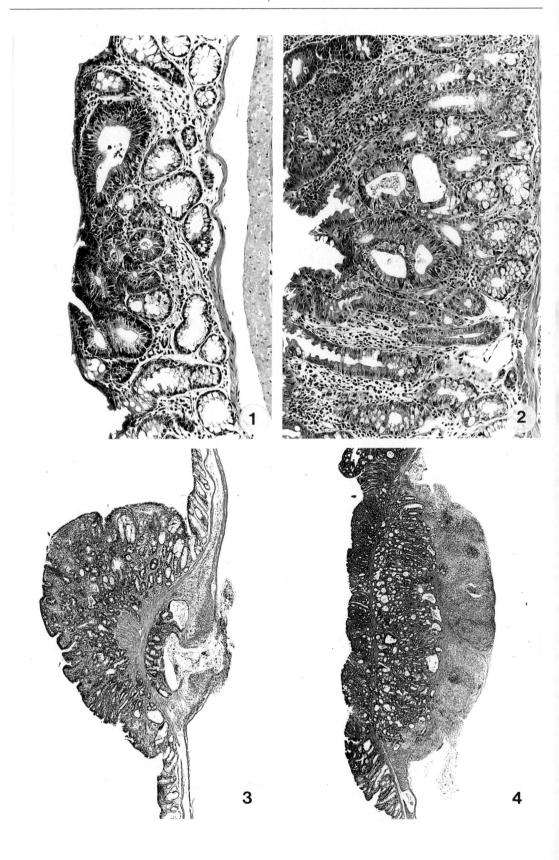

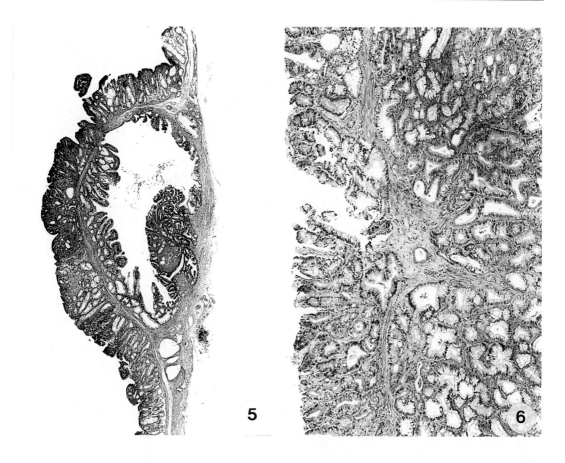

Figure 1. Intramucosal carcinoma of the large intestine. This tumour, composed of markedly dysplastic cells, is probably an early stage of adenocarcinoma. H & E; × 120

Figure 2. Intramucosal carcinoma of the large intestine. Atypical glands are evident. H & E; 120

Figure 3. Well differentiated adenocarcinoma of the large intestine. The polypoid pattern is accompanied with diverticulation through the submucosal layer penetrating to serosa. H & E; × 40

Figure 4. Well differentiated adenocarcinoma of the large intestine. Marked infiltration into the submucosal and muscular layers. H & E; × 40

Figure 5. Well differentiated adenocarcinoma of the large intestine. Cystic diverticulation in the submucosal layer. H & E × 40

Figure 6. Well differentiated adenocarcinoma of the large intestine. Neoplastic glands consist of mucous cells. H & E; × 60

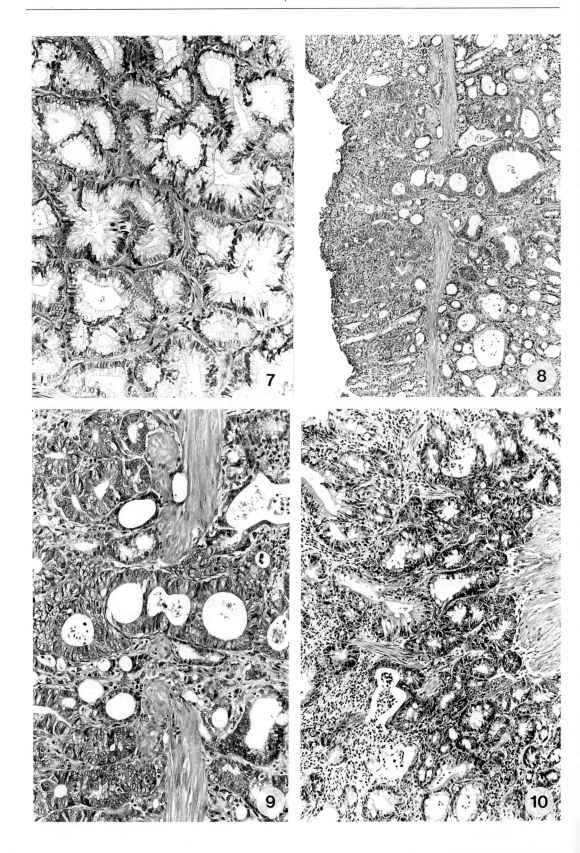

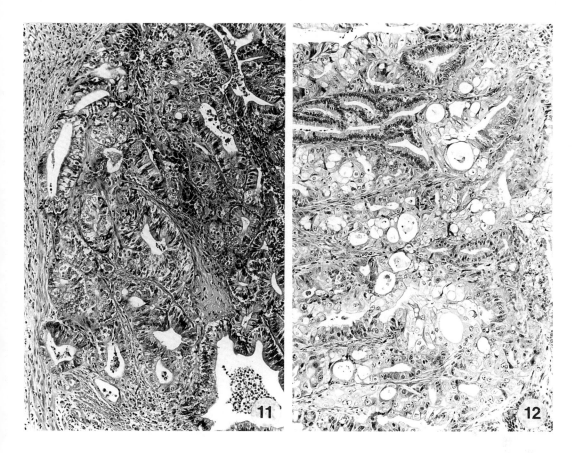

Figure 7. Higher magnification of Figure 6. Frequent mitotic figures with slight atypia can be seen × 150

Figure 8. Well differentiated adenocarcinoma of the large intestine. The tumour cells have invaded the submucosal layer. H & E; × 60

Figure 9. Higher magnification of Figure 8. Dilated glands are lined by atypical epithelial cells. × 150

Figure 10. Well differentiated adenocarcinoma of the large intestine. Some goblet cells can be seen.   H & E ; × 120

Figure 11. Moderately differentiated adenocarcinoma of the large intestine. Note atypical neoplastic glands. Cellular debris can be seen in the lumina. H & E; × 150

Figure 12. Moderately differentiated adenocarcinoma of the large intestine. Some of the glands show small cystic dilatation, while others are tubular with columnar cells. H & E; × 120

Tumours of the pancreas

P.M. POUR AND T. TOMIOKA

NORMAL STRUCTURE

The hamster pancreas is composed of three well defined segments or lobes forming a λ-shaped organ. The short segment, the duodenal lobe, is located medially to the descending duodenum and the two larger shanks extend posteriorly (splenic lobe) and anteriorly (gastric lobe) to the stomach towards the spleen and are connected to each other through a fatty string to the left of the stomach. These three shanks join at the level of the proximal duodenum and form the head of the organ (Figure 1).

Each pancreatic lobe usually has one main duct, except for the gastric lobe, which sometimes presents two main ducts. The duodenal duct enters the common bile duct directly, whereas the gastric and splenic ducts join in the head region to form a common pancreatic duct (Figure 1), which opens into the common bile duct shortly before it enters the duodenum; the common bile duct passes for some distance through the head of the pancreas.

For a description of the arterial and venous blood supply of the hamster pancreas, readers are referred to Takahashi *et al.* (1977a).

The basic histology of the hamster pancreas is similar to that of other animals. The exocrine pancreas is composed of acini and a complex of excretory conduits. The acini are formed by pyramidal or polyhedral acinar cells containing round nuclei in the basal basophilic cytoplasms and eosinophilic zymogen granules in supra-nuclear region (Figure 2a).

The ductal system begins with centroacinar cells which have faint, almost invisible cytoplasm and oval or spindle-shaped hypochromatic nuclei without distinct nucleoli (Figure 2a). Centroacinar cells merge imperceptibly into intercalated (terminal ductular) cells, which have elongated nuclei lying parallel to the axis of the lumen (Figure 2b). These intercalated ductules communicate with interlobular and the peri-insular ductules. The latter often form a circuit around some islets into which several neighbouring intercalated ductules enter.

The cells of the peri-insular ductules are usually small and hardly distinguishable from the alpha cells that populate the peripheral zone of the islet in this species. They can be demonstrated by injection of dye into pancreatic ducts (Figure 3a) or after treatment of hamsters with pancreatic carcinogens that cause hyperplasia of these ductules (Figure 3b). There is no connective tissue between islet and periductular cells, but these two cell types interdigitate (Figure 3c). From the peri-insular ductules, fine, branching (intra-insular) ductules penetrate into the islet (Figure 3a,b). These intra-insular ductules may have a large lumen visible at microscopic and scanning electron microscopic levels (Figure 3d); the presence of cilia in ductular cells distinguishes these ductules from blood vessels. Similar cilia are present in all ductal and ductular cells (Althoff *et al.*, 1976). A single row of flat or low cuboidal cells lines the interlobular (small) ducts (Figure 4). The delicate periductal connective tissue and larger lining cells distinguish these ducts from ductules.

The common pancreatic duct, a collecting conduit of the gastric and splenic lobes, is characterized by its larger lumen (150 μmm), relatively thicker periductal connective tissue and larger cell size; the cells usually lie parallel to the axis of the lumen (Figure 4). There are no mucin-producing cells in any pancreatic ductules and ducts, unlike the common bile duct which has the largest lumen, thickest periductal connective tissue and low cuboidal or cylindric mucin-producing epithelial cells (Figure 5).

MORPHOLOGY AND BIOLOGY OF TUMOURS

Grossly, adenomas present as small (<1–2 mm in diameter) cystic glistening lesions. Carcinomas exhibit either solid cystic patterns or present grey nodules of up to 30 mm diameter (Figure 6). These nodules, upon sectioning, sometimes show dull or glistening surface cystic areas. Necrosis and haemorrhage may be present in large tumours.

Tumours may occur in any pancreatic segment. However, the tail of the splenic lobe is the commonest area, partly because of the larger size of this segment, compared to other pancreatic lobes in this species (Takahashi *et al.*, 1977a,b). Once the tumour reaches a critical size (usually 10 mm in diameter), it breaks into the surrounding tissues and invades rapidly. The perineural lymphatic and the parapancreatic lymph nodes are the primary invasion sites. Later, tumours saturate the neighbouring tissues such as the spleen, stomach, duodenum, kidneys, peritoneum and pelvic cavity. Liver involvement, in most cases, is by continuous growth and only occasionally *via* blood circulation. Distant metastases to other organs, such the lungs, are uncommon.

There is no sex difference in the incidence, pattern and localization of tumours.

Weight loss, diarrhoea, ascites and, in some cases, vascular thrombosis are observed in hamsters bearing large or multiple small cancers. Jaundice occurs occasionally in hamsters with tumours from, or around, the common pancreatic duct or common duct obstructing the lumen. The particular relationship between the common duct and common pancreatic ducts in this species and the relatively low incidence of tumours in the head region of the pancreas could explain the rare occurrence of obstructive jaundice in hamsters.

Histological types of tumour

Microscopically, induced tumours present a wide spectrum of histological patterns. The evaluation of over 10 000 induced pancreatic lesions, and especially sequential studies on animals during tumorigenesis, led us to propose the following classification of hamster tumours. This classification uses the terminology and histopathology of human pancreatic tumours (Cubilla & Fitzgerald, 1984) as far as possible. This classification is based purely on histological appearance of tumours and, therefore, differs from the recent classification of human pancreatic tumours (Pour *et al.*, 1994), which is based on biological behavior of tumours).

I. *Duct-ductular lesions*
A. *Adenomas*
    a) serous (micro)cystic adenoma
    b) mucinous cyst adenoma
    c) papillary adenoma
    d) papillary cystic adenoma
    e) eosinophilic cell adenoma
    f) clear cell adenoma
    g) oncocytic cell adenoma
    h) ductular-insular adenoma

B. *Carcinomas*
   a) tubular adenocarcinoma
      cuboidal type
      cylindrical type
      clear cell type
      oncocytic type
      micro-glandular type
      desmoplastic type
   b) mucinous adenocarcinoma
   c) papillary carcinoma
   d) papillary cystic carcinoma
   e) adenosquamous carcinoma
   f) signet ring cell carcinoma
   g) giant cell carcinoma
      pleomorphic type
      multinucleated (osteoclastoid) type
   h) ductular-insular carcinoma

II. *Acinar cell lesions*
    acinar cell nodules

III. *Connective tissue lesions*
   a) neurogenic tumour
   b) angiogenic tumour
   c) fibrogenic tumour

IV. *Undifferentiated (anaplastic) tumours*
   a) spindle cell type
   b) myxoid cell type

V. *Embryonic tumours*
    pancreaticoblastoma

Tumours of ductal/ductular cell origin

Adenomas

Most adenomas derive from ductules and only a few from ducts. The distinction between hyperplasia and adenoma of ductular cells presents a problem because of the overlap between ductular proliferation (tubular or pseudo-ductular formation) and adenoma formation. In general, adenoma is defined as a lesion that shows signs of expansive growth into the surrounding tissue and is composed exclusively of ductular elements without any intervening acinar cells. However, since many adenomas appear to originate from the ductules around (peri-insular ductules) or within (intra-insular ductules) the islets, many adenomas contain foci of islet cells (Figure 7). Most adenomas have the size of a pancreatic lobule (Pour, 1978, 1980; Pour & Wilson, 1980).

The epithelial lining cells of adenomas vary from flat to cylindric mucin-producing cells. Most common types of adenoma have a micro-glandular structure lined with flattened uniform epithelial cells (Figure 7) lying parallel to the axis of the lumen which usually contains serous fluid (*serous (microcystic) adenoma*). A few or many of the ductules or glands can show cystic distension compatible with the term microcystic adenoma (*serous cystic adenoma*). A characteristic of ductular adenoma is the presence of cilia in each cell (Figure 8).

The cells lining the glands may be larger, and the lumen may contain mucigen. In this case *mucinous cyst adenoma* is diagnosed.

Papillary configuration may arise from a large pancreatic duct (Figures 9 and 10) or within a cystic ductular structure. These *papillary adenomas* are composed of cuboidal or cylindrical cells, usually in a single row. *Papillary cystic adenomas* (Figure 10), in contrast to their malignant counterpart (papillary cystic adenocarcinomas), present no signs of malignancy, such as nuclear atypia, mitotic activities and invasion. However, *papillary cystic adenomas* may contain foci of malignant cells, implying the potential of these neoplasms for malignant alteration.

Depending on the predominant type of epithelial cells lining an adenoma, *eosinophilic cell* (Figure 11), *clear cell* (Figure 12) and *oncocytic cell adenoma* (Figure 13) can be distinguished. Clear cells usually contain glycogen with the nuclei centred within the cytoplasm. These types of adenoma are relatively rare and seem to have potential for malignant alteration.

As stated above, foci of islet cells can often be found within adenomas. In cases where the tumour contains equal amounts of ductular and insular elements and there are signs of endocrine cell proliferation, a mixed *ductular-insular cell adenoma* (Figure 14) is diagnosed. Focal or multi-focal proliferation of endocrine cells from ducts and ductules (nesidioblastosis) is a common phenomenon during pancreatic carcinogenesis (Pour, 1978, 1980; Pour & Wilson, 1980) and should not be considered a mixed tumour.

Carcinomas

The pattern of carcinomas may vary with size. Small (micro) carcinomas, are generally composed of uniform malignant glandular structures, whereas large tumours may show regional variations in histocytological patterns. Overall, the peripheral portion of large carcinomas shows less differentiation as the tumours grow. The classification of such heterogeneously structured cancers is based on the predominant type.

Tubular adenocarcinomas are the most common type of induced pancreatic tumours (over 80%). Most micro-carcinomas have tubular structures, which are, in part or predominantly, retained during tumour growth. Depending on the type of tumour cells or the appearance of the lesions, six subtypes can be distinguished (see above). In large lesions, tubular carcinomas can show different subtypes in different regions of the same tumour or present a mixture of one or more subtypes or different cancer types, including giant cell and anaplastic cancers.

Most tubular carcinomas are composed of cuboidal (Figure 15) or cylindrical cells, usually interspersed with goblet-like cells (Figure 16).

Clear cell carcinomas are composed of light polygonal or cylindrical cells, which usually contain PAS-positive material and glycogen (Figure 17). The appearance of these cells mimics those of clear cell adenomas (see above).

Oncocytic carcinomas are characterized by the presence of large cells with eosinophilic fine granular cytoplasm, and fairly hypochromatic centrally located nuclei (Figure 18). These differ from oncocytic adenomas by their pleomorphic cell size and invasive behaviour.

Micro-glandular adenocarcinomas are composed of small glands with thin connective tissue septae between them (Figure 19).

Almost all pancreatic carcinomas have more or less fibrous connective tissue stroma; however, if the desmoplastic pattern is abundant and glandular structures are encased, these lesions are described as being of desmoplastic type (Figure 20).

Mucinous carcinomas represent a type of tubular carcinoma with mucous production. Although tubular adenocarcinoma could produce a minute or moderate amount of mucin, mucinous adenocarcinoma is characterized by exaggerated mucin production occasionally with formation of mucous lakes (Figure 21).

Papillary carcinomas, in general, originate from large pancreatic ducts. They are characterized by papillary projections of the stroma lined by a single row or often by multiple layers of malignant cells (Figure 22a,b). Cystic dilatation of glandular structures, probably owing to the excess formation and congestion of secreted mucous material within the glandular lumen, results in formation of *papillary cystic adenocarcinoma* (Figure 23).

Pure squamous cell carcinomas have not been observed in our material, nor been reported by others in hamsters. In two cases we have seen patterns consistent with the term *adenosquamous carcinoma* (Figure 24). In both cases the tumour had invaded and destroyed duodenal tissue, so that the squamous cell component may have been metaplastic and due to the effects of intestinal contents on the exposed cancer. It must be emphasized that neither in untreated hamsters nor in hamsters treated with pancreatic carcinogens has squamous cell metaplasia of ducts been observed, in contrast to the situation in humans.

The rare *signet ring cell carcinomas* are one group of mucus-producing adenocarcinomas. They are composed of round or oval cells filled with mucinous material pushing the nuclei away towards the cell membrane (Figure 25).

Giant cell carcinomas are also relatively rare. They exhibit pleomorphic giant cells of mononuclear (Figure 26) or multinucleated (osteoclastoid type) cells (Figure 27). Foci of giant cell carcinomas are sometimes seen in the vicinity of poorly differentiated tubular carcinomas.

Tumours composed of a mixture of ductular and insular elements (ductular-insular carcinomas) are not uncommon. The islet cell components could be well differentiated or present solid mass of cells with a few or no cytoplasmic granules. Insulin-, glycogen- and/or somatostatin-containing cells can be identified in these tumours as well as in their metastases (Figure 28).

Tumours of acinar cell origin

Acinar cell tumours have not been observed in routine laboratory experiments. Acinar cell foci and nodules have been induced in hamsters fed a high level of dietary fat (Birt & Pour, 1983) and show small foci of enlarged acinar cells which may or may not be delineated from the surrounding tissue. Although the incidence of these lesions was high in carcinogen-treated animals fed a high-fat diet, their occurrence also in hamsters fed only the high-fat diet (Birt & Pour, 1983, 1985; Birt *et al.*, 1983) and their lack of invasive behaviour argues against a malignant nature. Some of these nodules are generally well circumscribed, show cell pleomorphisms and increased mitotic figures (Figure 29), but no signs of invasion. On the basis of these findings, we believe that these lesions present an

adaptive rather than a neoplastic process, and this is reinforced by our more recent observations of similar lesions induced in less than 1% of hamsters fed a high-fat diet (Birt *et al.*, 1990).

Connective tissue origin

Benign or malignant connective tissue tumours of the pancreas are rare. Our tumour archive contains a neurogenic-like tumour (Figure 30), an angiogenic tumour (Figure 31) and a malignant fibrous tumour (Figure 32).

Undifferentiated (anaplastic) tumours

There is a small group of tumours which on purely morphological grounds can be considered as unclassified or anaplastic carcinomas. The spindle cell or myxoid tumours are large lesions that either lack any differentiation or contain small foci of abortive glandular structures. Fewer neoplasms exhibit a lymphoma-like pattern (Figure 33). However, immunohistochemically, many cells of such 'anaplastic' tumours show the presence of blood group A antigen, which is a marker for transformed ductal/ductular cells in hamsters (Pour, 1986), suggesting that these neoplasms originate from ductal/ductular cells.

Embryonic tumours

Exposure of pregnant hamsters to a pancreatic carcinogen (*N*-nitrosobis(2-oxopropyl)amine) resulted in induction of pancreatic tumours in the offspring when they reached 46 weeks of age (Pour, 1986). The induced adenomas and carcinomas were histologically similar to those seen in adult hamsters. However, in two of the 15 male offspring, an unusual lesion not seen in any of our previous studies with adult hamsters was found. Both of these tumours exhibited a few primitive glandular structures embedded in a bulk of undifferentiated cells resembling altered islet cells (Figure 34). A few somatostatin- and insulin-containing cells were scattered among them, as were a few abortive ductular structures expressing blood group A antigen. Focal calcification was present in the stroma. These findings suggest that these tumours had their origin in the embryological pancreas and correspond to pancreaticoblastomas described in humans (Cubilla & Fitzgerald, 1984; Morohoshi *et al.*, 1987).

SPONTANEOUS TUMOURS

Ductal/ductular adenomas and adenocarcinomas are occasionally seen in some strains of hamsters with an incidence of 0.3–2% (Fortner, 1957; Takahashi & Pour, 1978).

Papillary proliferation of pancreatic common duct epithelium, with goblet cell metaplasia (intestinalization), is not uncommon and usually is an age-related change. Squamous cell metaplasia has never been seen or reported, nor have acinar cell lesions.

INDUCTION OF TUMOURS

Numerous carcinogenic nitrosamines have been shown to induce pancreatic ductal/ductular neoplasms in the Syrian hamster. Our studies have shown that certain molecular features are required for neoplastic action of an aliphatic nitrosamine on the hamster pancreas. It appears that hydroxylation or a carbonyl group at the beta position of at least one of the aliphatic chains of a propyl-nitrosamine is necessary for pancreatotropic effects. Elongation of the chain, i.e., addition of a methyl group to the aliphatic chain (as in N-nitrosomethyl(2-oxobutyl)amine) reduces the potency of the carcinogen for pancreatic tumour induction and replacement of propyl chain with a methyl group (as in N-nitrosomethyl(2-oxopropyl)amine) reduces the specificity for the pancreas and causes induction of tumours in many other tissues. Moving the carbonyl group from the beta to gamma position (e.g., N-nitrosomethyl(3-oxobutyl)amine) abolishes the pancreatic carcinogenicity. Overall, N-nitrosobis(2-oxopropyl)amine is the most potent and specific pancreatic carcinogen found so far (Pour, 1989).

Pancreatic carcinogens are effective by either oral, subcutaneous or percutaneous application. Simply dropping the carcinogen on the shaved hamster skin leads to induction of pancreatic cancer in a high incidence (Pour *et al.*, 1977). There were no differences in the patterns of pancreatic tumours induced by any of these carcinogens.

Islet cell pancreatic tumours have been induced by intravenous administration of human BK polyomavirus (Uchita *et al.*, 1976).

Antigenicity of induced tumors

Lectin binding: The binding pattern of nine lectins (*Arachis hypogaea* (PNA), *Dolichos biflorus* (DBA), Griffonia simplicifolia (GS-I), *Helix aspersa* (HAA), *Helix pomatia* (HPA), *Sophora japonica* (SJA), *Ricinus communis* I (RCA- I), *Triticum vulgaris* (WGA) and *Ulex europaeus* I (UEA-I)) were examined in induced pancreatic lesions (Pour *et al.*, 1985). All of these lectins reacted in untreated hamsters to varying intensities with acinar cells. GS-I, HPA, RCA-I and UEA-I bound to the basolateral surface and PNA, HAA and HPA to the luminal surface of these cells. Some ductal cells bound PNA, HAA and RCA-I. Ductular cells did not react with any of these lectins. Islet cells showed reactivity to all but GS-I, RCA-I and UEA-I. In carcinogen-treated hamsters, the induced ductal and ductular lesions bound all of the nine lectins with different patterns and intensities (Figure 35). The reactivity of UEA-I was most consistent and specific. The results indicated heterogeneity of the carbohydrate structure of the glycoproteins produced by pancreatic cells during carcinogenesis.

Blood group-related antigens: Polyclonal and monoclonal antibodies against blood group antigens, ABH, Le[a], Le[b], Le[x] and Le[y] did not react with any pancreatic cells of untreated hamsters. However, all of these antibodies, except for Le[a], showed reactivity with hyperplastic, premalignant and malignant lesions (Figure 36). The reactivity of anti-A was comparable to that of UEA-I and was almost 100% in each case. Because these antigens are expressed only during carcinogenesis, they constitute cancer-associated antigens in this species. Presence of these antigens also in the anaplastic tumours (Pour, 1985) indicates that all induced neoplasms in hamsters derive from ductal/ductular cells.

Among other human cancer-associated antigens, 17-1A, TAG-72, CA125 and, to a lesser extent, DU-PAN-2 were expressed in induced hamster pancreatic cancer in patterns similar to that seen in human pancreatic cancer cells, but CA19-9 was lacking (Takiyama *et al.*, 1990). None of these antigens was detectable in the normal hamster pancreas, except for 17-1A which was expressed only in acinar and islet cells, as it is in the human pancreas (Takiyama *et al.*, 1990b).

COMPARATIVE ASPECTS

There are remarkable similarities between pancreatic cancer in man and that induced in Syrian hamsters, in their morphological, clinical and immunological aspects. Morphologically, hyperplastic, metaplastic, dysplastic and premalignant alterations of ducts and ductules are similar in these two species (Pour *et al.*, 1975). Squamous cell metaplasia and neoplasia is an exception.

As in humans, the biological behaviour of induced pancreatic cancers depends on the origin, site and size of the tumours. In both species, tumours are extremely aggressive and show a remarkable tendency for perineural invasion and for causing vascular thrombosis and ascites.

With regard to the anatomical location of tumours, there is a significant difference between the two species. Over 60% of human pancreatic cancer is found in the head of the gland (Tsuchiya *et al.*, 1986), whereas most tumours in hamsters develop in the splenic lobe (Pour *et al.*, 1981; Pour, 1989), the largest segment of the pancreas in hamsters, suggesting an effect of blood-borne carcinogen(s) in the hamster (Pour *et al.*, 1981). Whether this mode of action is different from the human situation is not yet known.

Lesions resembling the pancreaticoblastomas which occur in young and adolescent humans are also inducible in hamsters by intrauterine exposure of the fetuses to a pancreatic carcinogen during the later stages of gestation (Pour, 1986). This observation let assume that development of these neoplasms in humans is also related to transplacental exposure to some oncogenic agent(s).

Pancreatic tumours in hamsters and man also share certain immunological characteristics. Pancreatic cancer cells in hamsters, like those in humans, produce antigens related to the blood group substances, including A, B, H, Le[b], Le[x] and Le[y]. However, unlike most human pancreatic cancer cells which express Lea and CA19-9, hamster pancreatic cells lack these two related antigens (Pour *et al.*, 1986). On the other hand, in contrast to findings in man, whose normal pancreatic cells express compatible blood group antigens (Pour *et al.*, 1988; Philipsen *et al.*, 1988), normal hamster pancreatic cells do not produce these substances at detectable levels. Therefore, except for 17-1A, which is found in normal acinar and islet cells, the expression of these antigens in hamsters may be regarded as a marker for pancreatic cancer (Egami *et al.*, 1989).

Among other antigens commonly expressed in human pancreatic cancer, 17-1A, CA125, TAG-72 and DU-PAN-2 can be demonstrated immunohistochemically in induced hamster pancreatic cancers (Takiyama *et al.*, 1990a) in a pattern similar to that seen in human pancreatic cancer (Table 1).

Table 1. Immunoreactivity of human tumour-associated antigens in normal and malignant pancreatic cells in hamster model

	Acinar cell	Islet cell	Ductular cell	Cancer cell
CEA				
CO19-9				
DU-PAN-2				+/-
CO17-1A	++	++	+	++
OC 125				++
B72.3				++

Finally, in both humans and hamsters, pancreatic tumours develop from ductal/ductular cells, with only a few lesions deriving from the acinar cells. However, in contrast to the findings in man, acinar cell carcinoma is non-existent in hamsters, a situation which is also significantly different from pancreatic tumours seen in other species, including rats, mice, guinea-pigs, dogs and other mammals (Rowlatt, 1967).

REFERENCES

Althoff, J., Pour, P.M., Malick, L. & Wilson, R.B. (1976) Pancreatic neoplasms induced in Syrian golden hamsters. I. Scanning electron microscopic observations. *Am. J. Pathol.*, 83, 517–530

Birt, D.F. & Pour, P.M. (1983) Increased tumorigenesis induced by N-nitrosobis(2-oxopropyl)amine in Syrian golden hamsters fed high-fat diet. *J. Natl Cancer Inst.*, 70, 1135–1138Birt, D.F., Stepan, K.R. & Pour, P.M. (1983) Interaction of dietary fat and protein on pancreatic carcinogenesis in Syrian golden hamsters. *J. Natl Cancer Inst.*, 71, 355–360

Birt, D.F. & Pour, P.M. (1985) Effects of the interaction of dietary fat and protein on N-nitrosobis(2-oxopropyl)amine-induced carcinogenesis and spontaneous lesions in Syrian golden hamsters. *J. Natl Cancer Inst.*, 74, 1121–1127

Birt, D.F., Julius, A.D., Dwork, E., Hanna, T., White, T. & Pour, P.M. (1990) Comparison of the effects of dietary beef tallow and corn oil on pancreatic carcinogenesis in the hamster model. *Carcinogenesis*, 11, 745–748

Cubilla, A.L. & Fitzgerald, P.J. (1984) *Atlas of Tumor Pathology*. Second series, fascicle 19. *Tumors of the Exocrine Pancreas*, Washington, DC, Armed Forces Institute of Pathology

Egami, H., Takiyama, Y., Cano, M., Houser, W.H. & Pour, P.M. (1989) Establishment of hamster pancreatic ductal carcinoma cell line (PC-1) producing blood group-related antigens. *Carcinogenesis*, 10, 861–869

Fortner, J.G. (1957) Spontaneous tumors, including gastrointestinal neoplasms and malignant melanomas in the Syrian hamster. *Cancer*, 10, 1153–1156

Morohoshi, T., Kanda, M., Horie, A., Chott, A., Dreyer, T., Kloppel, G. & Heitz, P.U. (1987) Immunocytochemical markers of uncommon pancreatic tumors. *Cancer*, 59, 739–747

Philipsen, E.K., Clausen, H., Dabelsteen, E. & Graem, N. (1988) Part A: Blood group related carbohydrate antigen in human fetal pancreas. *Acta Pathol. Microbiol. Immunol. Scand.*, 96, 1109–1117

Pour, P.M. (1978) Islet cell as a component of pancreatic ductal neoplasms. *Am. J. Pathol.*, 90, 295–316

Pour, P.M. (1980) Experimental pancreatic ductal (ductular) tumors. In: Fitzgerald, P.J., ed., *The Pancreas*, Baltimore, Williams & Wilkins, pp. 111–139

Pour, P.M. (1985) Induction of unusual pancreatic neoplasms with morphologic similarity to human tumors and evidence for their ductal/ductular cell origin. *Cancer*, 55, 2411–2416

Pour, P.M. (1986) Induction of exocrine pancreatic, bile duct and thyroid gland tumors in offspring of Syrian hamsters treated with N-nitrosobis(2-oxopropyl)-amine during pregnancy. *Cancer Res.*, 43, 3663–3666

Pour, P.M. (1989) Experimental pancreatic cancer. *Am. J. Surg. Pathol.*, 13, 96–103

Pour, P.M. & Wilson, R.B. (1980) Experimental tumors of the pancreas. In: Moosa, A.R., ed., *The Tumors of the Pancreas*, Baltimore, Williams & Wilkins, pp. 37–158

Pour, P.M., Mohr, U., Cardesa, A., Althoff, J. & Kruger, F.W. (1975) Pancreatic neoplasms in an animal model: morphologic, biological and comparative studies. *Cancer*, 35, 379–389

Pour, P.M., Althoff, J. & Nagel, D. (1977) Induction of epithelial neoplasms by local application of N-nitrosobis(2-hydroxy-propyl)amine and N-nitrosobis(2-acetoxy-propyl)amine. *Cancer Lett.*, 3, 109–115

Pour, P.M., Birt, D. & Nagel, D. (1981) Current knowledge of pancreatic carcinogenesis in the hamster and its relevance to the human disease. *Cancer*, 47, 1573–1587

Pour, P.M., Burnett, D. & Uchida, E. (1985) Lectin binding affinities of induced pancreatic lesions in the hamster model. *Carcinogenesis*, 6, 1775–1780

Pour, P.M., Uchida, E., Burnett, D.A. & Steplewski, Z. (1986) Blood-group antigen expression during pancreatic cancer induction in hamsters. *Int. J. Pancreatol.*, 1, 327–340

Pour, P.M., Tempero, M.M., Takasaki, H., Uchida, E., Takiyama, Y., Burnett, D.A. & Steplewski, Z. (1988) Expression of blood group-related antigen ABH, Lewis A, Lewis B, Lewis X, Lewis Y and CA19-9 in pancreatic cancer cells in comparison with the patient's blood group type. *Cancer Res.*, 48, 5422–5426

Pour, P.M. Konishi, Y., Klöppel, G. Longnecker, D.S. Atlas of Endocrine Pancreatic Tumours. Morphology, Biology and Diagnosis with an International Guide for Tumour Classification. Springer-Verlag, 1994

Rowlatt, U (1967) Spontaneous epithelial tumours of the pancreas of mammals. *Br. J. Cancer*, 21, 82–107

Takahashi, M. & Pour, P.M. (1978) Spontaneous alterations in the pancreas of the aging Syrian golden hamster. *J. Natl. Cancer Inst.*, 60, 355–364

Takahashi, M., Pour, P.M., Althoff, J. & Donnelly, T. (1977a) The pancreas of the Syrian hamster. I. Anatomical study. *Lab. Anim. Sci.*, 27, 336–342

Takahashi, M., Pour, P.M., Althoff, J. & Donnelly, T. (1977b) Sequential alteration of the pancreas during carcinogenesis in Syrian hamster by N-nitrosobis(2-oxo-propyl)amine. *Cancer Res.*, 37, 4602–4607

Takiyama, Y., Egami, H. & Pour, P.M. (1990) Expression of human tumor-associated antigens in pancreatic cancer induced in Syrian hamsters. *Am. J. Pathol.*, 136, 707–715

Takiyama, Y., Tempero, M.A., Takasaki, H., Onda, M., Tsuchiya, R., Buchler, M., Ness, M., Colcher, D., Schlom, J. & Pour, P.M. (1989) Reactivity of CO17-1A and B72.3 in benign and malignant pancreatic diseases. *Human Pathol.*, 20, 832–838

Tsuchiya, R., Tomioka, T. & Tsunoda, T. (1986) Collective review of small carcinoma of the pancreas. *Ann. Surg.*, 203, 77–81

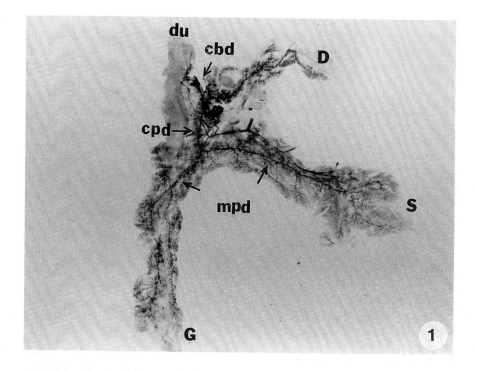

Figure 1. Pancreas of Syrian hamster after injection of Indian ink into pancreatic duct. du: duodenum; D: duodenal lobe; G: gastric lobe; S: splenic lobe; cbd: common bile duct; cpd: common pancreatic duct; mpd: main pancreatic duct. Duodenal lobe is turned 180°. × 2.5

Figure 2.

(a) Electron micrograph (EM) of the pancreas of a newborn hamster showing centroacinar cells (C) surrounded by several acinar cells with zymogen granules (Z). Tight junctions and desmosomes are presented between the acinar and centroacinar cells (arrows). Part of the lumen (L) is seen. × 2400

(b) Histological appearance of the normal pancreas in hamsters. T = terminal (intercalated) ductule; D = interlobular ductule. C = centroacinar cell. H & E; × 210

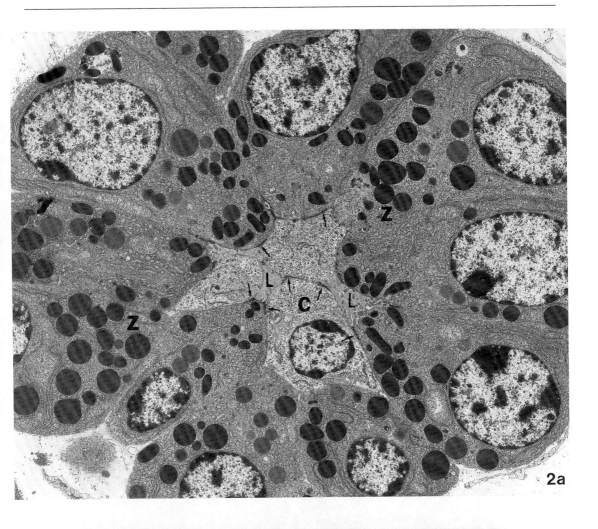

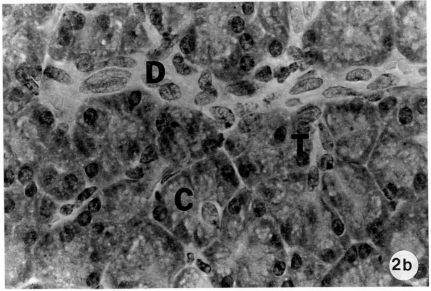

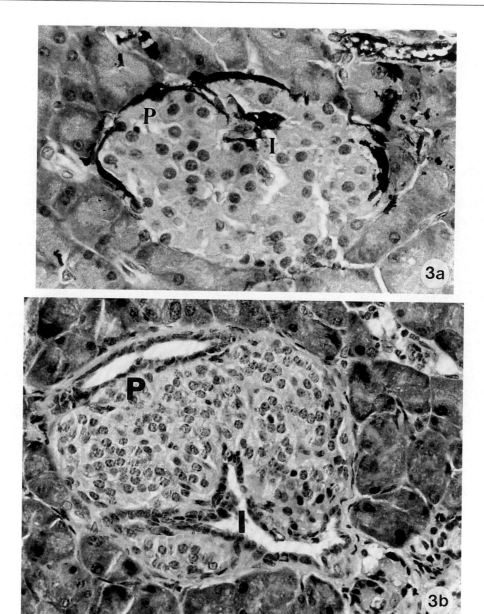

Figure 3. (a) Demonstration of peri-insular and intra-insular ductules after Indian ink injection (black in photo). P = peri-insular ductule; I = intra-insular ductule. H & E; × 210

(b) Islet cell with peri-insular ductules (P) and intra-insular ductules (I) in hamster treated with *N*-nitrosobis(2-oxopropylamine). In untreated hamsters, these ductules are invisible histologically. They become pronounced during carcinogenesis or by injection of Indian ink into the pancreatic duct (see Figure 3a). H & E; × 210

(c) Electron microscopic demonstration of two peri-insular ductular cells with microvilli and junctional complex (arrow) and a portion of a beta cell with typical granules (left bottom). Note the interdigitation (ID) of the ductular cells and the lack of any connective tissue between these and the beta cell. R = ribosomes; M = mitochondria; ER = endoplasmic reticulum. × 57 450

(d) Scanning electron microscopy of the hamster pancreas depicting peri-insular ductule (P) and an intra-insular ductule (I). B = blood vessels, A = acinar cells. × 400

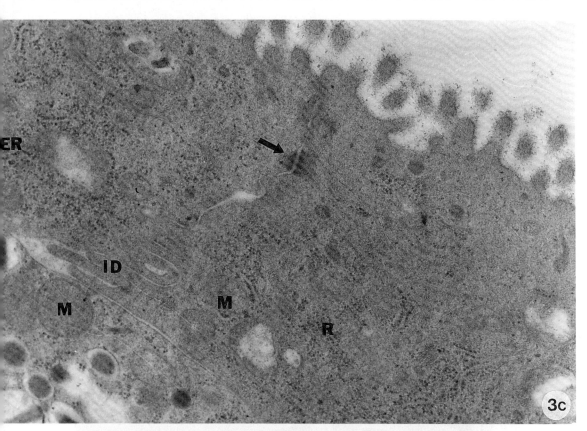

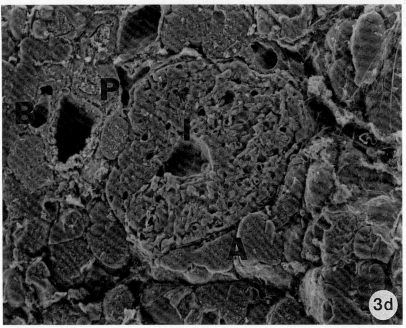

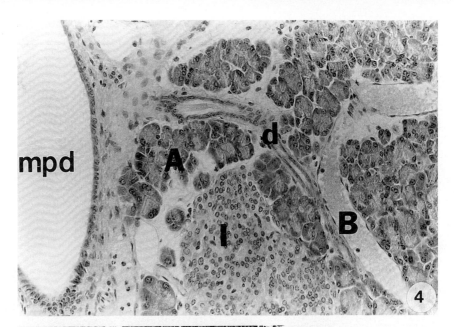

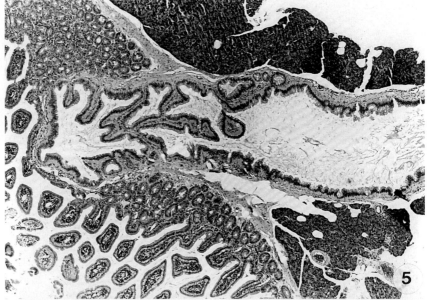

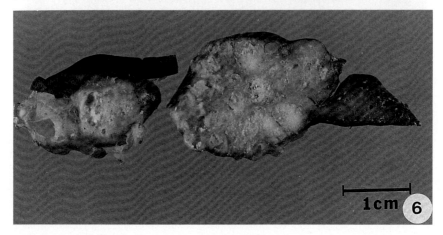

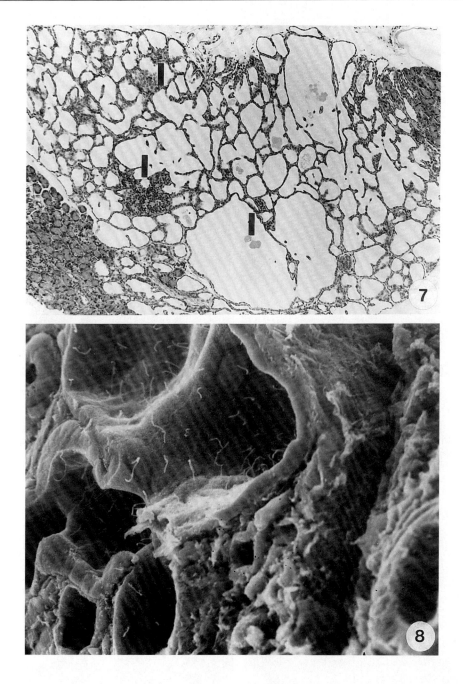

Figure 4. Histology of the normal hamster pancreas demonstrating main pancreatic duct (mpd) with periductal connective tissue, interlobular duct (d) and an islet (I). B = blood vessels, A = acinar cells. H & E; × 210

Figure 5. Common bile duct merging into the duodenum showing large lumen and papillary projections. H & E; × 40

Figure 6. Pancreatic cancer with invasion of the spleen (left) and liver (right). Areas of necrosis and cysts are seen. This and the following tumours were induced with *N*-nitrosobis(2-oxopropyl)-amine or *N*-nitrosobis(2-hydroxypropyl)amine

Figure 7. Serous cyst adenoma with foci of islet cells (I). Note fairly uniform pattern of glands, some with distension. H & E; × 40

Figure 8. Scanning electron micrograph of a ductular adenoma showing ductular cells with cilia. × 400

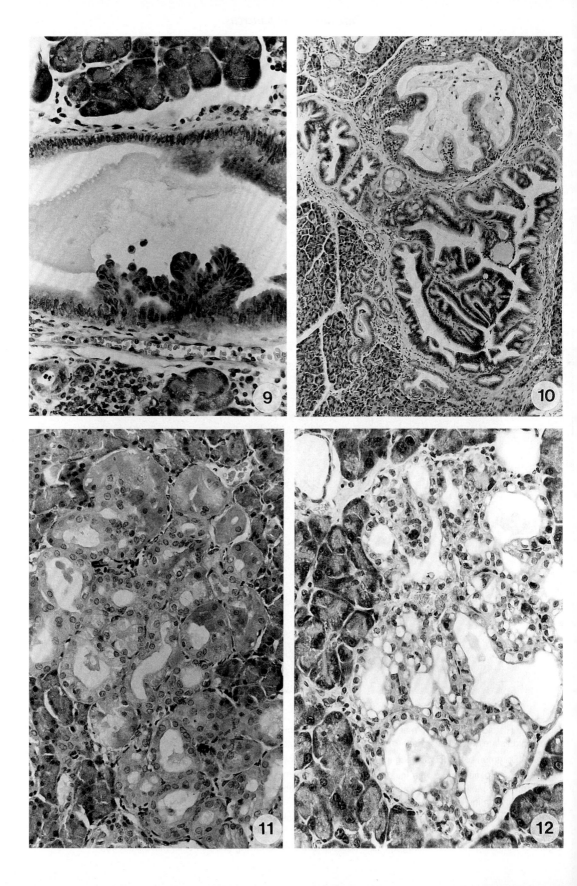

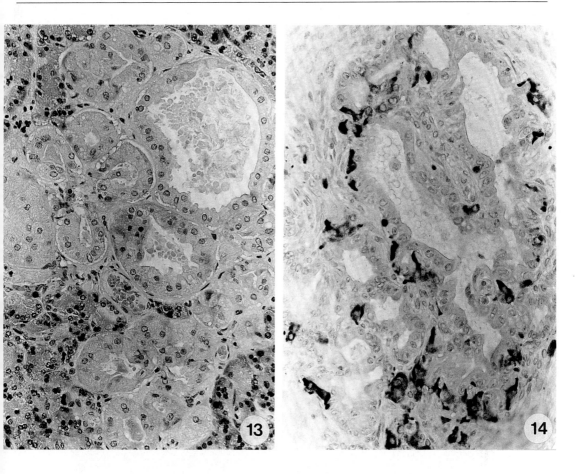

Figure 9. Papillary adenoma of a large pancreatic duct. H & E; × 210

Figure 10. Papillary cystic adenoma (top) and papillary adenoma (bottom). The cyst is partially lined with columnar mucinous epithelium. A few small papillae are present, but epithelium is benign in appearance. H & E; × 72

Figure 11. Eosinophilic cell adenoma composed of glands with eosinophilic cells. Note the central location of the nuclei. H & E; × 210

Figure 12. Clear cell adenomas are composed of glycogen-containing cells of various sizes and shapes. H & E; × 210

Figure 13. Oncocytic adenoma has large eosinophilic and finely granulated cytoplasm with centrally located nuclei. H & E; × 210

Figure 14. Mixed ductular–insular adenoma in which both components are intermingled. Dark cells represent alpha cells. Delta and beta cells may also be found. PAP method with anti-glucagon; × 210

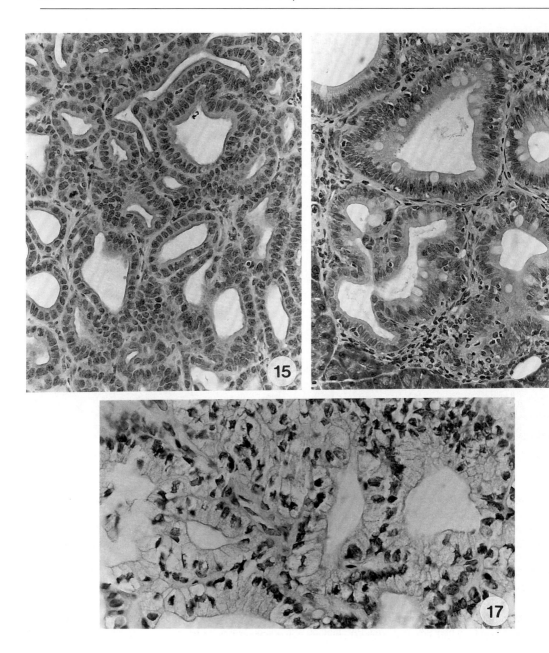

Figure 15. Tubular carcinoma showing irregular glands lined with cuboidal cells. H & E; × 210

Figure 16. Tubular carcinomas composed of high columnar epithelial cells interspersed with goblet-like cells. H & E; × 210

Figure 17. Tubular adenocarcinoma of clear cell type. The cells are rich in glycogen. H & E; × 210

Figure 18. Tubular carcinoma of oncocytic cell type showing eosinophilic fine granular cell cytoplasm and round or oval nuclei. A mitotic figure is seen (arrow). H & E; × 210

Figure 19. Micro-glandular adenocarcinomas are composed of many small irregular glands with flat or cuboidal epithelia and separated by connective tissue septae. H & E; × 72

Figure 20. Tubular carcinoma of desmoplastic type showing abundant connective tissue stroma. H & E; × 210

Figure 21. Mucinous carcinomas with formation of mucus lakes. The tumour is composed primarily of mucin-producing cells and ruptured glands. H & E; × 90

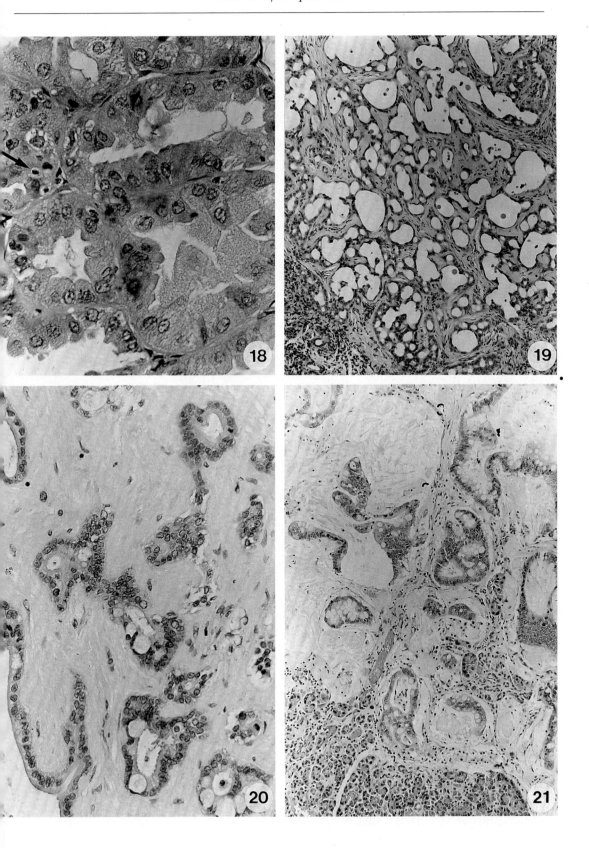

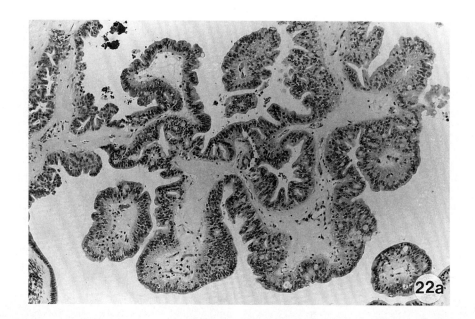

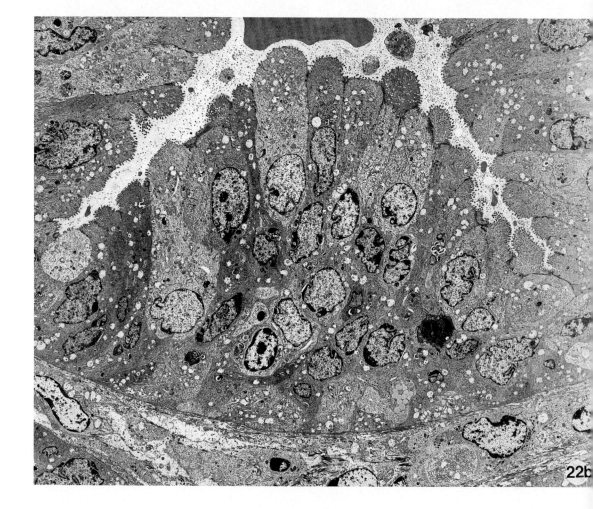

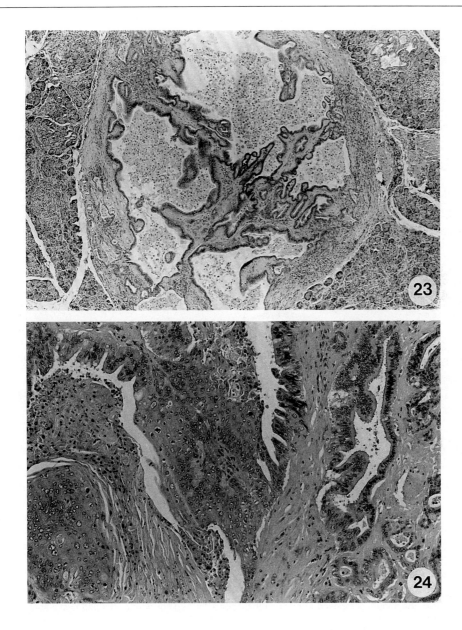

Figure 22. (a) Papillary carcinoma arising from large duct. The lining epithelium is composed of single or multiple rows of cells. H & E; × 90.

(b) Electron microscopic pattern of a papillary carcinoma showing a focal piling up of irregularly sized tumour cells with increased number of microvilli on the cell surface. × 1200

Figure 23. Low-power view of a papillary-cystic adenocarcinoma demonstrating cyst formation and papillary fronds lined with cylindrical cells. H & E; × 72

Figure 24. Adenosquamous carcinoma composed of a mixture of glandular structures and squamous epithelium. Sclerosis of the stroma encasing glandular structures. H & E; × 90

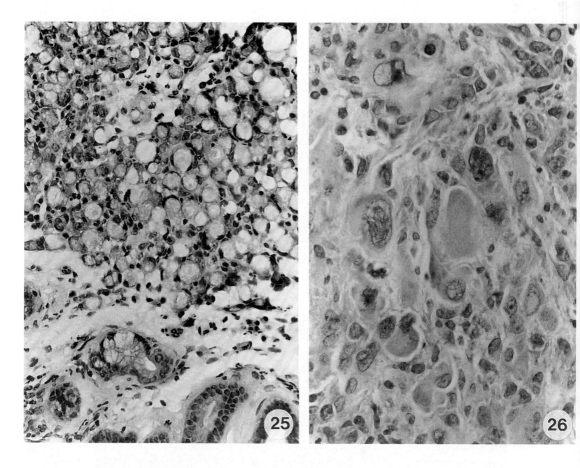

Figure 25. Signet ring cell carcinoma with cells filled up with mucin. Note the presence of mucin-containing cells in the adjacent duct (left). H & E; × 210

Figure 26. Giant cell carcinoma of pleomorphic type. Note bizarre giant cells with mono- or multi-nucleated irregular hyperchromatic nuclei with prominent nucleoli and deeply stained large cytoplasm. H & E; × 210

Figure 27. Giant cell carcinoma of osteoclastoid type. There are osteoclast-like giant cells surrounded by spindle or round pleomorphic cells. The osteoclast-like cells are relatively uniform in size. H & E; × 90

Figure 28. (a) Mixed ductular–insular carcinoma. × 90

(b) Higher magnification of the lesion is shown in Figure 28a depicting both cell components. H & E; × 400

Figure 29. Acinar cell nodule composed of pleomorphic cells with irregular dark nuclei and cystic space (C). I = an intact islet. H & E; × 210

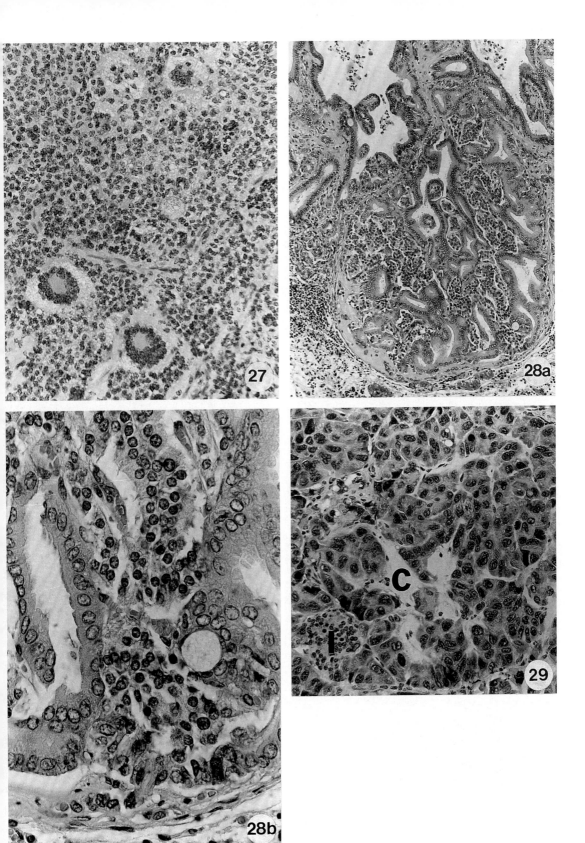

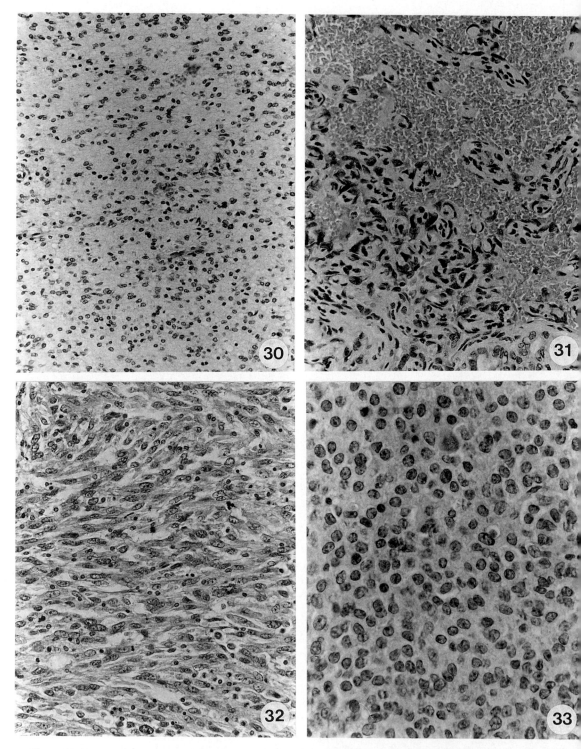

Figure 30. Neurogenic-like tumour composed of spindle-shaped cells with fairly uniform oval nuclei. H & E; × 210

Figure 31. Angiogenic tumour demonstrating many vascular cavities with endothelial septae. H & E × 210

Figure 32. Fibrogenic-like tumour. Note irregularly arranged spindle-shaped nuclei. H & E; × 210

Figure 33. Anaplastic lymphocytic-type tumour with oval, fairly monotonous nuclei. H & E; × 210

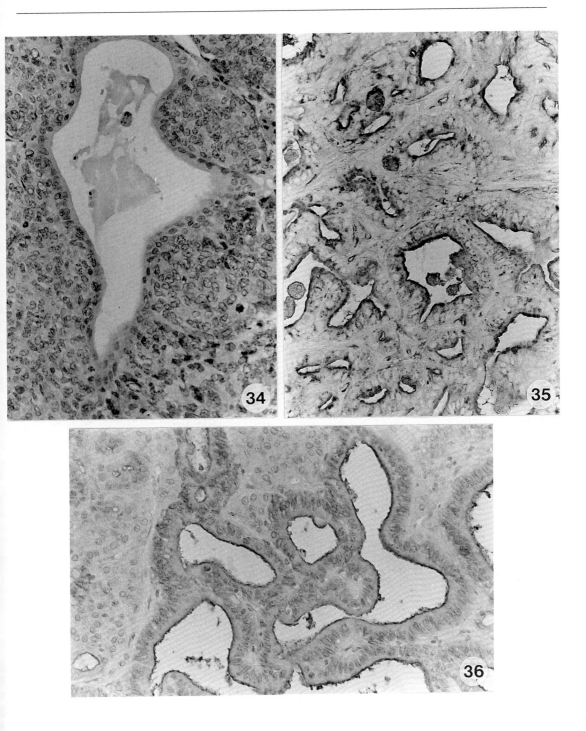

Figure 34. Pancreaticoblastoma composed of a gland-like structure within an undifferentiated cell mass. The cells have light cytoplasm and hypochromatic nuclei. H & E; × 210

Figure 35. A tubular adenocarcinoma stained with *Griffonia simplicifolia* I (GS-I) lectin. Note glycocalyx pattern of the staining. × 210

Figure 36. Tubular adenocarcinoma. All glands are stained with monoclonal anti-A in a glycocalyx pattern. PAP technique; × 210

Tumours of the nasal cavity

H.M. Schuller

The nasal cavity is an important bio-assay system to test agents which represent a potential carcinogenic hazard to man. Inhaled particles which, because of the larger diameter of the human airways, reach the lungs in people, are trapped in the narrow and more complex nasal passages of small rodents. Moreover, the relatively large olfactory origin of the rodent nasal cavity provides abundant target cells for systemic compounds with a specific carcinogenic effect on cell types comprising this type of epithelium.

For reasons not quite understood, the respiratory tract, including the nasal cavities, of the Syrian golden hamster appears to be highly sensitive to the carcinogenic actions of systemically administered *N*-nitroso compounds (Reznik-Schüller, 1983). This may be the reason why most information available on the histopathology and pathogenesis of hamster nasal cavity tumours is derived from studies using chemical carcinogens of this class.

occasional neuroendocrine cells. The most caudal part of the nasal cavities is formed by the ethmoturbinates which comprise the olfactory region. The ethmoturbinates consist of four ectoturbinates and three endoturbinates (Reznik, 1983) and are lined with olfactory epithelium (Figure 2) comprising basal cells, olfactory sensory cells, sustentacular cells and a few neuroendocrine cells. The respiratory and olfactory regions of the nasal cavity demonstrate submucous glands which are particularly prominent around the ostium of the maxillary sinus.

The maxillary sinus is approximately 15 mm long and extends into the nasal lumen through an ostium bounded by the anterior atrioturbinates and the ethmoturbinates (Pour, 1976). At the level of the maxillary sinus ostium, the nasopharyngeal duct begins behind the vomeronasal organs. Like the maxillary sinus, the nasopharyngeal duct is coated by respiratory epithelium.

NORMAL STRUCTURE

The nasal cavities are composed of the atrioturbinates, nasal turbinates, maxillary turbinates and ethmoturbinates. The atrioturbinates form the most apical portion of the nasal cavity and make up a non-keratinizing squamous epithelium. The intermediate portion of the nasal cavities consists of naso- and maxillo-turbinates which are lined by a pseudo-stratified respiratory epithelium (Figure 1) comprising ciliated, mucous, basal and

MORPHOLOGY AND BIOLOGY OF TUMOURS AND PRENEOPLASTIC LESIONS

Histological types of tumours and preneoplastic lesions

Tumours

Squamous cell papilloma/papillary polyp
Adenoma
Squamous cell carcinoma

Adenocarcinoma

Mixed (adenosquamous) carcinoma

Olfactory carcinoma (esthesioneuroepithelioma)

Neuroendocrine carcinoma

Preneoplastic lesions

Epithelial hyperplasia

Squamous cell metaplasia

Epithelial dysplasia

Squamous cell papilloma/papillary polyp

Like all neoplastic and preneoplastic lesions of the nasal cavity, squamous cell papilloma/papillary polyp is a rare spontaneous lesion in the hamster (Pour *et al.*, 1976). This benign lesion is induced by many chemical carcinogens in the most apical portion of the nasal cavity (which is lined by squamous epithelium), as well as in the respiratory portion (coated by respiratory epithelium) including the maxillary sinus, while it is uncommon in the olfactory region of the nasal cavity. By definition, squamous cell papillomas are composed of squamous cells with a distinct connective tissue stalk or core, while papillary polyps contain either ciliated and/or mucous cells in addition to the squamous cells. By electron microscopy (which yields a higher resolution than light microscopy), the majority of investigated squamous cell papillomas (so classified by histopathology) have to be reclassified as papillary polyps because of the occasional presence of ciliated and/or mucous cells. It is therefore advisable to collectively classify such lesions as squamous cell papilloma/papillary polyp unless unequivocal proof for some type of lesion is provided by electron microscopy, immunocytochemistry or special stains.

Adenoma

Adenomas (Figure 3) represent a rare spontaneous lesion in the hamster nasal cavity (Pour *et al.*, 1976). However, numerous chemical carcinogens can induce this lesion experimentally.

Adenomas may occur in the respiratory (including maxillary sinus) and olfactory regions of the nasal cavity. They may originate either from the lining epithelium itself or from submucous glands. Unlike in other organs, adenomas in the nasal cavity seldom demonstrate compression of surrounding tissues. However, their generally smooth outlines without indication of infiltrative tumour growth, in conjunction with a low mitotic index, allow their distinction from adenocarcinomas. Depending on their anatomical localization, adenomas of the hamster nasal cavity may be composed of cell types commonly found in respiratory epithelium or of basal cells and sustentacular cells (olfactory region). Typically, adenomas demonstrate a glandular growth pattern. Occasionally, they may contain focal areas of early squamous differentiation.

Squamous cell carcinoma

Squamous cell carcinomas (Figure 4) of the nasal cavity have not been reported as spontaneous lesions in hamsters (Pour *et al.*, 1976). This malignant tumour type is inducible experimentally by a variety of chemical carcinogens.

With respect to their degree of differentiation, these neoplasms can be subclassified into well differentiated and poorly differentiated squamous cell carcinomas. The morphological hallmark of both these variants is the production of keratin by the tumour cells. Such keratin synthesis will lead to the deposition of mature and occasionally excessive keratin (detectable by routine histopathology) in well differentiated squamous cell carcinomas. On the other hand, in poorly differentiated squamous cell carcinomas, keratin synthesis is generally minimal, leading to a less mature product such as keratohyalin granules or cytoplasmic tonofilament bundles. These may at times be beyond the resolution of histo-pathology, so that diagnosis requires application of techniques such as electron microscopy or immunocytochemistry.

Squamous cell carcinomas may occur in all three major regions of the nasal cavity, but are most common in the respiratory portion. Depending on their anatomical localization they may arise from the lining epithelium of the nasal apex, respiratory or olfactory region, as well as from maxillary glands and sub-mucous glands.

Squamous cell carcinomas may exhibit a very malignant growth pattern which often results in extensive infiltration and destruction of surrounding cartilage, bones and the brain. However, metastasis to distant organs is very rare.

Adenocarcinoma

Adenocarcinomas have not been reported as spontaneous tumours in the hamster nasal cavity (Pour *et al.*, 1976). However, they are commonly induced experimentally by a variety of chemical carcinogens.

Adenocarcinomas may develop in the respiratory (including maxillary sinuses) and olfactory regions of the nasal cavity, where they may originate either from the lining epithelium or submucous glands (Figure 5). Depending on their anatomical localization, they may be composed of basal, ciliated and mucous cells (respiratory region), or basal and sustentacular cells (olfactory region). Differentiated adenocarcinomas demonstrate a distinct glandular growth pattern (Figure 5) while poorly differentiated adenocarcinomas are generally more compact with only occasional gland-like patterns (Figure 6). This category of tumour may at times be difficult to distinguish from olfactory carcinomas.

Mixed (adenosquamous) carcinoma

Carcinomas composed of areas with an adenomatous growth pattern and

simultaneously exhibiting areas with squamous differentiation are very common in the respiratory region of the nasal cavity, but occur less frequently in the olfactory region. These tumours are commonly referred to as 'mixed' carcinomas. This may be the result of different pathways of differentation; the majority of cases are observed during a late stage of tumour development.

Olfactory carcinoma (esthesioneuroepithelioma)

Olfactory carcinomas are located in the olfactory region of the nasal cavity. Well differentiated tumours of this type demonstrate a characteristic growth pattern of rosettes and pseudorosettes (Figure 7), although individual tumour cells may vary considerably in size and shape. Neurotubules and axons are usually difficult to detect by histopathology. Even by electron microscopy, they are detectable only in a small proportion of such tumours. Poorly differentiated tumours (Figure 8) of this category may be difficult to distinguish from poorly differentiated adenocarcinomas. In particular, rosettes and pseudorosettes are generally absent. Most olfactory carcinomas demonstrate aggressive biological behaviour characterized by extensive invasion of brain (Figure 8) and adjacent bones.

Neuroendocrine carcinoma

Neuroendocrine carcinoma is a malignant tumour, largely composed of cells which express one or several neuroendocrine markers. The major diagnostic tools to identify this tumour type are transmission electron microscopy (identification of neuroendocrine secretion granules) and immunocytochemistry (identification of neuroendocrine secretory products such as mammalian bombesin or calcitonin). However, because of the cost, electron microscopy has rarely been applied in hamster experiments. Moreover, the commonly used methods for decalcification of the skull for histo-pathological processing destroy most antigens, precluding the use of immunocytochemistry. Nevertheless, a few investigations on nitrosamine-induced nasal cavity tumours in hamsters and rats have provided evidence that neuro-endocrine carcinoma may in fact develop in the respiratory and olfactory regions of the nasal cavities in rodents including the hamster (Reznik-Schüller, 1983). The tumours usually demonstrate a glandular growth pattern similar to adenocarci-nomas when localized in the respiratory portion of the nasal cavity, while they exhibit a much poorer differentiation when localized in the olfactory region. Electron microscopy reveals the presence of dense-cored cytoplasmic secretion granules which in other organs have been shown to store neuropeptides such as calcitonin.

Preneoplastic lesions

Epithelial hyperplasia, dysplasia and squamous metaplasia may occur in the squamous epithelium which lines the apical portion of the nasal cavity, in the respiratory and olfactory epithelium, as well as in submucous glands. Although such lesions often occur simultaneously with squamous cell carcinomas and may also precede the development of this tumour type, their precise association with carcinoma is not known. It is well established that such preneoplastic lesions can be induced by a large variety of irritants without ever progressing into neoplasia. Hyperplasia is generally multi-focal and is characterized by a thickening of the normally one-layered pseudo-stratified lining epithelia, thus forming multiple layers of cells. Squamous metaplasia (Figure 9) is characterized by the forma-tion of mature or immature keratin. Dysplasia (Figure 10) is characterized by abnormalities in size, shape and orientation of epithelial cells and is generally observed in hyperplastic

and metaplastic foci as well as in nasal cavity tumours.

SPONTANEOUS TUMOURS

The incidence of spontaneous tumours in the nasal cavity of Syrian golden hamsters is less than 0.1% (Pour *et al.*, 1976). In view of this, the experimental induction of even low incidences of tumours in this organ can be regarded as evidence for a potential carcinogenic risk posed by the agent under study.

INDUCTION OF TUMOURS

The vast majority of experimentally induced nasal cavity tumours in hamsters has been caused by nitrosamines (Table 1), all of which were administered by a series of systemic injections. Very few inhalation experiments have been conducted with Syrian golden hamsters, but cigarette smoke inhalation resulted in the development of an adenocarcinoma in the respiratory part of the nasal cavity in one out of 10 hamsters (Bernfeld *et al.*, 1974). In addition, inhalation experiments with dimethylcarbamoyl chloride, an intermediate in the production of some carba-mate pesticides, yielded moderately to well differentiated squamous cell carci-nomas in the respiratory portion of the nasal cavity in 50% of the exposed hamsters (Sellakumar *et al.*, 1980).

Chronic inhalation of high levels of acetaldehyde induced squamous cell carci-nomas in the respiratory portion of the nasal cavity of very few hamsters (Feron & Woutersen, 1980).

A large number of nitrosamines have been reported to induce tumours in the nasal cavity of Syrian golden hamsters (Table 1). Nitrosamines and their pre-cursors are ubiquitous in our environment and some are present in tobacco products. The induced tumours were generally found in all three portions of the nasal cavity and involved the entire spectrum of

Table 1. Carcinogenic agents which induce nasal cavity tumours in Syrian golden hamsters.

Carcinogen	Diagnosis of nasal cavity tumours	References
N-Nitrosodimethylamine	Esthesioneuroepithelial tumours	Herrold, 1964a,b, 1967
N-Nitrosodiethylamine	Olfactory neuroepithelium tumours; carcinomas derived from neuroblasts; adenocarcinomas derived from basal cells and sustentacular cell carcinomas; neuroepithelial tumours;squamous cell papillomas	Montesano & Saffiotti, 1968 Reznik-Schüller, 1978, Stenbäck, 1973
N-Nitrosodiethanolamine	Poorly differentiated adenocarcinomas	Hilfrich *et al.*, 1978
N-Nitroso-di-n-propylamine	Carcinomas originating in the olfactory epithelium (composed of basal cells and sustentacular cells);mucoepidermoid carcinomas	Pour *et al.*, 1974
N-Nitroso-β-hydroxypropyl-n-propylamine	Carcinomas originating in the olfactory epithelium (composed of basal cells and sustentacular cells); mucoepidermoid carcinomas	Pour *et al.*, 1974
N-Nitroso-β-oxopropyl-n-propylamine	Carcinomas originating in the olfactory epithelium (composed of basal cells and sustentacular cells); mucoepidermoid carcinomas	Pour *et al.*, 1974
N-Nitrosomethyl-n-propylamine	Carcinomas originating in the olfactory epithelium (composed of basal cells and and sustentacular cells); mucoepidermoid carcinomas	Pour *et al.*, 1974, 1979
N-Nitroso-1-oxopropyl-propylamine	No histological diagnosis	Althoff, 1977
N-Nitroso-bis(2-hydroxypropyl)amine	Papillomas, tumours, squamous cell carcinomas, adenocarcinomas	Althoff, 1977
N-Nitroso(2-hydroxypropyl)-(2-oxopropyl)amine	Squamous cell papillomas, mucoepidermoid tumours, squamous cell carcinomas, adenocarcinomas	Pour *et al.*, 1979
N-Nitrosomethyl-n-propylamine	Adenocarcinomas and poorly differentiated carcinomas of posterior region of nasal cavity	Pour *et al.*, 1979
N-Nitrosomorpholine	Olfactory neuroepitheliomas, mixed tumours, adenocarcinomas, anaplastic adenocarcinomas, squamous carcinomas, squamous papillomas	Haas *et al.*, 1973

Table 1 (Contd)

Carcinogen	Diagnosis of nasal cavity tumours	References
N-Nitroso-2,6-dimethylmorpholine	Adenocarcinoma in posterior region of nasal cavity papillomas, papillary polyps in anterior region of nasal cavity	Althoff *et al.*, 1973 Reznik *et al.*, 1978
N-Nitrosopiperidine	Adenocarcinomas, squamous carcinomas, olfactory neuroepitheliomas	Haas *et al.*, 1973
N-Nitrosopyrrolidine	Not specified	McCoy *et al.*, 1980
N-Nitrosohexamethyleneimine	Adenocarcinomas, carcinomas, esthesio-neuroepitheliomas, papillomas	Althoff *et al.*, 1973
N-Nitrosoheptamethyleneimine	Polyps, adenosquamous carcinomas,	Lijinsky *et al.*, 1970
N-Nitrosonornicotine	Papillomas, adenocarcinomas	Hilfrich *et al.*, 1977, Rivenson *et al.*, 1980
N-Nitrosodiallylamine	Adenocarcinomas, papillary polyps	
4-(Methylnitrosamino)-1-(3-pyridyl)-1-butanone (NNK)	Squamous cell carcinomas, adenocarcinomas, esthesioneuroepithelioma	Rivenson *et al.*, 1983
Cigarette smoke (inhalation)	Adenocarcinoma	Schreider, 1983
Dimethylcarbamoyl chloride (inhalation)	Squamous cell carcinomas	Herrold, 1964a
Acetaldehyde (inhalation)	Squamous cell carcinoma	Feron & Woutersen, 1980

histopathological tumour types listed above. Some of these agents (e.g., *N*-nitrosodiethylamine) yielded a tumour incidence of 100% in the nasal cavity of hamsters (Reznik-Schüller, 1983).

COMPARATIVE ASPECTS

The nasal cavity in man is generally shorter, less complex and has a smaller surface area than that of laboratory rodents including the hamster (Schreider, 1983). Moreover, humans do not have a clear-cut separation between the respiratory and olfactory portions of the nasal cavity (Mohr, 1982). With respect to the anatomical differences, the response to inhaled noxious agents is likely to be quite different in man and hamster, while responses to systemic exposure may be similar because basically the same cell types are present in both species.

Identical histological tumour types are found in the nasal cavities of man and hamster, although their frequency and localization may differ (Mohr, 1982). Among the laboratory rodents, the hamster nasal cavity appears to be particularly sensitive to the carcinogenic effects of *N*-nitrosamines, while it seems considerably less sensitive to inhaled carcinogens than that of the rat.

REFERENCES

Althoff, J., Cardesa, A., Pour, P. & Mohr, U. (1973) Carcinogenic effect of *N*-nitrosohexamethyleneimine in Syrian golden hamsters. *J. Natl Cancer Inst.*, 73, 323–329

Althoff, J., Grandjean, C., Gold, B. & Runge, P. (1977) Carcinogenicity of 1-oxopropylpropylnitrosamine in Syrian hamsters. *Z. Krebsforsch. Klin. Oncol.*, 90, 221–225

Althoff, J., Grandjean, C. & Gold, B. (1978) Carcinogenic effect of subcutaneously administered *N*-nitroso-2,6-dimethyl-morpholine in Syrian golden hamsters. *J. Natl Cancer Inst.*, 60, 197

Bernfeld, P. Homburger, F. & Russfield, A.B. (1974) Strain differences of inbred Syrian hamsters to cigarette smoke inhalation. *J. Natl Cancer Inst.*, 53, 1141–1157

Feron, V. & Woutersen, R. (1980) Respiratory tract tumours in hamsters exposed to formaldehyde vapour alone or simultaneously with benzo(a)pyrene. Abstracts of Symposium on Co-carcinogenesis and Biological Effects of Tumour Promoters, Klais, West Germany

Haas, H., Mohr, U. & Krüger, F.W. (1973) Comparative studies with different doses of *N*-nitrosomorpholine, *N*-nitrosopiperidine, *N*-nitrosomethylurea, and dimethylnitrosamine in Syrian golden hamsters. *J. Natl Cancer Inst.*, 51, 1295–1301

Herrold, K.M. (1964a) Induction of olfactory neuroepithelium tumours in Syrian hamsters by diethylnitrosamine. *Cancer*, 17, 114–121

Herrold, K.M. (1964b) Epithelial papillomas of the nasal cavity. Experimental induction in Syrian hamsters. *Arch. Pathol.*, 78, 189–195

Herrold, K.M. (1967) Histogenesis of malignant liver tumours induced by dimethylnitrosamine. An experimental study with Syrian hamsters. *J. Natl Cancer Inst.*, 39, 1099–1111

Hilfrich, J., Hecht, S.S. & Hoffman, D. (1977) A study of tobacco carcinogenesis. XV. Effects of N'-nitrosonornicotine and N'-nitrosoanabasine in Syrian golden hamsters. *Cancer Lett.*, 2, 169–176

Hilfrich, J., Schmeltz, T. & Hoffmann, D. (1977) Effects of *N*- nitrosodiethanolamine and 1,1-diethanolhydrazine in Syrian golden hamsters. *Cancer Lett.*, 4, 55–60

Lijinsky, W., Ferrero, A., Montesano, R. & Wenyon, C.E. (1970) Tumorigenicity of cyclic nitrosamines in Syrian golden hamsters. *Z. Krebsforsch.*, 74, 185–189

McCoy, G.D., Hecht, S.S., Chen, C.B., Katayama, S., Rivenson, A., Hoffman, D. & Wynder, E.L. (1980) Influence of chronic ethanol consumption on the metabolism and carcinogenicity of *N*-nitrosopyrrolidine and *N*-nitrosonornicotine in Syrian golden hamsters. *Proc. Am. Assoc. Cancer Res.*, 21, 100

Mohr, U. (1982) Tumours of the respiratory tract. In: Turusov, V.S., ed., *Pathology of Tumours in Laboratory Animals*, Vol. III, *Tumours of the Hamster* (IARC Scientific Publications No. 34), Lyon, IARC, pp. 115–146

Montesano, R. & Saffiotti, U. (1968) Carcinogenic response of the respiratory tract of Syrian golden hamsters in different doses of diethylnitrosamine. *Cancer Res.*, 28, 2197–2210

Pour, P., Cardesa, A., Althoff, J. & Mohr, U. (1974) Tumorigenesis in the nasal olfactory region of Syrian golden hamsters as a result of di-n-propylnitrosamine and related compounds. *Cancer Res.*, 34, 16–26

Pour, P., Mohr, U., Cardesa, A., Althoff, J. & Kmoch, N. (1976a) Spontaneous tumours and common diseases in two colonies of Syrian hamsters. II. Respiratory tract and digestive system. *J. Natl Cancer Inst.*, 56, 937–948

Pour, P., Stanton, M.F., Kuschner, M., Laskin, S. & Shabad, L.M. (1976b) Tumours of the respiratory tract. In: Turusov, V.S., ed., *Pathology of Tumours in Laboratory Animals*, Vol. 1, *Tumours of the Rat* (IARC Scientific Publications No. 6), Lyon, International Agency for Research on Cancer, pp. 1–37

Pour, P., Wallcave, L., Gingell, R. & Mohr, U. (1979) Carcinogenic effect of N-nitroso-(2-hyroxypropyl)(2-oxypropyl)amine, a postulated proximate pancreatic carcinogen in Syrian hamsters. *Cancer Res.*, 39, 3828–3833

Reznik, G. (1983) Comparative anatomy and histomorphology of the nasal and paranasal cavities in rodents. In: Reznik, G. & Stinson, S.F., eds, *Nasal Tumours in Animals and Man*, Vol. III, Boca Raton, CRC Press, pp. 35–44

Reznik, G., Mohr, U. & Lijinsky, W. (1978) Carcinogenic effect of N-nitroso-2,6-dimethylmorpholine in Syrian golden hamsters. *J. Natl Cancer Inst.*, 60, 371–378

Reznik-Schüller, H.M. (1978) Ultrastructure of N-diethylnitrosamine-induced tumours in the nasal olfactory region of the Syrian golden hamster. *J. Pathol.*, 124, 161–164

Reznik-Schüller, H.M. (1983) Nitrosamine-induced nasal cavity carcinogenesis. In: Reznik, G. & Stinson, S.F., eds, *Nasal Tumours in Animals and Man*, Vol. III, Boca Raton, CRC Press, pp. 47–78

Rivenson, A., Ohmori, T., Hecht, S.S. & Hoffmann, D. (1980) Organotropic carcinogenicity of tobacco specific N-nitrosamines. Proc. 5th Meeting Eur. Ass. Cancer Res., Vienna, Abstracts, Vienna, Kugler Publications, p. 51

Rivenson, A., Furguya, K., Hecht, S.S. & Hoffmann, D. (1983) Experimental nasal cavity tumours induced by tobacco-specific nitrosamines. In: Reznik, G. & Stinson, S.F., eds, *Nasal Tumours in Animals and Man*, Vol. III, Boca Raton, CRC Press, pp. 79–114

Schreider, J.P (1983) Nasal airway anatomy and inhalation deposition in experimental animals and people. In: Reznik, G. & Stinson, S.F., eds, *Nasal Tumours in Animals and Man*, Vol. III, CRC Press, Boca Raton, pp. 1–26

Sellakumar, A.R., Laskin, S., Kuschner, M., Rusch, G.., Katz, G.V., Snyder, C.A. & Albert, R.E. (1980) Inhalation carcinogenesis by dimethylcarbamoyl chloride in Syrian golden hamsters. *J. Environ. Pathol. Toxicol.*, 4, 107–115

Stenbäck, F. (1973) Glandular tumours of the nasal cavity induced by diethylnitrosamine in Syrian golden hamsters. *J. Natl Cancer Inst.*, 50, 895–898

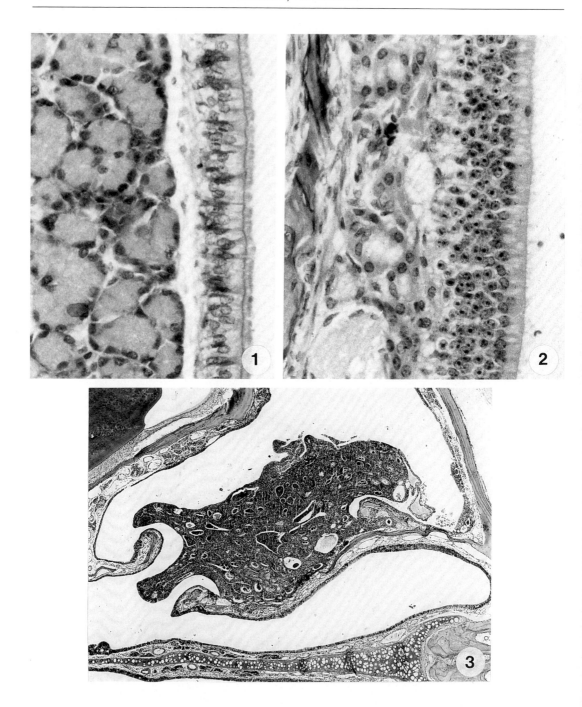

Figure 1. Normal epithelium in the respiratory portion of the nasal cavity: the pseudostratified epithelium consists of ciliated cells, mucous cells and basal cells. H & E; × 450

Figure 2. Normal epithelium in the olfactory region of the nasal cavity: the pseudostratified epithelium consists of olfactory sensory cells, sustentacular cells, and basal cells. H & E; × 350

Figure 3. Adenoma in the nasoturbinal of the respiratory portion of the nasal cavity: the tumour demonstrates a gland-like growth pattern and does not invade adjacent tissues. H & E; × 40

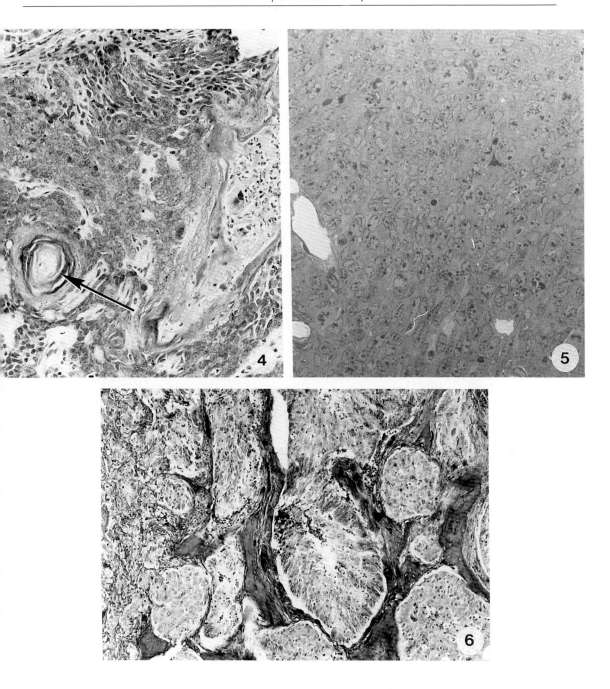

Figure 4. Part of a squamous cell carcinoma in the respiratory portion of the nasal cavity: the tumour cells invade muscle tissues and demonstrate formation of keratin (arrowed). H & E; × 160

Figure 5. Well differentiated adenocarcinoma arising from submucous glands in the respiratory portion of the nasal cavity: tall columnar tumour cells grow in a glandular pattern. H & E; × 160

Figure 6. Poorly differentiated adenocarcinoma in the olfactory portion of the nasal cavity: the tumour is highly cellular and compact with only occasional gland-like structures and invades the nasal bones. H & E; × 160

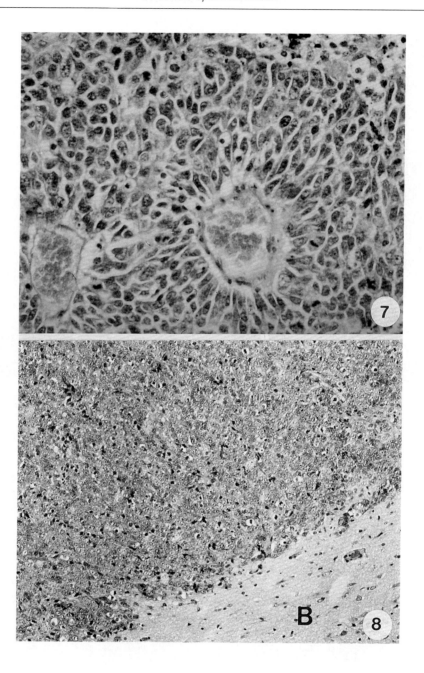

Figure 7. Part of a well differentiated carcinoma in the olfactory portion of the nasal cavity: the tumour cells grow in a rosette-like pattern which allows to classify this tumour as esthesioneuroepithelioma. H & E; × 600

Figure 8. Poorly differentiated olfactory carcinoma: the tumour is highly cellular and does not form rosette-like structures while invading the brain (B). H & E; × 160

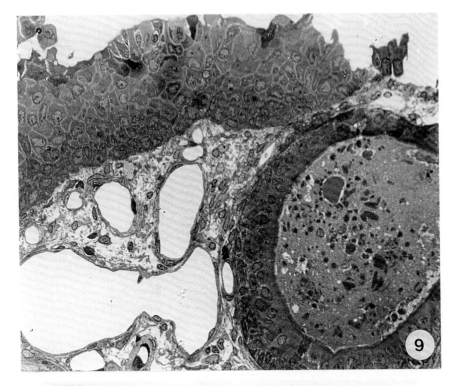

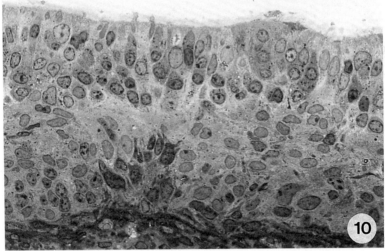

Figure 9. Hyperplasia and squamous metaplasia of the respiratory epithelium: the epithelium is multilayered with prominent intercellular bridges between cells and keratin formation at the surface. H & E; × 250

Figure 10. Hyperplasia and dysplasia of the olfactory epithelium: note that the altered epithelial focus is located in the basal part of the epithelium, while the olfactory epithelium at the surface remains intact. H & E; × 450

Tumours of the lower respiratory tract

U. MOHR, M. EMURA, D.L. DUNGWORTH AND H. ERNST

In attempts to find appropriate animal models for human lung cancer, many experimental studies have used rats or mice treated with chemicals, viruses or radiation. Since the successful induction of tumours in the respiratory system of the Syrian golden hamster (Della Porta *et al.*, 1958), however, this species has also been used for lung carcinogenesis research. Carcinogenic responsiveness of the respiratory tract differs greatly between species, and this has been best documented between the rat and hamster (Mohr & Dungworth, 1988); these differences are crucial considerations in the design and interpretation of experimental studies.

This chapter updates the one which appeared in the first edition of this monograph. Recent work has been focused mainly on two topics. One is the development of proliferative foci of pulmonary neuroendocrine cells in hamsters treated with nitrosamines or nitroquinoline oxide and exposed to hyperoxic atmospheres (Schuller *et al.*, 1988, 1990; Nylen *et al.*, 1990; Ito *et al.*, 1992; Sunday & Willett, 1992). The other topic relates to detailed pathogenetic studies of bronchiolo-alveolar carcinomas induced by N-nitrosomethyl-n-heptylamine (Rehm *et al.*, 1993; Rehm & Lijinsky, 1994).

NORMAL STRUCTURE

The skeleton of the larynx is formed by cartilage, connective tissue and muscles.

The lumen extends from the epiglottis to the plica laryngica and the trachea, and continues into that of the trachea. The trachea consists of 16–20 incomplete hyaline cartilaginous rings connected to each other by the ligamentum interanulare. The dorsal extremities of the cartilage are closed by the pars membranacea, which also contains smooth muscle fibres inserting into the cartilage. The structure of the stem and main bronchi is similar in character, but the cartilaginous rings in the main bronchi are often irregular. The intrapulmonary bronchi are free of cartilage and have a muscular ring structure.

Histologically, the respiratory epithelium has the same basic pattern: a basement membrane separates the vascularized connective tissue from pseudostratified or one-layered epithelium. The columnar cells lining the surface are ciliated cells, and various types of non-ciliated secretory goblet cells. Pseudostratified epithelium is seen in the nasal cavities, larynx, trachea and bronchi (Ehard, 1973).

Mucus glands are found in the subepithelial connective tissue and are of tubuloacinary type in the trachea. Where glands are prominent, secretory cells in the epithelium appear to be fewer in number.

Non-ciliated brush cells, which were described in the rat tracheal epithelium by Rhodin and Dalham (1956), are rarely seen among the cells lining the surface of the Syrian hamster trachea.

Neuroendocrine cells have been identified as solitary cells in the epithelium of trachea, extrapulmonary bronchi and intrapulmonary airways of neonatal and adult hamsters (see review by Sorokin & Hoyt, 1989). They have also been found in the submucosal glands of trachea and bronchi. They also form so-called neuroepithelial bodies in the fetal hamster trachea and in the intrapulmonary airways of fetal, neonatal and adult hamsters (see review by Sorokin & Hoyt, 1989). Association with nerve endings has been observed.

Additional details on the architecture of the tracheobronchial tree, and on the cells lining it, can be found in the comparative reviews by Mariassy (1992) and McBride (1992).

The histological patterns of the respiratory epithelium change strikingly in the alveoli. Two main epithelial cell types are found forming a mosaic. Attenuated lining cells (type I) are interspersed among occasional cuboidal cells (type II) and both are supported by thin septa of connective tissue containing the alveolar capillaries (Weibel, 1973).

Although the basic structures of respiratory epithelium are similar in various mammalian species, including the Syrian hamster, important cytochemical, immunocytochemical and ultrastructural differences have been described by several authors (Plopper *et al.*, 1983; Plopper & Dungworth, 1987; Massaro, 1989). Additional details on gross and microscopic features are provided by Bivin *et al.* (1987).

MORPHOLOGY AND BIOLOGY OF TUMOURS

The first classification of respiratory tract tumours, the so-called 'proposal B' (Nettesheim *et al.*, 1970; Mohr, 1982), was later modified in the light of various sets of data (Stünzi *et al.*, 1974; Pour *et al.*, 1976b; Jones *et al.*, 1985; Mohr & Dungworth, 1988). Basically, lower respiratory tract tumours in the Syrian golden hamster can be classified in a similar manner to those of rats (Mohr *et al.*, 1990), except for the cystic squamous cell tumours in the bronchiolo-alveolar region, which have not been observed in the hamster as yet. Listed below are the main types of tumours in the hamster according to the modified classification.

Squamous cell tumours

    Squamous cell papilloma (laryngeal/ tracheobronchial region)

    Squamous cell carcinoma (laryngeal-tracheobronchial/bronchiolo-alveolar region)

    Spindle-cell variants

Adenomas and adenocarcinomas

    Adenoma and adenocarcinoma (tracheobronchial region)

    Bronchiolo-alveolar tumour (Clara cells and/or type II pneumocytes)

Adenosquamous carcinomas

    Adenosquamous carcinoma

Neuroendocrine cell tumours

    'Clear cell' tumour

    Neuroendocrine tumour of bronchiolo-alveolar region

Undifferentiated/poorly differentiated tumours

    Small cell carcinoma

    Large cell carcinoma

    Mixed tumours (carcinosarcomas)

Mesenchymal tumours

Tumours of neurogenic tissues

Gross appearance

Larynx, trachea, extrapulmonary bronchi

Papillary tumours of the larynx, trachea and extrapulmonary bronchi occur as single or multiple neoplasms. Pedunculated nodules up to 8 mm in diameter may occasionally be found and the neoplasms frequently originate in the membranous part. The pearly white or grey, often cauliflower-like nodules have a coarse granular surface and frequently occlude the lumen. In such instances, the lungs can have various patterns of hyper-inflation and atelectasis. Concurrent acute bronchitis or pneumonia can be observed and bleeding can occur. Macroscopically, invasive growth can sometimes be seen, since malignant tumours destroy the cartilage and invade the paratracheal tissue and the mediastinum, or the adjacent pulmonary lobes.

Lungs

Neoplasms in the lungs of hamsters are often visible at the lung surface. Small, white, sometimes multiple nodules are usually seen. On section, they are found to encroach on or invade the underlying lung parenchyma. Distinct, round, single (or multiple), yellow-grey nodules at the surface and in the lung parenchyma, similar to those found in human pulmonary 'adenomatosis', are rarely found (Herrold, 1967). Tumours have been observed to develop from the small bronchi or the bronchiolo-alveolar region as small nodular lesions invading the lung parenchyma (Montesano & Saffiotti, 1968a,b; Rehm *et al.*, 1989, 1993; Rehm & Lijinsky, 1994). Large tumours may be seen originating in the central parts of the lung. Small neoplasms are difficult or impossible to identify macroscopically; larger white nodules with glistening cut surfaces or containing cystic cavities filled with reddish-brown fluid are readily detected. Haemorrhagic masses may be present at the pleural surface, with invasion of the diaphragm and mediastinum.

Histological types of tumour

Squamous cell papillomas

Papillary or villous neoplasms (papillomas) occur in the larynx, trachea and bronchi of Syrian golden hamsters. Usually they originate from the airway surface lining epithelium (Figure 1). It is uncertain whether these types of tumour can also originate in the epithelium of submucosal glands.

Papillary tumours usually have a well vascularized, ramiform or stem-like stalk composed of a loose, poorly cellular connective tissue (Figure 2). The vessels are thin-walled and apparently develop from the subepithelial vessels. The subepithelial connective tissue continues into the tumour stalk without any clear demarcation. Signs of oedema may be observed. In some instances, lymphocytic, plasmacytic or polymorphonuclear cells infiltrate the stalk and the connective tissue of the tumours (Herrold & Dunham, 1962). A clear basal lamina separates the connective tissue from the tumour epithelium. At the base of the papillary neoplasms this basal lamina continues, without change in morphological appearance, into the lamina basalis of the non-tumorous parts of the respiratory epithelium. The basal lamina is interrupted by downgrowth of small cords of undifferentiated epithelial neoplastic cells only on relatively rare occasions (Dontenwill & Mohr, 1962a; Herrold & Dunham, 1963; Montesano & Saffiotti, 1968a). Towards the lumen of the airway, the lamina basalis of the papillary tumours is lined by a dense layer of ovoid basal cells, followed by 1–7 layers of intermediate, less-differentiated cells. Well differentiated cells, however, can be seen in the surface lining layers. In squamous cell papillomas, the surface lining cells undergo a metaplastic change into stratified squamous epithelium (Figure 3). The superficial cells sometimes show intensively stained keratohyaline granules, and keratinization and pearl formation might be found. These characteristics are frequently seen in papillary tumours of the larynx. In other parts of the respiratory system, mixed cell papillomas are more common. These papillomas have an epithelial lining formed by polygonal or sometimes by cuboidal or columnar cells. They occasionally assume an adenomatous appearance with the cells frequently containing mucus granules

(PAS-positive) and intracytoplasmic lumina filled with PAS-positive material (Wahnschaffe *et al.,* 1987). Well differentiated goblet cells are sometimes seen in the intermediate layers, admixed with a population of variously differentiated cells. Adenomatous areas alternate with less differentiated cells. Ciliated cells may be detected in these papillary tumours, both at the surface and in the intermediate zone. Invasive patterns have never been reported.

At the base of the stalks of papillary tumours, a clear boundary between the normal respiratory epithelium and the tumour epithelium can only rarely be seen. In most instances, the adjacent respiratory epithelium has also undergone extensive changes (hyperplasia, dysplasia, metaplasia).

Squamous cell carcinomas

These tumours can be induced by various carcinogenic agents in the larynx, trachea, bronchi, bronchioli and bronchiolo-alveolar areas (Rabson *et al.,* 1960; Herrold & Dunham, 1962; Dontenwill & Mohr, 1962b; Saffiotti *et al.,* 1964, 1966, 1967, 1968, 1972a,b; Gross *et al.,* 1965; Saffiotti, 1970; Henry & Kaufmann, 1973; Henry *et al.,* 1973, 1975; Schreiber *et al.,* 1974; Reznik-Schüller & Mohr, 1974a,b, 1975; Rehm & Lijinsky, 1994). The tumours consist of interdigitating masses and cords of cells manifesting various degrees of squamous differentiation. Abundant keratin and pearl formation are sometimes seen (Figures 4 and 5), but moderate amounts of keratinization (Figures 6 and 7) and less differentiated patterns are usual (Figures 8 and 9). The tumour cells show polymorphism and have hyperchromatic or large vesicular nuclei with prominent nucleoli. They are sometimes anaplastic. Cell boundaries are usually distinct. Keratohyaline granules and keratin are seen in the surface lining areas and in the tumour 'pearls'. Mitotic figures are frequent. The amount of

connective tissue and vascularization varies. Tumours originating in bronchiolo-alveolar regions tend to destroy alveolar framework by forming nodules which are often multilobular.

Carcinomas of a spindle cell type found in larynx or trachea consist of an exophytic portion and an infiltrating portion which grows in a circumferential pattern between the tracheal or laryngeal mucosa and the cartilage rings (Stinson *et al.,* 1983). The epithelium overlying the neoplasms is mostly intact and varies from having a relatively normal morphological appearance over the infiltrating portion to being dysplastic or anaplastic over the exophytic portion. The tumour cells have oval nuclei and the cytoplasm is elongated and attenuated. Nests of anaplastic epithelial cells are surrounded by sheets of the spindle cells. An apparent transition can be seen from the overlying epithelial cells into the spindle cells. Electron-microscopically, the tumours consist of squamous cells with various degrees of differentiation. They are linked by numerous desmosomes and their cytoplasm contains bundles of tonofilaments and various quantities of keratohyaline granules. Hence, the tumours are considered to be a variant of squamous cell carcinomas. Mature keratin is lacking, however. The endoplasmic reticulum is generally poorly developed, and neither formation of mucus nor granules of endocrine type are detected.

Squamous cell carcinomas may also arise from benign papillary tumours. Small basaloid or spindle-cell-like foci in squamous cell papillomas may invade their own stroma or the subepithelial layers of the airway. The basal lamina is destroyed, and even cartilage sometimes invaded. Neoplastic spread to more peripheral tissues is rarely observed. Tumour cells are mainly found in small nests and cords. The degree of differentiation is usually low, and keratin formation is unusual.

Adenomas

Adenomas of the lower respiratory tract develop either spontaneously or, in relatively few instances, after application of chemical carcinogens or inhalation of radionuclides (Hahn, 1985). The tumours appear to develop from the tracheobronchial epithelium, including submucosal glands, or from the bronchiolo-alveolar region. The low incidence makes it difficult to investigate their origin properly and to classify them accurately.

The morphological pattern of bronchiolo-alveolar adenomas is often similar to that seen in mice (Kauffman & Sato, 1985a, b). The growth is nodular (Figures 10 and 12), or sometimes papillary (Figure 11). In certain adenomas cells are vacuolized (Figures 12 and 13). A true capsule is absent. The surrounding lung parenchyma is often compressed to form a pseudocapsule in immersion-fixed lung specimens, but this is mainly an artifact of post-mortem collapse and contraction. Small neoplasms occasionally have poorly defined edges. One or two layers of tumour cells are separated by a delicate, capillarized connective-tissue stroma. The tumour cells form tubulo-papillary, alveolar or solid structures and lumina are sometimes filled with condensed mucus. The cells are uniform and cuboidal, and the spherical nuclei are centrally placed and show very few cytological abnormalities. Mitosis is rare. One observation of benign tumours with squamous and adenomatous differentiation has been reported (Montesano *et al.*, 1970).

The term 'pulmonary adenomatosis', as used in the earlier literature on experimental pulmonary carcinogenesis, lumped together bronchiolo-alveolar neoplasms (both benign and malignant) and the hyperplastic changes in bronchiolar and alveolar type II cells associated with carcinogen-induced injury and inflammation. Since the neoplasms appear to arise from the background of hyperplastic changes, it is not possible to make a clean separation between hyperplasia and neoplasia by routine histological methods. The use of the term pulmonary adenomatosis should be discontinued, however, because it merely confuses the issue.

Adenocarcinomas

Adenocarcinomas originate in the tracheobronchial epithelium (including submucosal glands) or bronchiolo-alveolar epithelium. The neoplasms in the tracheobronchial region form nodules without demarcation from the surrounding tissue. Neoplastic cells have pleomorphic, sometimes hyperchromatic, and foamy nuclei. Giant cells are occasionally seen. The cells frequently form irregular, tubular or trabecular patterns and papillary growth has been observed. PAS-positive mucus can be abundant in the lumina of acinar structures and in the cells themselves.

Bronchiolo-alveolar adenocarcinomas can be seen forming nodules (Figure 14) with distorted tubulo-papillary (Figures 15 and 16), alveolar or solid patterns. The neoplastic cells (Figure 17) are often columnar with large, pleomorphic, vesicular and hyperchromatic nuclei. The cytoplasm is pale and slightly eosinophilic. The cells in certain cases show a positive PAS reaction and cover the walls of adjacent alveoli. Lumina, when present, are frequently filled with one or more of mucus, macrophages and cell debris (Figure 15). Dontenwill and Mohr (1962c) have described cuboidal or columnar cells, and occasionally also ciliated and mucus-producing cells, lining the spaces of the alveoli, bronchioli and bronchi in an irregular manner. The connective tissue appears to be thickened and invaded by neoplastic cells. Inflammatory cell infiltrations are frequent. The lumina are filled with mucus and cell debris.

The most precise information on the origin of bronchiolo-alveolar tumours in hamsters comes from the *N*-nitroso-methyl-n-heptylamine model (Rehm *et al.*,

1993). Using histological, ultrastructural, immunohistochemical and immuno-cytochemical examinations of sequentially sampled pulmonary tissue, these investigators concluded that the bronchiolo-alveolar carcinomas were derived from proliferating and distally-migrating Clara cells. Rehm and associates furthermore concluded that neoplastic Clara cells, or undifferentiated cells derived from them, were capable of differentiating into ciliated or mucous cells. This would account for the mixed cell types occasionally seen by themselves and others (Dontenwill & Mohr, 1962c). The role of alveolar type II cells in giving rise to bronchiolo-alveolar tumours in hamsters is still unclear. Reznik-Schuller and Reznik (1979) provided ultrastructural evidence that some of the bronchiolo-alveolar tumours might be of type II cell origin. Rehm *et al.* (1993), on the other hand, considered type II cells in the tumours they examined to be entrapped, non-neoplastic components. Two general observations seem to be in order. One is that because of the variety of evidence indicating phenotypic lability of both Clara and alveolar type II cells, it would be dangerous to make sweeping statements about the cell of origin of bronchiolo-alveolar tumours in any species. The second observation is that the relative importance of Clara cells and alveolar type II cells in giving rise to bronchiolo-alveolar tumours almost certainly will depend on the carcinogenic agent and the mechanisms by which it induces cancer.

Adenosquamous carcinomas

Adenosquamous carcinomas develop in the larynx, trachea, bronchi and pulmonary parenchyma. They frequently show adenomatous structural patterns, less differentiated squamous cell features, and sometimes clusters of anaplastic cells (Figure 18). These three components are often found together in large tumours. Some of the cells have intracellular PAS-positive material. Giant cells with bizarre-shaped nuclei are occasionally found. Scattered areas of glandular structure and spindle-cell patterns are also seen. Parts of the tumour may show marked keratinization, but this is rare; however, epidermoid elements are an integral component.

This category of tumours merges with adenocarcinomas containing inconspicuous foci of squamous differentiation (Mohr *et al.*, 1990). A diagnosis of 'adenosquamous carcinoma' is justified only when substantial portions of the tumour consist of neoplastic squamous cells. Otherwise, the tumours should be considered as adenocarcinomas with squamous metaplasia. In the hamster tracheobronchial epithelium, several lines of evidence have been presented that metaplastic (squamous) and neoplastic lesions can arise as a direct consequence of modulation of the structure and function of fully differentiated mucous cells (Becci *et al.*, 1978, 1980; McDowell & Trump, 1983).

The origin of the squamous portions of pulmonary adenosquamous carcinomas induced by *N*-nitrosomethyl-n-heptyl-amine was shown by Rehm and Lijinsky (1994) to be by squamous differentiation of neoplastic Clara cells or undifferentiated neoplastic cells in bronchiolo-alveolar carcinomas, particularly those with an acinar adenocarcinomatous pattern. It is worth noting that the squamous components seemed to be poorly or non-keratinizing.

Neuroendocrine cell tumours

So-called 'clear cell' carcinomas and their precursor lesions have been reported to occur spontaneously at incidences of up to 9% in the larynx of Syrian hamsters (Pour, 1985). Recent observations in our laboratory indicate that these tumours are composed of neuroendocrine cells and that they occur also in the proximal trachea (Ernst *et al.*, 1995). There seems to be a continuum from minute intraepithelial neuroendocrine cell hyperplasia (Figure 19) to malignant neuroendocrine tumour (Figures 20 and 21). The overall frequency of neuroendocrine cell proliferations in the larynx and trachea of up to 25-month-old Han:AURA hamsters from a chronic inhalation toxicity study was 62/798 (7.8%). Sixteen cases were detected in the larynx, but the majority (46 cases) were located in the proximal trachea. There were no sex differences and no relationship to the treatment of the animals. Neuroendocrine cell proliferations occurred in old hamsters and were first observed at 15 months of age. Separation of the proliferative lesions into hyperplasia, adenoma or carcinoma is somewhat arbitrary. Since there is no pronounced cytological difference between hyperplasias and tumours, the diagnosis has to depend on criteria such as size of the lesion, depth of invasion into the submucosal tissues and metastases. The cells have abundant pale, nearly translucent cytoplasm with an irregular shape (Figure 21). The large nuclei are centrally located, round to ovoid and contain finely distributed chromatin and occasionally a large nucleolus. Mitotic figures are rare, even in invasive tumours. Ultrastructurally, the cytoplasm of the tumour cells contains dense-cored neuroendocrine granules and the nuclei show a characteristic marginal distribution pattern of heterochromatin. Immunohistochemical investigations revealed a positive reaction of the tumour cells to calcitonin and calcitonin gene-related peptide (CGRP), neuron-specific enolase (NSE) and serotonin (Ernst *et al.*, 1995). The benign neuroendocrine tumours exhibit a predominantly exophytic growth with no invasion into the submucosa. The malignant ones usually deeply invade the submucosal tissue. Occasionally, neuroendocrine tumours obliterate the laryngeal or tracheal lumen. The tumours may also include large amounts of a homogeneous eosinophilic

secretory product. Local spread of the tumours into the paralaryngeal and paratracheal tissue as well as distant metastases to the lungs are quite common.

Experimental induction of what were interpreted to be neuroendocrine cell tumours was first reported by Schuller *et al.* (1988). They occurred in hamsters treated with *N*-nitrosodiethylamine and simultaneously exposed to hyperoxia (70% oxygen atmosphere). Similar proliferations were produced in a repeat experiment with 60% oxygen atmosphere and *N*-nitrosodiethylamine (Nylen *et al.*, 1990) and with hyperoxia and NNK (Schüller *et al.*, 1990). The proliferations do not demonstrate the oat cell histology characteristic of small cell lung cancer in humans (Figure 22). They are always multiple, compact and highly cellular. Large areas of the proliferating cells are immunopositive for mammalian bombesin and calcitonin (Figure 23). Ultrastructurally, the majority of proliferating cells have numerous dense-cored granules that are characteristic of neuroendocrine cells (Figure 24). Currently, there is uncertainty as to the nature of the neuroendocrine cell proliferation in the hyperoxia/nitrosamine model. There is a strong possibility that the cells are hyperplastic rather than neoplastic (Sunday & Willett, 1992). In any event, evidence is lacking that truly malignant neuroendocrine cells have been induced.

Pulmonary small cell anaplastic carcinomas were reportedly also induced by intratracheal instillation of benzo[*a*]-pyrene or arsenic (Pershagen *et al.*, 1984), but there was no information as to whether neuroendocrine cells were involved.

Undifferentiated/poorly differentiated tumours

Undifferentiated and poorly differentiated tumours have been observed in the larynx, trachea and bronchi, and usually consist of a relatively large cell type (Montesano & Saffiotti, 1968a,b). Anaplastic tumours of the small-cell type have been found in animals treated with carcinogens as newborns or via the placenta *in utero* (Saffiotti, 1970; Montesano *et al.,* 1970). Histologically, the neoplasms vary greatly in phenotypic differentiation.

The neoplastic cells often possess all the characteristics of undifferentiated cells. They are usually polygonal in shape and small-cell areas are intermingled with large-cell areas. The cytoplasm is often pale and vacuolated. The nuclei are oval, sometimes bizarre and granular, and show one or two distinct nucleoli. The tumours do not usually develop any distinct pattern or architecture, but cords of tumour cells occasionally enclose tiny spaces.

Mixed tumours (carcinosarcomas)

Both carcinomatous and sarcomatous patterns, intricately mixed, have been reported in a tumour of the tracheal wall (Saffiotti *et al.,* 1968). The present definition of this tumour type is that both epithelial and mesenchymal neoplastic elements must be present.

Mesenchymal tumours

Sarcoma. Malignant mesenchymal neoplasms are rarely seen in the respiratory system of Syrian golden hamsters, but the characteristic patterns of fibrosarcomas and spindle-cell sarcomas of the lung have been reported following viral infection (Eddy *et al.,* 1958; Chesterman & Negroni, 1961). One round-cell sarcoma originating in the tracheal tissue after treatment with nitroso compounds has been described (Lijinsky *et al.,* 1970). Fibrosarcomas of the trachea were seen after BP application (Gross *et al.,* 1965; Saffiotti *et al.,* 1968; Stenbäck *et al.,* 1975).

Mesotheliomas have been induced by polyomavirus (Rabson *et al.,* 1960) and asbestos (Smith *et al.,* 1964). These tumours develop from the mesothelial cells of the pleura. They fill the pleural cavities and invade the diaphragm. Tumour cells are pleomorphic with nuclear hyperchromatism, and are arranged in nests and clusters; interspersed giant cells with vesicular or very bizarre nuclei are sometimes present. The possibility of distant metastasis cannot be eliminated (Rabson *et al.,* 1960).

Since there are few published reports of mesotheliomas in hamsters, a systematic classification as has been done for rats (see Mohr *et al.,* 1990) is difficult. Nonetheless, a tentative classification has been proposed, in which three histological types, epithelioid (Figure 25), fusiform (Figure 26) and mixed, are designated (Cardesa & Bombi, 1985).

The epithelioid type, most common in hamsters, consists of large polyhedral cells with abundant amphophilic cytoplasm and sharply defined cell contours. Tumours of this type frequently assume a papillary form but some have a nodular, tubular or gland-like form. The epithelioid cells contain diastase-labile, PAS-positive materials as well as hyaluronidase-labile, alcian blue-positive substances.

The fusiform cell type mainly contains cells with spindle-shaped cytoplasm, poorly defined cell contours and elongated nuclei. Tumours of this type are able to form collagen, imitating a fibrosarcoma-like pattern and sometimes mimicking malignant fibrous histiocytomas.

The mixed type has areas of a characteristic epithelioid pattern alternating with other areas of fusiform pattern.

Other mesenchymal tumours. One chondroma was reported in hamsters treated with dimethylbenz[*a*]anthracene (DMBA) (Della Porta *et al.,* 1958).

Biological behaviour

Papillary tumours of the larynx, trachea and bronchi in Syrian golden hamsters rarely invade adjacent tissues. Evidence of facultative malignancy in the case of these often well differentiated tumours has been obtained by successful transplantation of papillomas into hamster hosts (Herrold, 1964c). Papillomas are the commonest tumours to develop after treatment with various carcinogenic compounds. This shows that the tracheobronchial tree is particularly susceptible to the carcinogenic effects of different substances and is the main target organ.

Hamsters often develop large obstructive papillary tumours fairly soon after treatment has been started and die from suffocation. Many animals, therefore, do not live long enough for carcinomatous progression to be manifest. This may explain the relatively low frequency of bronchial carcinomas (Dontenwill & Mohr, 1961a, b; Montesano & Saffiotti, 1968a, b). Tracheal or bronchial carcinomas may invade the fat tissue around the lung hilus. Emboli and clusters of neoplastic cells can be found in the lumina of both small and large vessels. One report describes distant metastases in which tumour cells were found in the regional lymph nodes (Saffiotti *et al.*, 1966).

The frequency and localization of tumour development varies slightly after administration of different carcinogenic substances. Intratracheal application of BP/ferric oxide suspended in saline induces tumours of the larynx and trachea as well as bronchogenic neoplasms, but the stem and main bronchi were the main targets (Saffiotti *et al.*, 1966, 1968, 1972a, b; Saffiotti, 1969; Harris *et al.*, 1972; Farrell *et al.*, 1972; Farrell & Davis, 1974). These parts of the tracheobronchial tree are particularly exposed to the carcinogen, as shown by fluoroscopic studies.

Intratracheal instillation of other carcinogens (e.g., DMBA, tobacco tar or BP in mineral oil) leads to more reactions in the proximal part of the respiratory tree than in the distant lung parenchyma.

Non-neoplastic and atypical lesions

After treatment with carcinogens, Syrian golden hamsters develop acute and chronic inflammatory reactions and sometimes also necrosis and haemorrhages in the tracheobronchial tree. Hyperplasia of

basal cells and conversion into a multilayered epithelium is observed. Squamous metaplasia, together with nuclear polymorphism and cell atypia, is sometimes seen. Since these changes are also seen in the process of regeneration, it is difficult to be certain whether preneoplastic growth has taken place. Morphologically, it may be impossible to detect where normal epithelium, or epithelium that has already undergone certain changes, turns into neoplastic epithelium. It can only be assumed that loss of cell organization and orientation, in conjunction with cellular atypia, may be followed by neoplastic growth. In addition, inflammatory reactions, regenerative changes and atypical lesions may occur simultaneously. Tumours may also develop without previous changes in the epithelium.

Inflammatory reactions (laryngitis, tracheitis, bronchitis, pneumonia, abscesses, fibrosis) were commonly seen after intratracheal instillation of hydrocarbons (Della Porta *et al.*, 1958; Herrold & Dunham, 1962; Herrold, 1963, 1970; Gross *et al.*, 1965). However, administration of BP was reported to result only in a phagocytic reaction. The inflammatory reactions found in the animals were related to tumours causing obstruction of the tracheal and bronchial lumina (Saffiotti *et al.*, 1966, 1968).

Parenteral administration of nitroso compounds does not usually result in inflammatory reactions of the lower respiratory system (Dontenwill & Mohr, 1961a, b, 1962a; Montesano & Saffiotti, 1968a, b; Lijinsky *et al.*, 1970; Mohr, 1970; Mohr *et al.*, 1970; Althoff *et al.*, 1971a, b, 1973a, b, 1974; Feron *et al.*, 1972; Haas *et al.*, 1973), although some have been described (Rehm *et al.*, 1993). Changes in the epithelial lining were frequently found to be reversible and were classified as 'regenerative' (Herrold & Dunham, 1962). Basal cell hyperplasia and increase in mucus-producing cells were reversible changes, and even well differentiated squamous cell metaplasia in this part of the respiratory system of hamsters was found to be reversible.

However, with long-term exposure to cigarette smoke, a sequence of atypical changes was induced in the laryngeal epithelium, namely multi-layered epithelial hyperplasia (pachydermia) and leukoplakia (verrucous, papillomatous, pseudo-epitheliomatous) with atypical changes in the cell nuclei and proliferation of the basal layers (Dontenwill, 1970; Dontenwill *et al.*, 1973; Bernfeld *et al.*, 1974; Wehner *et al.*, 1974, 1976). Acanthosis, hyperkeratosis, parakeratosis or dyskeratosis were observed in these lesions. The final step in this sequence of changes was early invasive carcinoma. Some of the changes may have been irreversible and precancerous, especially in the presence of an increased mitosis rate and atypia (Della Porta *et al.*, 1958).

Non-invasive, proliferative lesions of the tracheal and bronchial epithelium were generally observed after administration of BP (Herrold & Dunham, 1962; Herrold, 1963) and treatment with nitroso compounds (Dontenwill & Mohr, 1962b; Dontenwill, 1964; Dontenwill & Wiebecke, 1964). Cellular differentiation was sometimes absent, and loss of cell orientation was seen. Polymorphous cells showed variations in nuclear size, shape and chromatin content, and a change in their nucleus:cytoplasm ratio.

Subcutaneous injection of NDEA led to induction of pulmonary neuroendocrine cell hyperplasias, which were detected by the presence of immunoreactive calcitonin, a marker of APUD-cells (Linnoila *et al.*, 1984). Hyperplasias of similar cell type also occur spontaneously in laryngeal and tracheal regions (see Figure 19).

In contrast to the epithelial changes seen in the larynx, trachea and large bronchi (hyperplasia, dysplasia, metaplasia) (Dontenwill & Mohr, 1962a), the epithelium of the small bronchi often had more widespread lesions together with

squamous cell metaplasia. The changes also involved the respiratory bronchioles and the adjacent alveolar ducts and spaces. Epithelial proliferations consisted of 'adenomatoid' structures made up of uniform cuboidal or columnar cells. The lesions were reported as 'bronchiolar proliferations with an adenomatous pattern' (Della Porta *et al.*, 1958; Herrold & Dunham, 1962) and as 'bronchiolar adenomatoid lesions' (Saffiotti *et al.*, 1966, 1967, 1968). A progression of hyperplasia and dysplasia of Clara cells to bronchioalveolar carcinoma, accompanied by evidence of Clara cell migration, has been described by Rehm *et al.* (1993). As mentioned previously, use of the term pulmonary adenomatosis to cover the range of lesions from bronchiolo-alveolar hyperplasia to neoplasia should be avoided. Use of 'adenomatoid' also leads to confusion and should be avoided. Preferable terms for non-neoplastic proliferations of bronchiolo-alveolar epithelium in response to injury are bronchioloalveolar hyperplasia (Figure 27) as used, for instance, by Marshall *et al.* (1987) or bronchiolization (Figure 28) as used by Dagle and Wehner (1985) and Ito (1985). Precise definitions of bronchiolo-alveolar hyperplasia and bronchiolization still need to be formulated, however, because we believe that, though overlapping, the two terms are not absolutely synonymous.

Irradiation of the lungs (De Villiers & Gross, 1966; Little *et al.*, 1970, 1973; Kennedy & Little, 1974a, b; Liscon *et al.*, 1974; Little & O'Toole, 1974; McGandy *et al.*, 1974) seemed to result in a well defined sequence of changes. Apart from typical radiation injury, there were hyperplastic lesions of conspicuous alveolar cellularity, clusters of cells with small, densely stained nuclei, and cells with basophilic cytoplasm and large nuclei. Nuclear atypia and small papillary formations developed from these hyperplastic changes.

SPONTANEOUS TUMOURS

The prevalence of naturally occurring ('spontaneous') lung tumours in the Syrian golden hamster is estimated to be not more than 0.1–0.5% (Mohr & Ketkar, 1980). These tumours are associated with minimal inflammatory lesions and histologically they can be separated from experimentally induced neoplasms (Homburger *et al.*, 1983). The hamster's respiratory tract has been considered an appropriate model system for studies of respiratory carcinogenesis (Mohr & Ketkar, 1980). Later, however, the hamster lung was proven particularly resistant to inhaled materials known to be carcinogenic in the rat (Mohr & Dungworth, 1988). As is the case with animal models generally, therefore, the suitability of the hamster for studies of respiratory carcinogenesis depends on the questions being asked in the study. Only a few adenocarcinomas have been seen among several thousand untreated hamsters (Fortner, 1957; Herrold & Dunham, 1962; Dontenwill & Mohr, 1962b). Tumours of the stem bronchi, trachea, larynx and nasal cavities have been reported occasionally in untreated hamsters (Pour *et al.*, 1976b). Of particular interest are the spontaneous clear cell tumours found in the larynx (Pour, 1985) and neuroendocrine cell tumours in the larynx and trachea (Ernst *et al.*, 1995). It appears that their frequency varies considerably between colonies of hamsters.

INDUCTION OF TUMOURS

Polycyclic hydrocarbons

A suspension of DMBA in 1% gelatin given to hamsters intratracheally induced tumours with various differentiation patterns from the larynx to the bronchi (Della Porta *et al.*, 1958). Similar results were seen with DMBA in mineral oil applied in the same way (Gross *et al.*, 1965).

Steel gauze impregnated with 3-methylcholanthrene (MC) was surgically implanted as a pellet into the stem bronchus.

Lung tumours were reported. Repeated weekly intratracheal instillation of MC in aqueous or colloidal suspension also led to lung tumours in hamsters (Laskin *et al.*, 1970).

Intratracheal administration of BP in Tween-60 to hamsters induced neoplasms of the trachea and bronchi (Herrold & Dunham, 1962). Oral application of BP in sesame oil resulted in tumours only in the trachea (Dontenwill & Mohr, 1962b). Intratracheal instillation of BP in mineral oil or suspended in gelatin led to lung tumours (Gross *et al.*, 1965). BP attached to ferric oxide and suspended in saline was given to hamsters intratracheally. Tumours of the trachea and the lungs were observed (Saffiotti *et al.*, 1966, 1968). Additional treatment with vitamin A after BP/ferric oxide application increased the latency period and decreased tumour incidence (Saffiotti *et al.*, 1967). A cumulative analysis of the results obtained from experiments with intrabronchial instillation of BP/ferric oxide has been made (Montesano *et al.*, 1970). Malignant neoplasms of the lung were also found after surgical implantation of pelleted gauze impregnated with BP into the bronchi (Laskin *et al.*, 1970).

Combined effects of arsenic and BP were studied after intratracheal instillation (Pershagen *et al.*, 1984). No marked potentiation was observed between the two compounds in the induction of either 'adenomatous' lesions or carcinomas. An increase in tumour frequency in the respiratory system was reported when hamsters were treated first with NDEA, and then with BP/ferric oxide in saline (Montesano & Saffiotti, 1968b).

Recently, a hypothesis has been developed that local retention of BP in the respiratory tract may be a critical factor in initiating a neoplastic process in the epithelial cells. This concept is based upon findings such as the fact that coarse BP particles instilled intratracheally clear less rapidly from the respiratory tract, causing higher incidences of respiratory tumours than the fine ones (Stenbäck & Roland, 1978; Feron *et al.*, 1980). When the hamsters were subjected to inhalation of BP instead of instillation, however, no tumours developed in the lower respiratory tract (Thyssen *et al.*, 1980). This is in sharp contrast to results with rats similarly subjected to BP inhalation, which developed a high incidence of respiratory tumours (Mohr *et al.*, 1990). The rats also have extensive inflammatory lesions with proliferative epithelial responses, whereas hamsters do not (Mohr & Dungworth, 1988). This difference in pathological reaction between hamsters and rats suggests a crucial association of BP-induced inflammation and epithelial proliferation in the rat with the subsequent development of epithelial neoplasms.

Urethane

Pulmonary 'adenomatosis' was found in hamsters receiving urethane in drinking-water (Toth *et al.*, 1961).

Isonicotinic acid hydrazide

Pulmonary 'adenomatosis' was also found when isonicotinic acid hydrazide was added to drinking-water (Toth & Boreisha, 1969).

Nitroso compounds

Oral application of NDEA led to neoplasms of the trachea and bronchi (Dontenwill & Mohr, 1961a,b). Similar results were obtained when NDEA was administered by inhalation (spray) or by subcutaneous injection (Dontenwill *et al.*, 1962). In addition to the neoplasms of the lower respiratory tract, tumours of the nasal cavities were observed after oral and intratracheal application of NDEA (Herrold & Dunham, 1963; Herrold, 1964b, c, d). Similar effects on the respiratory system were reported after intraperitoneal, intradermal or topical application of NDEA (Herrold, 1964d). A single dose of NDEA led to papillary tumours of

the trachea (Mohr *et al.*, 1966b). Implantation of pieces of trachea in the spleen resulted in tracheal tumours after treatment with NDEA (Dontenwill & Rucker, 1967; Mohr *et al.*, 1976). When the carcinogen was given subcutaneously to pregnant hamsters, the offspring developed tumours of the trachea 8–25 weeks after birth (Mohr *et al.*, 1966a, 1975). A cumulative analysis of experiments with subcutaneous injections of NDEA in Syrian golden hamsters has been made by Montesano *et al.* (1970).

In hamsters kept under hyperoxia, NDEA induced a high incidence of pulmonary neuroendocrine proliferations (Schuller *et al.*, 1988; Nylen *et al.*, 1990; Sunday & Willett, 1992).

Nitrosodibutylamine (NDBA) was given to hamsters intragastrically and tumours of the respiratory system were found (Mohr *et al.*, 1970). The same effect was observed after subcutaneous treatment (Althoff *et al.*, 1971). Nitrosobutylmethylamine was given subcutaneously and induced tumours of the respiratory system (Dontenwill, 1968). Subcutaneously injected *N*-nitrosovinylethylamine induced a high incidence of respiratory tract tumours (Green & Althoff, 1982).

4-(Methylnitrosamino)-1-(3-pyridyl)-1-butanone (NNK), a nitrosamine formed from nicotine during tobacco processing, storage and smoking, is also highly carcinogenic for the respiratory tract of the Syrian golden hamster after subcutaneous injection (Hecht *et al.*, 1983). NNK was also proven to be a potent inducer of pulmonary neuroendocrine cell proliferations when applied (subcutaneously) to hamsters under hyperoxia (Schüller *et al.*, 1990).

Nitrosopyrrolidine was found to induce tumours of the lower respiratory system (Dontenwill, 1968). Chronic alcohol consumption appears to enhance the carcinogenicity of this compound in the respiratory tract, while it scarcely affected the carcinogenicity of nitrosonornicotine in the same organ (McCoy *et al.*, 1981).

Of *N*-nitrosobis(2-hydroxypropyl)amine (NDHPA), *N*-nitrosobis(2-oxopropyl)amine (NDOPA), *N*-nitroso(2-hydroxypropyl)-(2-oxopropyl)amine (NHOPA) and *N*-nitroso-2,6-dimethylmorpholine (Me2NM), Me2NM appeared the most potent carcinogen in the hamster lung. NDHPA and NDOPA were next in potency and NHOPA was the least potent (Lijinsky *et al.*, 1984).

Both nitrosomorpholine and nitroso-piperidine administered in the drinking water for a lifetime induced squamous cell carcinomas and squamous cell papillomas in the larynx (Cardesa *et al.*, 1990). The former bore morphological and biological similarities to laryngeal squamous cell carcinomas in adult humans, but the latter were not similar to the squamous papillomas of infants and children. The mucoepidermoid papillomas induced in the trachea in the same experiment are considered to be a neoplasm peculiar to the Syrian hamster (Cardesa *et al.*, 1990).

Intratracheal application of *N*-methyl-*N*-nitrosourea gave rise to tumour development in the respiratory tract (Herrold, 1970; Grubbs *et al.*, 1981; Stinson *et al.*, 1983). By contrast, *N*-ethyl-*N*-nitrosourea applied in the same way was ineffective in inducing tracheal carcinomas (Grubbs *et al.*, 1981). Nitroso-methylurethane given to hamsters subcutaneously led only to pulmonary 'adeno-matosis' (Herrold, 1967).

Repeated administration of *N*-nitroso-methyl-n-heptylamine by gavage has been used as a model to study the pathogenesis of bronchio-alveolar carcinomas, adeno-squamous and squamous cell carcinomas in pulmonary parenchyma (Rehm *et al.*, 1993; Rehm & Lijinsky, 1994).

Cigarette smoke and tobacco tar

Tracheal neoplasms were found after exposure of hamsters to cigarette smoke for one year in inhalation chambers (Dontenwill & Mohr, 1962c; Dontenwill, 1964; Wynder & Hoffmann, 1969). Tumours of the larynx were found after inhalation of cigarette smoke for more than 24 months (Dontenwill, 1970; Dontenwill *et al.*, 1973; Wehner *et al.*, 1976; Bernfeld *et al.*, 1979). However, there have been no reports of tumour development due to cigarette smoke inhalation alone in regions of the respiratory tract distal to the trachea (Ketkar *et al.*, 1977; Bernfeld *et al.*, 1979, 1983; Reznik-Schüller, 1980).

The treatment of hamsters with NDEA followed by exposure in inhalation chambers to cigarette smoke or to various volatile aldehydes or acids resulted in various incidences of tracheal tumours (Wynder & Hoffmann, 1969). Inhalation experiments with cigarette smoke impregnated with methanolic solutions of NDEA, nitrosobutylmethylamine or nitrosopiperidine also showed similar effects on the respiratory system (Dontenwill, 1968).

Tobacco tar in sesame oil, applied as an oral spray to hamsters, caused tumours of the trachea (Dontenwill & Mohr, 1962c).

Radiation and radionuclides

Irradiation of the chest with X-rays (total dose 3912–4094 r), was reported to induce bronchogenic carcinomas of various morphologies including squamous cell carcinomas (De Villiers & Gross, 1966).

It appears difficult to induce lung tumours in Syrian golden hamsters with radionuclides, except with intratracheal instillation of polonium-210 plus haematite (Hahn, 1985) or saline (Shami *et al.*, 1982). Combined treatment by repeated intratracheal instillation of ^{210}Po and exposure to hyperoxia also led to induction of tumours (Witschi & Schuller, 1991). Another type of particle, zirconium dioxide ceramic, induced much higher incidences of pulmonary tumours when applied simultaneously with inhalation of plutonium (Thomas & Smith, 1979) than appeared after inhalation of plutonium-239 dioxide particles alone (Thomas *et al.*,

1981). Inhalation of a beta-emitter, cerium-141 dioxide, was also weakly carcinogenic to the lung of hamsters (Hahn, 1985).

Metals, minerals and fibres

As regards the respiratory carcinogenicity of beryllium, chromium and cadmium in Syrian hamsters, either no data are available or the experiments carried out do not allow a reliable judgement to be made (see Wilbourn *et al.*, 1986). Nickel and silica have been proven to be carcinogenic in rats, but results were negative in hamsters after inhalation or intratracheal instillation (see Mohr & Dungworth, 1988; Mohr *et al.*, 1990). Intratracheally instilled ferric oxide particles (without any other carcinogen simultaneously applied) can be carcinogenic to epithelium injured mechanically by cannulation, although these particles themselves are not tumorigenic (Keenan *et al.*, 1989).

Mesotheliomas of the pleura were reported after local application or single injection into the right pleural cavity of amosite or of hard or soft chrysotile (Smith *et al.*, 1964).

Intratracheal instillation of glass fibres and crocidolite led to development of no tumours of the respiratory tract in one study (Feron *et al.*, 1985), whereas there was a low incidence of lung carcinomas and a moderate number of mesotheliomas in another study (Mohr *et al.*, 1984).

After similar application, chrysotile and amphibole induced a relatively high incidence of pulmonary and pleural tumours (Pylev, 1980). By contrast, inhalation of pulverized asbestos pipe covering failed to induce pulmonary neoplasms in hamsters (Leong *et al.*, 1978). BP given intratracheally with chrysotile or amosite in Tween-60 induced tumours in the lower respiratory system (Miller *et al.*, 1966).

Other inhalants

Arsenic was found weakly carcinogenic to the hamster respiratory tract after intratracheal instillation. It also slightly enhanced carcinogenicity of BP (Pershagen *et al.*, 1984).

Diesel exhaust after chronic inhalation did not induce any tumours of the respiratory tract in the Syrian hamster (Heinrich *et al.*, 1986). Combined application of diesel exhaust (inhaled) and NDEA (subcutaneous injection) provided insufficient evidence that diesel exhaust or its components have cotumorigenic effects on the tumour induction by NDEA (Heinrich *et al.*, 1989).

Acetaldehyde vapour induced laryngeal carcinomas after inhalation and it slightly enhanced carcinogenic activity of intratracheally instilled BP (Feron *et al.*, 1982).

Viruses

Lung tumours were found when supernatants from tissue cultures treated with mouse tumour extracts were injected subcutaneously into hamsters (Eddy *et al.*, 1958). Bronchogenic and alveolar-cell carcinomas developed when polyomavirus was given to hamsters by tracheotomy (Rabson *et al.*, 1960). Squamous cell carcinomas appeared to have originated in the bronchioli; various degrees of squamous cell differentiation and pleomorphism were noted in a tumour.

Mesenchymal tumours (spindle-cell sarcomas, angiosarcomas) of the lung were found as early as six days after intraperitoneal or subcutaneous inoculation of newborn hamsters with polyomavirus (Chesterman & Negroni, 1961).

COMPARATIVE ASPECTS

Some differences exist between tumours of the hamster's lower respiratory system (larynx, trachea and stem bronchi) and the corresponding human tumours. In man, papillary tumours of the larynx are more frequent than those of the trachea, but in hamsters tumours of the trachea predominate. Human tumours, which occur mainly in young patients, may be multiple or even diffuse and involve the entire tracheobronchial tree. Single papillary tumours develop predominantly in the stem bronchi and carina, but also occasionally in the main and segmental bronchi (Liebow, 1952). In hamsters, the commonest site of origin is the pars membranacea of the upper bronchi and lower third of the trachea and, with decreasing frequency, the other bronchi, larynx and remainder of the trachea. Papillary tumours are very rarely seen in the hamster's small bronchi.

Malignant tumours of the larynx and trachea seem to be more frequent in humans than in hamsters. The tumour types are similar in both species. Squamous cell carcinomas are most common, whereas adenocarcinomas and sarcomas are rare. Experimentally induced bronchogenic carcinomas in Syrian golden hamsters show a morphology similar to that seen in man. The tumour type induced depends on the substance given and the method of administration. After treatment with polycyclic hydrocarbons (e.g., BP, MC, DMBA), squamous cell carcinomas develop. Nitrosamines tend to induce adenomas and adenocarcinomas. Anaplastic carcinomas in man are classified according to their predominant cell types (Saffiotti, 1970). In hamsters, large-cell types are usually seen, but some cases of small-cell anaplastic carcinomas have been reported (Montesano *et al.*, 1970; Pershagen *et al.*, 1984). Quite recently a very high frequency of neuroendocrine tumours was reproducibly induced in this species. These tumours had ultrastructural and functional features corresponding to those of man (Schuller *et al.*, 1988). Areas of squamous or adenomatous differentiation are occasionally found in anaplastic carcinomas in man and hamster; bronchogenic carcinomas may spread and invade the regional lymph nodes and blood vessels. Distant metastases have not been described in hamsters.

Bronchiolo-alveolar carcinoma in man (also known under numerous synonyms) includes diffuse or focally distributed, usually bilateral tumours in which the neoplastic cells line the walls of alveolar-type airspaces. In a recent investigation using immunohistochemical techniques, a Clara cell antigen has been demonstrated in tumours of bronchiolar origin that developed after NDEA administration to Syrian hamsters (Rehm *et al.*, 1989). More detailed studies with bronchiolo-alveolar tumours induced by *N*-nitrosomethyl-n-heptylamine have confirmed the Clara cell as the source in this model (Rehm *et al.*, 1993; Rehm & Lijinsky, 1994). Bronchiolo-alveolar tumours are one of the categories of tumours induced by a variety of agents in hamsters, as described in the preceding section of this chapter. There are still several unsolved questions concerning the histogenesis of bronchiolar and alveolar cell carcinomas in man and in hamsters. However, a number of the histological parallels of these multicentric, peripheral, neoplastic lesions in hamsters are similar to the morphological characteristics observed in man, making the hamster a suitable animal model for further investigations.

In the case of pleural tumours (Williamson *et al.*, 1968), information on the pathology of this type of neoplasm is inadequate for comparative purposes.

ACKNOWLEDGEMENTS

The authors thank Mr Marcel Tauscher for photographic assistance and Ms Gillian Teicke for editing the manuscript.

REFERENCES

Althoff, J., Wilson, R. & Mohr, U. (1971a) Diethylnitrosamine-induced alteration in the tracheobronchial system of the Syrian golden hamster. *J. Natl Cancer Inst.*, 46, 1067–1071

Althoff, J., Kruger, F.W., Mohr, U. & Schmahl, D. (1971b) Dibutylnitrosamine carcinogenesis in Syrian golden and Chinese hamsters. *Proc. Soc. Exp. Biol.* (N.Y.), 136, 168–173

Althoff, J., Kruger, F.W. & Mohr, U. (1973a) Carcinogenic effect of dipropylnitro-samine and compounds related by β-oxidation. *J. Natl Cancer Inst.*, 51, 287–288

Althoff, J., Cardesa, A., Pour, P. & Mohr, U. (1973b) Carcinogenic effect of *N*-nitroso-hexamethyleneimine in Syrian golden hamsters. *J. Natl Cancer Inst.*, 50, 323–329

Althoff, J., Wilson, R., Cardesa, A. & Pour, P. (1974) Comparative studies of neoplastic response to a single dose of nitroso compounds. 3. The effect of *N*-nitroso-piperidine and *N*-nitrosomorpholine in Syrian golden hamsters. *Z. Krebsforsch.*, 81, 251–259

Becci, P.J., McDowell, E.M. & Trump, B.F. (1978) The respiratory epithelium. VI. Histogenesis of lung tumors induced by benzo[a]pyrene-ferric oxide in the hamster. *J. Natl Cancer Inst.*, 61, 607–618

Becci, P.J., Thompson, H.J., Grubbs, C.J. & Moon, R.C. (1980) Histogenesis and dose dependence of *N*-methyl-*N*-nitrosourea-induced carcinoma in a localized area of the hamster trachea. *J. Natl Cancer Inst.*, 64, 1135–1140

Bernfeld, P., Homburger, F. & Russfield, A.B. (1974) Strain differences in the response of inbred Syrian hamsters to cigarette smoke inhalation. *J. Natl Cancer Inst.*, 53, 1141–1157

Bernfeld, P., Homburger, F., Soto, E. & Pai, K.J. (1979) Cigarette smoke inhalation studies in inbred Syrian golden hamsters. *J. Natl Cancer Inst.*, 63, 675–689

Bernfeld, P., Homburger, F. & Soto, E. (1983) Subchronic cigarette smoke inhalation studies in inbred Syrian golden hamsters that develop laryngeal carcinoma upon chronic exposure. *J. Natl Cancer Inst.*, 71, 619–623

Bivin, W.S., Olsen, G.H. & Murray, K.A. (1987) Morphophysiology. In: Van Hoosier, G.L., Jr & McPherson, C.W., eds, *Laboratory Hamsters*, London, Academic Press, pp. 9–41

Cardesa, A. & Bombi, J.A. (1985) Pleural mesothelioma, Syrian hamster. In: Jones *et al.* (1985), pp. 133–137

Cardesa, A., Garcia-Bragado, F., Ramirez, J. & Ernst, H. (1990) Histological types of laryngo-tracheal tumors induced in Syrian golden hamsters by nitrosomorpholine and nitrosopiperidine. *Exp. Pathol.*, 40, 267–281

Chesterman, F.C. & Negroni, G. (1961) Tumours and other lesions induced in golden hamsters by a polyoma virus (Mill Hill strain): Induction time and dose response. *Br. J. Cancer*, 15, 790–797

Dagle, G.E. & Wehner, A.P. (1985) Fly ash pneumoconiosis, hamster. In: Jones *et al.* (1985), pp. 180–183

Della Porta, G., Kolb, L & Shubik, P. (1958) Induction of tracheobronchial carcinomas in the Syrian golden hamster. *Cancer Res.*, 18, 592–597

De Villiers, A.J. & Gross, P. (1966) Morphological changes induced in the lungs of hamsters and rats by external radiation (X-rays). A study in experimental carcinogenesis. *Cancer*, 19, 1399–1410

Dontenwill, W. (1964) Experimentelle Untersuchungen zur Genese des Lungencarcinoms. *Arzneimittelforschung*, 14, 774–780

Dontenwill, W. (1968) Experimental studies on the organotropic effect of nitrosamines in the respiratory tract. *Food Cosmet. Toxicol.*, 6, 571

Dontenwill, W. (1970) Experimental investigations on the effect of cigarette smoke inhalation on small laboratory animals. In: Hanna, M.G., Nettesheim, P. & Gilbert, J.R., eds, *Inhalation Carcinogenesis* (AEC Symposium Series No. 18), Oak Ridge, TN, USAEC, Division of Technical Information Extension, pp. 389–412

Dontenwill, W. & Mohr, U. (1961a) Carcinome des Respirations-traktes nach Behandlung von Goldhamstern mit Diäthylnitrosamin. *Z. Krebsforsch.*, 64, 305–312

Dontenwill, W. & Mohr, U. (1961b) Über Tracheal- und Bronchialcarcinome bei Goldhamstern nach Behandlung mit Diäthylnitrosamin. *Klin. Wschr.*, 39, 493

Dontenwill, W. & Mohr, U. (1962a) Die organotrope Wirkung der Nitrosamine. *Z. Krebsforsch.*, 65, 166–167

Dontenwill, W. & Mohr, U. (1962b) Vergleichende Untersuchungen an metaplastischen und malignen Epithelwucherungen des Respirationstraktes im Tier-experiment. *Z. Krebsforsch.*, 65, 168–170

Dontenwill, W. & Mohr, U. (1962c) Experimentelle Untersuchungen zum Problem der Carcinomentstehung im Respirationstrakt. II. Die Wirkung von Tabakrauch-kondensaten und Zigarettenrauch auf die Lunge des Goldhamsters. *Z. Krebsforsch.*, 65, 62–68

Dontenwill, W. & Rücker, K. (1967) Erzeugung von Papillomen durch Diäthylnitrosamin in der in die Milz implantierten Trachea. *Z. Krebsforsch.*, 69, 270–274

Dontenwill, W. & Wiebecke, B. (1964) Autoradiographische Untersuchungen wahrend der experimentellen Carcinomentstehung im Respirationstrakt des Goldhamsters nach Behandlung mit Diäthylnitrosamin. *Z. Krebsforsch.*, 66, 321–332

Dontenwill, W., Mohr, U. & Zagel, M. (1962) Über die unterschiedliche Lungencarcinogene Wirkung des Diäthylnitrosamin bei Hamster und Ratte. *Z. Krebsforsch.*, 64, 499–502

Dontenwill, W., Chevalier, H.-J., Harke, H.-P., Lafrenz, U., Reckzeh, G. & Schneider, B. (1973) Investigations on the effects of chronic cigarette-smoke inhalation in Syrian golden hamsters. *J. Natl Cancer Inst.*, 51, 1781–1832

Eddy, B., Stewart, S.E., Young, R. & Mider, G.B. (1958) Neoplasms in hamsters induced by mouse tumor agent passed in tissue culture. *J. Natl Cancer Inst.*, 20, 747–761

Ehard, H. (1973) *Vergleichende Untersuchungen zur Anatomie der Lungen von kleinen Versuchstieren (Kaninchen, Meerschweinchen, Albino-Ratten, Syrische Goldhamster)* (thesis, Hannover School of Veterinary Medicine)

Ernst, H. Heinrichs, M., Bargsten, G., Kittel, B., Rittinghausen, S., Dungworth, D.L. & Mohr, U. (1995) Neuroendocrine hyperplasias and tumors, larynx and trachea, Syrian hamster. In: Jones, T.C., Mohr, U. & Hunt, R.D., eds, *Respiratory System*, 2nd edition (Monographs on Pathology of Laboratory Animals), Berlin, Heidelberg, New York, Springer-Verlag (in press)

Evans, R.W. (1966) *Histological Appearances of Tumors*, 2nd ed., Baltimore, Williams and Wilkins

Farrell, R.L. & Davis, G.W. (1974) Effect of particulate benzo[a]pyrene carrier on carcinogenesis in the respiratory tract of hamsters. In: Karbe, E. & Park, J.F., eds, *Experimental Lung Cancer, Carcinogenesis and Bioassays*, Berlin, Heidelberg, New York, Springer-Verlag, pp. 219–233

Farrell, R.L., Davis, G.W. & Shadduck, J.A. (1972) Studies on the role of vehicles and particulates in respiratory carcinogenesis bioassays. In: *Proceedings of the First Annual Collaborative Conference of the Carcinogenesis Program*, Bethesda, MD, National Cancer Institute

Feron, V.J., Emmelot, P. & Vossenaar, T. (1972) Lower respiratory tract tumors in Syrian golden hamsters after intratracheal instillations of diethylnitrosamine alone and with ferric oxide. *Eur. J. Cancer*, 8, 445–449

Feron, V.J., Van den Heuvel, P.D., Koeter, H.B.W.M. & Beems, R.B. (1980) Significance of particle size of benzo[a]pyrene for the induction of respiratory tract tumours in hamsters. *Int. J. Cancer*, 25, 301–307

Feron, V.J., Kruysse, A. & Woutersen, R.A. (1982) Respiratory tract tumours in hamsters exposed to acetaldehyde vapour alone or simultaneously to benzo[a]pyrene or diethylnitrosamine. *Eur. J. Cancer Clin. Oncol.*, 18, 13–31

Feron, V.J., Kuper, C.F., Spit, B.J., Reuzel, P.G.J. & Woutersen, R.A. (1985) Glass fibers and vapor phase components of cigarette smoke as cofactors in experimental respiratory tract carcinogenesis. In: Mass, M.J., Kaufman, D.G., Siegfried, J.M., Steele, V.E. & Nesnow, S., eds, *Carcinogenesis: A Comprehensive Survey*, Vol. 8, *Cancer of the Respiratory Tract: Predisposing Factors*, New York, Raven, pp. 93–118

Fortner, J.G. (1957) Spontaneous tumors, including gastrointestinal neoplasms and malignant melanomas, in the Syrian hamster. *Cancer*, 10, 1153–1156

Green, U. & Althoff, J. (1982) Carcinogenicity of vinylethyl-nitrosamine in Syrian golden hamsters. *J. Cancer Res. Clin. Oncol.*, 102, 227–233

Gross, P., Tolker, E., Babyak, M.A. & Kaschak, M. (1965) Experimental lung cancer in hamsters. *Arch. Environ. Hlth.*, 11, 59–65

Grubbs, C.J., Becci, P.J., Thompson, H.J. & Moon, R.C. (1981) Carcinogenicity of *N*-methyl-*N*-nitrosourea and *N*-ethyl-*N*-nitrosourea when applied to a localized area of the hamster trachea. *J. Natl Cancer Inst.*, 66, 961–965

Haas, H., Mohr, U. & Kruger, F.W. (1973) Comparative studies with different doses of *N*-nitrosomorpholine, *N*-nitrosopiperidine, *N*-nitrosomethylurea, and dimethylnitrosamine in Syrian golden hamsters. *J. Natl Cancer Inst.*, 51, 1295–1301

Hahn, F.F. (1985) Radiation-induced squamous cell carcinoma, lung of rodents. In: Jones, *et al.* (1985), pp. 127–133

Harris, C.C., Sporn, M.B., Kaufman, D.G., Smith, J.M., Baker, M.S. & Saffiotti, U. (1971) Acute ultrastructural effects of benzo[a]pyrene and ferric oxide on the hamster tracheobronchial epithelium. *Cancer Res.*, 31, 1977–1989

Hecht, S.S., Adams, J.D., Numoto, S. & Hoffmann, D. (1983) Induction of respiratory tract tumors in Syrian golden hamsters by a single dose of 4-(methyl-nitrosamino)-1-(3-pyridyl)-1-butanone (NNK) and the effect of smoke inhalation. *Carcinogenesis*, 4, 1287–1290

Heinrich, U., Muhle, H., Takenaka, S., Ernst, H., Fuhst, R., Mohr, U., Pott, F. & Stober, W. (1986) Chronic effects on the respiratory tract of hamsters, mice and rats after long-term inhalation of high concentrations of filtered and unfiltered diesel engine emissions. *J. Appl. Toxicol.*, 6, 383–395

Heinrich, U., Mohr, U., Fuhst, R. & Brockmeyer, C. (1989) Investigation of a potential cotumorigenic effect of the dioxides of nitrogen and sulfur, and of diesel engine exhaust, on the respiratory tract of Syrian golden hamsters. *Health Effects Inst. Res. Report* No. 26, Cambridge, MA, Health Effects Institute, pp. 1–27

Henry, M.C. & Kaufman, D. (1973) Clearance of benzo[a]pyrene from hamster lungs after administration on coated particles. *J. Natl Cancer Inst.*, 51, 1961–1964

Henry, M.C., Port, C.D., Bates, R.R. & Kaufman, D.G. (1973) Respiratory tract tumors in hamsters induced by benzo[a]pyrene. *Cancer Res.*, 33, 1585–1592

Henry, M.C., Port, C.D. & Kaufman, D.G. (1975) Importance of physical properties of benzo[a]pyrene-ferric oxide mixtures on lung tumor induction. *Cancer Res.*, 35, 207–217

Herrold, K.M. (1963) The effects of benzo[a]pyrene, cigarette smoke condensate and atmospheric pollutants on the respiratory system of Syrian hamsters. *Acta Un. Int. Cancr.*, 19, 710–714

Herrold, K.M. (1964a) Induction of olfactory neuroepithelial tumors in Syrian hamsters by diethylnitrosamine. *Cancer*, 17, 114–121

Herrold, K.M. (1964b) Epithelial papillomas of the nasal cavity. *Arch. Pathol.*, 78, 189–195

Herrold, K.M. (1964c) Effect of the route of administration on the carcinogenic action of diethylnitrosamine. *Br. J. Cancer*, 18, 763–767

Herrold, K.M. (1964d) Comparative carcinogenic effects of diethylnitrosamine by different routes of administration to Syrian hamsters. *Proc. Am. Assoc. Cancer Res.*, 5, 26

Herrold, K.M. (1967) Fibrosing alveolitis and atypical proliferative lesions of the lung. An experimental study in Syrian hamsters. *Am. J. Pathol.*, 50, 639–651

Herrold, K.M. (1970) Upper respiratory tract tumors induced in Syrian hamsters by *N*-methyl-*N*-nitrosourea. *Int. J. Cancer*, 6, 217–222

Herrold, K.M. & Dunham, L.J. (1962) Induction of carcinoma and papilloma of the tracheobronchial mucosa of the Syrian hamster by intratracheal instillation of benzo[a]pyrene. *J. Natl Cancer Inst.*, 28, 467–476

Herrold, K.M. & Dunham, L.J. (1963) Induction of tumors in the Syrian hamster with diethylnitrosamine (N-nitrosodiethylamine). *Cancer Res.*, 23, 773–777

Homburger, F., Adams, R.A., Bernfield, P., Van Dongen, C.G. & Soto, E. (1983) A new first-generation hybrid Syrian hamster, B10F1D Alexander, for *in vivo* carcinogenesis bioassay, as a third species or to replace the mouse. *Surv. Synth. Pathol. Res.*, 1, 1

Ito, T. (1985) An ultrastructural study of the acute effects of 4-nitroquinoline 1-oxide on the hamster lung. *Exp. Mol. Pathol.*, 42, 220–233

Ito, T., Kawabe, R., Kitamura, H., Inayama, Y. & Kanisawa, M. (1992) Modulation of the incidence of hamster pulmonary endocrine cell hyperplasia by unilateral collapse of the lung. *Exp. Toxic. Pathol.*, 44, 209–213

Jones, T.C., Mohr, U. & Hunt, R.D., eds (1985) *Respiratory System* (Monographs on Pathology of Laboratory Animals), Berlin, Heidelberg, New York, Springer-Verlag

Kauffman, S.L. & Sato, T. (1985a) Alveolar type II cell adenoma, lung, mouse. In: Jones *et al.* (1985), pp. 102–107

Kauffman, S.L. & Sato, T. (1985b) Bronchiolar adenoma, lung, mouse. In: Jones *et al.* (1985), pp. 107–111

Keenan, K.P., Saffiotti, U., Stinson, S.F., Riggs, C.W. & McDowell, E.M. (1989) Multifactorial hamster respiratory carcinogenesis with interdependent effects of cannula-induced mucosal wounding, saline, ferric oxide, benzo[a]pyrene and *N*-methyl-*N*-nitrosourea. *Cancer Res.*, 49, 1529–1540

Kennedy, A.R. & Little, J.B. (1974a) Cellular localization of intratracheally administered ^{210}Po in the hamster lung using autoradiography of thin sections from plastic embedded tissue. In: Karbe, E. & Park, J.F., eds, *Experimental Lung Cancer Carcinogenesis and Bioassays*, Berlin, Heidelberg, New York, Springer-Verlag, pp. 475–484

Kennedy, A.R. & Little, J.B. (1974b) The transport and localization of benzo[a]pyrene-hematite and hematite ^{210}Po in the hamster lung following intratracheal instillation. *Cancer Res.*, 34, 1344–1352

Ketkar, M.B., Reznik, G. & Mohr, U. (1977) Pathological alterations in Syrian golden hamster lungs after passive exposure to cigarette smoke. *Toxicology*, 7, 265–273

Kimura, N. (1923) Artificial production of a cancer in the lungs following the intra-bronchial insufflation of coal-tar. *Jap. Med. Wld*, 3, 45–47

Kreyberg, L., (1981) International histological classification of tumours, No. 1. In: *Histological Typing of Lung Tumours*, 2nd ed., Geneva, World Health Organization

Laskin, S., Kuschner, M. & Drew, R.T. (1970) Studies in pulmonary carcinogenesis. In: Hanna, M.G., Nettesheim, P. & Gilbert, J.R., eds, *Inhalation Carcinogenesis* (AEC Symposium Series No. 18), Oak Ridge, TN, USAEC, Division of Technical Information Extension, pp. 321–351

Leong, B.K.J., Kociba, R.J., Pemell, H.C., Lisowe, R.W. & Rampy, L.W. (1978) Induction of pulmonary carcinoma in rats by chronic inhalation of dust from pulverized asbestos pipe covering. *J. Toxicol. Environ. Hlth*, 4, 645–659

Liebow, A.A. (1952) Tumors of the lower respiratory tract. In: *Atlas of Tumor Pathology*, Washington, D.C., Armed Forces Institute of Pathology, Section 5, fascicle 17

Lijinsky, W., Ferrero, A., Montesano, R. & Wenyon, C.E.M. (1970) Tumorigenicity of cyclic nitrosamines in Syrian golden hamsters. *Z. Krebsforsch.*, 74, 185–189

Lijinsky, W., Saavedra, J.E., Knutsen, G.L. & Kovatch, R.M. (1984) Comparison of the carcinogenic effectiveness of *N*-nitrosobis-(2-hydroxypropyl)amine, *N*-nitrosobis(2-oxopropyl)amine, *N*-nitroso(2-hydroxypropyl)-(2-oxopropyl)amine and *N*-nitroso-2,6-dimethylmorpholline in Syrian hamsters. *J. Natl Cancer Inst.*, 72, 685–688

Linnoila, R.I., Becker, K.L., Silva, O.L., Snider, R.H. & Moore, C.F. (1984) Calcitonin as a marker for diethylnitrosamine-induced pulmonary endocrine cell hyperplasia in hamsters. *Lab. Invest.*, 51, 39–45

Liscon, H., Kennedy, A.R. & Little, J.B. (1984) Histologic observations on the pathogenesis of lung cancer in hamster following administration of polonium-210. In: Karbe, E. & Park, J.F., eds, *Experimental Lung Cancer, Carcinogenesis and Bioassays*, Berlin, Heidelberg, New York, Springer-Verlag, pp. 468–474

Little, J.B. & O'Toole, W.F. (1974) Respiratory tract tumors in hamsters induced by benzo[a]pyrene and polonium-210 alpha radiation. *Cancer Res.*, 34, 3026–3039

Little, J.B., Grossman, B.N. & O'Toole, W.F. (1970) Respiratory carcinogenesis in hamsters induced by polonium-210 alpha radiation and benzo[a]pyrene. In: Nettesheim, *et al.* (1970), pp. 383–392

Little, J.B, Grossman, B.N. & O'Toole, W.F. (1973) Factors influencing the induction of lung cancer in hamsters by intratracheal administration of polonium-210. In: Sanders, C.L., Busch, R.H., Ballou, J.E. & Mahlum, D.D., eds, *Radionuclide Carcinogenesis* (AEC Symposium Series No. 29), Oak Ridge, TN, USAEC Division of Technical Information Extension, pp. 119–137

Mariassy, A.T. (1992) Epithelial cells of trachea and bronchi. In: Parent, R.A., ed., *Treatise on Pulmonary Toxicology. Comparative Biology of the Normal Lung*, Boca Raton, FL, CRC Press, pp. 63-76

Marshall, H.E., III, Keenan, K.P. & McDowell, E.M. (1987) The stathmokinetic and morphological response of the hamster respiratory epithelium to intralaryngeal instillations of saline and ferric oxide in saline. *Fund. Appl. Toxicol.*, 9, 705–714

Massaro, D., ed. (1989) *Lung Cell Biology*, New York, Marcel Dekker

McBride, J.T. (1992) Architecture of the tracheobronchial tree. In: Parent, R.A., ed., *Treatise on Pulmonary Toxicology. Comparative Biology of the Normal Lung*, Boca Raton, FL, pp. 49-61

McCoy, G.D., Hecht, S.S., Katayama, S. & Wynder, E.L. (1981) Differential effect of chronic ethanol consumption on the carcinogenicity of N-nitrosopyrrolidine and N'-nitroso-nornicotine in male Syrian golden hamsters. *Cancer Res.*, 41, 2849–2854

McDowell, E.M. & Trump, B.F. (1983) Histogenesis of preneoplastic and neoplastic lesions in tracheobronchial epithelium. *Surv. Synth. Pathol. Res.*, 2, 235–279

McGandy, R.B., Kennedy, A.R., Terzaghi, M. & Little, J.B. (1974) Experimental respiratory carcinogenesis: Interaction between alpha radiation and benzo[a]pyrene in hamsters. In: Karbe, E. & Park, J.F., eds, *Experimental Lung Cancer, Carcinogenesis and Bioassays*, Berlin, Heidelberg, New York, Springer-Verlag, pp. 485–491

Miller, L., Smith, W.E. & Berliner, S.W. (1966) Tests for effect of asbestos on benzo[a]-pyrene carcinogenesis in the respiratory tract. *Ann. N.Y. Acad. Sci.*, 132, 489–500

Mohr, U. (1970) Effects of diethylnitrosamine in the respiratory system of Syrian golden hamsters. In: Nettesheim, *et al.* (1970), pp. 255–265

Mohr, U. (1982) Tumours of the respiratory tract. In: Turusov, V.S., ed., *Pathology of Tumours in Laboratory Animals*. Vol. 3. *Tumours of the Hamster* (IARC Scientific Publications No. 34), Lyon, IARC, pp. 115–145

Mohr, U. & Ketkar, M.B. (1980) Animal model: spontaneous carcinoma of the lung in hamsters. *Am. J. Pathol.*, 99, 521–524

Mohr, U. & Dungworth, D.L. (1988) Relevance to humans of experimentally induced pulmonary tumors in rats and hamsters. In: Mohr, U., Dungworth, D.L., Kimmerle, G., Lewkowski, J., McClellan, R. & Stober, W., eds, *Inhalation Toxicology*, Berlin, Heidelberg, New York, Springer-Verlag, pp. 209–232

Mohr, U., Althoff, J. & Authaler, A. (1966a) Diaplacental effect of the carcinogen diethylnitrosamine in the golden hamster. *Cancer Res.*, 26, 2349–2352

Mohr, U., Wieser, O. & Pielsticker, K. (1966b) Die Minimaldosis fur die Wirkung von Diäthylnitrosamin auf die Trachea beim Gold-hamster. *Naturwissenschaften*, 53, 229

Mohr, U., Althoff, J., Schmähl, D. & Kruger, F.W. (1970) The carcinogenic effect of dibutylnitrosamine in Syrian and Chinese hamsters. *Z. Krebsforsch.*, 74, 112–113

Mohr, U., Reznik-Schuller, H., Reznik, G. & Hilfrich, J. (1975) Transplacental effect of diethylnitrosamine in Syrian hamsters as related to different days of administration during pregnancy. *J. Natl Cancer Inst.*, 55, 681–683

Mohr, U., Reznik, G. & Emminger, E. (1976) Intrasplenic tumour formation in the Syrian golden hamster (Mesocricetus auratus) after tracheal implants and treatment with diethylnitrosamine. *J. Natl Cancer Inst.*, 56, 811–818

Mohr, U., Pott, F. & Vonnahme, F.-J. (1984) Morphological aspects of mesotheliomas after intratracheal instillations of fibrous dusts in Syrian golden hamsters. *Exp. Pathol.*, 26, 179–183

Mohr, U., Rittinghausen, S., Takenaka, S., Ernst, H., Dungworth, D.L. & Pylev, L.N. (1990) Tumours of the lower respiratory tract and pleura in the rat. In: Turusov, V.S. & Mohr, U., eds, *Pathology of Tumours in Laboratory Animals*. Vol. 1. *Tumours of the Rat* (IARC Scientific Publications No. 99), Lyon, IARC, pp. 149–163

Montesano, R. & Saffiotti, U. (1968a) Carcinogenic response of the respiratory tract of Syrian golden hamsters to different doses of diethylnitrosamine. *Cancer Res.*, 28, 2197–2210

Montesano, R. & Saffiotti, U. (1968b) Synergistic effect of diethylnitrosamine (DEN) and benzo[a]pyrene (BP) on respiratory carcinogenesis in hamsters. *Proc. Am. Assoc. Cancer Res.*, 9, 51

Montesano, R., Saffiotti, U. & Shubik, P. (1970) The role of topical and systemic factors in experimental respiratory carcinogenesis. In: Hanna, M.G., Nettesheim, P. & Gilbert, J.R., eds, *Inhalation Carcinogenesis* (AEC Symposium Series No. 18), Oak Ridge, TN, USAEC, Division of Technical Information Extension, pp. 353–371

Nettesheim, P., Hanna, M.G. & Deatherage, J.W., eds (1970) *Morphology of Experimental Respiratory Carcinogenesis* (AEC Symposium Series No. 21), Oak Ridge, TN, USAEC, Division of Technical Information Extension, pp. 353–371

Nylen, E.S., Becker, K.L., Joshi, P.A., Snider, R.H. & Schuller, H.M. (1990) Pulmonary bombesin and calcitonin in hamsters during exposure to hyperoxia and diethylnitrosamine. *Am. J. Respir. Cell. Mol. Biol.*, 2, 25-31

Och, R. (1959) *Beitrag zur Anatomie des Respirationsapparates des Syrischen Gold-hamsters (Mesocricetus auratus W.)* (thesis, Leipzig University)

Pershagen, G., Nordberg, G. & Bjorklund, N.-E. (1984) Carcinomas of the respiratory tract in hamsters given arsenic trioxide and/or benzo[a]pyrene by the pulmonary route. *Environ. Res.*, 34, 227–241

Plopper, C.G. & Dungworth, D.L. (1987) Structure, function, cell injury and cell renewal of bronchiolar-alveolar epithelium. In: McDowell, E.M., ed., *Lung Carcinomas*, Edinburgh, New York, Churchill Livingstone, pp. 94–128

Plopper, C.G., Mariassy, A.T., Wilson, D.W., Alley, J.L., Nishio, S.J. & Nettesheim, P. (1983) Comparison of nonciliated tracheal epithelial cells in six mammalian species: ultrastructure and population densities. *Exp. Lung Res.*, 5, 281–294

Pour, P.M. (1985) Clear cell carcinoma, larynx, Syrian hamster. In: Jones *et al.* (1985), pp. 75–77

Pour, P., Althoff, J., Cardesa, A., Kruger, F.W. & Mohr, U. (1974) Effects of beta-oxidized nitrosamines on Syrian golden hamsters. II. 2-oxo-propyl-*N*-propyl-nitrosamine. *J. Natl Cancer Inst.*, 52, 1869–1874

Pour, P., Kmoch, N., Greiser, E., Mohr, U., Althoff, J. & Cardesa, A. (1976a) Spontaneous tumours and common diseases in two colonies of Syrian golden hamsters. Part I. Incidences and sites. *J. Natl Cancer Inst.*, 56, 931–935

Pour, P., Kruger, F.W., Cardesa, A., Althoff, J. & Mohr, U. (1973) Carcinogenic effect of di-*N*-propylnitrosamine in Syrian golden hamsters. *J. Natl Cancer Inst.*, 51, 1019–1027

Pour, P., Mohr, U., Cardesa, A., Althoff, J. & Kmoch N. (1976b) Spontaneous tumours and common diseases in two colonies of Syrian golden hamsters. Part II. Respiratory tract and digestive system tumours. *J. Natl Cancer Inst.*, 56, 937–948

Pylev, L.N. (1980) Pretumorous lesions and lung and pleural tumours induced by asbestos in rats, Syrian golden hamsters and Macaca mulatta (rhesus) monkeys. In: Wagner, J.C., ed., *Biological Effects of Mineral Fibres* (IARC Scientific Publications No. 30), Lyon, IARC, pp. 343–355

Rabson, A.S., Branigan, W.J. & Legallais, F.Y. (1960) Lung tumors produced by intratracheal inoculation of polyoma virus in Syrian hamsters. *J. Natl Cancer Inst.*, 25, 937–946

Rehm, S. & Lijinsky, W. (1994) Squamous metaplasia of bronchiolar cell-derived adenocarcinoma induced by *N*-nitrosomethyl-n-heptylamine in Syrian hamsters. *Vet. Pathol.*, 31, 561–571

Rehm, S., Takahashi, M., Ward, J.M., Singh, G., Katyal, S.L. & Henneman, J.R. (1989) Immunohistochemical demonstration of Clara cell antigen in lung tumors of bronchiolar origin induced by *N*-nitrosodiethylamine in Syrian golden hamsters. *Am. J. Pathol.*, 134, 79–87

Rehm, S., Lijinsky, W., Thomas, R.G. & Kasprzak, B.H. (1993) Clara cell antigen in normal and migratory dysplastic Clara cells, and bronchioloalveolar carcinoma of Syrian hamsters induced by *N*-nitroso-methyl-*N*-heptylamine. *Virchows Arch B. Cell Pathol.*, 64, 181–190

Reznik-Schuller, H.M. (1980) Acute effects of cigarette smoke-inhalation on the Syrian hamster lungs. *J. Environ. Pathol. Toxicol.*, 4, 285–291

Reznik-Schuller, H. & Mohr, U. (1974a) Investigations on the carcinogenic burden by air pollution in man. IX. Early pathological alterations of the bronchial epithelium in Syrian golden hamsters after intratracheal instillation of benzo[a]pyrene. 1. Morphological studies from semi-thin sections. *Zbl. Bakt. Hyg. I. Abt. Orig. Reihe B*, 159, 493–502

Reznik-Schuller, H. & Mohr, U. (1974b) Investigations on the carcinogenic burden by air pollution in man. X. Morphological changes of the tracheal epithelium in Syrian golden hamsters during the first 20 weeks of benzo[a]pyrene instillation: an ultrastructural study. *Zbl. Bakt. Hyg. I. Abt. Orig. Reihe B*, 159, 503–522

Reznik-Schuller, H. & Mohr, U. (1975) Investigations on the carcinogenic burden by air pollution in man. XII. Early pathological alterations of the bronchial epithelium in Syrian golden hamsters after intratracheal instillation of benzo(a)pyrene. *Zentralbl. Bakteriol* [Orig. B], 160, 108–129

Reznik-Schuller, H. & Reznik, G. (1979) Experimental pulmonary carcinogenesis. *Int. Rev. Exp. Pathol.*, 20, 211–281

Rhodin, J. & Dalham, T. (1956) Electron microscopy of the tracheal ciliated mucosa in rat. *Z. Zellforsch.*, 44, 345–412

Saffiotti, U. (1969) Experimental respiratory tract carcinogenesis. *Prog. Exp. Tumor Res.*, 11, 302–333

Saffiotti, U. (1970) Experimental respiratory tract carcinogenesis and its relation to inhalation exposures. In: Hanna, M.G., Nettesheim, P. & Gilbert, J.R., eds, *Inhalation Carcinogenesis* (AEC Symposium Series No. 18), Oak Ridge, TN, USAEC, Division of Technical Information Extension, pp. 27–54

Saffiotti, U., Cefis, F. & Kolb, L.H. (1964) Bronchogenic carcinoma induction by particulate carcinogens. *Proc. Am. Assoc. Cancer Res.*, 5, 55

Saffiotti, U., Cefis, F. & Shubik, P. (1966) Histopathology and histogenesis of lung cancer induced in hamsters by carcinogens carried by dust particles. In: Severi, L., ed., *Lung Tumors in Animals*, Perugia, Division of Cancer Research, University of Perugia, pp. 537–546

Saffiotti, U., Montesano, R., Sellakumar, A.R. & Borg, S.A. (1967) Experimental cancer of the lung. Inhibition by vitamin A of the induction of tracheobronchial squamous metaplasia and squamous cell tumors. *Cancer*, 20, 857–864

Saffiotti, U., Cefis, F. & Kolb, L.H. (1968) A method for the experimental induction of bronchogenic carcinoma. *Cancer Res.*, 28, 104–124

Saffiotti, U., Montesano, R., Sellakumar, A.R., Cefis, F. & Kaufman, D.G. (1972a) Respiratory tract carcinogenesis in hamsters induced by different numbers of administrations of benzo[a]pyrene and ferric oxide. *Cancer Res.*, 32, 1073–1081

Saffiotti, U., Sellakumar, A.R. & Kaufman, D.G. (1972b) Respiratory tract carcinogenesis induced in hamsters by different dose levels of benzo[a]pyrene and ferric oxide. *J. Natl Cancer Inst.*, 49, 1199–1204

Schreiber, H., Saccomanno, G., Martin, D.H. & Brennan, L. (1974) Sequential cytological changes during development of respiratory tract tumors induced in hamsters by benzo[a]pyrene ferric oxide. *Cancer Res.*, 34, 689–698

Schuller, H.M., Becker, K.L. & Witschi, H.-P. (1988) An animal model for neuro-endocrine lung cancer. *Carcinogenesis*, 9, 293–296

Schuller, H.M., Witschi, H.-P., Nylen, E., Joshi, P.A., Correa, E. & Becker, K.L. (1990) Pathobiology of lung tumors induced in hamsters by 4-(methylnitrosamino)-1-(3-pyridyl)-1-butanone and the modulating effect of hyperoxia. *Cancer Res.*, 50, 1960–1965

Shami, S.G., Thibodeau, L.A., Kennedy, A.R. & Little, J.B. (1982) Proliferative and morphological changes in the pulmonary epithelium of the Syrian golden hamster during carcinogenesis initiated by $^{210}Po^{\alpha}$ α-radiation. *Cancer Res.*, 42, 1405–1411

Shubik, P., Della Porta, G., Pietra, G., Tomatis, L., Rappaport, H., Saffiotti, U. & Toth, B. (1962) Factors determining the neoplastic response induced by carcinogens. In: *Biological Interactions in Normal and Neoplastic Growth*, Boston, MA, Little, Brown, pp. 285–297

Smith, W.E., Miller, L., Churg, J. & Selikoff, I.J. (1964) Pleural reaction and mesothelioma in hamsters injected with asbestos. *Proc. Am. Assoc. Cancer Res.*, 5, 59

Sorokin, S.P. (1970) The cells of the lungs. In: Nettesheim *et al.* (1970), pp. 3–43

Sorokin, S.P. & Hoyt, R.F., Jr (1989) Neuroepithelial bodies and solitary small-granule cells. In: Massarro, D., ed., *Lung Cell Biology*, New York, Marcel Dekker, pp. 191–344

Stenbäck, F. & Rowland, J. (1978) Role of particle size in the formation of respiratory tract tumors induced by benzo[a]pyrene. *Eur. J. Cancer*, 14, 321–326

Stenbäck, F., Sellakumar, A. & Shubik, P. (1975) Magnesium oxides as carrier dust in benzo[a]pyrene-induced lung carcinogenesis in Syrian hamsters. *J. Natl Cancer Inst.*, 54, 861–867

Stinson, S.F., Reznik-Schuller, H.M., Reznik, G. & Donahoe, R. (1983) Spindle cell carcinoma of the hamster trachea induced by N-methyl-N-nitrosourea. *Am. J. Pathol.*, 111, 21–26

Stunzi, H., Head, K.W. & Nielsen, S.W. (1974) Tumours of the lung. *Bull. World Health Org.*, 50, 9–19

Sunday, M.E. & Willett, C.G. (1992) Induction and spontaneous regression of intense pulmonary neuroendocrine cell differentiation in a model of preneoplastic lung injury. *Cancer Res.*, 52, 2677s-2686s

Thomas, R.G. & Smith, D.M. (1979) Lung tumors from $PuO_2.ZrO_2$ aerosol particles in Syrian hamsters. *Int. J. Cancer*, 24, 594–599

Thomas, R.G., Drake, G.A., London, J.E., Anderson, E.C., Prine, J.R. & Smith, D.M. (1981) Pulmonary tumours in Syrian hamsters following inhalation of [239]PuO_2. *Int. J. Radiat. Biol.*, 40, 605–611

Thyssen, J., Althoff, J., Kimmerle, G. & Mohr, U. (1980) Inhalation studies with benzo[a]pyrene in Syrian golden hamsters. *J. Natl Cancer Inst.*, 66, 575–577

Toth, B. & Boreisha, I. (1969) Tumorigenesis with isonicotinic acid hydrazide and urethan in the Syrian golden hamster. *Eur. J. Cancer*, 5, 165–171

Toth, B., Tomatis, L. & Shubik, P. (1961) Multipotential carcinogenesis with urethan in the Syrian golden hamster. *Cancer Res.*, 21, 1537–1541

Wahnschaffe, U., Emura, M. & Mohr, U. (1987) Development of intracytoplasmic lumina in diethylnitrosamine-induced tracheal papillomas of Syrian golden hamster. *Virchows Arch. B*, 54, 59–66

Wallenborn, W.M., Fitz-Hugh, G.S. & Wilkerson, J.A. (1963) Olfactory esthesioneuroepithelioma, report of case. *Ann. Otol. Rhin. Laryng.*, 72, 149–156

Wehner, A.P., Busch, R.H. & Olson, R.J. (1974) Effect of chronic exposure to cigarette smoke on tumor incidence in the Syrian golden hamster. In: Karbe, E. & Park, J.F., *Experimental Lung Cancer, Carcinogenesis and Bioassays*, Berlin, Heidelberg, New York, Springer-Verlag, pp. 360–368

Wehner, A.P., Busch, R.H. & Olson, R.J. (1976) Effects of diethylnitrosamine and cigarette smoke on hamsters. *J. Natl Cancer Inst.*, 56, 749–756

Weibel, E.R. (1973) Morphological basis of alveolar capillary gas exchange. *Physiol. Rev.*, 53, 419–495

Wilbourn, J., Haroun, L., Heseltine, E., Kaldor, J., Partensky, C. & Vainio, H. (1986) Response of experimental animals to human carcinogens: an analysis based upon the IARC monographs programme. *Carcinogenesis*, 7, 1853–1863

Williamson, M., Leestma, J.E. & Black, W.C., eds (1968) *Histological Patterns in Tumor Pathology*, New York, Evanston, London, Hoeber Medical Division, Harper & Row

Witschi, H. & Schüller, H.M. (1991) Diffuse and continuous cell proliferation enhances radiation-induced tumorigenesis in hamster lung. *Cancer Lett.*, 60, 193–197

Wynder, E.L. & Hoffmann, D. (1969) Bioassays in tobacco carcinogenesis. *Prog. Exp. Tumor Res.*, 11, 163–193

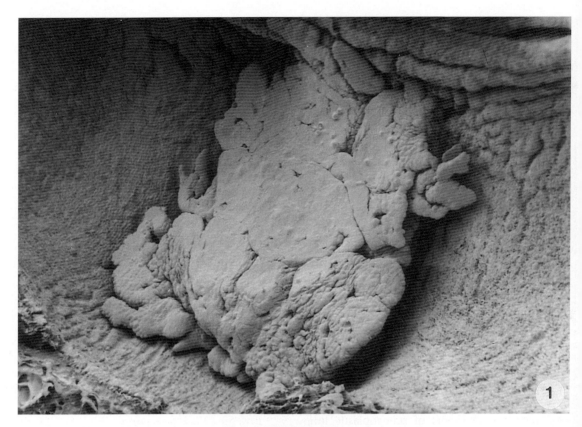

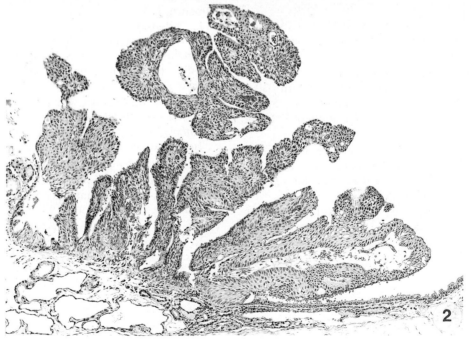

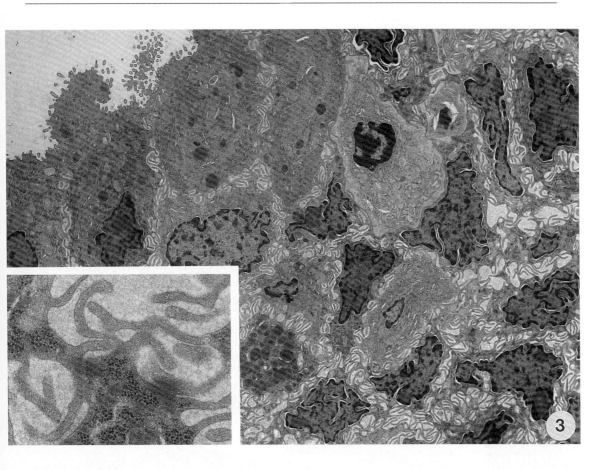

Figure 1. Papilloma of the trachea growing exophytically from the surface lining epithelium. Scanning electron microscopy; × 170

Figure 2. Papilloma of the trachea with well vascularized, ramified stalks composed of loose, poorly cellular connective tissue. H & E; × 80

Figure 3. Papilloma of the trachea demonstrating highly squamous features with extensively developed cellular interdigitation in the stratified surface area. Transmission electron microscopy, uranyl acetate and lead citrate; × 2800. Insert × 35 000

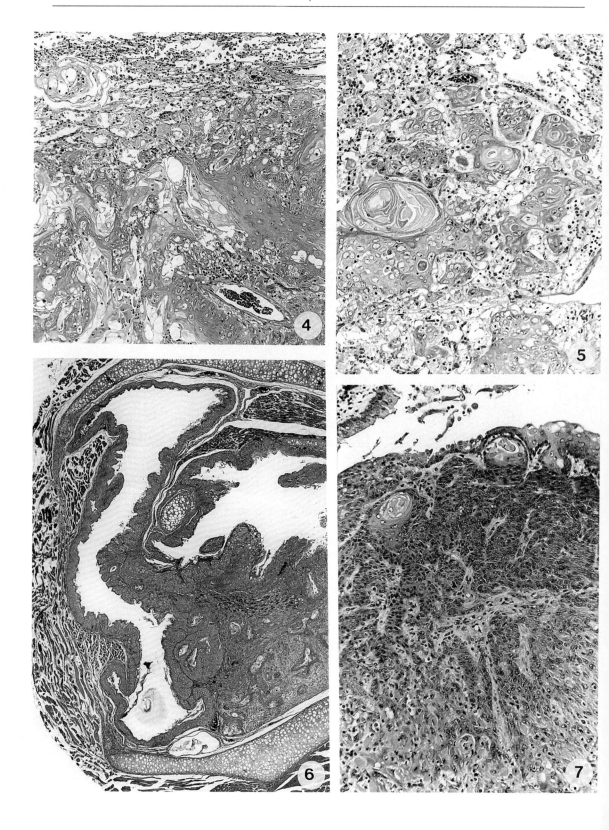

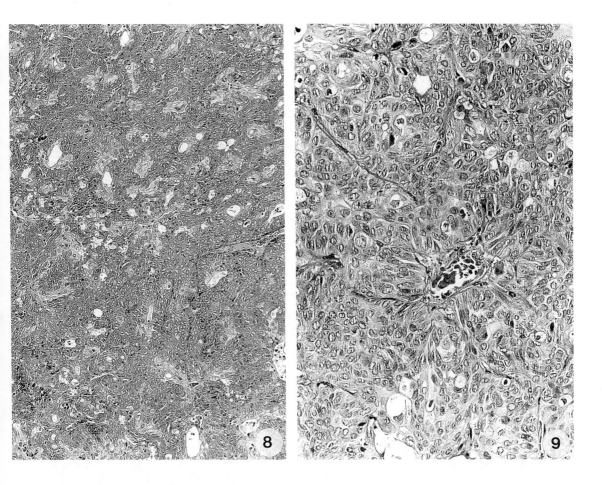

Figure 4. Squamous cell carcinoma of the lung with strong keratinization (cornification). H & E; × 80

Figure 5. Squamous cell carcinoma of the lung with keratinization. H & E; × 130

Figure 6. Squamous cell carcinoma of the larynx. H & E; x 30

Figure 7. Squamous cell carcinoma in a laryngeal/tracheal region. H & E; ×180

(Picture courtesy of Dr P.M. Pour, Eppley Institute for Research in Cancer, University of Nebraska Medical Center, Omaha, Nebraska, USA)

Figure 8. Squamous cell carcinoma of the lung, non-keratinizing type. H & E; × 80

Figure 9. Squamous cell carcinoma of the lung, non-keratinizing type. H & E; × 210

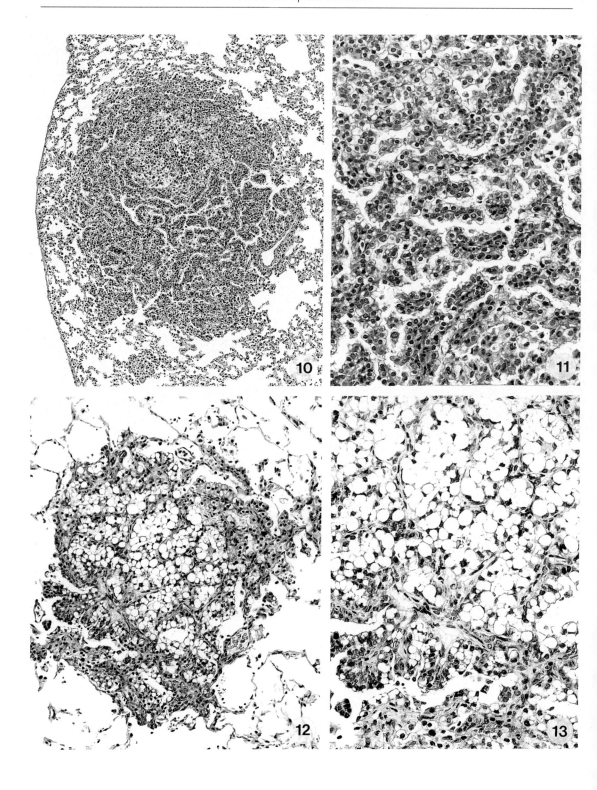

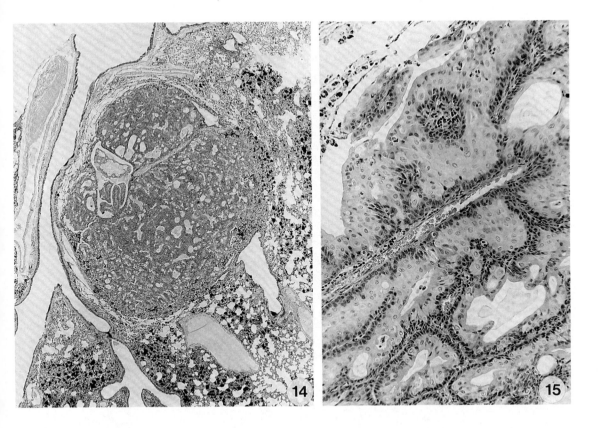

Figure 10. Adenoma of the lung. H & E; x 100

(Paraffin block courtesy of Dr Y. Konishi, Cancer Center, Nara Medical College, Nara, Japan)

Figure 11. Same as in Figure 10. H & E; x 140

Figure 12. Adenoma of the lung, consisting of vacuolized cells. H & E; x 130

Figure 13. A higher magnification of Figure 12. Note the nuclei located in the cellular periphery. H & E; x 250

Figure 14. Adenocarcinoma of the lung in a nodular form. H & E; x 30

Figure 15. Adenocarcinoma of the lung with a papillary growth pattern. H & E; x 200

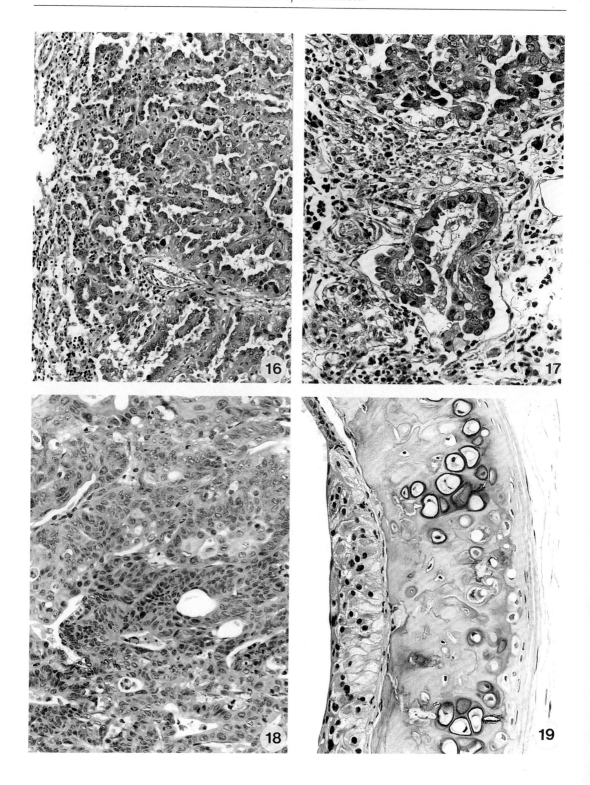

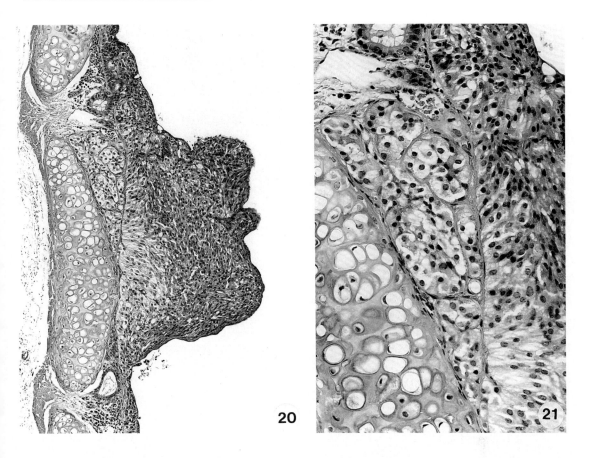

Figure 16. Adenocarcinoma of the lung with yet another papillary growth pattern than the one in Figure 15. H & E; ×160

Figure 17. Adenocarcinoma of the lung showing vascular invasion. H & E; ×250

Figure 18. Adenosquamous carcinoma of the lung. H & E; × 210

Figure 19. Neuroendocrine cell hyperplasia in the trachea. H & E; × 230

Figure 20. Malignant neuroendocrine cell tumour of the trachea. H & E; ×90

Figure 21. High-power view of Figure 20. H & E; ×250

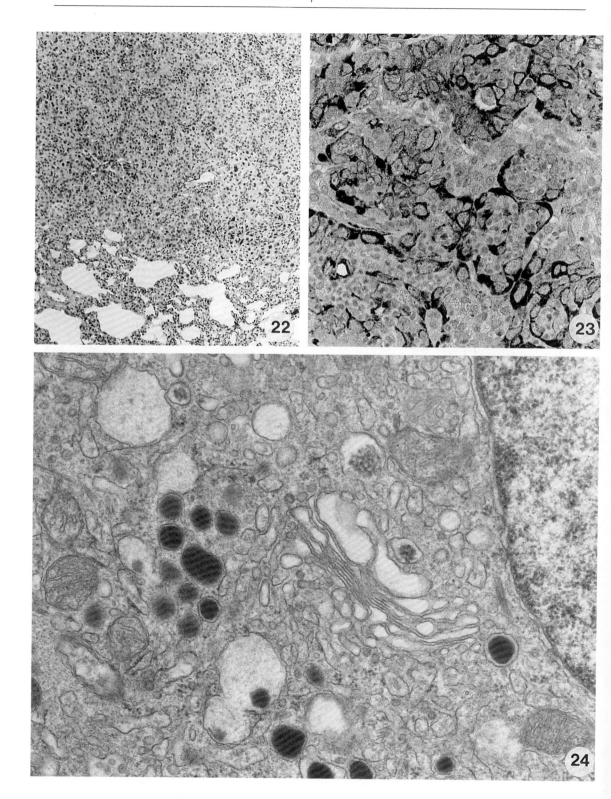

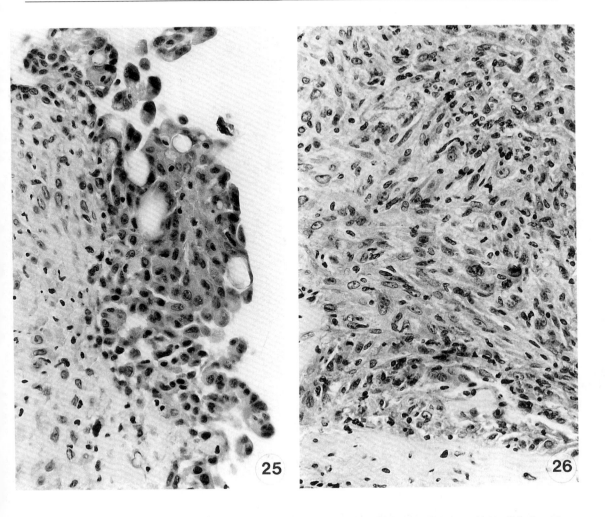

Figure 22. Neuroendocrine cell proliferation of the lung. Note absence of glandular growth pattern, high cellularity and faint stain. H & E; x 160

(Picture courtesy of Dr. H.M. Schuller, College of Veterinary Medicine, University of Tennessee, Knoxville, TN, USA)

Figure 23. Immunocytochemical demonstration of mammalian bombesin in the same lesion as in Figure 22. Dark-stained areas indicate sites of positive immunoreaction following exposure to a primary antiserum. Vectastain ABC-kit, diaminobenzidine; x 250

(Picture courtesy of Dr H.M. Schuller, College of Veterinary Medicine, University of Tennessee, Knoxville, TN, USA)

Figure 24. Ultrastructure of a cell from the neuroendocrine proliferation shown in Figure 22. Note dense-cored neuroendocrine secretory granules. Uranyl acetate and lead citrate; x 30 000

(Picture courtesy of Dr H.M. Schuller, College of Veterinary Medicine, University of Tennessee, Knoxville, TN, USA)

Figure 25. Mesothelioma of the lung; epithelial type. H & E; x 220

(Histological slide courtesy of Dr A. Cardesa, Facultad de Medicina, Universidad de Barcelona, Barcelona, Spain)

Figure 26. Mesothelioma of the lung; fusiform type. H & E; x 220

(Histological slide courtesy of Dr A. Cardesa, Facultad de Medicina, Universidad de Barcelona, Barcelona, Spain)

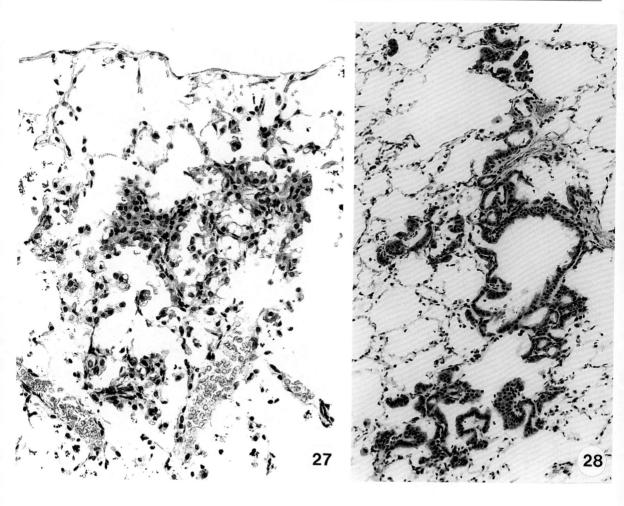

Figure 27. Hyperplasia of alveolar epithelium in the lung. Note vacuolized cells. H & E; x 210
Figure 28. Alveolar bronchiolization in the lung. H & E; x 140

Tumours of the kidney

H. TSUDA, D.J. KIM, T. KATO, K. HAKOI AND A. HAGIWARA

Naturally occurring kidney tumours are uncommon in rodents, including the Syrian golden hamster. This is in contrast to the relatively high yields of spontaneous liver, mammary or lung tumours seen in certain strains of rats and mice.

However, the kidney of various species is susceptible to a variety of carcinogenic insults, either chemical or viral, and the hamster is no exception. Indeed, apart from the generally nitrosamine-induced tubular lesions shared in common with other rodents, the Syrian golden hamster is unique in responding to estrogenic stimulus by development of hormone-dependent kidney tumours of uncertain origin.

MORPHOLOGY AND BIOLOGY OF TUMOURS
Histological types of tumour

Epithelial tumours

    Altered tubules
    Renal cell adenoma
    Renal cell carcinoma
Epithelial–mesenchymal
    (controversial) tumours
Mesenchymal tumours

Nephroblastomas

Epithelial tumours

As with renal neoplastic lesions in the rat, epithelial tumours of the kidney in hamsters are classified into clear, granular and basophilic types on a cytological basis,

and papillary, solid and cystic types on a structural basis. Since clear distinction between benign and malignant lesions appears to be difficult, the term 'renal cell adenoma' is generally given to non-invasive lesions. Diagnosis of 'renal cell carcinoma' is made when local invasion or metastatic lesions are found. However, the latter term is also used for lesions showing obvious cellular atypia and frequent mitotic figures, even without obvious invasion.

Before the development of adenomas and carcinomas, single or groups of a few tubules demonstrating atypical, basophilic or clear cell morphology are frequently observed. This type of tubular lesion, designated as altered, atypical or dysplastic tubules, is considered to be the preneoplastic stage from which renal cell tumours develop.

Since most renal cell tumours develop in the cortex, when the tumours reach a diameter of approximately 0.5 mm, they can usually be easily seen as whitish nodular lesions through the capsular tissue.

When exposure to a carcinogen and the length of observation period are sufficient, tumour development is often multiple and bilateral. Larger nodules are occasionally palpable through the abdominal wall before autopsy.

Cut surfaces of small tumours show a whitish colour with occasional cyst formation in the central areas. The tumour is clearly defined from the surrounding normal renal tissue. Larger tumours often have haemorrhagic or softened areas in the centre and their borders are often ill-defined.

Altered (atypical, dysplastic) tubules. The term 'altered tubules' is given to small lesions comprising a single or small group of tubules lined by a single layer of normal to slightly atypical epithelial cells with enlarged and basophilic nuclei. Their cytoplasm is usually either basophilic (basophilic cell tubules) or clear (clear cell tubules) in appearance. The diagnosis of altered tubules is only made when the lesion retains obvious tubular structure (Figure 1).

According to the characteristics of the constituent cells, altered tubules are divided into two types, basophilic (Figure 1 and 2) and clear (Figure 3). Cells in the basophilic tubules have slightly more basophilic cytoplasm as compared to surrounding tubules, whereas the clear cell tubules have clear scant cytoplasm due to accumulation of glycogen (Bannasch *et al.*, 1978, 1980, 1986, 1989; Tsuda *et al.*, 1985, 1986, 1987).

Adenomas. The term renal cell adenoma is given to focally proliferative, well defined epithelial lesions distorting the structural integrity of a single tubule with obvious compression of the surrounding tissues. As with altered tubules, they are classified into basophilic, clear and, less commonly, granular cell types. They can also be categorized as papillary, solid or cystic according to their structural characteristics.

The most frequent type is the basophilic papillary adenoma which has branching epithelial elements lined by cuboidal to basophilic columnar tumour cells and supported by a fibrous stroma (Bannasch *et al.*, 1980; Pour *et al.*, 1976; Pour, 1986a). In contrast, solid adenomas are composed of tumour cells without the fibrous stroma. This latter lesion is prone to development of central necrosis, even when only of small size, possibly due to insufficient blood supply caused by lack or occlusion of capillaries. Occasionally papillary (Figure 4) and solid (Figure 5) adenomas are composed of clear cells. Cystic adenomas consist of dilated tubules lined by proliferated single layers of cuboidal or flattened tumour cells of basophilic (Figure 6) or clear appearance with some atypia. Occasionally there is serous fluid in the lumen. Transitions between papillary and solid structure are also observed, diagnosis in such cases usually being based on the morphology of the major constituent.

Cell types comprising renal cell adenomas are similar to those observed in altered tubules, i.e. basophilic and clear cells. In contrast to the rat (Nogueira & Bannasch, 1988), oncocytic cell adenomas have not been reported in the hamster.

Carcinomas. Malignant renal epithelial lesions are often called renal cell carcinomas rather than adenocarcinomas. The term renal cell carcinoma is given when the cells exhibit nuclear atypia and more frequent mitotic figures, and there is obvious invasion of the surrounding tissue or, less commonly, remote metastasis (Pour, 1986b). Cyst formation or necrosis is often observed in the centre of large tumours. Histological and cytological appearance is basically similar to that in adenomas, making differential diagnosis often difficult. However diagnosis of carcinoma is occasionally given when the lesion cell has obvious atypia (Figure 7) without invasive morphology. A diagnosis of 'malignant adenomas', which is liable to cause confusion of nomenclature, has even been used (Kirkman & Bacon, 1950). Renal cell adenomas induced by nitrosamines in hamsters do not differ from those caused by other chemicals or hormones (Kirkman, 1974). Renal cell carcinomas in hamsters are not characterized by the vast variation in morphological patterns one finds with rat tumours induced by the same carcinogen (Pour, 1986b).

With regard to enzyme-histochemical and immunohistochemical phenotypes, no data are available.

Epithelial–mesenchymal (controversial) tumours

Natural and synthetic estrogenic hormones have been shown to induce renal tumours in male Syrian hamsters. Even though extensive investigations have been made (Kirkman & Robbins, 1959; Llombardt-Bosch & Peydró-Olaya, 1986), the classification and histogenesis of these estrogen-induced tumours remain controversial. Their histological appearance does not directly correspond to spontaneous renal epithelial cell tumours in either hamsters or rats, although several investigators have described a possible origin from the proximal tubule (Kirkman & Bacon, 1950; Horning & Whittick, 1954), stromal cells or juxtaglomerular apparatus (Dodge & Kirkman, 1981; Dodge et al., 1988). Tumour cells as well as normal tubular cells were shown to be positive for binding with estrogen (Caviezel et al., 1984) and possess sex hormone receptors (Li & Li, 1978, 1981; Li et al., 1976, 1977, 1979; Tse et al., 1989).

Recent investigations using combined histochemical, immunohistochemical and/or electron microscopic approaches have indicated possible histogenesis from vascular smooth muscle cells (Hacker et al., 1988, 1991) or from precursor cells in the epithelial cell differentiation pathway (Gonzalez et al., 1989).

Macroscopically, tumours appear as single or more often multiple whitish nodules within the same kidney. Size varies from tiny dots to palpable masses that can reach 3 cm in diameter. Cut surfaces have whitish or slightly yellow colour and solid or partly cystic character with occasional haemorrhagic foci. The tumours are usually reasonably well defined but not clearly encapsulated. Multiple metastases to the abdominal cavity, liver, pancreas and spleen may be found. Metastasis to the cervical lymph nodes has also been reported (Kirkman, 1959a, b).

The most common histological type of estrogen-induced tumour is composed of spindle-shaped poorly differentiated or so-called blastemal cells. The lesions are formed by solid arrangement of elongated or spindle-shaped tumour cells. Nuclei are usually elongated or oval in shape. Cytoplasm is moderately abundant and eosinophilic to clear. Perivascular radiating patterns formed by more spindle-shaped cells are often observed (Figures 8 and 9). In some areas, tumour cells are arranged to form a large blood space lined by a single layer of endothelial-like cells (Figure 10) and pseudorosette patterns also can be seen (Figure 11). Borders with surrounding parenchymal tissue are not clearly defined. Tumour cells infiltrate the surrounding tissue, as occurs with nephroblastomas, and metastasis to the peritoneal cavity occurs even when the lesion is small (Figure 12). The early lesions (foci) consist of small clusters of spindle-shaped cells forming solid blocks or cords penetrating between tubules (Hacker et al., 1988). Transition between apparently epithelial lesions, mostly altered or cystic tubules, and small blastemal foci can be found.

Attention has concentrated on biochemical, histochemical and immunohistochemical analysis of estradiol-induced tumours for the purpose of establishing histogenesis (Murthy & Russfield, 1968; Dodge, 1977; Dodge et al., 1988; Hacker et al., 1988, 1991). Tumour tissue has been shown to demonstrate high activities of glycogen synthetase, glycogen phosphorylase, adenylate cyclase, glucose-6-phosphate dehydrogenase, glyceraldehyde-3-phosphate dehydrogenase and alkaline phosphatase. These enzymes indicate aberrant glycogen metabolism and increased flow along glycolysis pathways possibly linked to nucleic acid synthesis and energy production. Lipid-containing or glycogen-rich cells are often observed

(Ising, 1956; Arcadi, 1963). These results are generally in line with findings for epithelial tumours in the rat kidney except for the high activity of alkaline phosphatase, which can therefore be used as a marker enzyme for this tumour (Figure 13).

Immunohistochemical studies using cytokeratin have given conflicting results. A positive finding has been taken to suggest epithelial differentiation (González *et al.*, 1989; Cortés-Vizcaíno *et al.*, 1994), while negative staining for cytokeratin, but positive for vimentin and desmin localization, indicated non-epithelial nature (Hacker *et al.*, 1988) (Figure 14). The same phenotype was found to be expressed from early small lesions through large lesions (Hacker *et al.*, 1988, 1991).

Induction of drug-metabolizing enzymes by estrogens leading to enhanced neoplastic development, similar to that observed in the rat liver, has been reported (Roy & Liehr, 1988, 1989; Wu, 1979).

Ultrastructurally, blastemal, epithelial-like and mesenchymal cells can all be distinguished, with considerable intermingling. Epithelial-like cells lining tubules or cysts are rich in well organized cilia on the luminal surface. In contrast to blastemal cells, scattered organelles such as mitochondria, ribosomes and rough endoplasmic reticulum in close contact with Golgi complexes are evident.

Blastemal cells are characterized by relatively intimate intercellular contact, by poorly developed organelles and by irregular nuclei with one to three well developed nucleoli (Figures 15 and 16). Such mesenchymal cells may demonstrate obvious transition to epithelial-like cells (Llombardt-Bosch & Peydro-Olaya, 1986; Cortés-Vizcaíno *et al.*, 1994).

Mesenchymal tumours

Mesenchymal tumours arising in the kidneys of Syrian hamsters are fibromas or fibrosarcomas. Tumours of other mesenchymal tissues have not been reported.

The histogenesis of mesenchymal tumours in hamsters remains unclear. No information exists concerning induction of mesenchymal renal neoplasms by chemical carcinogens. A histopathological sequence, however, has been established for virus-induced tumours (Ham *et al.*, 1960).

After virus inoculation (Toronto polyomavirus), moderate stromal cell proliferation is observed in the corticomedullary junction. Cells are closely packed in areas between tubules and some nuclei appear damaged. Then, along with appearance of intranuclear inclusion bodies, mitotic figures become frequent. Subsequently as the degenerative response decreases, altered stromal cells proliferate progressively so that invasive tumour formation is evident as early as day 11.

The rapid development of kidney tumours induced by Stewart–Eddy polyomavirus (Stewart & Eddy, 1958) is essentially similar. However, the tumour cells have no alkaline phosphatase activity. Nodular tumours are reported to appear four weeks after polyomavirus infection, and large tumours (20–30 mm in diameter) show local invasion (Stanton & Otsuka, 1963). Virus-induced renal mesenchymal tumours are usually multiple and bilateral.

Characteristic findings are hard nodular masses in the renal area, which are sometimes palpable in living hamsters and, at autopsy, massive intraperitoneal haemorrhage into the abdominal cavity is often present. The kidneys are frequently enlarged and contain nodular, mostly multiple, solid masses of varying size which are grey-white in colour. Small neoplasms diagnosed in the first few weeks after viral treatment are not visible grossly. With large neoplasms invasive growth into the renal pelvis or directly through the capsule into the abdominal cavity may be observed.

At the microscopic level, renal sarcomas induced by several different species of polyomaviruses have all been found to consist of spindle-shaped tumour cells, occasionally interspersed with areas of abundant fibrous matrix but little collagen. Palisading arrangements may be apparent. Some regions may contain polygonal anaplastic or bizarre giant cells. Abundant mitotic figures are often seen in fibrosarcomas. Central necroses occur in large tumours (Althoff & Chesterman, 1982). The only haemangioendothelioma reported in the literature consisted of blood-filled cavernous spaces lined by single layers of poorly differentiated endothelial cells and separated by variable amounts of connective tissue; mitotic figures were common (Kesterson & Carlton, 1970).

Nephroblastomas

Nephroblastomas are not as common in hamsters as some other types of tumour. This may be due to the absence of a suitable experimental model or of carcinogens capable of inducing them. They appear as whitish indistinct lesions, and therefore are easily distinguishable from epithelial tumours which show clear demarcation from surrounding renal tissue.

Packed blastema tissue with varying degrees of epithelial differentiation is characteristic. Rosette-like, pseudoglandular, glomeruloid, tubular and papillary arrangements can be found. Occasionally, nephroblastomas are predominantly composed of epithelial elements with papillary structure (Figure 17).

TRANSPLANTATION OF TUMOURS

Transplantation of estrogen-induced epithelial or mesenchymal (including controversial) tumours has been successful only in orchidectomized or diethylstilbestrol (DES)-implanted hamsters. However, transplant take was 30 to 40%. Autonomous growth was observed after serial passage (Kirkman, 1974). Transplantation failed in intact and gonadectomized

untreated hamsters. A regression of transplants was observed after removal of DES implants, but treatment with testosterone did not cause regression of transplanted tumours (Ising, 1956; Horning, 1956; Kirkman, 1959b; Dontenwill & Ranz, 1960b; Fortner *et al.* 1961; Bloom *et al.*, 1963; Streggles & King, 1968; Dodge & Kirkman, 1970; Arcadi, 1971; El-Fiky & Abdo, 1971; El-Fiky *et al.*, 1971a, 1971b; Althoff & Chesterman, 1982).

SPONTANEOUS TUMOURS

Spontaneous development of kidney tumours in the Syrian hamster is very rare. In a group of 301 animals, one malignant renal neoplasm resembling a Wilms' tumour developed in a female (Fortner, 1957). In another group of 181 hamsters of both sexes, one renal tubular carcinoma was reported in a male (Fortner, 1961a), and a female in a group of 200 controls had an adenocarcinoma (Toth, 1967). In 4757 hamsters, one adenocarcinoma and one nephroblastoma type A, as classified according to Bodian and Rigby (1964), were observed (Kirkman & Algard, 1968). In another colony, 4762 hamsters were examined but no kidney neoplasms were detected (Chesterman, 1972).

No kidney neoplasms have been described in the large hamster colony at the Hannover Medical School (Chesterman, 1972; Pour *et al.*, 1976). However, in the Eppley Institute in Omaha, Nebraska, a small incidence of renal tumours has been found. For example, in one group of 313 hamsters in the Eppley colony, a tubular adenoma was recorded in a female, while in another female from a separate group of 200 hamsters one adenocarcinoma was diagnosed (Toth & Shimizu, 1973; Pour *et al.*, 1976). However, in 6 of 154 albino hamsters maintained in the same facility, renal neoplasms including cystic or tubular adenomas developed in one male and three females, and nephroblastomas were found in two females (Althoff & Chesterman, 1982). Nevertheless, it can be generally estimated that the incidence of spontaneous renal tumours is less than one in 1000 for the Syrian hamster (Althoff & Chesterman, 1982).

INDUCTION OF TUMOURS

Epithelial tumours

Epithelial kidney tumours have been induced by 7-methyl-bis-dihydroxy-synolic acid (Kirkman, 1959a, b; Kirkman & Bacon, 1952b), N-nitroso-N-(2-oxo-propyl)propylamine (Pour et al., 1974, 1980), N-nitrosobis(2-hydroxypropyl)-amine (Pour et al., 1975; Pour & Salmas, 1982), nitrosomorpholine (Althoff et al., 1985), N-nitrosodimethylamine (Tomatis et al., 1964), N-ethyl-N-nitrosourea plus phenacetin (Mennel & Zülch, 1972), ethylurea plus sodium nitrite (Rustia, 1974), urethane (Toth et al., 1961) and potassium bromate (Takamura et al., 1985).

Renal adenomas and carcinomas also occur after subcutaneous implantation of estradiol benzoate, treatment with DES, repeated injections of human bile (Vazquez-Lopez, 1944; Fortner et al., 1961), administration of betel quid extracts and intragastric application of cycasin (Dunham & Herrold, 1962; Hirono et al., 1971). Adenomatous proliferation of the renal tubules and adenomas were additionally observed in hamsters injected with polyomavirus suspensions obtained from a malignant hamster lymphoma (Stanton & Otsuka, 1963; Toth, 1967).

Epithelial–mesenchymal (controversial) tumours

This category of tumours has been induced by the following estrogen analogues: diethylstilbestrol (Matthews et al., 1947; Kirkman, 1951, 1960; Kirkman & Bacon, 1950, 1952a, b; Horning, 1954; Horning & Whittick, 1954; Pol'kina, 1959, 1961; Dontenwill & Eder, 1959; (Matthews

et al., 1947; McGregor et al., 1960; Dodge & Kirkman, 1970; de Kernion & Fraley, 1971; Llombart-Bosch & Peydró, 1975; Reznik-Schüller, 1979; Saluja et al., 1981; Liehr et al., 1984; Dodge et al., 1988; Gladek & Liehr, 1989). DES propionate (Mannweiller & Bernhard, 1957; Rivière et al., 1960; Dontenwill & Eder, 1959), DES dimethyl ester (Lacomba & Galbaldon, 1971), estradiol (Kirkman & Bacon, 1952b; Bacon & Kirkman, 1955; Kirkman, 1959a, b; Liehr, 1984; Liehr et al., 1984, 1986a, b, c; Lu et al., 1988), ethinyl-estradiol (Kirkman, 1959a; Kirkman & Bacon, 1952b; Li et al., 1980;1983; Li & Li, 1984; Liehr et al., 1992), and estrol (Kirkman, 1959a). However, a direct interaction between these estrogenic hormones and normal or tumorous kidney tissue has not been established (Liehr et al., 1989; Roy & Liehr, 1990).

Nephroblastomas

Nephroblastomas were reported to develop after intravenous injection of N-nitrosoethylurea (Mennel & Zülch, 1972; Nakamura et al., 1989) or transplacental administration of ethylurea and sodium nitrite (Rustia & Shubik, 1974).

Mesenchymal tumours

Mesenchymal tumours have been induced by DES (Matthews et al., 1947; Dontenwill & Eder, 1959), benzo[a]pyrene (Dontenwill & Ranz, 1960a, 1960b), and by different strains of polyomavirus and simian virus 40.

The following polyomavirus strains are able to induce mesenchymal tumours: Stewart–Eddy strain (Stewart & Eddy, 1958; Eddy et al., 1958, 1961, 1962; Stanton & Otsuka, 1963; Georgii & Ludwig, 1965), Toronto strain (McCulloch et al., 1959; Axelrad et al., 1960), and Mill Hill strain (Negroni & Chesterman, 1960; Chesterman, 1961). The incidence of mesenchymal tumours observed depends on age of administration of the virus (newborn versus older ages) and also on the virus strain and type of preparation used (Althoff & Chesterman, 1982).

COMPARATIVE ASPECTS

Available information concerning the characteristics of epithelial tumours and their precursor lesion, altered tubules, induced in hamsters by nitrosamines is not sufficient to allow detailed comparison with those generated in rats or mice. However, haematoxylin and eosin-stained sections of hamster tumours are similar to neoplastic lesions in kidneys of rats and man.

The high yields of characteristic tumours in response to estrogenic hormone administration appears to provide an interesting model for the analysis of hormone-dependent neoplasia. While many investigations have already been performed, the mechanisms of tumour development are not fully understood. Endogenous DNA adducts may be considered to mediate carcinogenic processes in the kidney of hamsters. Three different classes of covalent DNA alteration are induced by estrogens *in vivo* during hormonal renal carcinogenesis in the hamster:

(*a*) estrogen-DNA adducts formed by reactive estrogen quinone metabolites (Liehr *et al.*, 1986b, 1986c, 1987, 1988, 1993; Gladek & Liehr, 1989; Roy & Liehr, 1989; Han & Liehr, 1994);

(*b*) enhanced endogenous DNA modification (Liehr *et al.*, 1986a, 1987, 1988, 1993; Han & Liehr, 1994a; Wang & Liehr, 1995);

(*c*) 8-hydroxyguanine bases formed by free radicals generated by redox cycling of estrogen (Roy & Liehr, 1989, 1992; Han & Liehr, 1994b); A further action of relevance to carcinogenesis is destruction of cytochrome P450 enzymes in the hamster kidneys by reactive estrogen metabolites or lipid peroxides (Roy & Liehr, 1992).

ACKNOWLEDGEMENTS

The authors express their sincere gratitude to Dr Nobuyuki Ito, of the First Department of Pathology, Nagoya City University Medical School, for kind assistance and valuable advice during the preparation of this manuscript. Thanks are also due to Drs Keisuke Ozaki, Shuji Yamagachi and Malcolm A. Moore, of the First Department of Pathology, Nagoya City University Medical School, for assistance in the animal experiments and preparation of slides and photographs and to Drs Yuzo Hayashi and Yuji Kurokawa, of the National Institute of Hygienic Sciences, Tokyo, and Dr Yoichi Konishi, of Nara Medical University, for kindly providing histological slides.

REFERENCES

Althoff, J., Mohr, U. & Lijinsky, W. (1985) Comparative study on the carcinogenicity on *N*-nitroso-2,6-dimethylmorpholine in the European hamster. *J. Cancer Res. Clin. Oncol.*, 109, 183–187

Althoff, J. & Chesterman, F.C. (1982) Tumours of the kidney. In: Turusov, V.S. ed., *Pathology of Tumours in Laboratory Animals*. Vol. III, *Tumours of the Hamster*, (IARC Scientific Publications No. 34), Lyon, IARC, pp. 147–155

Arcadi, J.A. (1963) Glycogen-containing cells of estrogen-induced renal tumours of hamster. *Science*, 142, 592–593

Arcadi, J.A. (1971) Mast cells in the estrogen-induced transplantable renal tumour of the hamster. *J. Surg. Oncol.*, 3, 553–557

Axelrad, A.A., McCulloch, E.A., Howatson, A.F., Ham, A.W. & Siminovitch, L. (1960) Induction of tumours in Syrian hamsters by a cytopathogenic virus derived from a C3H mouse mammary tumour. *J. Natl Cancer Inst.*, 24, 1095–1112

Bacon, R.L. & Kirkman, H. (1955) The response of the testis of the hamster to chronic treatment with different estrogens. *Endocrinology*, 5, 255–271

Bannasch, P., Krech, R. & Zerban, H. (1978) Morphogenese und Mikromorphologie epithelialer Nierentumoren bei Nitrosomorpholin-vergifteten Ratten: II. Tubuläre Glykogenose und die Genese von klar- oder acidophilzelligen Tumouren. *Z Krebsforsch.*, 92, 63–86

Bannasch, P., Krech, R. & Zerban, H. (1980) Morphogenese und Mikromorphologie epithelialer Nierentumouren bei Nitroso-morpholine-vergifteten Ratten. IV. Tubulare Läsionen and basophile Tumoren. *J. Cancer Res. Clin. Oncol.*, 98, 248–265

Bannasch, P., Hacmer, H.J., Tsuda, H. & Zerban, H. (1986) Aberrant regulation of carbohydrate metabolism and metamorphosis during renal carcinogenesis. *Adv. Enzyme Regul.*, 25, 279–296

Bannasch, P., Nogueira, E. & Zerban, H. (1989) Zytologie und Zytogenese experimenteller epithelialer Nierentumoren. *Verh. Deutsch. Ges. Path.*, 73, 301–313

Bloom, H.J.G., Baker, W.H., Dukes, C.E. & Mitchely, B.C.V. (1963) Hormone dependent tumours of the kidney. II. Effect of endocrine ablation procedures on the transplanted oestrogen-induced renal tumour of the Syrian hamster. *Br. J. Cancer*, 17, 646–656

Bodian, M. & Rigby, C.C. (1964) The pathology of nephroblastoma. In: Riches, E., ed., *Neoplastic Disease of Various Sites*, Baltimore, Williams and Wilkins, pp. 219–234

Caviezel, M., Lutz, W.K., Minini, U. & Schlatter, C. (1984) Interaction of estrone and estradiol with DNA and protein of liver and kidney in rat hamster in vivo and vitro. *Arch. Toxicol.*, 55, 97–103

Chesterman, F.C. (1961) The pathological effects of the Mill Hill polyoma virus (MHP). *Med. Press*, 245, 350–355

Chesterman, F.C. (1972) Background pathology in a colony of golden hamsters. *Prog. Exp. Tumour Res.*, 16, 50–67

Cortés-Vizcaíno, V., Peydró-Olaya, A. & Llombart-Bosch, A. (1994) Morphological and immunohistochemical support for the interstitial cell origin of oestrogen-induced kidney tumours in the Syrian golden hamster. *Carcinogenesis*, 15, 2155–2162

deKernion, J.B. & Fraley, E. E. (1971) Growth characteristics of the stilbestrol-induced hamster kidney tumour. *J. Surg. Oncol.*, 3, 507–515

Dodge, A.H. (1977) Fine structural, G-6-PD isoenzyme, and HaLV g antigen studies of poly I/C and antiestrogen treated DES-induced hamster renal tumours. *Eur. J. Cancer*, 13, 1377–1387

Dodge, A.H. & Kirkman, H. (1981) A secretory stilbestrol-induced renal tumour of the Syrian hamster. *Proc. Am. Ass. Cancer Res.*, 22, 134

Dodge, A.H., Brownfield, M., Reid, I.A. & Inagami, T. (1988) Immunohistochemical renin study of DES-induced tumour in the Syrian hamster. *Am. J. Anat.*, 182, 347–352

Dontenwill, W. & Eder, M. (1959) Histogenese und biologische Verhaltensweise hormonell ausgelöster Geschwülste. *Beitr. Path. Anat.*, 120, 270–301

Dontenwill, W. & Ranz, H. (1960a) Experimentelle Untersuchungen zur Genese von Nierengeschwülsten beim Goldhamster. *Beitr. Path. Anat.*, 122, 381–389

Dontenwill, W. & Ranz, H. (1960b) Untersuchungen über die hormonale Abhängigkeit des durch Follikelhormon erzeugten Nierentumours des Goldhamsters bei der Transplantation. *Klin. Wschr.*, 38, 828

Dunham, L.J. & Herrold, K.M. (1962) Failure to produce tumours in the hamster cheek pouch by exposure to ingredients of betel quid: histopathologic changes in the pouch and other organs by exposure to known carcinogens. *J. Natl Cancer Inst.*, 29, 1047–1067

Eddy, B.E., Borman, G.S., Berkeley, W.H. & Young, R.D. (1961) tumours induced in hamsters by injection of rhesus monkey kidney cell extracts. *Proc. Soc. Exp. Biol. (N.Y.)*, 107, 191–197

Eddy, B.E., Borman, G.S., Berkeley, W.H. & Young, R.D. (1962) Identification of the oncogenic substance in rhesus monkey kidney cell cultures as simian virus 40. *Virology*, 17, 65–75

Eddy, B.E., Stewart, S.E., Young, R. & Mider, G.B. (1958) Neoplasms in hamsters induced by mouse tumour agent passed in tissue culture. *J. Natl Cancer Inst.*, 20, 747–761

El-Fiky, S.M. & Abdo, S.E. (1971) Karyometrical and cytochemical studies of Harding-Passey melanoma and Horning-Mitcheley kidney tumour. I. Karyometrical studies. *Acta Histochem.*, 41, 84–91

El-Fiky, S.M. Fahmy, T.Y. & Abdo, S.E. (1971a) Karyometrical and cytochemical studies on Harding-Passey melanoma and Horning-Mitcheley kidney tumour. II. Cytochemistry of nucleic acids and proteins. *Acta Histochem.*, 41, 92–101

El-Fiky, S.M. Fahmy, T.Y. & Abdo, S.E. (1971b) Karyometrical and cytochemical studies of Harding-Passey melanoma and Horning-Mitcheley kidney tumour. III. Cytochemistry of some hydrolytic enzymes. *Acta Histochem.*, 41, 102–107

Fortner, J.G. (1957) Spontaneous tumours, including gastrointestinal neoplasms and malignant melanomas, in the Syrian hamster. *Cancer*, 10, 1153–1156

Fortner, J.G. (1961a) The influence of castration on spontaneous tumorigenesis in the Syrian golden hamster. *Cancer Res.*, 21, 1491–1498

Fortner, J.G., Mahy, A.G. & Cotran, R.S. (1961b) Cancer chemotherapy screening data X, Part II: tumours of the hematopoietic tissues, genitourinary organs, mammary glands and sarcomas. Renal adenocarcinoma No.1. *Cancer Res.*, 21, 206–207

Georgii, A. & Ludwig, B. (1965) Nierenveränderungen durch SE-Polyoma virus. *Verh. Deutsch. Ges. Path.*, 49, 212–214

Gladek, A. & Liehr, J.G. (1989) Mechanism of genotoxicity of diethylstilbestrol in vitro. *J. Biol. Chem.*, 264, 16847–16852

González, A., Oberley, T.D. & Li, J.J. (1989) Morphological and immunohistochemical studies of the estrogen-induced Syrian hamster renal tumour: Probable cell of origin. *Cancer Res.*, 49, 1020–1028

Hacker, H.J., Bannasch, P. & Liehr, J.G. (1988) Histochemical analysis of the development of estradiol-induced kidney tumours in male Syrian hamsters. *Cancer Res.*, 48, 971–976

Hacker, H.J., Vollmer, G., Chiquet-Ehrismann, R., Bannasch, P. & Liehr, J.G. (1991) Changes in the cellular phenotype and extracellular matrix during progression of estrogen-induced mesenchymal kidney tumors in Syrian hamsters. *Virchows Arch.* (B), 60, 213–223

Ham, A.W., McCulloch, E.A., Axelrad, A.A., Siminovitch, L. & Howatson, A.F. (1960) The histopathological sequence in viral carcinogenesis in the hamster kidney. *J. Natl Cancer Inst.*, 24, 1113–1129

Han, X. & Liehr, J.G. (1994a) DNA single-strand breaks in kidneys of Syrian hamsters treated with steroidal estrogens: hormone-induced free radical damage preceding renal malignancy. *Carcinogenesis*, 15, 997–1000

Han, X. & Liehr, J.G. (1994b) 8-Hydroxylation of guanine bases in kidney and liver DNA of hamsters treated with estradiol: role of free radicals in estrogen-induced carcinogenesis. *Cancer Res.*, 54, 5515–5517

Hirono, I., Hayashi, K., Mori, H. & Miwa, T. (1971) Carcinogenic effects of cycasin in Syrian golden hamsters and the transplantability of induced tumours. *Cancer Res.*, 31, 283–287

Horning, E.S. (1954) The influence of unilateral nephrectomy on the development of stilbestrol-induced renal tumours in the male hamster. *Br. J. Cancer*, 8, 627–634

Horning, E.S. (1956) Observations on the hormone-dependent renal tumours in the golden hamster. *Br. J. Cancer*, 10, 678–687

Horning, E.S. & Whittick, J.W. (1954) The histogenesis of stilbestrol-induced renal tumours in the male golden hamster. *Br. J. Cancer*, 8, 451–457

Ising, U. (1956) The effect of unilateral ureterectomy on the development of estrogen-induced renal tumours in male hamsters. *Acta Pathol. Microbiol. Scand.*, 39, 168–180

Kesterson, J.W. & Carlton, W.W. (1970) Multiple malignant neoplasms in a golden hamster. A case report and literature survey. *Lab. Anim. Care*, 20, 220–225

Kirkman, H. (1974) Autonomous derivatives of estrogen-induced renal carcinomas and spontaneous renal tumours in the Syrian hamster. *Cancer Res.*, 34, 2728–2744

Kirkman, H. (1951) Relation of sex hormones to the induction and solution of renal tumours in the golden hamster. *Anat. Rec.*, 109, 311

Kirkman, H. (1959a) Estrogen-induced tumours of the kidney. III. Growth characteristics in the Syrian hamster. *Natl Cancer Inst. Monogr.*, 1, 1– 57

Kirkman, H. (1959b) Estrogen-induced tumours of the kidney. IV. Incidence in female Syrian hamsters. *Natl Cancer Inst. Monogr.*, 1, 59–91

Kirkman, H. & Algard, F.T. (1968) Spontaneous and non-viral induced neoplasms. In: Hoffman, R.A., Robinson, P.F. & Magalhaes, H., eds, *The Golden Hamster, its Biology and Use in Medical Research*, Ames, Iowa State University Press, pp. 227–240

Kirkman, H. & Bacon, R.L. (1950) Malignant renal tumours in male hamsters (*Cricetus auratus*) treated with estrogen. *Cancer Res.*, 10, 122–123

Kirkman, H. & Bacon, R.L. (1952a) Estrogen-induced tumours of the kidney. I. Incidence of renal tumours in intact and gonadectomized male golden hamsters treated with diethylstilbestrol. *J. Natl Cancer Inst.*, 13, 745–755

Kirkman, H. & Bacon, R.L. (1952b) Estrogen-induced tumours of the kidney. II. Effect of dose, administration, type of estrogen and age on the induction of renal tumours in the intact male golden hamster. *J. Natl Cancer Inst.*, 13, 757–771

Kirkman, H. & Robbins, M. (1959) Estrogen-induced tumours of the kidney. V. Histology and histogenesis in the Syrian hamster. *Natl Cancer Inst. Monogr.*, 1, 93–139

Lacomba, T. & Galbaldon, M. (1971) Biochemical studies of diethylstilbestrol-induced kidney tumours in the Syrian golden hamster. *Cancer Res.*, 31, 1251–1256

Li, S.A. and Li, J.J. (1978) Estrogen-induced progesterone receptor in the Syrian hamster kidney. I. Modulation by anti-estrogens and androgens. *Endocrinology*, 103, 2119–2128

Li, J.J. & Li, S.A. (1981) Estrogen-induced progesterone receptor in the Syrian hamster kidney. II. Modulation by synthetic progestins. *Endocrinology*, 108, 1751–1756

Li, J.J. & Li, S.A. (1984) Estrogen-induced tumourigenesis in hamsters: roles for hormonal and carcinogenic-activities. *Arch. Toxicol.*, 55, 110–118.

Li, J.J., Talley, D.J., Li, S.A. (1976) Receptor characteristics of specific estrogen binding in the renal adenocarcinoma of the golden hamster. *Cancer Res.*, 36, 1127–1132

Li, S.A., Li, J.J. & Villee, C.A. (1977) Significance of the progesterone receptor in the estrogen-induced and -dependent renal tumor of the Syrian golden hamster. *Ann. N.Y. Acad. Sci.*, 286, 369–383

Li, J.J., Li, S.A. & Cuthbertson, T.L. (1979) Nuclear retention of all steroid hormone receptor classes in the hamster renal carcinoma. *Cancer Res.*, 39, 2647–2651

Li, J.J., Cuthbertson, T.L. & Li, S.A. (1980) Inhibition of estrogen tumorigenesis in the Syrian golden hamster kidney by anti-estrogens. *J. Natl Cancer Inst.*, 64, 795–800

Li, J.J., Li, S.A., Klicka, J.K., Parsons, J.A. & Lam, L.K.T. (1983) Relative carcinogenic activity of various synthetic and natural estrogens in the Syrian hamster kidney. *Cancer Res.*, 43, 5200–5204

Liehr, J.G. (1984) Modulation of estrogen-induced carcinogenesis by chemical modifications. *Arch. Toxicol.*, 55, 119–122

Liehr, J.G., Ballatore, A.M., McLachlan, J.A. & Sirbasku, D.A. (1984) Mechanisms of diethylstilbestrol carcinogenicity as studies with the fluorinated analogue E-3'-3",5'5"-tetrafluorodiethylstilbestrol. *Cancer Res.*, 43, 2678–2682

Liehr, J.G., Avitts, T.A., Randerath, E. & Randerath, K. (1986a) Estrogen-induced endogenous DNA adduction: possible mechanism of hormonal cancer. *Proc. Natl Acad. Sci. USA*, 83, 5301–5305

Liehr, J.G., Fang, W.F. & Sirbasku, D.A. (1986b) Carcinogenicity of catechol estrogens in Syrian hamsters. *J. Steroid Biochem.*, 24, 353–356

Liehr, J.G., Stancel, G.M., Chorich, L.P. & Bousfield, G.R. (1986c) Hormonal carcinogene-sis: separation of estrogenicity from carcinogenicity. *Chem. Biol. Interact.*, 59, 173–184

Liehr, J.G., Hall, E.R., Avitts, T.A., Randerath, E. & Randerath, K. (1987) Localization of estrogen-induced DNA adducts and cytochrome P-450 activity at the site of renal carcinogenesis in the hamster kidney. *Cancer Res.*, 47, 2156–2159

Liehr, J.G., Sirbasku, D.A., Jurka, E., Randerath, K. & Randerath, E. (1988) Inhibition of estrogen-induced renal carcinogenesis in male Syrian hamsters by tamoxifen without decrease in DNA adduct levels. *Cancer Res.*, 48, 779–783

Liehr, J.G., Roy, D. & Gladek, A. (1989) Mechanism of inhibition of estrogen-induced renal carcinogenesis in male Syrian hamsters by vitamin C. *Carcinogenesis*, 10, 1983–1988

Liehr, J.G., Han, X. & Bhat, H.K. (1993) 32P-postlabelling in studies on hormonal carcinogenesis. In: Phillips, D.H., Castegnaro, M. & Bartsch, H., eds, *Postlabelling Methods for Detection of DNA Adducts* (IARC Scientific Publications No. 124), Lyon, IARC, pp. 149–155

Llombardt-Bosch, A. & Peydró, A. (1975) Morphological, histochemical and ultra-structural observations of diethylstilbestrol-induced kidney tumours in the Syrian golden hamster. *Eur. J. Cancer*, 11, 403–412

Llombardt-Bosch, A. & Peydro-Olaya, A. (1986) Estrogen-induced malignant tumour, kidney, Syrian hamsters. In: T.C. Jones, U. Mohr & R.D. Hunt eds., *The Urinary System* (Monographs on Pathology of Laboratory Animals), Berlin, Heidelberg, New York, Springer-Verlag, pp. 141–152

Lu, L.J., Liehr, J.G., Sirbasku, D.A., Randerath, E. & Randerath, K. (1988) Hypomethylation of DNA in estrogen-induced and -dependent hamster kidney tumours. *Carcinogenesis*, 9, 925–929

Mannweiler, K. & Bernhard, W. (1957) Recherches ultrastructurales sur une tumeur rénale expérimentale du hamster. *J. Ultrastruct. Res.*, 1, 158–169

Matthews, V.S., Kirkman, H. & Bacon, R.L. (1947) Kidney damage in the golden hamster following chronic administration of diethylstilbestrol and sesame oil. *Proc. Soc. Exp. Biol. (N.Y.)*, 66, 195–196

McCulloch, E.A., Howatson, A.F., Siminovitch, L., Axelrad, A.A. & Ham, A.W. (1959) A cytopathogenetic agent from a mammary tumour in a CH mouse that produces tumours in Swiss mice and hamsters. *Nature*, 183, 1535–1536

McGregor, R.F., Putsch, J.D. & Ward, D.N. (1960) Estrogen-induced kidney tumours in the golden hamster. I. Biochemical composition during tumorigenesis. *J. Natl Cancer Inst.*, 24, 1057–1066

Mennel, H.D. & Zülch, K.J. (1972) Zur Morphologie transplacentar erzeugter neurogener tumoren beim Goldhamster. *Acta Neuropathol. (Berlin)*, 21, 194–203

Murthy, A.S.K. & Russfield, A.B. (1968) Dehydrogenases in diethylstilbestrol-induced kidney tumours of the Syrian hamster. *Experientia*, 24, 60–61

Nakamura, T., Hara, M. & Kasuga, T. (1989) Transplacental induction of peripheral nervous tumour in the Syrian golden hamster by *N*-nitroso-*N*-ethylurea. A new animal model for von Recklinghausen's neurofibromatosis. *Am. J. Pathol.*, 135, 251–258

Negroni, G. & Chesterman, F.C. (1960) Virus-cell relationship in kidney tumours induced in golden hamsters by Mill Hill polyoma virus. *Br. J. Cancer*, 14, 672–678

Nogueira, E. & Bannasch, P. (1988) Cellular origin of renal oncocytoma. *Lab. Invest.*, 59, 337–343

Pol'kina, R.F. (1959) An experimental morphological investigation of tumours of the kidneys in golden hamsters caused by diethylstilbestrol. *Vop. Onkol.*, 5, 32–37

Pol'kina, R.J. (1961) Kidney tumours induced by sinestrol and diethylstilbestrol in hamsters. *Vop. Onkol.*, 7, 35–41

Pour, P.M. & Salmasi, S.Z. (1982) Comparative studies of compounds. The effect of *N*-nitrosobis(2-hydroxypropyl)amine on Syrian golden hamsters. *J. Cancer Res. Clin. Oncol.*, 102, 265–269

Pour, P., Althoff, J., Cardesa, A., Krüger, F.W. & Mohr, U. (1974) Effect of beta-oxidized nitrosamine on Syrian golden hamsters. II. 2-oxopropyl-*N*-propylnitrosamine. *J. Natl Cancer Inst.*, 52, 1869–1874

Pour, P., Krüger, F.W., Althoff, J., Cardesa, A., & Mohr, U. (1975) Effect of oxidized nitrosamines on Syrian hamsters. III. 2,2'-dihydroxy-di-*N*-propylnitrosamine. *J. Natl Cancer Inst.*, 54, 141

Pour, P.M., Mohr, U., Althoff, J., Cardesa, A. & Kmoch, N. (1976) Spontaneous tumours and common diseases in two colonies of Syrian hamsters. III. Urological system and endocrine glands. *J. Natl Cancer Inst.*, 56, 949–961

Pour, P., Gingell, R., Langenback, R., Nagel, D., Grandjean, C., Lawson, T. & Salmasi, S. (1980) Carcinogenicity of *N*-nitroso-methyl-(2-oxopropyl)amine in Syrian hamsters. *Cancer Res.*, 40, 3585–3590

Pour, P.M. (1986a) Adenoma, kidney, Syrian hamster. In: Jones, T.C., Mohr, U. & Hunt, R.D. eds, *The Urinary System* (Monographs on Pathology of Laboratory Animals), Berlin, Heidelberg, New York, Springer-Verlag, pp. 101–107

Pour, P.M. (1986b) Adenocarcinoma, kidney, Syrian hamster. In: Jones, T.C., Mohr, U. & Hunt, R.D. eds, *The Urinary System* (Monographs on Pathology of Laboratory Animals), Berlin, Heidelberg, New York, Springer-Verlag, pp. 107–112

Reznik-Schüller, S.H. (1979) Carcinogenic effects of diethylstilbestrol in male Syrian golden hamsters and European hamsters. *J. Natl Cancer Inst.*, 62, 1083–1088

Rivière, M.R., Chouroulinkov, I. & Guérin, M. (1960) Action inhibante de la désoxy-corticostérone sur la production de tumeurs rénales chez le hamster male traité par un oestrogène. *C. R. Séanc. Soc. Biol.*, 154, 1415–1418

Roy, D. & Liehr, J.G. (1988) Characterization of drug metabolism enzymes in estrogen-induced kidney tumours in male Syrian hamsters. *Cancer Res.*, 48, 5726–5729

Roy, D. & Liehr, J.G. (1989) Changes in activities of free radical detoxifying enzymes in kidneys of male Syrian hamsters treated with estradiol. *Cancer Res.*, 49, 1475–1480

Roy, D. & Liehr, J.G. (1990) Inhibition of estrogen-induced kidney carcinogenesis in Syrian hamsters by modulators of estrogen metabolism. *Carcinogenesis*, 11, 567–570

Roy, D. & Liehr, J.G. (1992) Target organ-specific inactivation of drug metabolizing enzymes in kidney of hamsters treated with estradiol. *Mol. Cell. Biochem.*, 110, 31–39

Rustia, M. (1974) Multiple carcinogenic effects of the ethylnitrosourea precursors ethylurea and sodium nitrite in hamsters. *Cancer Res.*, 27, 3232–3244

Rustia, M. and Shubik, P. (1974) Prenatal induction of neurogenic tumours in hamsters by precursors ethylurea and sodium nitrite. *J. Natl Cancer Inst.*, 52, 605–608

Saluja, P.G. Hamilton, J.M. & Thody, A.J. (1981) Hormonal induction of kidney tumours in male hamsters. Inhibition of growth by a phenothiazine derivative (perphenazine). *Eur. J. Cancer Clin. Oncol.*, 17, 767–773

Stanton, M.F. & Otsuka, H. (1963) Morphology of the oncogenic response of hamsters to polyoma virus infection. *J. Natl Cancer Inst.*, 31, 365–409

Stewart, S.E. & Eddy, B.E. (1958) A review on the biological properties of SE polyoma virus. In: Proceedings, VI World Congress on Haematology (Rome), pp. 596–601

Streggles, A.W. & King, R.J.B. (1968) The uptake of 6,7-^{3}H-oestradiol by oestrogen dependent and independent hamster's kidney tumours. *Eur. J. Cancer*, 4, 395–401

Takamura, N., Kurokawa, Y., Matsushima, Y., Imazawa, T., Onodera, H. & Hayashi, Y. (1985) Long-term oral administration of potassium bromate in male Syrian golden hamsters. *Sci. Rep. Res. Inst. Tohoku Univ.*, 32, 43–46

Tomatis, L., Magee, P.N. & Shubik, P. (1964) Induction of liver tumours in the Syrian hamster by feeding dimethylnitrosamine. *J. Natl Cancer Inst.*, 33, 341–346

Toth, B. (1967) Studies on the incidence, morphology, transplantation, and cell-free filtration of malignant lymphomas in the Syrian golden hamster. *Cancer Res.*, 27, 1430–1442

Toth, B. & Shimizu, H. (1973) Methylhydrazine tumorigenesis in Syrian golden hamsters and the morphology of malignant histocytomas. *Cancer Res.*, 33, 2744–2753

Toth, B., Tomatis, L. & Shubik, P. (1961) Multipotential carcinogenesis with urethan in the Syrian golden hamster. *Cancer Res.*, 21, 1537–1541

Tse, J., Golfarb, S. & Pugh, T.D. (1989) Autoradiographic evidence of estrogen binding sites in nuclei of diethylstilbestrol induced hamster renal carcinomas. *Carcinogenesis*, 10, 957–959

Tsuda, H., Moore, M.A., Asamoto, M., Satoh, K., Tsuchida, S., Sato, K., Ichihara, A. & Ito, N. (1985) Comparison of the various forms of glutathione S-transferase with glucose-6-phosphate preneoplastic and neoplastic lesions in rat kidney induced by *N*-ethyl-*N*-hydroxyethylnitrosamine. *Jpn. J. Cancer Res.*, 76, 919–929

Tsuda, H., Hacker, H.J., Katayama, H., Masui, T., Ito, N. & Bannasch, P. (1986) Correlative histochemical studies on preneoplastic lesions in the kidney of rats treated with nitrosamines. *Virchows Arch.* (B), 51, 385–484

Tsuda, H., Moore, M.A., Asamoto, M., Inoue, T., Fukushima, S., Ito, N., Satoh, K., Amelizad, Z. & Oesch, F. (1987) Immunohistochemically demonstrated altered expression of cytochrome P-450 molecular forms and epoxide hydrolase in *N*-ethyl-*N*-hydroxy-ethyl-nitrosamine-induced rat kidney and liver lesions. *Carcinogenesis*, 8, 711–717

Vazquez-Lopez, E. (1944) The reaction of the pituitary gland and related hypothalamic centres in the hamster to prolonged treatment with oestrogens. *J. Pathol. Bacteriol.*, 56, 1–15

Wang, M.Y. & Liehr, J.G. (1995) Lipid hydroperoxide-induced endogenous DNA adducts in hamsters: possible mechanism of lipid hydroperoxide-mediated carcinogenesis. *Arch. Biochem. Biophys.*, 316, 38–46

Wu, C. (1979) Estrogen receptor translocation and ornithine aminotransferase induction by estradiol in rat kidney. *Biochem. Biophys. Res. Commun.*, 89, 769–776

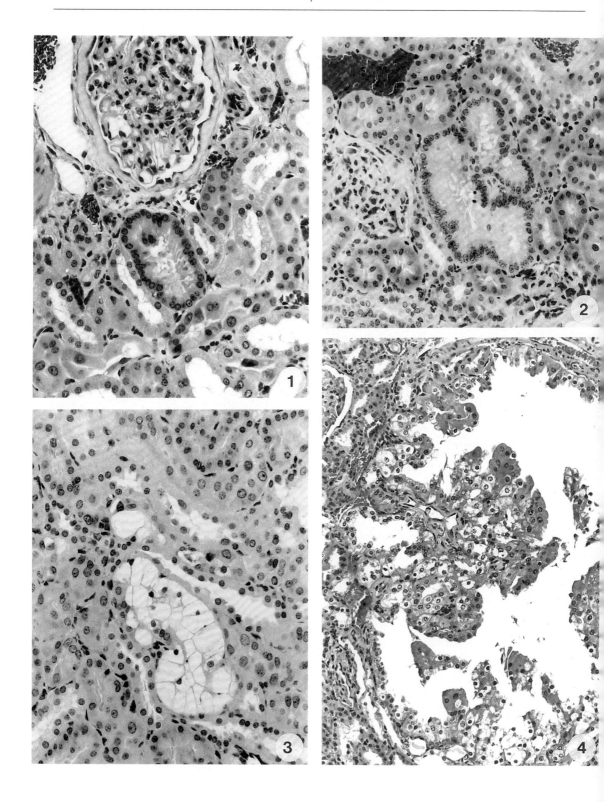

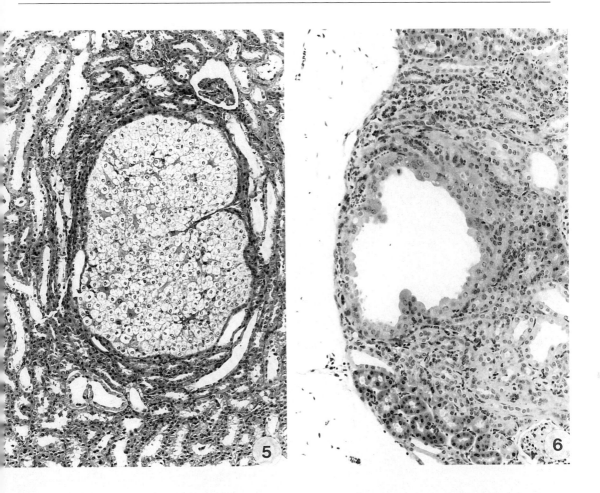

Figure 1. Basophilic cell tubule in a male Syrian golden hamster given *N*-nitrobis(2-hydroxypropyl)amine (NDHPA). H&E; × 80

Figure 2. Basophilic cell tubules in a male hamster after NDHPA treatment. The alteration involves a large part of the proximal tubules. H&E; ×66

Figure 3. Clear cell tubule in a male Syrian hamster given NDHPA. Note clear cytoplasm and hyperchromatic round nuclei. H&E; ×80

Figure 4. Papillary adenoma in a male Syrian hamster after NDHPA treatment. Epithelial cells in papillary formations are observed projecting into the lumen. H&E; ×50

Figure 5. Clear cell solid adenoma in a male hamster given potassium bromate. The lesion does not have any obvious stromal element. H&E; ×33

Figure 6. Basophilic cystic adenoma in a male hamster given NDHPA. Single or double layers of cells are arranged around a dilated lumen. H&E; ×40

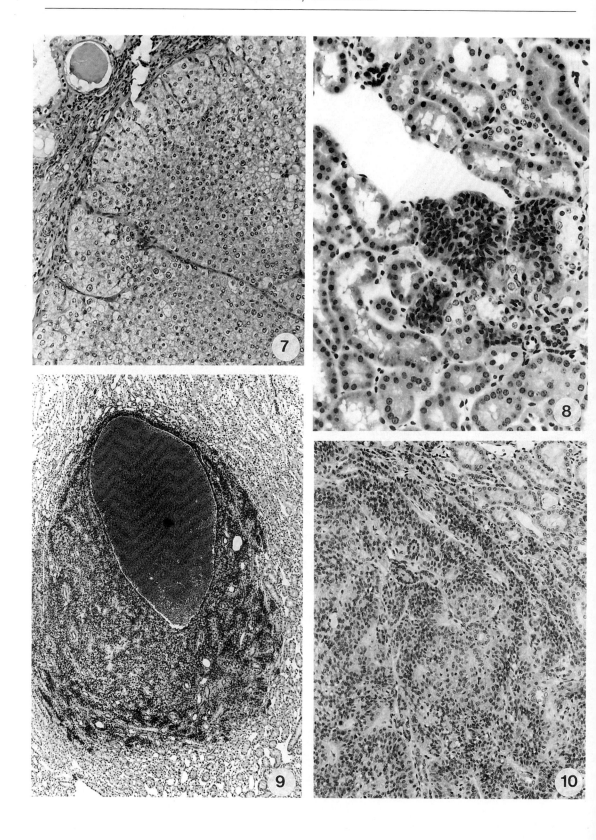

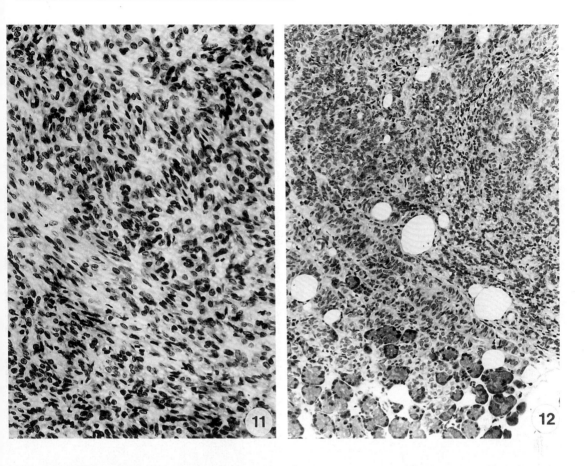

Figure 7. Clear/granular cell carcinoma in a male golden hamster given potassium bromate. Note obvious cellular and nuclear atypia. H&E; ×50

Figure 8. Early focus formation of mesenchymal tumour in the cortex of a male golden hamster kidney after subcutaneous implantation of 17β- estradiol. H&E; ×80

Figure 9. Mesenchymal tumour in a male Syrian hamster given 17β-estradiol. Tumour cells are strongly positive for alkaline phosphatase activity. The tumour contains a large dilated blood space. Note the infiltrative mode of growth in the periphery of the lesion. Alkaline phosphatase histochemistry plus haematoxylin; ×13

Figure 10. Histopathological detail of a part of the tumour shown in Figure 9 (semi-serial section). H&E; ×33

Figure 11. High-power magnification of the tumour in Figure 10. Round to spindle-shaped tumour cells are arranged in rosette-like or pseudo-palisade patterns. H&E; ×80

Figure 12. Metastatic focus of a mesenchymal tumour in the pancreas of a Syrian hamster given 17β-estradiol. H&E; ×50

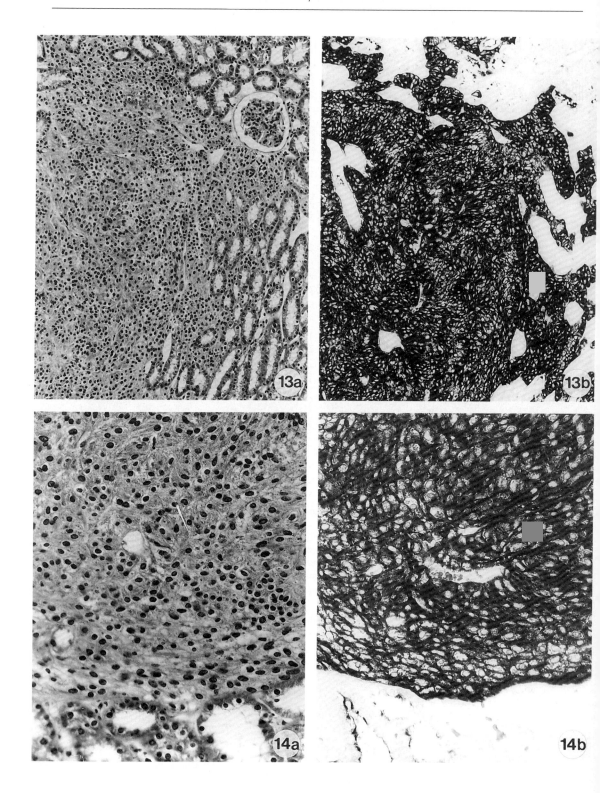

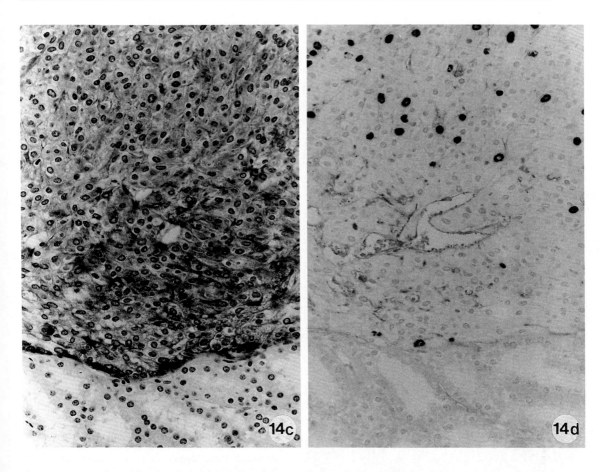

Figure 13. Mesenchymal tumour in a male Syrian hamster receiving 17β-estradiol (serial section). Tumour cells infiltrate into the surrounding tubular tissue. a, H&E; b, alkaline phosphatase activity; ×33

Figure 14. Serial sections through a mesenchymal tumour in a Syrian hamster given 17β-estradiol. a, H&E; b, alkaline phosphatase (histochemistry); c, vimentin (immunostaining); d, nuclear BrdU incorporation by S-phase cells; ×80

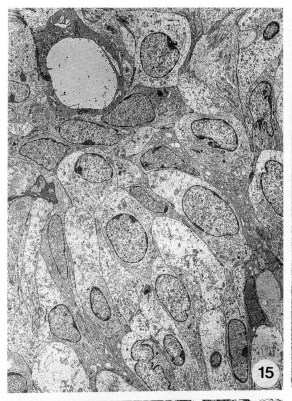

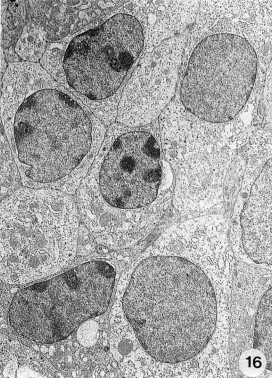

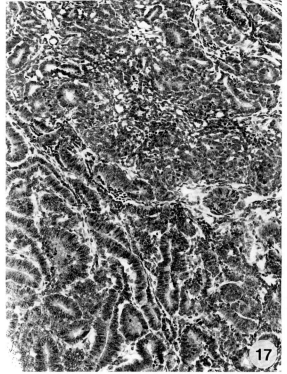

Figure 15. Electron microscopic appearance of mesenchymal tumour cells. Spindle-shaped cells are arranged some degree of polarity. Gland-like lumen (lower left) may indicate epithelial differentiation. ×1000

Figure 16. Electron microscopic appearance of a mesenchymal tumour at higher magnification. Tumour cells are round to oval shape and devoid of cell-to-cell adhesion organelles. ×5000

Figure 17. Nephroblastoma (epithelial type) in a male golden hamster given NDHPA. Note presence of both epithelial and mesenchymal components. H&E; ×40

Tumours of the urinary bladder, renal pelvis, ureter and urethra

S. Fukushima, Y. Kurata and M.-A. Shibata

Chemicals such as 2-naphthylamine, 4-aminobiphenyl, cyclophosphamide and benzidine have been identified as carcinogens for the human urinary bladder, and their carcinogenicity has been confirmed experimentally (IARC, 1987). Other agents that have been found to be strongly carcinogenic for the urinary bladder of experimental animals include N-butyl-(4-hydroxybutyl)nitrosamine (BBN) (Druckrey et al., 1964; Ito et al., 1969), N-ethyl-(4-hydroxybutyl)nitrosamine (EHBN) (Hashimoto et al., 1972), N-[4-(nitro-2-furyl)-2-thiazolyl]formamide (FANFT) (Ertürk et al., 1967), 2-acetylaminofluorene (AAF) (Littlefield et al., 1975) and N-methyl-N-nitrosourea (MNU) (Hicks & Wakefield, 1972). The tumours induced by chemicals in rodents closely resemble human bladder cancers both grossly and histologically. Studies of such tumours, especially in rats and mice, have thus contributed not only to analysis of the histogenesis of urothelial neoplasms, but also to selection of drugs for systemic and intravesical chemotherapy and to detection of modifiers of urinary bladder carcinogenesis.

However, the question of how to extrapolate the results of laboratory studies to man, given the species differences in metabolic activation and susceptibility, has received increasing attention. Thus, demand for suitable animal species, other than the rat and mouse, for toxicological assessment has lent weight to use of the hamster as an experimental animal.

NORMAL STRUCTURE

The normal structure of the hamster urinary tract is almost the same as that of other rodent species. Urine is conveyed from the kidney to the exterior through the minor and major calyxes, the renal pelvis, the ureter, the urinary bladder and the urethra. The mucosa lining these organs, except for the latter part of the urethra, is transitional cell epithelium (urothelium). This epithelial lining is basally supported by two layers, the submucosal layer and the muscle layer in the ureter, urinary bladder and urethra.

Urinary bladder

The thickness of the transitional epithelium comprises two to three cell layers under conditions of inflation with fixative, but depends on the urine volume. In the empty urinary bladder, the multilayer epithelium forms prominent folds. The normal epithelium is made up of a superficial cell layer, one or more layers of intermediate cells, and a basal cell layer resting on a basement membrane. The upper layers of epithelial cells become progressively larger in size, the uppermost superficial elements, however, being flattened and therefore called 'umbrella cells'. On transmission electron microscopy, the luminal membrane of surface cells appears as a triple layer, asymmetrical unit membrane, and the cells demonstrate numerous fusiform vesicles. The basement membrane is composed of a lamina lucida and a lamina densa. The basal cells of the epithelium are attached to the lamina densa by hemidesmosomes. The region of the trigone, where both right and left ureters open and the urethra is located, lacks the submucosal elements, but has a thick muscular layer. The epithelium in the trigone is especially thick in the hamster.

Under the scanning electron microscope (SEM), the epithelial luminal surface demonstrates a network of fine-peaked microridges, formed by regularly arranged cells that are mainly hexagonal, but partly pentagonal or rhombic in shape, with no microvilli (Ito 1976; Shirai *et al.,* 1977) (Figure 1).

Ureter

The epithelium of the ureter is three to six cells thick, a capillary network being located beneath the basal layer. The submucosa contains abundant fine collagenous fibres and elastic fibres. The muscular layer consists of two opposed layers of smooth muscle, the inner being longitudinal and the outer circular. An additional longitudinal muscle outer layer is seen in the portion of the ureter close to the urinary bladder.

Urethra

The male urethra is longer than that of the female and can be divided into three parts: the pelvic, bulbo-urethral and penile regions. The pelvic zone is further divided into prostatic and membranous parts. The urethra from the pelvic to the bulbo-urethral parts is lined by transitional, but the penile part by stratified squamous epithelium.

The mucosa of the female consists mainly of transitional epithelium, with only a short final section having stratified squamous epithelium.

MORPHOLOGY AND BIOLOGY OF TUMOURS

Gross appearance

For optimal observation of neoplastic lesions, the urinary bladder should be inflated by intraluminal injection of fixative. The distended normal luminal surface of the urinary bladder has a smooth surface and the wall is whitish and translucent. Simple hyperplastic changes are difficult to recognize, but focal nodules are visible as small white spots and/or irregular thickened areas on the bladder mucosa. Tumour occurrence is not associated with any particular site in the urinary bladder. Exophytic, sessile or pedunculated types of growth are seen.

Thickening of the urinary bladder wall is often observed. Surfaces of larger lesions are discoloured and irregular with areas of a haemorrhage and ulceration. Gross haematuria is observed occasionally. Sometimes, neoplastic thickened areas appreciably reduce the lumen space.

Histological types of tumour

Epithelial hyperplasia

    Simple hyperplasia
    Papillary or nodular (PN) hyperplasia

Benign tumour

    Transitional cell papilloma
    Squamous cell papilloma
    Haemangioma
    Others

Malignant tumour

    Transitional cell carcinoma (TCC)
    Squamous cell carcinoma
    Adenocarcinoma
    Haemangiosarcoma
    Others

The hamster urinary bladder gives rise mainly to transitional cell papillomas or carcinomas and the occurrence of other tumour types is uncommon.

Microscopic appearance of transitional cell tumours

The morphological features of preneoplastic or neoplastic lesions derived from transitional epithelium in the hamster are similar, whether they occur in the urinary bladder, urethra, ureter or renal pelvis.

Epithelial hyperplasia. The first visible transformation stage is a simple hyperplasia consisting of a diffuse or focal thickening of the epithelium with 4 to 8 layers of transitional epithelial cells (Figure 2). Generally, normal cell differentiation from basal to superficial cells is essentially maintained and mitotic figures are quite rare. However, in the hamster, large and dysplastic cells are frequently observed (Figure 3). Cytoplasmic vacuoles presumably reflecting apoptosis are commonly noted in the upper parts of the hyperplastic area. Under the SEM, short uniform microvilli, or ropy or leafy microridges, are seen on the luminal cell surfaces of early hyperplastic areas in the hamster (Ito, 1976; Shirai *et al.*, 1977) (Figure 4).

The next advanced stage is papillary or nodular (PN) hyperplasia. This lesion has been recognized as a preneoplastic lesion in rats and mice (Fukushima *et al.*, 1982; Tamano *et al.*, 1991), and in the hamster, most neoplasia seems to occur from areas of PN hyperplasia. It is localized and of two types: papillary proliferation of epithelial cells supported by thin stromal tissue elements including neovascularization and nodular proliferation showing downward growth. In the hamster, the latter type is frequently observed involving dysplastic change (Figure 5). Its development precedes the appearance of carcinoma. However, it is difficult to distinguish between reversible and irreversible forms of PN hyperplasia. Under the SEM, various microvilli are observed on the luminal surface of proliferative areas in the bladder. SEM lesions are more marked on bladder tumour cell surfaces.

Transitional cell papilloma. This tumour is composed of epithelial cells with slightly hyperchromatic nuclei and oval form. Mitotic figures are quite few and cell shape is relatively uniform. Althoff and Chesterman (1982) previously reported that some surface-lining cells have basally oriented nuclei and show mucus formation (periodic acid–Schiff reaction and Kreyberg's and Alcian blue staining). Papillomas also show downward growth, without invasion, forming bulges along the basal cell layer. The degree of cellular atypia is an important issue for differential diagnosis from carcinoma when there is no apparent infiltration or metastasis.

Transitional cell carcinoma (TCC). Typical TCCs have high levels of cellular atypia (enlargement and hyperchromasia) and many mitotic figures. Small cell nests with marked cellular atypia which develop within the epithelial layer can be interpreted as carcinoma *in situ* (Figure 6). Early-stage TCCs form nests and strands of atypical cells and penetrate the basement membrane and invade as if taking root in the submucosa (Figure 7). The invasive cell nests sometimes demonstrate pseudoglandular patterns (Figure 8) and/or squamous cell metaplasia (Althoff & Chesterman, 1982). Inflammatory changes become more common in areas surrounding neoplastic tissues (Figure 9). The classification of TCC based on growth pattern according to human pathology (Koss, 1975; Mostofi & Sesterhenn, 1983) divides them into two types: papillary and non-papillary. The papillary type shows exophytic growth into the lumen , while the non-papillary type which is frequently observed exhibits endophytic growth highly accompanied by invasion (Figures 10 and 11). Non-papillary, non-invasive carcinomas which are confined to the mucosa are diagnosed as carcinomas *in situ*.

Microscopic appearance of other urinary bladder tumours

Squamous cell carcinoma. The morphology of squamous cell carcinomas in the hamster urinary bladder does not differ from equivalent lesions in other tissues. The presence of keratinization, intercellular bridges and other features of normal squamous cell elements provides the diagnostic criteria. Squamous cell carcinomas presumably develop from transformed transitional cells, since squamous metaplasia always occurs in areas of transitional cell hyperplasia.

Adenocarcinoma. Carcinomas which show glandular patterns with mucus production and secretion into the lumina, and in which the epithelial cells possess brush borders, are diagnosed as adenocarcinomas. Their pathogenesis is unknown. However, Tomatis *et al.* (1961) reported adenocarcinomas in the urinary bladder of the hamster to closely resemble those observed in man and suggested an origin from the urachus or remnants of the allantoic duct which connect the dome or adjacent anterior wall of the bladder to the allantois via the umbilicus during early embryonal life.

Haemangioma or haemangiosarcoma. Vascular tumours arise from the urinary bladder wall of the hamster. Microscopically, cavernous haemangioma (Figure 12) shows many spacious vascular channels lined by a single cell layer of endothelial cells. Haemangiosarcoma or haemangioendothelioma contain many small irregular vascular spaces. The channels are lined by endothelial cells which exhibit atypical features including mitotic figures. These vascular tumours are haemorrhagic.

Staging and grading of urinary bladder carcinomas

The histological stages and grades of urinary bladder carcinomas in the hamster have not yet been established. There are some reports which attempt to evaluate the carcinogenicity of certain chemicals according to strict criteria (Althoff & Lijinsky, 1977; Croft & Bryan, 1973; Oyasu, 1973). If it is necessary to make comparisons with

human bladder carcinomas, staging according to the UICC modification (1989) of the TNM classification of bladder tumours is recommended. The following classification scheme is based on these proposals. TCC can be classified into five stages; pTa – papillary, non-invasive carcinoma or pTis – carcinoma *in situ*, a non-papillary carcinoma confined to the mucosa with high-grade cellular atypia (pre-invasive carcinoma); pT1 – invasion into the sub-mucosa; pT2 – invasion into muscle; pT3 – invasion into serosa (Figure 13) or perivesicular adipose tissue; and pT4 – invasion into adjacent or distant organs.

TCC can also be graded on a scale of 1 to 3 on the basis of the degree of cellular and structural atypia (Figures 14–16). Cellular atypism is morphological difference from normal cells based on the sizes of the nucleus (N) and cytoplasm (C), the N:C ratio, shape and staining intensity of the nucleus, mitotic figures or cellular pleomorphism. Structural atypism means disorders of cell arrangement including epithelial thickness, superficial cell differentiation or cellular polarity. Features of grade 1 (G1) are slight loss of polarity and hyperchromatism of the nuclei (Figure 14), amounting to slight atypia of both structure and cellularity. Grade 2 (G2) is characterized by moderate atypia of either structure or cells (Figure 15). Grade 3 (G3) represents severe atypia of either structure or cellularity, nuclear pleomorphism being a striking feature of the tumour cells (Figure 16).

SPONTANEOUS TUMOURS

Since 1937, one of the main reasons for the use of hamsters in carcinogenesis studies has been the low incidence of spontaneous tumours. No naturally occurring epithelial neoplasm of the urinary bladder has been reported in the literature reviewed (Pour *et al.*, 1976a,b). Two cases of malignant lymphoma have been found as the only neoplastic lesions developing in the urinary bladder of non-treated hamsters (Schmidt *et al.*, 1983).

INDUCTION OF TUMOURS

Tumours of the urinary bladder

A summary of published reports (1961–1988) of urinary bladder carcinoma induction by various chemicals in the hamster is presented in Table 1. More than 99% of induced bladder carcinomas have been found to be of transitional cell type, the remainder being squamous cell carcinomas. With many regimens only one case of adenocarcinoma developed within the area of TCC (Tomatis *et al.*, 1961). Carcinoma *in situ* may be sometimes seen, but no undifferentiated carcinomas have been reported so far. Generally, experimental induction of urinary bladder tumours requires relatively long periods of time. As shown in Table 1, the hamster urinary bladder is no exception, with carcinoma induction usually requiring more than 30 weeks. Indeed, 2-acetylaminofluorene (AAF) produces a high incidence of urinary bladder tumours in the hamster only if simultaneous administration of indole is used to indirectly inhibit its hepatocarcinogenicity and therefore prolong survival (Oyasu *et al.*, 1970). To a certain extent, organ- or tissue-specific chemical carcinogens are thus required for generation of urinary bladder carcinomas. Various authors have reported only benign tumours or early neoplastic lesions in the hamster urinary bladder (Pour *et al.*, 1974; Rustia, 1974; Ito, 1976; Shirai *et al.*, 1977).

Vascular tumours of the hamster urinary bladder have been induced by intragastric administration of *n*-octylamine (7.4 mg/week, males, haemangiosarcoma, 8%; haemangioma, 17%), cyclohexylamine (2.5 mg/week, females, haemangioma, 8%) (Lijinsky & Kovatch, 1988) or *N*-nitroso-*N*-methyl-*N*-dodecylamine (60 mg/kg/week, haemangioendothelioma; incidence not reported) (Althoff & Lijinsky, 1977). The tumours were usually found in the submucosa (subepithelial connective tissue) (Figure 12) (Althoff & Lijinsky, 1977).

Tumours of the renal pelvis

The renal pelvis as well as areas of the urinary tract other than the urinary bladder are unlikely sites for tumour induction by chemicals because the transitional cell epithelium is not sufficiently exposed to the ultimate carcinogens. Thus tumours of the renal pelvis in the hamster are rare, although one transitional cell papilloma was found in an animal treated with AAF and indole (Oyasu *et al.*, 1970). A TCC of the renal pelvis was also described in a hamster treated with nitrosodiethylamine and cigarette smoke (Dontenwill *et al.*, 1973). In addition, two cases of renal pelvic TCCs, one from a hamster treated with *N*-[4-(5-nitro-2-furyl)-2-thiazolyl]acetamide and the other from an animal receiving formic acid 2-[4-(5-nitro-2-furyl)-2-thiazolyl]hydrazide, were observed in another study (Croft & Bryan, 1973).

Tumours of the ureter

Two invasive TCCs were found in hamsters treated with AAF alone or in combination with indole (Oyasu *et al.*, 1972). Two hamsters treated with *N*-butyl-*N*-(4-hydroxybutyl)nitrosamine (BBN) also developed transitional cell tumours in the ureter (Althoff, 1975).

Tumours of the urethra

One transitional cell papilloma of the urethra was seen in a female hamster treated with 2-oxopropyl-*n*-propylnitrosamine (Pour *et al.*, 1974).

Table 1. Summary of experimental induction of urinary bladder tumours in hamsters

Compound	Treatment (duration)	No. (Sex)	Incidence TP	TCC	Reference
o-Aminoazotoluene	0.1% in the diet (49 weeks)	25 (m) 15 (f)	– 2	15 3	Tomatis *et al.* (1961)
2-Naphthylamine	1% w/w in the diet (600 mg/week/animal) (45 weeks, m; 49 weeks,f)	23 (m) 16 (f)	– –	10 8	Saffiotti *et al.* (1967)
o-Dianisidine	0.1% in the diet (?)	60 (m&f)	–	1	Sellakumar *et al.* (1969)
3,3'-Dichlorobenzidine	0.3% in the diet (?)	? (?)	–	4	Sellakumar (1969)
2-Acetylaminofluorene (AAF)	AAF+indole[a] (12 months)	16 (m) 10 (f)	– –	16 10	Oyasu (1970)
AAF	0.03% AAF+ indole[b] 0.03% AAF 0.06% AAF + indole 0.06% AAF 0.06% AAF+ tryptophan 0.06% AAF + indole[c] (8 months)	27 (m) 26 (m) 58 (m) 42 (m) 28 (m) 34 (m)	– – – – – –	24 13 48 30 19 27	Oyasu (1972)
3',2'-Diethyl-4-aminobiphenyl	s.c. injection (52 weeks)	3 (m) 15 (f)	1 3	2 9	So & Wynder (1972)
AAF	AAF+indole[d] AAF	25 (m & f) 23 (m & f)	- -	8 10	Oyasu (1973)
N-[4-5-Nitro-2-furyl)-2-thiazolyl]formamide (FANFT)	0.1% in diet (48 weeks)[e]	24 (m)	-	23	Croft & Bryan (1973)
N-[4-(5-Nitro-2-furyl)-2-thiazolyl]acetamide (NFTA)	0.1% in diet (48 weeks)[e]	24 (m) 24 (m)	-	16	Croft & Bryan (1973)
Formic acid 2-[4-(5-nitro-2-furyl)-2-thiazolyl]-hydrazide (FNT)	0.1% in the diet (48 weeks)[e]	24 (m)	-	9	Croft & Bryan (1973)
Dibutylnitrosamine (DBN)	s.c. injections 0.05 of the LD_{50} 0.10 of the LD_{50} 0.20 of the LD_{50}	10 (f) 10 (f) 10 (f)	1 2 2	6[g] 1 1[g]	Althoff *et al.* (1974)

Table 1 (Contd)

Compound	Treatment (duration)	No. (Sex)	Incidence TP	Incidence TCC	Reference
	0.02 of the LD_{50}	5 (m)	2	0	
	0.04 of the LD_{50}	5 (m)	2	0	
	0.08 of the LD_{50}	5 (m)	1	1	
	0.16 of the LD_{50}	5 (m)	1	2	
	0.32 of the LD_{50}	5 (m)	1	1[g]	
N-Butyl-N-(4-hydroxy-butyl)nitrosamine (BBN)	s.c. injection[h] 0.1 g/kg/b.w. 0.3 g/kg/b.w.	24 (m) 25 (m) 29 (m)	7 5 1	2 8 6	Althoff (1975)
N-ethyl-N-(4-hydroxy-butyl nitrosamine (EHBN)	0.025% in drinking water	22 (m)	12	3	Hirose *et al.* (1976)
N-Butyl-N-(3-carboxy-propyl)nitrosamine (BCPN)	0.025% in drinking water (40 weeks)[i]	14 (m)	2	-	Hirose *et al.* (1976)
N-nitroso-N-methyl-N-dodecylamine	Intragastric adminis-tration[j] 15 mg/kg 30 mg/kg 30 mg/kg 60 mg/kg 60 mg/kg	15 (m) 15 (f) 15 (m) 15 (f) 15 (m)	- - - - -	3 4 5 13 13	Althoff & Lijinsky (1977)
N-Nitrosomethyl-*n*-hexylamine	6.2 mg/week Intragastric administration[j]	12 (m) 20 (f)	3 2	1 3	Lijinsky & Kovatch (1988)
N-nitrosomethyl-*n*-octylamine	6.2 mg/week Intragastric administration[j]	12 (m)	2	-	Lijinsky & Kovatch (1988)

No. = No. of hamsters; TP = transitional cell papilloma; TCC = transitional cell carcinoma

[a] i.p. injection of AAF (5 mg/100 g b.w.) to neonates followed by feeding diet containing AAF with or with 1.6% indole or 2.0% DL-tryptophan

[b] i.p. injection of AAF (5 mg/100 g b.w.) to neonates followed by feeding diet containing AAF with or with 1.6% indole or 2.0% DL-tryptophan

[c] Without i.p. injection of AAF to neonates followed by feeding diet containing AAF and 1.6% indole

[d] Intratracheal instillation of AAF followed by feeding diet containing 1.6% indole

[e] In the diet for 48 weeks then controlled diet for an additional 22 weeks

[f] Once a week for life

[g] One case was squamous cell carcinoma

[h] Once a week for 75 weeks

[i] In the drinking water for 20 weeks then tap water without carcinogen for an additional 20 weeks

[j] Once a week for life

COMPARATIVE ASPECTS

Comparison with human urinary bladder carcinomas

More than 90% of human bladder cancers are of transitional cell type, other tumours being rare, although a relatively high incidence of squamous cell carcinoma occurs in the Middle East. Similarly, in the hamster, the majority of induced bladder cancers are TCCs (99%). Although glandular-like patterns and squamous metaplasia sometimes develop in areas of TCCs in the hamster (Althoff & Lijinsky, 1977), primary adenocarcinomas, squamous cell carcinomas and undifferentiated carcinomas of the urinary bladder are exceedingly rare. Generally, a sex difference regarding urinary bladder carcinomas has been reported, the incidence of TCCs being higher in males than in females while squamous cell carcinomas are more prevalent in females (Friedell *et al.*, 1983; Ito *et al.*, 1989). However, no consistent sex difference in tumour incidences has been evident in hamster studies (Tomatis *et al.*, 1961; Althoff *et al.*, 1974). Growth patterns of TCC in man are mainly of papillary non-invasive or papillary invasive types, metastasis occurring to the lung, liver, bone and lymph nodes, particularly those situated in the retro-peritoneum and para-aortic regions (Babaian, 1980). In the hamster, the growth pattern is mainly of non-papillary, invasive type, although distant metastases are very rare. Only two reports have described metastasis, to the lung, perirenal tissues and serosal surface of the large intestine (Croft & Bryan, 1973) and in the other to the lung and liver (Althoff *et al.*, 1974).

A positive correlation between histological grading and staging of carcinoma has been demonstrated in man (Mostofi *et al.*, 1973; Kakizoe *et al.*, 1984), the tendency for invasion clearly increasing with histological grading. While TCCs in hamsters can similarly be classified by stage and grade, no firm evidence of a correlation has been reported.

Comparison with the other rodent urinary bladder carcinomas

BBN induces a high incidence of bladder tumours in rats and mice (Akagi *et al.*, 1973). With regard to the histogenesis of bladder cancers in rats and mice, the first transformation stage of transitional epithelium is simple hyperplasia. PN hyperplasia appears following simple hyperplasia after a variable latent period. Two types of PN hyperplasia exist, one reversible and the other irreversible (preneoplasia). Some of the latter become papillomas or carcinomas (non-invasive or invasive), while reversible lesions revert to normal epithelium (Fukushima *et al.*, 1982). However, carcinoma *in situ* can also arise from simple hyperplasia through dysplastic change. In rats treated with a bladder carcinogen for a long period or at high concentration, squamous metaplasia or glandular metaplasia is more frequently observed within bladder tumours. In mice given a bladder carcinogen for a long period, squamous cell carcinomas predominate (Tamano *et al.*, 1991) and the remaining tumours are mostly TCC. Adenocarcinomas are rarely seen. Most mouse bladder tumours are non-papillary and invasive carcinomas.

The endophytic growth patterns of TCCs in the hamster are similar to those in mice, but different from rat lesions where exophytic growth predominates. Carcinoma *in situ*, which is frequently observed in mice and relatively often in hamster, is uncommon in rats.

The susceptibility of hamster urinary bladder epithelium to carcinogens appears to vary from low to high depending on the individual agent. For example, hamsters are as susceptible as other species to the carcinogenicity of 5-nitrofurans (Croft & Bryan, 1973), but this is the only rodent species demonstrating a positive response to the bladder carcinogenicity of aromatic amines such as 2-naphthylamine (Saffiotti *et al.*, 1967) which are known to be carcinogenic to man. On the other hand, when Hirose *et al.* (1976) examined the susceptibility of four species to BBN, the hamster proved less susceptible than rats and mice, and guinea-pigs were least responsive. Species differences were confirmed ultrastructurally by using transmission and scanning electron microscopy (Ito, 1976). Thus, after BBN treatment, microvilli were also seen on the surface cells in rats, mice and hamsters, but not in guinea-pigs. The numbers of fusiform vesicles were shown by transmission electron microscopy to be decreased in rats and mice but not in hamsters or guinea-pigs.

REFERENCES

Akagi, G., Akagi, A., Kimura, M. & Otsuka, H. (1973) Comparison of bladder tumors induced in rats and mice with N-butyl-N-(4-hydroxybutyl)nitrosamine. *Gann,* 64, 331–336

Althoff, J. (1975) Carcinogenicity of 4-hydroxybutyl-butylnitrosamine in Syrian hamsters. *Cancer Lett.,* 1, 15–19

Althoff, J. & Chesterman, F.C. (1982) Tumours of the urinary bladder, renal pelvis and urethra. In: Turusov, V.S., ed., *Pathology of Tumours in Laboratory Animals,* Vol. 3, *Tumours of the Hamster* (IARC Scientific Publications No. 34), Lyon, IARC, pp. 163–168

Althoff, J. & Lijinsky, W. (1977) Urinary bladder neoplasms in Syrian hamsters after administration of N-nitroso-N-methyl-N-dodecylamine. *Z. Krebsforsch.,* 90, 227–231

Althoff, J., Mohr, U., Page, N. & Reznik, G. (1974) Carcinogenic effect of dibutylnitrosamine in European hamsters (*Cricetus cricetus*). *J. Natl Cancer Inst.,* 53, 795–880

Babaian, R.J., Johnson, D.E., Llamas, L. & Ayala, A.G. (1980) Metastases from transitional cell carcinoma of urinary bladder. *Urology,* 16, 142–144

Croft, W.A. & Bryan, G.T. (1973) Production of urinary bladder cancer in male hamsters by N-[4-(5-nitro-2-furyl)-2-thiazolyl]-formamide, N-[4-(5-nitro-2-furyl)-2-thiazolyl]-acetamide, or formic acid 2-[4-5-nitro-2-furyl]-2-thiazolyl]-hydrazide. *J. Natl Cancer Inst.,* 51, 941–949

Dontenwill, W., Chevalier, H.J., Harke, H.P., Lafrenz, U. & Reckzeh, G. (1973) Spontantumoren des syrischen Goldhamsters. *Z. Krebsforsch.,* 80, 127–158

Druckrey, H., Preussmann, R., Ivankovic, S. & Schmidt, C.H. (1964) Selektive Erzeugung von Blasenkrebs an Ratten durch Dibutyl-und N-Butyl-N-butano(4)nitrosamine. *Z. Krebsforsch.,* 66, 280–290

Ertürk, E., Price, J.M., Morris, J.E., Cohen, S.M., Leith, R.S., von Esch, A.M. & Crovetti, A.J. (1967) The production of carcinoma of the urinary bladder in rats by feeding N-[4-(5-nitro-2-furyl)-2-thiazolyl]-formamide. *Cancer Res.,* 27, 1988–2002

Friedell, G.H., Nagy, G.K. & Cohen, S.M. (1983) Pathology of human bladder cancer and related lesions. In: Bryan, G.T. & Cohen, S.M., eds, *The Pathology of Bladder Cancer,* Vol. 1, Boca Raton, FL, CRC Press, pp. 11–42

Fukushima, S., Mursaki, G., Hirose, M., Nakanishi, K., Hasegawa, R. & Ito, N. (1982) Histopathological analysis of pre-neoplastic changes during N-butyl-N-(4-hydroxybutyl)nitrosamine-induced urinary bladder carcinogenesis in rats. *Acta Pathol. Jpn.,* 32, 243–250

Hicks, R.M. & Wakefield, J.St.J. (1972) Rapid induction of bladder cancer in rats with N-methyl-N-nitrosourea. I. Histology. *Chem. Biol. Interact.,* 5, 139–152

Hirose, M., Fukushima, S., Hananouchi, M., Shirai, T., Ogiso, T., Takahashi, M. & Ito, N. (1976) Different susceptibilities of the urinary bladder epithelium of animal species to three nitroso compounds. *Gann,* 67, 175–189

Ito, N. (1976) Early changes caused by N-butyl-N-(4-hydroxybutyl)nitrosamine in the bladder epithelium of different animal species. *Cancer Res.,* 36, 2528–2531

Ito, N., Hiasa, Y., Tamai, A., Okajima, E. & Kitamura, H. (1969) Histogenesis of urinary bladder tumors induced by N-butyl-N-(4-hydroxybutyl)nitrosamine in rats. *Gann,* 60, 401–410

Ito, N., Fukushima, S. & Hasegawa, R. (1989) Bladder cancers, their process of development and its modification. *Acta Pathol. Jpn.,* 39, 1–14

IARC (1987) *IARC Monographs on the Evaluation of Carcinogenic Risks to Humans,* Supplement 7, *Overall Evaluations of Carcinogenicity: An Updating of IARC Monographs Volumes 1 to 42,* Lyon, IARC

Kakizoe, T., Matsumoto, K., Nishio, Y. & Kishi, K. (1984) Analysis of 90 step-sectional cystectomized specimens of bladder cancer. *J. Urol.*, 131, 467–472

Koss, L.G. (1975) *Tumors of the Urinary Bladder*, Second series. Washington, DC, Armed Forces Institute of Pathology, pp. 9–43

Lijinsky, W. & Kovatch, R.M. (1988) Comparative carcinogenesis by nitromethylalkylamine in Syrian hamsters. *Cancer Res.*, 48, 6648–6652

Littlefield, N.A., Cuesto, C., Jr, Davis, A.K. & Medlock, K. (1975) Chronic dose-response studies in mice fed 2-AAF. *J. Toxicol. Environ. Health*, 1, 25–37

Mostofi, F.K. & Sesterhenn, I.A. (1983) Pathology of epithelial tumors and carcinoma *in situ* of bladder. In: Küss, R., Khoury, S., Denis, L.J., Murphy, G.P. & Karr, J.P., eds, *Bladder Cancers*, Part A, *Pathology, Diagnosis, and Surgery*, New York, Alan R. Liss, pp. 55–74

Mostofi, F.K., Sobin, L.H. & Torboni, H. (1973) *International Biological Classification of Tumors*, No. 10, *Histological Typing of Urinary Bladder Tumors*, Geneva, World Health Organization

Oyasu, R., Kitajima, T., Hopp, M.L. & Sumie, H. (1972) Enhancement of urinary bladder tumorigenesis in hamsters by coadministration of 2-acetylaminofluorene and indole. *Cancer Res.*, 32, 2027–2033

Oyasu, R., Kitajima, T., Hopp, M.L. & Sumie, H. (1973) Induction of bladder cancer in hamsters by repeated intratracheal administration of 2-acetylaminofluorene. *J. Natl Cancer Inst.*, 50, 503–506

Oyasu, R., Sumie, H. & Burg, H.E. (1970) Neoplasms of urinary bladders of hamsters treated with 2-acetylaminofluorene and indole. *J. Natl Cancer Inst.*, 45, 853–860

Pour, P., Althoff, J., Cardesa, A., Kruger, F.W. & Mohr, U. (1974) Effect of beta-oxidated nitrosamines on Syrian golden hamsters. II. Oxopropyl-n-propylnitrosamine. *J. Natl Cancer Inst.*, 52, 1869–1874

Pour, P., Kmoch, N., Greiser, E., Mohr, U., Althoff, J. & Cardesa, A. (1976a) Spontaneous tumours and common diseases in two colonies of Syrian hamsters. I. Incidence and sites. *J. Natl Cancer Inst.*, 56, 931–935

Pour, P., Mohr, U., Althoff, J., Cardesa, A. & Kmoch, N. (1976b) Spontaneous tumours and common diseases in two colonies of Syrian hamsters. III. Urogenital system and endocrine glands. *J. Natl Cancer Inst.*, 56, 949–961

Rustia, M. (1974) Multiple carcinogenic effects of the ethylnitrosourea precursors ethylurea and sodium nitrite in hamsters. *Cancer Res.*, 34, 3232–3244

Saffiotti, U., Cefis, F., Montesano, R. & Sellakumar, A.R. (1967) Induction of bladder cancer in hamsters fed aromatic amines. In: *Bladder Cancer, A Symposium*, Birmingham, Alabama, Aesculapius Publishing Co., pp. 129–135

Schmidt, R.E., Eason, R.L., Hubbard, G.B., Young, J.T. & Eisenbrandt, D.L. (1983) *Pathology of Aging Syrian Hamsters,* Boca Raton, FL, CRC Press, pp. 88–106

Sellakumar, A.R., Montesano, R. & Saffiotti, U. (1969) Aromatic amine carcinogenicity in hamsters. *Proc. Am. Ass. Cancer Res.*, 10, 78

Shirai, T., Murasaki, G., Tatematsu, M., Tshuda, H., Fukushima, S. & Ito, N. (1977) Early surface changes of the urinary bladder epithelium of different animal species induced by *N*-butyl-*N*-(4-hydroxybutyl)-nitrosamine. *Gann*, 68, 203–212

So, B.T. & Wynder, E.L. (1972) Induction of hamster tumors of the urinary bladder by 3,2-dimethyl-4-aminobiphenyl. *J. Natl Cancer Inst.*, 48, 1733–1748

Tamano, S., Hagiwara, A., Suzuki, E., Okada, M., Shirai, T. & Fukushima, S. (1991) Time- and dose-dependent induction of invasive urinary bladder cancers by *N*-ethyl-*N*-(4-hydroxybutyl)nitrosamine in B6C3F1 mice. *Jpn. J. Cancer Res.*, 82, 650–656

Tomatis, L., Della Porta, G. & Shubik, P. (1961) Urinary bladder and liver cell tumors induced in hamsters with o-amino-azotoluene. *Cancer Res.*, 21, 1513–1517

UICC (Union Internationale Contre le Cancer) (1989) Urinary bladder. In: Spiessl, B., Beahrs, O.H., Hermanek, P., Hutter, R.V.P., Scheibe, O., Sobin, L.H. & Wagner, G., eds, *TNM Atlas, Illustrated Guide to the TNM/pTNM-Classification of Malignant Tumours*, Berlin, Heidelberg, New York, Springer-Verlag, pp. 245–250

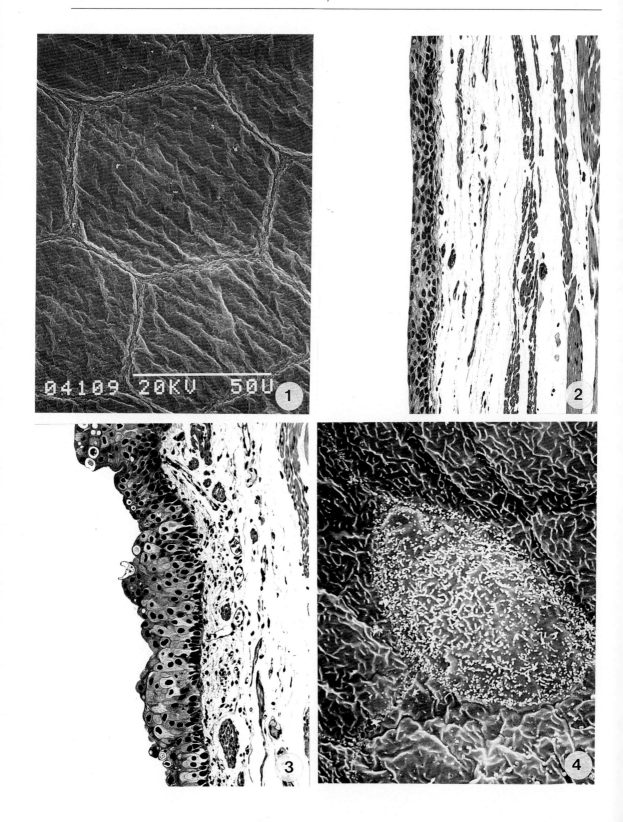

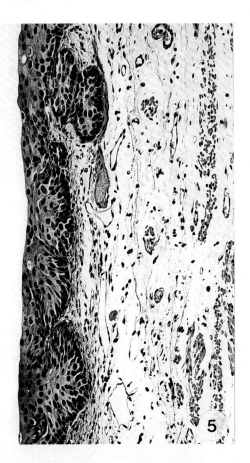
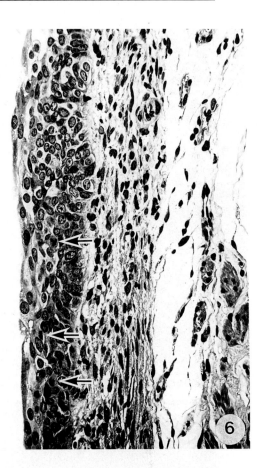

Figure 1. Scanning electron microscopy of the luminal surface of normal urinary bladder epithelium demonstrates large polygonal cells with fine peaked microridges. 99-day-old untreated male. × 1900

Figure 2. Simple hyperplasia showing an increased number of cell layers. The nuclei of component cells are slightly enlarged and occasionally hyperchromatic. These nuclear features are commonly seen even in very early proliferative lesions of the urinary bladder in the hamster. 407-day-old female received intravesical instillation of MNU (1.5 mg/animal, once a week for 10 weeks). H & E; × 109

Figure 3. Dysplasia demonstrating moderate cellular atypia. 281-day-old male received intragastric administration of *N*-nitrosomethyl-n-hexylamine (6.2 mg/animal, once a week) for 252 days and then no treatment for 29 days. H & E; ×109

Figure 4. Scanning electron microscopic appearance of an area of hyperplasia, illustrating development of short uniform microvilli and ropy or leafy microridges on the luminal surface of a cell in the centre. 99-day-old male given 0.05% BBN in drinking water for 56 days. × 3500

Figure 5. Nodular hyperplasia of the urinary bladder exhibiting dysplastic change. Cells exhibit marked downward growth with formation of small nests. 321-day-old male given 0.025% BCPN in drinking water for 140 days and then no treatment for 141 days. H & E; × 109

Figure 6. Carcinoma *in situ*. Note nuclear mitoses (arrows) and disorderly epithelial growth. 407-day-old male given 0.05% BBN in drinking water for 364 days. H & E; × 109

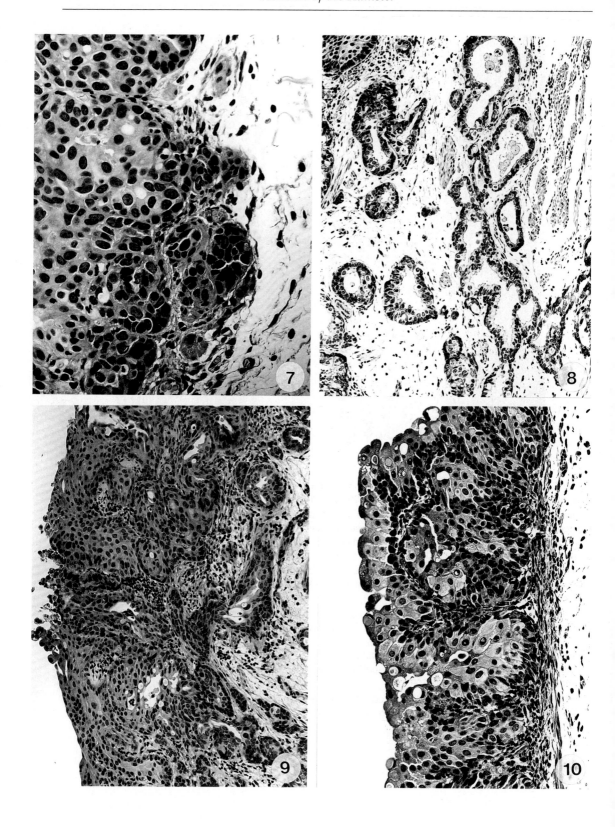

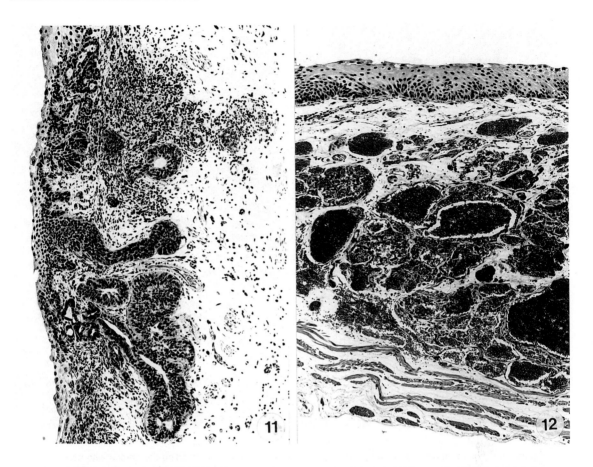

Figure 7. Transitional cell carcinoma with microinvasion. Small nests of tumour cells are seen in the submucosa. 321-day-old male given 0.025% EHBN in drinking water for 140 days and then no treatment for 141 days. H & E; × 435

Figure 8. An area of transitional cell carcinoma showing invasion into the muscular layer. The invading cells demonstrate pseudoglandular patterns. 321-day-old male given 0.025% EHBN in drinking water for 140 days and then no treatment for 141 days. H & E; × 218

Figure 9. Invasive transitional cell carcinoma showing a small superficial erosion. Inflammatory cell infiltration is prominent. 407-day-old male given 0.05% BBN in drinking water for 364 days. H & E; × 109

Figure 10. Non-papillary transitional cell carcinoma showing endophytic growth pattern. 321-day-old male given 0.025% EHBN in drinking water for 140 days and then no treatment for 141 days. H & E; × 109

Figure 11. Transitional cell carcinoma showing endophytic growth, invasion into the submucosa. Inflammation is prominent surrounding the neoplastic tissue. 407-day-old male given 0.05% BBN in drinking water for 364 days. H & E; × 109

Figure 12. Cavernous haemangioma of the hamster urinary bladder. Large, irregular, vascular spaces containing erythrocytes are seen in the submucosa. 407-day-old male given 0.05% BBN in drinking water for 364 days. H & E; × 63

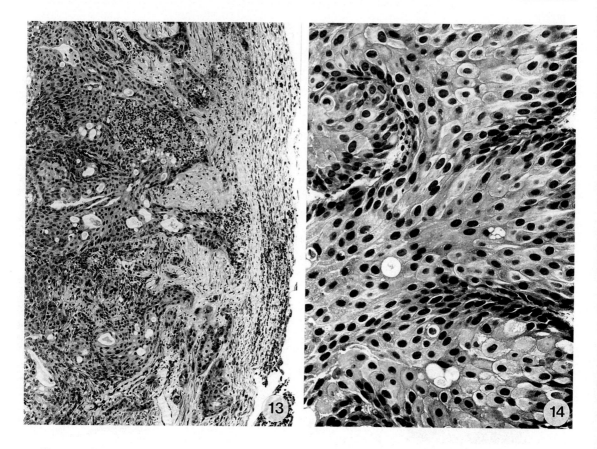

Figure 13. Transitional cell carcinoma penetrating the muscular layer and invading the serosa with accompanying inflammatory infiltration. The serosa is observed to be almost destroyed. 321-day-old male given 0.025% EHBN in drinking water for 140 days and then no treatment for 141 days. H & E; × 109

Figure 14. Transitional cell carcinoma (grade 1). Cell polarity is relatively well maintained and nuclear hyperchromatism is visible. 407-day-old male given 0.05% BBN in drinking water for 364 days. H & E; × 500

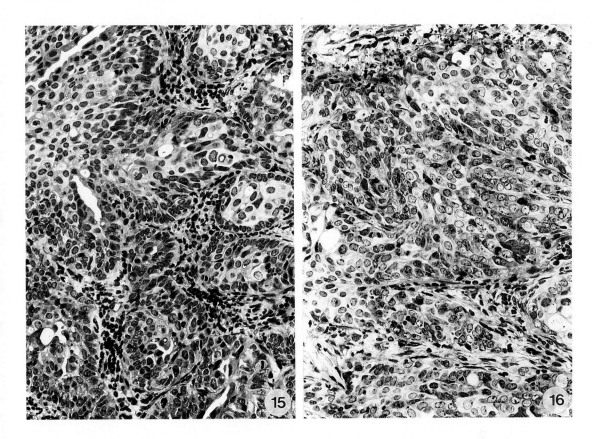

Figure 15. Transitional cell carcinoma (grade 2). Moderate loss of cell polarity and hyperchromatic enlarged nuclei are prominent. 321-day-old male given 0.025% EHBN in drinking water for 140 days and then no treatment for 141 days. H & E; × 320

Figure 16. Transitional cell carcinoma (grade 3). The tumour shows obvious nuclear pleomorphism and random cell alignment. 321-day-old male given 0.025% EHBN in drinking water for 140 days and then no treatment for 141 days. H & E; × 320

Tumours of the testis and accessory male sex glands

J.L. RIBAS AND F.K. MOSTOFI

Despite extensive study of the hamster, spontaneous tumours of the testis and accessory sex glands have rarely been reported. In part, this may be due to the fact that in the laboratory hamster, as in other mammalian species, the incidence of neoplasia increases with advancing age but the life of an experimental animal is shortened by design. It may also reflect a lack of thoroughness in some pathological studies, particularly since many tumours cannot be detected grossly; some workers have attributed higher tumour incidences in their studies to the intensive histological examination of step sections in multiple organs (Pour *et al.*, 1976).

This chapter provides an update of the chapter by Kirkman and Kempson in the first edition of this volume. It also compares the hamster tumours, when possible, to their human counterparts (Table 1), according to classifications based on the WHO Histological Typing of Testis Tumours (Mostofi & Sobin, 1977) and of Prostate Tumours (Mostofi *et al.*, 1980). It should be noted that the literature in this area is fragmentary and widely scattered, and it is occasionally anecdotal or buried in technical reports which are not usually included in standard bibliographic data-bases. More importantly, there has been a lack of uniformity in histological diagnosis in the literature.

NORMAL STRUCTURE

In the sexually mature male hamster (approximately 12 weeks of age), the testes within the scrotal sac protrude caudally, conferring a rounded appearance to the posterior end of the body. The cranial end of the testicle, the caput and part of the epididymis are covered by a thick fat pad. There is no mediastinum separating the testes within the scrotal sac. The intratesticular genital ducts are composed of *tubuli recti* (straight tubules), *rete testis* and the *ductuli efferentes*. The excretory genital ducts consist of the cauda epididymis, ductus (vas) deferens, and urethra. Intratesticular and excretory genital ducts have unique histological, histochemical and physiological characteristics. Accessory sex glands include seminal vesicles (vesicular gland), interior and exterior ampullary glands, coagulating glands, a three-lobed (cranial, caudal and central) prostate, and bulbourethral (Cowper's) gland (Figure 1). For more detailed information, the reader is referred to a review by Bivin *et al.* (1987).

MORPHOLOGY AND BIOLOGY OF TUMOURS

Histological types of tumour

The histological types of testicular, ductal and accessory glandular tumours that have been recognized in the male hamster are listed in Table 1. Their human counterparts (Mostofi & Sobin, 1977; Mostofi *et al.*, 1980) are also included for purposes of comparison.

Testis

Testicular tumours in the hamster are extremely rare. As pointed out by Kirkman (1972), it is debatable whether the few that have been reported as experimentally induced have resulted from treatment or arose spontaneously.

Spontaneous and induced seminomas have been reported in the hamster. The neoplasm consists of cells with scant cytoplasm, irregular cell outlines, large pleomorphic nuclei, and prominent nucleoli (Figure 2). There is moderate to marked nuclear atypia and the mitotic rate is increased. There is progressive efface-ment of seminiferous tubules by the infiltrating tumour cells, but residual seminiferous tubules are commonly seen (Figure 3). In some areas tumour cells may form nests and be separated by connective tissue stroma to mimic a lobular pattern. Multifocal areas of necrosis are common and they may be associated with a neutrophilic infiltrate. Metastatic deposits (Figure 3) and *in vivo* transplants (Figure 4) are histologically similar. Lymphocytes are conspicuously absent. The differential diagnosis includes histiocytic lymphoma and Leydig cell tumours.

Embryonal carcinoma has been repor-ted in treated male hamsters (Guthrie & Guthrie, 1974; Rustia, 1974), but its existence is in question since neither report includes a histological description. Histologically, neoplastic cells should have an embryonic epithelial appearance and should grow in glandular, alveolar, tubular or tubulopapillary patterns, but a pattern-less growth consisting of sheets of cells may be more typical of undifferentiated lesions. Although there may be consi-derable variation in cell and nuclear size, neoplastic cells tend to be large and have hyperchromatic, bizarre-looking nuclei with prominent nucleoli. Multinucleated tumour giant (syncytial) cells may be present.

Interstitial cell hyperplasia follows estrogen administration (Figure 5).

Sertoli cell tumour has been reported in estrogen-treated hamsters (Bacon & Kirk-man, 1955). Neoplastic cells are columnar or polyhedral, and they have abundant and vacuolated cytoplasm and a centrally located elongated nucleus. They tend to grow in cords, thus mimicking tubule formation, but they may also form sheets of cells (Figures 5, 6 and 7). Mitotic figures may be numerous, but visceral or skeletal metastasis has not been reported.

Spontaneous proliferative lesions of Leydig (interstitial) cell origin are exceedingly rare (Kirkman, 1972). Hyper-plastic lesions are probably more common than solid tumours. Hyperplastic and tumourous cells are remarkably similar to their progenitor cells, in that they are round or polygonal, and they also have indistinct cell boundaries, abundant granular eosinophilic cytoplasm and a round central nucleus (Figure 7). Metas-tasis has not been reported.

Epididymis, spermatic cord and ductus deferens

Cystadenomas have been observed only in the head of the epididymis (Figure 8) and are common in hamsters chronically stimulated with estrogen. As the name implies, they consist of cysts of various sizes (Figures 9 and 10) containing papillary stalks which are lined by cuboidal to columnar ciliated cells, and sheets of cells often forming gland-like spaces. Some cells, however, display stereocilia suggesting that they may arise from ductuli efferentes. The glandular and tubular spaces and lining epithelium often contain eosinophilic, PAS-positive secre-tory products (Figure 11). The solid areas are composed of spindle to cuboidal cells growing in sheets (Figures 12 and 13). Necrotic, hyalinized and haemorrhagic areas are common anywhere in the tumours. Areas of normal epididymis may be present (Figures 9 and 14).

Smooth muscle tumours of the *ductus efferentes* are induced by androgen/ estrogen treatment and begin as local areas

Table 1. Histological types of tumours of the hamster testis and accessory male sex glands, and their human counterparts.

HAMSTER (Revised after Kirkman & Kempson, 1982)	HUMAN (Abbreviated) (Mostofi *et al.* 1977; 1980)
TESTES	TESTES
Germ cell tumours	Germ cell tumours
Seminoma	Tumours of one histological pattern
Teratoma	Seminoma
Sex cord/stromal tumours	Spermatocytic seminoma
Leydig cell tumour	Embryonal carcinoma
Sertoli cell tumour	Yolk sac tumour
Spindle-cell sarcoma	Choriocarcinoma
	Teratomas
EPIDIDYMIS, SPERMATIC CORD AND	Tumours of more than one histological type
VAS DEFERENS	(name histological type)
Epithelial tumours	Sex cord/stromal tumours
Cystadenoma of the epididymal head	Leydig cell tumour
Adenocarcinoma of the epididymis	Sertoli cell tumour
Acanthotic squamous cell carcinoma	Granulosa cell tumour
of the inguinal canal	Mixed forms
Mesenchymal tumours	Germ cell/sex cord/stromal tumours
Leiomyosarcoma, epididymal tail–ductus	Gonadoblastoma
deferens complex	Miscellan eous tumours
Miscellaneous tumours	Carcinoid, others
Lymphoid & haematopoietic tumours	Lymphoid and haematopoietic tumours
Tumour-like lesion	
Sperm granuloma	TUMOURS OF COLLECTING DUCTS, RETE,
	EPIDIDYMIS, SPERMATIC CORD, ETC.
	TUMOUR-LIKE LESIONS
PROSTATE	PROSTATE
Epithelial tumours	Epithelial tumours
Adenocarcinoma	Benign
Mesenchymal tumours	Malignant
Leiomyoma	Adenocarcinoma
Leiomyosarcoma	Transitional cell carcinoma
	Squamous cell cacinoma
	Undifferentiated carcinoma
	Non-epithelial tumours
	Benign
	Malignant
OTHER ACCESSORY GLANDS	Rhabdomyosarcoma
Bulbo-urethral (Cowper's) gland	Leiomyosarcoma
Cystadenocarcinoma	Others
Seminal vesicles	Miscellaneous tumours
Adenocarcinoma	Secondary tumours
Haemangiosarcoma	Unclassified tumours
Tumour-like lesions	Tumour-like lesions

of hyperplasia (Algard, 1965; Kirkman & Algard, 1965, 1970), which then develop into large neoplastic masses (Figures 15 and 16). The tumours are transplantable and are initially hormone-dependent tumours, but eventually they become autonomous. Neoplastic cells are spindle-shaped and form interlacing bundles (Figure 17). The cytoplasm is eosinophilic. The nuclei are plumper and more rounded than in non-neoplastic smooth muscle and are mildly atypical. Mitoses are seldom present. The histological appearance of the primary tumour is of a leiomyoma, but after several serial transplant generations, it becomes histologically malignant. The neoplastic cells may then be cuboidal. Nuclei are markedly irregular and contain prominent and pleomorphic nucleoli (Figures 18 and 19), and mitoses become more abundant and atypical. Eventually, most transplanted tumours are histologically malignant (Figure 20).

Among tumour-like lesions, the epididymal sperm granuloma (Figure 21) occurs with some frequency in adult hamsters and it may be confused at necropsy with cystadenomas of the epididymis (Schmidt *et al.*, 1983).

Prostate

A variety of spontaneous and induced neoplasms of the hamster prostate have been reported including adenocarcinoma, angiofibroleiomyoma, carcinoma, fibrosarcoma, leiomyosarcoma, and sarcoma. Spontaneous, transplantable adenocarcinomas have been reported (Fortner, 1961; Fortner *et al.*, 1963), but they do not duplicate their human counterparts in either histological appearance or hormone sensitivity (Webber *et al.*, 1968; Kirkman & Kempson, 1982). Treatment of hamster prostatic tissue *in vitro* with SV40 virus induces the formation of malignant neoplasms when cultures are transplanted into untreated males (Paulson *et al.*, 1968). Tumours from the dorsal and ventral lobes resemble prostatic carcinomas, and those from the lateral lobe present as fibrosarcomas.

A fibroleiomyoma of the dorsal gland has also been reported (Kirkman & Algard, 1968). It was composed of interlacing spindle cells with elongated nuclei and tapered cytoplasm (Figures 22 and 23).

Bulbo-urethral (Cowper's) gland

Spontaneous and chemically induced adenocarcinomas, adenomas, and cystadenomas of the bulbo-urethral gland have been reported and histological descriptions are available.

SPONTANEOUS TUMOURS

In a review of over 13 000 hamster necropsies, several variables including gender, longevity, and the presence or absence of gonadectomy, hypophysectomy, adrenalectomy, hormone treatment (estrogen, androgen or combinations) and neoplasia were examined (Kirkman & Yau, 1972). In a subsequent review of this necropsy series, the incidence of neoplasia was reported by gender, by age, and by hormonal status (Kirkman & Kempson, 1982). For convenience, animals were age-grouped in 200-day increments from 200-day to 1400-day old. Tumour incidence in each of these seven age-groups was charted as a percentage of the total number of animals in each group, arranged according to gender and the presence or absence of experimentally induced hormonal imbalance. On the basis of the data reported, the following observations can be drawn: (*a*) general tumour incidence at any given age is higher in male than in female hamsters; (*b*) chronic hormonal imbalance increases tumour incidence, particularly in males; and (*c*) for both genders exposed to persistent hormonal imbalance, the incidence is dramatically increased in younger animals and starts to level off or drop at 600 days of age.

Testis

Spontaneous seminoma has been reported in the hamster (Althoff *et al.*, 1976, 1977b), including a transplantable seminoma (Kirkman, 1972; Kirkman & Chesterman, 1972). A single seminoma found in 39 hamsters treated with 2-aminoacetophenone was considered to be induced (Kharkovskaya, 1979), but until confirmed it is best listed with the spontaneous testicular tumours (Kirkman & Kempson, 1982). An extremely low incidence of spontaneous seminoma was reported to occur in the Stanford colony (Kirkman, 1962; Kirkman & Kempson, 1982).

A fibrosarcoma was found in a 657-day-old untreated hamster. No metastases were discovered. When the tumour was transplanted, the average survival time for the transplant-bearing hosts was 59 days (Yabe *et al.*, 1972). According to Kirkman and Kempson (1982), this tumour appears to be similar to a 3-methylcholanthrene-induced spindle cell sarcoma (Llombart & Peña, 1964).

Epididymis

Spontaneous adenomas of the head of the epididymis are quite rare. Pour *et al.* (1976b, c) found one adenoma in 77 untreated males. An even lower incidence rate (one adenoma) was reported for 7200 hamsters (Kirkman, 1962); malignant variants were absent. An adenocarcinoma was found among 60 males injected subcutaneously with bile from a human patient with carcinoma of the common bile duct (Fortner & Allen, 1958).

Prostate

Two spontaneous and transplantable adenocarcinomas of the prostate were reported (Fortner, 1961) among 94 males (mean age, 731 days); one of them was subsequently used in an experimental study of actinomycins (Goldin & Johnson, 1974). No malignant prostatic tumours were found in the Stanford colony.

Accessory glands

Bulbo-urethral (Cowper's) gland. The incidence of cystadenocarcinomas in one study (Fortner, 1961) was reported to be 7.45% (7 in 94 males with a mean age of 731 days). In subsequent studies (Sichuk *et al.*, 1966; Fortner *et al.*, 1966), similar tumours were reported in 24 of 108 control males (22%) and in two of 20 incompletely hypophysectomized animals (10%). Althoff *et al.* (1977b) reported one adenoma in 203 untreated males. In a subsequent paper the incidence was increased to 1 in 30 (Althoff & Likinsky, 1977). Pour *et al.* (1978) described seven adenomas in 20 untreated males.

Inguinal canal. A squamous cell carcinoma has been described by Lindt (1958).

Seminal vesicle. In a group of 182 untreated male Han:Chin hamsters (*Cricetulus criseus*) kept in a lifespan study from weaning to their natural death (Kaspareit-Rittinghausen & Deerberg, 1988), 10 adenocarcinomas and one haemangiosarcoma were reported. All the adenocarcinomas invaded the fibrous capsule, and one gave rise to distant metastases (Figures 24 and 25).

INDUCTION OF TUMOURS

Testis

The incidence of testicular tubular adenomas in estrogen-treated hamsters appears to be very low (Horning & Whittick, 1954; Fortner, 1957) and the tumour histology is variable (Bacon & Kirkman, 1955). The reported occurrence of interstitial cell adenoma in diethylstilbestrol (DES)-treated hamsters (Reznik-Schüller, 1979) has been interpreted as hyperplasia (Kirkman & Kempson, 1982).

Induced seminomas have also occurred infrequently with DES- and 2-aminoacetophenone-treated hamsters (Kharkovskaya, 1979; Rivière *et al.*, 1964).

Experimentally induced testicular embryonal carcinoma has been described in association with ethylurea plus sodium nitrite treatment (Rustia, 1974) and intra-testicular administration of zinc chloride (Guthrie & Guthrie, 1974). Unfortunately, neither report provided a histopatho-logical description.

A Sertoli cell tumour has been observed following long-term administration of estrogen (Bacon & Kirkman, 1955). Inter-stitial cell hyperplasia has been observed following chronic estrogen adminis-tration (Kirkman, 1972). A high incidence of Leydig cell adenoma (60%) has been described in hamsters with unilateral orchiectomy and intratesticular injection of methylcholanthrene. Some of these lesions progressed to solid tumours (Llombart & Peña, 1964); a spindle cell sarcoma was also present.

Epididymis, spermatic cord and ductus deferens

The excretory genital ducts differ histologically, histochemically, and phy-siologically from the adjoining intra-testicular genital ducts and the urethra. These differences may be reflected in the particular neoplastic phenotypic expres-sion of the excretory ducts.

Two types of neoplastic epididymal responses have been described in treated hamsters – epididymal head hyperplasia and cystadenoma, and leiomyosarcoma. Cystadenomas and epididymal head hyperplasia occur in young males treated for several months with estrogen pellets (estriol, DEC, estrone, or 17β-estradiol), subcutaneously implanted and replaced periodically. These are benign neoplasms characterized by the presence of haemor-rhagic cysts (Granados & Dam, 1948). The period of latency for neoplastic induction is variable and ranges from 300 to 500 days post-treatment. However, all male hamsters treated with DES for at least 500 days developed tumours. Of 41 estrogen-treated hamsters, enlarged epididymal heads were transplanted from 14 but only three were transplanted successfully in the first passage and all failed to grow in the second passage in untreated or DES-treated male hosts. Cystadenomas have been reported to occur in the epididymal head in hamsters chronically treated with estrogen (Kirkman, 1972). In another study, only two adenomas occurred among 55 males treated with DES (Llombart-Bosch & Peydro, 1975). The finding that in estrogen-treated male hamsters epididymal head carcinoma with renal metastasis developed in two out of five animals (Vasquez-Lopez, 1944) has been reinterpreted. The metastases are now believed to be primary estrogen-induced renal carcinomas (Kirkman & Bacon, 1952).

Multiple leiomyosarcomas occur in the epididymal tails of all adult males treated with androgen/estrogen pellets (testos-terone propionate/DES (Tpr/DES or 17β-estradiol, 30:20 mg), implanted sub-pannicularly, and reimplanted every 150 days for 300 days or longer (Kirkman, 1957). Androgen/estrogen treatment can induce neoplastic transformation of the smooth muscle of the ductus deferens into leiomyoma or leiomyosarcoma (Bacon, 1952; Kirkman & Bacon, 1958). These neoplasms are reported to begin as focal areas of hyperplasia and progress into tumourous masses (Algard, 1965; Kirkman & Algard, 1965; 1970; Rivière *et al.*, 1961, 1962a). A cloned cell line, DDT1, has been developed from one of these leiomyo-sarcomas (Norris *et al.*, 1974) and has been shown to contain an androgen receptor (Norris & Kohler, 1977).

Prostate

In contrast to the rat (Noble, 1980a,b), the hamster prostate appeared to be refractory to the development of car-cinoma. Intact male and gonadectomized hamsters have been treated with Tpr for 908 and 906 of the 958 and 956 days, respectively, of their existence. A com-bination treatment of DES/Tpr in intact males for as long as 747 days (age 811 days) and in orchiectomized ones for 458 days (age 518 days) was also unsuccessful.

It appears then that induced prostatic tumours are rare and that only two types have been well documented. One is the SV40-induced fibrosarcoma (Paulson *et al.*, 1968a,b; Abdalla & Oliver, 1971a,b,c; Fraley & Paulson, 1968, 1969) which, although not hormone-induced, is hormone-responsive, thus contrasting with Fortner's spontaneous carcinoma which is unresponsive to hormonal stimulation (McDonald, 1963; Webber *et al.*, 1968). The other (Norris *et al.*, 1977; Norris, 1980) is derived from cultured ventral prostate cells removed from an orchiectomized hamster which were transformed *in vitro* by methylchol-anthrene into a cell line of fibrosarcoma (HVP-B1) and another line (HVP-G3) containing both sarcomatous and epithelial components (carcinosarcoma). In their enzymology and responsiveness to sex hormones, both transformed cell lines show marked similarities to human prostatic carcinoma. Except for Fortner's spontaneous hamster carcinoma, which is no longer available, these cell lines are the best *in vitro* models for experimental studies of the prostatic carcinoma, particularly for studies of steroid hormone receptors.

Accessory glands

Induced tumours of the bulbo-urethral (Cowper's) gland, seminal vesicle, coagulating gland or preputial gland are rare. Several adenomas were reported in the bulbo-urethral gland of 11 of 20 hamsters treated with oxopropyl-nitrosamine (Althoff *et al.*, 1977a), 11 of 213 treated with nitrosopiperidine (Althoff *et al.*, 1977b), 3 of 15 treated with nitrosomethyl-*N*-dodecylamine (Althoff & Lijinsky, 1977), 1 of 159 treated with nitrosodipropylamine (Althoff *et al.*, 1977c), 23 of 74 treated with nitrosobis(2-oxopropyl)amine (Pour *et al.*, 1978), an unstated number of 957 treated with nitrosamines (Althoff & Granjean, 1979)

and 1 of 20 treated with nitroso-bis(2-acetoxypropyl)amine (Pour *et al.*, 1976a).

Preneoplastic changes

The nature of any preneoplastic changes associated with tumours of the male hamster reproductive tract is largely unknown. It is possible that estrogen-induced testicular involution may be associated with both the development of testicular tumours and the preneoplastic stages in the histogenesis of Leydig cell tumours (Llombart & Peña, 1964). Among 2776 estrogen-treated males over 99 days of age, 7 testicular tumours were found, but none in 2807 untreated males (Kirkman & Kempson, 1982). This represents a 0.25% incidence, but it is not known if it is significantly related to estrogen treatment and, thus, the estrogen-induced testicular involution may or may not be of etiological significance (Kirkman & Kempson, 1982). As pointed out by Kirkman & Kempson (1982), there is no reason to suspect that the epididymal cysts observed in hamsters (Granados & Dam, 1948) are related to the estrogen-induced papillary cystadenomas in the epididymal head (Kirkman, 1972; Kirkman & Kempson, 1982). Likewise, the prostatic hypertrophy observed in two lines of inbred hamsters (Homburger & Nixon, 1970; Wang & Schaffner, 1976) appears benign and it is not known to have progressed to neoplasia.

COMPARATIVE ASPECTS

Testicular tumours

Two important histological features distinguish the seminoma in the hamster from its human counterpart. The hamster seminoma lacks the scattered lymphocytes present in the human neoplasm, and the primary lesion in the hamster contains readily recognized remnants of seminiferous tubules which have usually been obliterated in the human lesion.

Sertoli cell tumours vary from well developed tubules to poorly differentiated areas of proliferating cords or sheets of cells without lumina.

Epididymal tumours

Cystadenomas of the epididymal head may eventually develop into papillary variants, as has been described in man (Sherrick, 1956). Bacon & Kirkman (1955) noted that since these tumours may be induced by estrogen treatment when started in very young animals, the estrogen-primed hamster may be an excellent experimental system to study the histogenesis of adenomatoid lesions in the area of the efferent ductules.

Ductus deferens tumours

The androgen/estrogen-induced leiomyosarcomas of the epididymus–vas deferens region are histologically similar to their counterparts in other mammals including humans, but differ in their hormonal sensitivity (Kirkman & Kempson, 1982).

Prostatic tumours

It appears that histologically confirmed spontaneous adenocarcinomas have not been reported. After reviewing Fortner's adenocarcinoma, several investigators have concluded that it has no resemblance to its human counterpart (for review see Kirkman & Kempson, 1982). It is not hormone-responsive and, based on karyotype studies, it may be composed of a mixed cell population (McDonald, 1963; Webber *et al.*, 1968).

ACKNOWLEDGEMENTS

We are indebted to CRC Press for permission to reproduce Figure 21 from Schmidt *et al.* (1982); Academic Press for permission to reproduce Figure 1 from Bivin *et al.* (1987); *Cancer Research* for permission to reproduce, from Kirkman & Algard (1965), Figures 15, 16 and 19 and, from Kirkman & Algard (1970), Figure 19; to *Cancer* for permission to reproduce Figure 17 from Kirkman (1957); and to S. Karger, Basel, for permission to reproduce Figures 3, 4, 6, 7, 8, 11, 12, 22 and 23 from Kirkman (1972).

REFERENCES

Abdalla, A.M. & Oliver, J.A. (1971a) SV40-transformed prostatic carcinoma in the hamster. Effect of hormonal manipulation on the growth rate. *Cancer*, 27, 468–470

Abdalla, A.M. & Oliver, J.A. (1971b) SV40-transformed prostatic carcinoma in the hamster: I. Comparisons of lactate dehydrogenase isoenzymes with human prostatic cancer. *Invest. Urol.*, 8, 442–447

Abdalla, A.M. & Oliver, J.A. (1971c) SV40-transformed prostatic carcinoma in the hamster: II. Comparisons of lactate dehydrogenase isoenzymes with human prostatic cancer. *Invest. Urol.*, 8, 488–493

Algard, F.T. (1965) Characteristics of an androgen/estrogen induced, dependent leiomyosarcoma of the ductus deferens of the Syrian hamster. II. *In vitro. Cancer Res.*, 25, 147–151

Althoff, J. & Grandjean, C. (1979) In vivo studies in Syrian golden hamsters: a transplacental bioassay of ten nitrosamines. *Natl Cancer Inst. Monogr.*, 51, 251–255

Althoff, J. & Lijinsky, W. (1977) Urinary bladder neoplasms in Syrian hamsters after administration of *N*-nitroso-*N*-methyl-*N*-dodecylamine. *Z. Krebsforsch.*, 90, 227–231

Althoff, J., Pour, P., Grandjean, C. & Eagen, M. (1976) Transplacental effects of nitrosamines in Syrian hamsters. I. Dibutylnitrosamine and nitrosohexamethyleneamine. *Z. Krebsforsch.*, 86, 69–75

Althoff, J., Grandjean, C., Gold, B. & Runge, R. (1977a) Carcinogenicity of 1-oxopropylpropylnitrosamine (*N*-nitroso-*N*-propylpropionamide) in Syrian hamsters. *Z. Krebsforsch.*, 90, 221–225

Althoff, J., Grandjean, C., Marsh, S., Pour, P. & Takahashi, M. (1977b) Transplacental effects of nitrosamines in Syrian hamsters. II. Nitrosopiperidine. *Z. Krebsforsch.*, 90, 71–77

Althoff, J., Pour, P., Grandjean, C. & Marsh, S. (1977c) Transplacental effects of nitrosamines in Syrian hamsters. III. Dimethyl and dipropylnitrosamine. *Z. Krebsforsch.*, 90, 78–86

Altman, P.L. & Katz, D.D. (1979) *Inbred and Genetically Defined Strains of Laboratory Animals*. Part 2. *Hamster, Guinea Pig, Rabbit and Chicken*, Bethesda, MD, Federation of American Societies for Experimental Biology (Handbook III)

Bacon, R.L. (1952) Tumors of the epididymis in hamsters treated with diethylstilbestrol and testosterone propionate. *Cancer Res.*, 12, 246

Bacon, R.L. & Kirkman, H. (1955) The response of the testis of the hamster to chronic treatment with different estrogens. *Endocrinology*, 57, 255–271

Bielschowsky, F. & Horning, E.S. (1958) Aspects of endocrine carcinogenesis. *Br. Med. Bull.*, 14, 106–115

Bivin, W.S., Olsen, G.A. & Murray, K.A. (1987) Morphophysiology. In: Van Hoosier, Jr, G.L. & McPherson, C.W., eds, *Laboratory Hamsters*, New York, Academic Press, pp. 9–41

Fortner, J.G. (1957) Spontaneous tumors, including gastrointestinal neoplasms and malignant melanomas, in the Syrian hamster. *Cancer*, 10, 1153–1156

Fortner, J.G. (1961) The influence of castration on spontaneous tumorigenesis in the Syrian (golden) hamster. *Cancer Res.*, 21, 1491–1498

Fortner, J.G. & Allen, A.C. (1958) Hitherto unreported malignant melanomas in the Syrian hamster; an experimental counterpart of human melanomas. *Cancer Res.*, 18, 98–10

Fortner, J.G., Funkhauser, J.W. & Cullen, M.R. (1963) A transportable, spontaneous adenocarcinoma of the prostate in the Syrian (golden) hamster. *Natl Cancer Inst. Monogr.*, 12, 371–379

Fortner, J.G., Mahy, A.G. & Cotran, R.S. (1961) Transplantable tumors of the Syrian (golden) hamster. II. Tumors of the hematopoietic tissues, genitourinary organs, mammary glands, and sarcomas. *Cancer Res.*, 21, 199–239

Fraley, E.E. & Paulson, D.F. (1968) Effects of hormones on the growth of virus transformed hamster prostatic tissue. *Surg. Forum*, 191, 544–545

Fraley, E.E. & Paulson, D.F. (1969) Morphological and biochemical studies of virus (SV40) transformed prostatic tissue. *J. Urol.*, 101, 735–740

Franks, L.M. (1967) Normal and pathological anatomy and histology of the genital tract of rats and mice. In: Cotchin, E. & Roe, F.J.C., eds, *Pathology of Laboratory Rats and Mice*, Philadelphia, Davis, pp. 469–499

Goldin, A. & Johnson, R.K. (1974) Evaluation of actinomycins in experimental systems. *Cancer Chemother. Rep.* (Part 1), 58, 63–77

Granados, H. & Dam, H. (1948) Testicular hypoplasia and epididymal cysts in the Syrian hamster. *Nature*, 162, 297

Guthrie, J. & Guthrie, O.A. (1974) Embryonal carcinomas in Syrian hamsters after intratesticular inoculation of zinc chloride during seasonal testicular growth. *Cancer Res.*, 34, 2612–2614

Handler, A.H. (1965) Spontaneous lesions of the hamster. In: Ribelin, W.E. & McCoy, J.R., eds, *The Pathology of Laboratory Animals*, Springfield, IL, Thomas, pp. 210–240

Homburger, F. (1969) Chemical carcinogenesis in the Syrian golden hamster: A review. *Cancer*, 23, 313–338

Homburger, F. & Nixon, C.W. (1970) Cystic prostatic hypertrophy in two inbred lines of Syrian hamsters. *Proc. Soc. Exp. Biol. (N.Y.)*, 134, 284–286

Homburger, F. & Russfield, A.B. (1970) An inbred line of Syrian hamsters with frequent spontaneous adrenal tumors. *Cancer Res.*, 30, 305–308

Horning, E.S. & Whittick, J.W. (1954) The histogenesis of stilbestrol-induced renal tumours in the male golden hamster. *Br. J. Cancer*, 8, 451–457

Jay, G.E., Jr (1963) Genetic strains and stocks. In: Burdette, W.J., ed., *Methodology in Mammalian Genetics*, San Francisco, Holden-Day, pp. 83–123

Kaspareit-Rittinghausen, J. & Deerberg, F. (1988) Spontaneous neoplasms of the seminal vesicles in aged Han:Chin hamsters (*Cricetelus criseus*). *Lab. Animals*, 22, 127–130

Kharkovskaya, N.A. (1979) Carcinogenic action of 2-aminoacetophenone in Syrian hamsters (in Russian). *Vop. Onkol.*, 25, 81–84

Kirkman, H. (1957) Steroid tumorigenesis. *Cancer*, 10, 757–764

Kirkman, H. (1962) A preliminary report concerning tumors observed in Syrian hamsters. *Stanford Med. Bull.*, 20, 163–166

Kirkman, H. (1972) Hormone-related tumors in Syrian hamsters. *Prog. Exp. Tumor Res.*, 16, 201–240

Kirkman, H. & Algard, F.T. (1965) Characteristics of an androgen/estrogen-induced, dependent leiomyosarcoma of the ductus deferens of the Syrian hamster. I. In vivo. *Cancer Res.*, 25, 141–146

Kirkman, H. & Algard, F.T. (1968) Spontaneous and nonviral-induced neoplasms. In: Hoffman, R.A., Robinson, P.E. & Magalhaes, H., eds., *The Golden Hamster, its Biology and Use in Medical Research*, Ames, Iowa State University Press, pp. 227–240

Kirkman, H. & Algard, F.T. (1970) Autonomous variants of an androgen/estrogen-induced and dependent ductus deferens leiomyosarcoma of the Syrian hamster. *Cancer Res.*, 30, 35–40

Kirkman, H. & Bacon, R.L. (1952) Estrogen-induced tumors of the kidney. I. Incidence of renal tumors in intact and gonadectomized male golden hamsters treated with diethylstilbestrol. *J. Natl Cancer Inst.*, 13, 745–755

Kirkman, H. & Bacon, R.L. (1958) Transplanted, estrogen-androgen-induced tumors of the uterus and vas deferens in Syrian hamsters. *Proc. Am. Ass. Cancer Res.*, 2, 315

Kirkman, H. & Chesterman, F.C. (1972) Additional data on transplanted tumours of the golden hamster. *Prog. Exp. Tumor Res.*, 16, 580–621

Kirkman, H. & Kempson, R.L. (1982) Tumours of the testis and accessory male sex glands. In: Turusov, V.S., ed., *Pathology of Tumours in Laboratory Animals*. Vol. III. *Tumours of the Hamster* (IARC Scientific Publications No. 34), Lyon, IARC, pp. 175–197

Kirkman, H. & Yau, P.K.S. (1969) Transplantable, Syrian hamster tumors, stored in liquid nitrogen. *Proc. Am. Assoc. Cancer Res.*, 10, 46

Kirkman, H. & Yau, P.K.S. (1972) Longevity of male land female, intact and gonadectomized, untreated and hormone-treated, neoplastic and non-neoplastic Syrian hamsters. *Am. J. Anat.*, 135, 205–220

Lindt, S. (1958) Uber Krankheiten des syrischen Goldhamsters (Mesocricetus auratus). *Schweiz. Arch. Tierheilk.*, 100, 86–97

Llombart, A., Jr & Sansano Peña, V. (1964) Tumores testiculares inducidos sobre el hamster dorado pro el 20-metilcolantreno, previa hemicastracióm y criptorchidia experimental. Estudio morfobiológico del sarcoma TTS. *Acta Oncol. (Madr.)*, 31, 88–106

Llombart-Bosch, A. & Peydro, A. (1975) Morphological, histochemical and ultrastructural observations of diethylstilbestrol-induced kidney tumors in the Syrian golden hamster. *Eur. J. Cancer*, 11, 403–412

Martan, J. (1969) Epididymal histochemistry and physiology. In: *Symposium on Male Reproductive Physiology*, New York, Academic Press, pp. 134–154

McDonald, D.F. (1963) Experimental therapy of the Fortner prostatic carcinoma in the hamster. *Invest. Urol.*, 1, 60–64

McGadey, J., Baillie, A.H. & Ferguson, M.M. (1966) Histochemical utilization of hydroxysteroids by the hamster epididymis. *Histochemie*, 7, 211–217

Mostofi, F.K. & Sobin, L.H. (1977) *Histological Typing of Testis Tumours*, Vol. 16. *International Histological Classification of Tumours*, Geneva, World Health Organization

Mostofi, F.K., Sesterhenn, I. & Sobin, L.H. (1980) *Histological Typing of Prostate Tumours*, Vol 22. *International Histological Classification of Tumours*, Geneva, WHO

Noble, R.L. (1964) Tumors and hormones. In: Pincus, G., Thimann, K.V. & Astwood, E.B., eds, *The Hormones*, Vol. V, New York, Academic Press, pp. 559–695

Noble, R.L. (1980a) Production of Nb rat carcinoma of the dorsal prostate and response of estrogen-dependent transplants to sex hormones and tamoxifen. *Cancer Res.*, 40, 3551–3554

Norris, J.S. (1980) Syrian hamster tumors in vitro: models for studying hormone action. In: Spring-Mills, E. & Hafez, E.S.E., eds, *Males Accessory Sex Glands, Biology and Pathology*, Amsterdam, Elsevier/North-Holland, pp. 609–616

Norris, J.S. & Kohler, P.O. (1976) Characterization of the androgen receptor from a Syrian hamster ductus deferens tumor cell line (DDT1). *Science*, 192, 898–900

Norris, J.S. & Kohler, P.O. (1977) The co-existence of androgen and glucocorticoid receptors in the DDT1, clones cell line. *Endocrinology*, 100, 613–618

Norris, J.S., Gorsky, J. & Kohler, P.O. (1974) Androgen receptors in a Syrian hamster ductus deferens tumour cell line. *Nature*, 248, 422

Norris, J.S., Bowden, C. & Kohler, P.O. (1976) Description of a new hamster ventral prostate cell line containing androgen receptors. *In Vitro*, 13, 108–114

Paulson, D.F., Rabson, A.S. & Fraley, E.E. (1968a) Viral neoplastic transformation of hamster prostatic tissue in vitro. *Science*, 159, 200–201

Paulson, D.F., Fraley, E.E., Rabson, A.S. & Ketcham, A.S. (1968b) SV40-transformed hamster prostatic tissue: a model of human prostatic malignancy. *Surgery*, 64, 241–247

Pour, P.M., Salmasi, S.Z. & Runge, R.G. (1978) Selective induction of pancreatic ductular tumors by single doses of *N*-nitrosobis(2-oxopropyl)amine in Syrian golden hamsters. *Cancer Lett.*, 4, 317–323

Pour, P., Althoff, J., Gingell, R., Kupper, R., Krüger, F.W. & Mohr, U. (1976a) A further pancreatic carcinogen in Syrian golden hamsters: *N*-nitroso-bis(2-acetooxypropyl)-amine. *Cancer Lett.*, 1, 197–202

Pour, P., Kmoch, N., Greiser, L., Mohr, U., Althoff, J. & Cardesa, A. (1976b) Spontaneous tumors and common diseases in two colonies of Syrian hamsters. I. Incidence and sites. *J. Natl Cancer Inst.*, 56, 931–935

Pour, P., Mohr, U., Althoff, J., Cardesa, A. & Kmoch, N. (1976c) Spontaneous tumors and common diseases in two colonies of Syrian hamsters. III. Urogenital system and endocrine glands. *J. Natl Cancer Inst.*, 56, 949–961

Pour, P.M., Salmasi, S.Z. & Runge, R.G. (1978) Selective induction of pancreatic ductular tumors by single doses of N-nitrosobis(2-oxopropyl)amine in Syrian golden hamsters. *Cancer Lett.*, 4, 317–323

Reznik-Schüller, H. (1979) Carcinogenic effects of diethylstilbestrol in male Syrian golden hamsters and European hamsters. *J. Natl Cancer Inst.*, 52, 1083–1088

Rivière, M.R., Chouroulinkov, I. & Guérin, M. (1960) Actions hormonales expérimentales de longue durée chez le hamster du point de vue de leur effet cancérigène. I. Etude de la testostérone. *Bull. Ass. franç. Cancer*, 47, 558–564

Rivière, M.R., Chouroulinkov, I. & Guérin, M. (1961) Actions hormonales expérimentales de longue durée chez le hamster du point de vue de leur effet cancérigène. II. Etude de la testostérone associée à un oestrogène. *Bull. Ass. franç. Cancer*, 48, 499–524

Rivière, M.R., Chouroulinkov, I. & Guérin, M. (1962a) Leiomyosarcomes de l'épididyme développés chez des hamsters dorés après un traitement simultané par la testostérone et un oestrogène. *C.R. Séanc. Soc. Biol. (Paris)* 156, 1033–1035

Rivière, M.R., Chouroulinkov, I. & Guérin, M. (1962b) Lésions et tumeurs du testicule apparues chez le hamster doré après un traitement oestrogénique prolongé. Quoted by Rivière *et al.* (1964)

Rivière, M.R., Chouroulinkov, I. & Guérin, M. (1964) Contribution à la carcinogenèse hormonale chez le hamster. *Acta Un. int. Cancer*, 20, 1509–1511

Robinson, R. (1968) Genetics and karyology. In: Hoffman, R.A., Robinson, P.F. & Magalhaes, H., eds, *The Golden Hamster, its Biology and Use in Medical Research*, Ames, Iowa State University Press, pp. 41–72

Robinson, F.R. (1976) *Hamsters*. In: Melby, E.C., Jr & Altman, N.H., eds, *Handbook of Laboratory Animal Science*, Vol. III, Cleveland, CRC Press, pp. 253–270

Russfield, A.B. (1966) *Tumors of Endocrine Glands and Secondary Sex Organs*. Washington, D.C., US Government Printing Office (Public Health Service Publication No. 1332)

Rustia, M. (1974) Multiple carcinogenic effects of the ethylnitrosourea precursors ethylurea and sodium nitrite in hamsters. *Cancer Res.*, 34, 3232–3244

Rustia, M. (1975) Inhibitory effect of sodium ascorbate on ethylurea and sodium nitrite carcinogenesis and negative findings in progeny after intestinal inoculation of precursors into pregnant hamsters. *J. Natl Cancer Inst.*, 55, 1389–1394

Rustia, M. (1979) Role of hormone imbalance in transplacental carcinogenesis induced in Syrian golden hamsters by sex hormones. *Natl Cancer Inst. Monogr.*, 51, 77–87

Rustia, M. & Shubik, P. (1976) Transplacental effects of diethylstilbestrol on the genital tract of hamster offspring. *Cancer Lett.*, 1, 139–146

Rustia, M. & Shubik, P. (1979) Effects of transplacental exposure to diethylstilbestrol in carcinogenic susceptibility during postnatal life in hamster progeny. *Cancer Res.*, 39, 4636–4644

Schmidt, R.E., Eason, R.L., Hubbard, G.B., Young, G.T. & Eisenbrandt, D.L. (1983) *Pathology of Aging Syrian Hamsters*, Boca Raton, FL, CRC Press

Sherrick, J.C. (1956) Papillary cystadenoma of the epididymis. *Cancer*, 9, 403–407

Sichuk, G., Fortner, G.J. and Der, B.K. (1967) Evaluation of the influence of norethynodrel with mestranol (Enovid) in middle-aged male Syrian (golden) hamsters, with particular reference to spontaneous tumours. *Acta Endocrinol. (Kbh.)*, 55, 97–107

Sichuk, G., Fortner, G.J., Der, B.K. & Russfield, A.B. (1966) Spontaneous tumorigenesis in hypophysectomized Syrian (golden) hamsters. *Cancer Res.*, 26, 2154–2164

Squire, R.A., Goodman, D.G., Valerio, M.G., Fredrickson, T.N., Strandberg, J.D., Levitt, M.H., Lingenman, C.H., Harschbarger, J.C. & Dawe, C.J. (1978) Tumors. In: Benirschke, K., Gerner, K.M. & Jones, T.C., ed., *Pathology of Laboratory Animals*, Vol. II, Berlin, Heidelberg, New York, Springer-Verlag, pp. 1051–1283

Strandberg, J.D. (1987) Neoplastic diseases. In: Van Hoosier, G.L., Jr & McPherson, C.W., ed., *Laboratory Hamsters*, New York, Academic Press, pp. 9–41, 157–168

Trentin, J.J. (1987) Experimental biology: Use in oncological research. In: Van Hoosier, G.L., Jr & McPherson, C.W., ed., *Laboratory Hamsters*, New York, Academic Press, pp. 201–214

Varvarakis, M.J., Sampson, D., Schoones, R., Goeta, J.F., Reynoso, G., Mirand, E.A. & Murphy, G.P. (1972) The effect of androgens and estrogens on induced prostatic tumor in the hamster. *J. Surg. Oncol.*, 4, 48–59

Vasquez-Lopez, E. (1944) The reaction of the pituitary gland and related hypothalamic centers in the hamster to prolonged treatment with oestrogens. *J. Pathol. Bacteriol.*, 56, 1–13

Wang, G.M. & Schaffner, C.P. (1976) Effect of candicidin and cholestipol on the testes and prostate glands of B1087.20 hamsters. *Invest. Urol.*, 14, 66–71

Webber, M.M., Joneja, M.G. & Connolly, J.G. (1968) Observations on Fortner tumour – a transplantable carcinoma of the hamster prostate. *Invest. Urol.*, 5. 348–357

Yabe, Y., Kataoka, N. & Koyama, H. (1972) Spontaneous tumors in hamsters; incidence, morphology, transplantation and virus studies. *Gann*, 63, 329–336

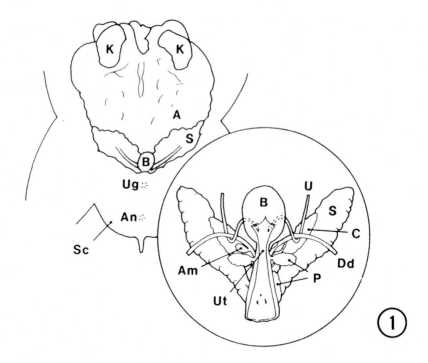

Figure 1. Ventral view of the urogenital system of the male hamster. The insert is also a ventral view of the accessory sex organs. The bladder and urethra have been opened to show entrances of ducts. A bulbo-urethral gland enters the urethra distally but its opening is not illustrated. Kidney (K), bladder (B), seminal vesicle (S), urogenital opening (Ug), anus (An, scrotum (Sc), adipose tissue (A), ureter (U), ductus deferens (Dd), urethra (Ut), coagulating gland (C), prostate (p), ampullary gland (Am). From Bivin *et al.* (1987)

Figure 2. Primary seminoma in right testis from an untreated 662-day-old hamster. H & E; × 94. From Kirkman (1972)

Figure 3. Renal metastasis from primary seminoma in Figure 2. H & E; × 468. From Kirkman (1972)

Figure 4. Fifty-seventh serial passage *in vivo* of seminoma in Figure 2. H & E; × 468. From Kirkman (1972)

Figure 5. Hyperplasia of testicular interstitial cells characteristic of hamster treated chronically with estrogen. From a 4-day-old hamster implanted with DES pellets for 350 days. (Same testis as that shown in Figure 14). H & E; × 94

Figure 6. A Sertoli cell tubular adenoma from a 563-day-old hamster implanted with estrone pellets for 516 days. H & E; 94. From Kirkman (1972)

Figure 7. A Sertoli cell adenoma from a 697-day-old hamster implanted with a Tpr pellet for 50 days followed by DES pellets for 597 days. H & E; × 468. From Kirkman (1972)

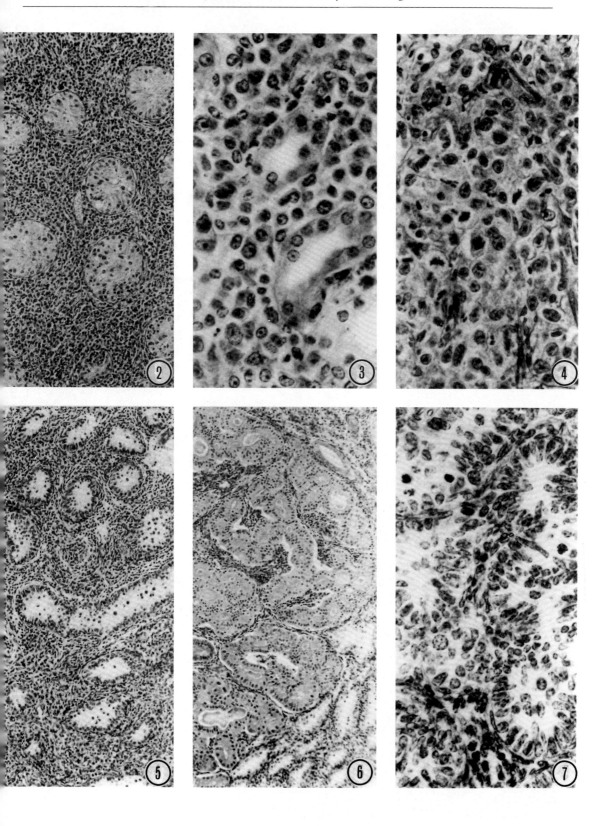

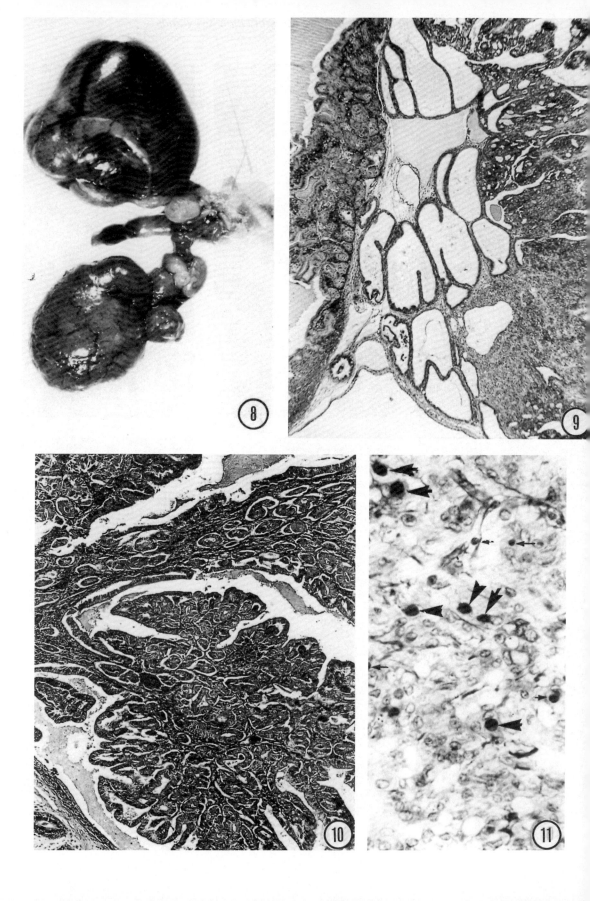

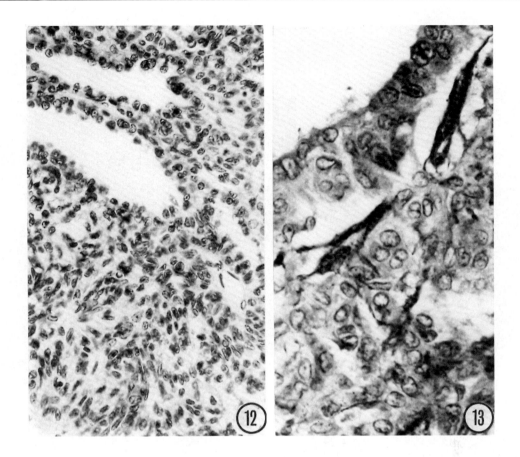

Figure 8. Epididymal head cystadenomas from a 458-day-old hamster implanted with DES pellets for 409 days. × 15. From Kirkman (1972)

Figure 9. Epididymal head cystadenoma from a 451-day-old hamster implanted with DES pellets for 402 days. H & E; × 40

Figure 10. Epididymal head cystadenomas from a 423-day-old hamster implanted with DES pellets for 373 days. H & E; × 65. From Kirkman (1972)

Figure 11. Epididymal head adenoma from a 448-day-old hamster implanted with DES pellet for 399 days. Arrows indicate PAS-positive droplets. PAS; × 500. From Kirkman (1972)

Figure 12. As for Figure 9. × 375

Figure 13. As for Figure 11; × 625. From Kirkman (1972)

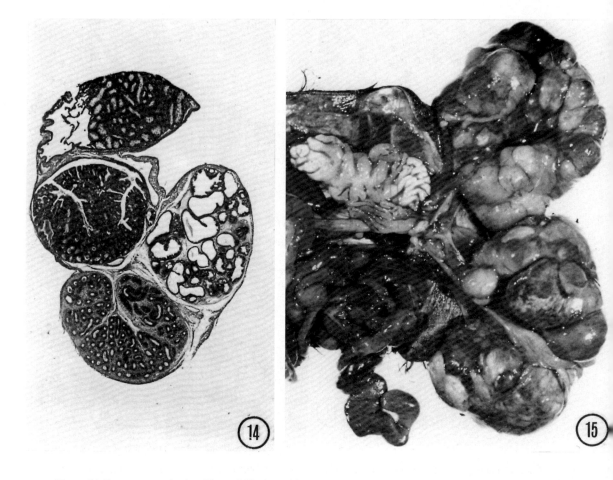

Figure 14. From same animal as Figure 5. Testis, epididymis and epididymal head adenoma. H & E; × 20

Figure 15. Paired, epididymal tail/ductus deferens leiomyosarcomas from a 572-day-old hamster implanted with pellets of Tpr/DES for 522 days. × 15. From Kirkman & Algard (1965)

Figure 16. Leiomyosarcomas in epididymal tail from a 450-day-old hamster implanted with pellets of Tpr/DES for 400 days. H & E; × 29. From Kirkman & Algard (1965)

Figure 17. Leiomyosarcoma in ductus deferens from a 500-day-old hamster implanted with pellets of Tpr/DES for 273 days. H & E; × 857. From Kirkman (1957)

Figure 18. Twenty-ninth serial subpannicular transplant of Tpr/DES-induced ductus deferens leiomyosarcoma. From a 151-day-old hamster transplanted with the tumour tissue and implanted with pellets of Tpr/DES for 93 days; H & E; × 620

Figure 19. As for Figure 18. From Kirkman & Algard (1970)

Figure 20. Intravascular pulmonary metastasis from 100th serial passage (32nd in untreated hosts) of autonomous derivative of an originally Tpr/DES-induced and dependent ductus deferens leiomyosarcoma. PTAH; × 570. From Kirkman & Algard (1965)

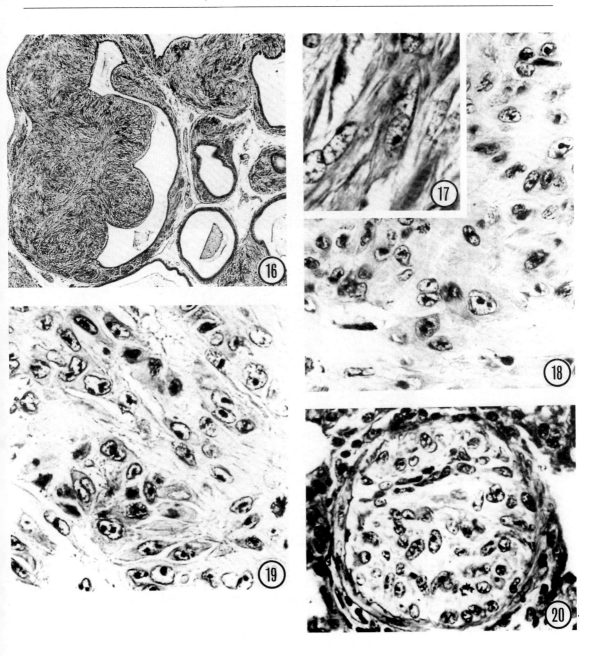

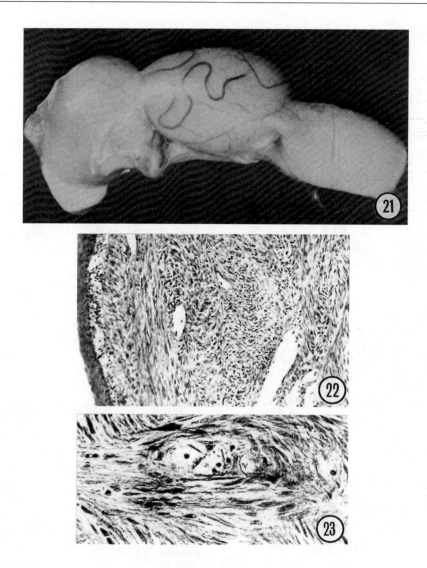

Figure 21. Gross appearance of epididymal sperm granuloma. From Schmidt *et al.* (1983)

Figure 22. Leiomyoma in wall of dorsal prostate; 698-day-old hamster treated with Tpr for 50 days followed with DES for 598 days. H & E; × 95. From Kirkman (1972)

Figure 23. As for Figure 21

Tumours of the female genital system

J.L. RIBAS AND J.M. PLETCHER

In the area of chemical carcinogenesis of the genital system, relatively few agents have been tested in the hamster, and only four have produced a significant yield of tumours. Spontaneous neoplasms of the reproductive tract of the female hamster are uncommon, although among different colonies the incidence may range from 3.5 to 11% and the pre-dilection site may also vary (Pour et al., 1976c). When a large number of untreated and estrogen-treated female hamsters in the Stanford colony (Kirkman & Kempson, 1982) were compared, the incidence of ovarian tumours in untreated animals was 0.12% as opposed to 0.28% for estrogen-treated ones, while the corresponding figures for uterine tumours were 0.22% and 1.40% (Tables 1 and 2). The low incidence of spontaneous genital tumours, coupled with the range of preneoplastic and neoplastic conditions that can be induced by some chemical carcinogens, makes the hamster a potentially valuable biological system for studying etiology and pathogenesis, hormone-dependence, autonomous growth, morphology, biological behaviour and treatment of induced tumours of the female reproductive tract.

In addition to reviewing the literature since 1965, this chapter includes comparisons, where possible, of the different tumours of the female reproductive tract of the hamster with their human counterparts. However, the WHO classification of human ovarian (Serov et al., 1973) and genital tract tumours (Poulsen et al., 1975) is complex due to the large numbers of different tumours arising from these organs. In contrast, relatively few spontaneous tumours arise from the genital tract of female hamsters, making a direct comparison between human and hamster neoplasms of limited value. Earlier literature on hamster tumours has been reviewed by various authors (Noble, 1964; Handler, 1965, 1976; Russfield, 1966; Homburger, 1968, 1969, 1972, 1979; Kirkman & Algard, 1968; Van Hoosier & Trentin, 1979; Van Hoosier et al., 1971; Robinson, 1976; Squire et al., 1978; Altman & Katz, 1979). Additional reviews on hormone-induced tumours of the reproductive tract of the female hamster (Kirkman, 1972) and its transplantable tumours (Kirkman & Chesterman, 1972) are also available.

NORMAL STRUCTURE

In the mature female hamster the external genitalia are located in the midline and ventrocaudally, with the introitus vaginae situated halfway between the urinary opening cranially and the anus caudally (Figure 1). The internal reproductive organs consist of the ovaries, the uterine horns, a duplex uterus, and vagina. The ovaries are located dorsolateral to the kidneys. They are oval-shaped and are enclosed within the bursae ovaricae. The oviducts are long and tightly coiled and the duplex uterus consists of an undivided

Table 1. Distribution and incidence of ovarian tumours among hamsters, with and without induced hormonal imbalances, in the Stanford colony

Hormonal state of animal	Total size of samples[a]	Number and percentage of animals with ovarian tumours	Mean age and range (in days) of animals with ovarian tumours	Right or left ovary	Classification of ovarian tumours	No. of tumours
Normal	4 166	5 (0.12)	660 (472–818)	4 in left 1 in right	Benign theca-granulosa-cell tumour	1
					Malignant thecomas	3
					Stromal luteoma (?)	1
Induced imbalance	1 786	5 (0.28)	568 (479-743)	4 in left 1 in right	Arrhenoblastoma	1
					Malignant theca-granulosa cell tumour	1
					Mucoid cystadenomas	2
					Tubular mesonephric adenoma	1
Total	5 952	10 (0.17)	614	8 in left 2 in right	Sex-cord mesenchymal tumours	7
					Surface epithelial tumours	3

[a] All females 472 or more days of age
[b] There were no bilateral tumours

Table 2. Distribution and incidence of uterine tumours among untreated and estrogen-treated hamsters in the Stanford colony

Hormonal state of animal[a]	Total size of sample	Mean age and range (in days) of sample	Number and percentage of animals with uterine tumours	Mean age and range (in days) of animal with uterine tumours	Tumours in cervix, or left or right horns[b]	Classification of uterine tumours	No of tumours
Untreated	523	631 (500–1200)	9 (0.22)	698 (555–847)	Cervix 3 Left horn 1 Right horn 5 Total 9	Carcinomas	4
						Stromal tumour (benign)	1
						Leiomyomas	2
						Leiomyo-sarcomas	2
Estrogen-treated	210	552 (501-900)	25 (1.40)	433 (325–680)	Cervix 9 Left horn 5 Right horn 9 Left or right horn 4 Total 27	Carcinomas	3
						Stromal tumours: Benign	4
						Malignant	1
						Leiomyoma	5
						Leiomyo-sarcomas	2
						Carcinosarcomas[c]	10

[a] Exclusive of S/T-induced leiomyosarcomas
[b] One animal with tumours in each horn. One animal with tumours in cervix and horns
[c] Uterine horn carcinosarcomas are estrogen-induced and estrogen-dependent. The role of estrogen in the induction of other uterine tumours found in estrogen-treated hamsters is uncertain.

(7–8 mm long) segment and a divided segment (or two uterine horns) measuring 20 mm in length. The cervix is dual in its cranial end, but it fuses into a single canal caudally as it continues into the vagina. The upper portion of the vagina extends craniodorsally to and beyond the os cervicis as it forms a crescent-shaped cul-de-sac. The lower or caudal portion of the vagina is flattened dorsoventrally and has a pair of vaginal pouches. The gross and microscopic anatomy of the female reproductive tract of the hamster has been reviewed in detail by Bivin *et al.* (1987).

MORPHOLOGY AND BIOLOGY OF TUMOURS

Histological types of tumours

The histological types of ovarian, oviductal, uterine, vaginal, clitoral and perineal skin tumours that have been recognized in the female hamster were listed in the corresponding chapter of the first edition of this volume (Kirkman & Kempson, 1982). Histopathological descriptions of the more common spontaneous and induced neoplasms are presented below; however, morphological descriptions of tumours well characterized in other species have not been included.

Ovary

Tumours of the ovary are usually unilateral. They commonly arise from granulosa or theca cells.

Surface epithelial tumours

Spontaneous and induced cystadenomas have been reported. Mucinous cystadenoma and tubular clear cell (mesonephric) adenoma in hormone-treated hamsters have been reported from the Stanford colony (Kirkman & Kempson, 1982). Mucinous cystadenoma may be solid or cystic. Mucinous cells may form gland-like structures of varying size (Figure 2). Cystic spaces are lined by neoplastic cuboidal or columnar cells (Figures 3 and 4). They contain abundant, foamy, alcian blue-positive cytoplasmic material, indicating the presence of mucopolysaccharides. The nuclei are usually basally located and are often compressed. However, in solid areas the nuclei may be more elongated, are centrally located, and show minimal atypia. Also, nuclei appear to be more closely packed since their cytoplasm is less abundant and does not have the foamy appearance typical of gland-forming cells. Mitoses are generally not found.

Tubular, clear cell (mesonephric) adenoma consists of irregular, branching tubules lined by a non-ciliated simple columnar epithelium (Figure 5). The epithelial cells have a vesicular, round to oval nucleus which is basally located. There is little nuclear pleomorphism and the stroma consists mainly of proliferating smooth muscle cells. The tumour is histologically benign and failed to grow when transplanted in untreated female hosts (Kirkman & Kempson, 1982).

Fibromas and thecomas

Fibromas are circumscribed neoplasms composed of collagen-producing, spindle-shaped cells. Neoplastic cells are well differentiated and mitotic figures are rare. Malignant variants have ill-defined margins and increased cellularity, and they may be arranged in a herringbone pattern in anastomosing narrow bundles (Figures 6 and 7) or in diffuse sheets. Mitoses may be sparse or numerous. Neoplastic cells may have ill-defined borders and are surrounded by an argyrophilic network of delicate collagenous fibres. Thecomas are ovarian tumours composed of spindle-shaped to rounded cells; the former cell is usually arranged in bundles and fascicles, while the latter contains abundant, eosinophilic cytoplasm and vesicular nuclei. Thecomas produce estrogen and are thought to be derived from stromal cells. Both benign and malignant as well as spontaneous and induced thecomas have been reported (Table 1). Unfortunately, it is not always possible to separate fibromas from thecomas on morphological features alone, since the latter is also a spindle-cell tumour with similar patterns. The more inclusive term of thecoma–fibroma has been proposed (Kirkman & Kempson, 1982). Two transplantable thecoma–fibrosarcomas were reported from the Stanford tumour bank (Kirkman & Kempson, 1982). One of these was a markedly lobulated ovarian neoplasm with no metastasis in a 726-day-old untreated hamster. It consisted of small, intermingling bundles of plump, spindle-shaped cells (Figure 8). Cell borders were ill-defined, and the nuclei ovoid and small. The connective tissue stroma was scant and areas of hyaline degeneration were present. Subpannicular transplants grew rapidly and, for the first 12 generations, masses were palpable within 60 days. A pulmonary metastasis from one of the transplant animals is shown in Figure 9. The other thecoma–fibrosarcoma also had no metastatic lesions and was present in the left ovary of a 653-day-old untreated hamster. It was composed of thick sheets or bundles of short, plump, spindle to cuboidal-shaped cells (Figure 10). Transplants (Figure 11) grew slowly and subpannicular masses were palpable for the first four *in vivo* generations at a mean latent period of 300 days.

Arrhenoblastoma (Sertoli–Leydig cell tumour)

Only one arrhenoblastoma has been reported in the literature (Kirkman, 1972). It was present in the left ovary of a 479-day-old hamster. Since the animal had been ovariectomized on the 60th day of life, this was initially thought to be a remnant of the left ovary, but histological studies disclosed a neoplasm composed of a mixture of tubular and interstitial elements (Figure 12). In well differentiated areas, the tubules were lined by cells with abundant cytoplasm and vesicular nuclei.

Sheets or cords of Leydig-like cells with round nuclei and acidophilic cytoplasm surrounded the tubular component. In less differentiated regions, focal collections of Leydig-like cells were interspersed among Sertoli-like cells forming primitive cords; mitoses were frequent.

Stromal luteoma

Kirkman & Kempson (1982) described a mass in the left ovary of a 596-day-old untreated virgin hamster that resembled a stromal luteoma (Figures 13 and 14), although they could not rule out stromal luteinization. Most of the tumour was characterized by massive luteinization of the stromal cells.

Granulosa cell tumours

Granulosa cells and theca-granulosa cell tumours (Figures 15 and 16) have been reported in the hamster. They have been seen in both control and treated animals. The tumours reported are histologically similar to those described in other laboratory animals.

Other tumours

Other tumours including haemangioma and a variety of other mesenchymal tumours have been reported sporadically.

Uterus

Adenocarcinoma

Endometrial adenocarcinomas can arise in the cervix, body of the uterus or the uterine horns as spontaneous or induced neoplasms. They show different histological patterns and degrees of differentiation. Well differentiated adenocarcinomas are composed of epithelial cells forming irregular, gland-like spaces which are lined by atypical endometrial cells and which are supported by a proliferating fibrovascular stroma (Figure 17) that may occasionally become scirrhous (Strandberg, 1987). Tumour cells have abundant eosinophilic, glassy cytoplasm and their nuclei contain prominent nucleoli. Cell differentiation can vary from one area in the tumour to another. The invasive characteristic of these tumours renders them easily recognizable regardless of their degree of differentiation. Less differentiated tumours may be composed of sheets of cuboidal cells which can organize focally into gland-like spaces. Adenocarcinomas have been successfully transplanted to the subpanniculus (Figure 18) and the transplants have produced metastases (Figure 19). Normal squamous cell epithelium is often seen adjacent to adenocarcinoma of the cervix (Figure 20); however, adenocarcinomas of the uterine horn can demonstrate squamous differentiation (Figure 21). Squamous metaplasia of the endometrium, often resulting in polyplike structures, must also be distinguished from neoplasia (Figure 22).

Endometrial stromal nodules

Endometrial stromal nodules are composed of closely packed endometrial stromal cells (Figures 23 and 24). They grow by expansion and are usually found just beneath the endometrial surface; in extreme cases they may approach the serosa. Mitoses are typically absent and there is no infiltration. They are considered benign lesions and must be differentiated from leiomyoma. This can be accomplished by means of trichrome or reticulin stains.

Papillary fibroepithelial polyps are occasionally seen arising from the endometrium (Figure 25). These are benign lesions.

Leiomyoma/leiomyosarcoma

Leiomyoma/leiomyosarcomas can be found throughout the tubular reproductive tract. Both spontaneous and induced smooth muscle tumours occur in hamsters. It is often difficult to determine whether a given smooth muscle tumour is

benign or malignant based on histopathology alone. In general, tumours with ten mitoses per ten high power fields are considered malignant regardless of their degree of differentiation. Tumours with fewer mitotic figures but showing marked atypia are also considered malignant. Those tumours with less than four mitoses per ten high power fields are usually considered benign. These criteria apply to spontaneous tumours and are useful in evaluating induced neoplasms. Tumours that are benign at induction can become aggressive with serial passage. It is interesting to note that metastatic lesions only occur from tumours which show histological evidence of malignancy. Leiomyomas are well circumscribed neoplasms which can range greatly in size (Figure 26). They are composed of well differentiated smooth muscle cells arranged in interlacing bundles (Figure 27). Leiomyosarcomas tend to be less differentiated and are also composed of interlacing bundles of spindle cells (Figure 28), a pattern that is retained in serial *in vivo* transplantation (Figure 29). Poorly differentiated leiomyosarcomas are difficult to differentiate from other spindle-cell sarcomas. Induction of smooth muscle tumours by diethylstilbestrol/testosterone propionate (DES/Tpr) often results in multiple neoplasms in both the uterine horns and body (Figure 30).

Malignant mixed tumours (carcinosarcoma)

Mixed (epithelial/mesenchymal) tumours are reported to occur following estrogen implantation. These tumours are composed of gland-like structures embedded in whorls of smooth muscle cells (Figure 31). In the primary tumours, mitoses are rare and there is mild cellular atypia. However, after passage in estrogen-treated hosts, histological features of malignancy develop in both the mesenchymal and epithelial components, prompting some to classify these tumours as carcinosarcomas. They are slow-growing tumours but they are transplantable as estrogen-dependent neoplasms. Some authors believe that they arise from the Müllerian ducts (Kirkman & Kempson, 1982).

Extensive cystic glandular hyperplasia of the endometrium, which often involves the myometrium (Figure 32), is commonly seen in estrogen-treated female hamsters. This lesion, as well as multiple uterine leiomyosarcomas and uterine carcinosarcomas, is associated with long-term estrogen treatment.

Vagina and clitoris

Very few vaginal tumours have been reported in untreated hamsters. Vaginal squamous cell papillomas are benign lesions and are histologically similar to cutaneous papillomas (Figure 33). Inverted papillomas with glandular differentiation have occasionally been reported (Figure 34).

Rustia (1974) has given a brief histological description of solid and follicular adenomas in the clitoris.

SPONTANEOUS TUMOURS

Kirkman and Yau (1972) discussed the relationship of hormonal imbalance to the incidence of spontaneous tumours in the female hamster.

Ovary

Spontaneous ovarian tumours are quite rare. The granulosa cell tumour (Chesterman, 1972; Dontenwill et al., 1973a; Rustia, 1974; Pour et al., 1976b; Cotchin & Marchant, 1977; Althoff & Lijinsky, 1977) appears to be the most common spontaneous neoplasm of the ovary. Very few ovarian tumours were observed in the Stanford colony (Kirkman & Kempson, 1982). Their distribution and incidence are shown in Table 2.

Uterus and oviduct

A variety of spontaneous uterine neoplasms have been described including

adenoma, papilloma, adenocarcinoma, leiomyoma, leiomyosarcoma and haemangioma. It is also probable that some uterine tumours that have been reported as induced may have been of spontaneous origin (Kirkman & Kempson, 1982). The incidence of spontaneous endometrial carcinoma appears to be low, but a 25% incidence was found to occur in Chinese hamsters (Ward & Moore, 1969; Squire et al., 1978). Table 2 summarizes data for uterine tumours found in the Stanford colony. A very few neoplasms arising spontaneously in the oviducts have been reported and include papillomas (Toth, 1969, 1970) and cystadenomas (Pour et al., 1976b).

Vagina

The incidence of spontaneous tumours of the vagina is exceedingly low and encompasses papilloma (Althoff et al., 1973; Pour et al., 1973, 1976b,c, 1979) and squamous cell carcinoma (Chesterman, 1972).

INDUCTION OF TUMOURS

As indicated earlier, relatively few studies on experimental tumorigenesis of the female genital system have been done using the hamster. Moreover, in most of these studies there has been no independent verification. Homburger et al. (1972) have shown the different susceptibilities of inbred and random-bred hamster lines to tumour induction by administration of 3-methylcholanthrene (MC). This is a particularly relevant concern here since in some studies the breed is not given. Kirkman and Kempson (1982) also questioned whether some of the 'induced' neoplasms of the female genital tract of the hamster may not be in fact spontaneous tumours, particularly since in some of the published studies the incidence of neoplasia in carcinogen-treated animals was almost as low as that reported in untreated animals.

Ovary

The hamster ovary appears to be refractory to chemical induction of neoplasms. This paucity of neoplasms has led Kirkman (1972) to state that 'no specific experimental treatment has yielded a consistently high harvest of ovarian tumors'. Despite this caveat, several types of neoplasm have been reported to occur in hamsters treated in a variety of ways. Of the chemical carcinogens that have been tested in the hamster, oral administration of MC to seven inbred hamster strains yielded the highest number (82) of ovarian neoplasms (Homburger, 1972). Unfortunately, the tumours were not identified histologically.

Oviducts

Urethane and dimethylbenz[*a*]anthracene (DMBA) have been reported to induce oviductal papillomas in hamsters (Toth, 1969, 1970). However, the low yield of papillomas has raised questions as to whether they were indeed induced or arose spontaneously. Life-long treatment with DES/Tpr induces oviductal leiomyomas (Kirkman & Kempson, 1982).

Uterus

A number of carcinogens, including X-ray irradiation (Homburger, 1968, 1969; Kirkman & Algard, 1968; Robinson, 1976), have resulted in the production of tumours of various types. However, the most reproducible method of inducing uterine tumours is hormonal treatment (Leavitt *et al.*, 1981; Kirkman & Kempson, 1982). Both epithelial and smooth muscle uterine neoplasms have been found in estrogen-treated hamsters (Table 2) in the Stanford colony and elsewhere (Kirkman & Kempson, 1982). They also tended to occur earlier in life in estrogen-treated animals as compared to controls. It appears that treatment with estrogen shortens the latency period for tumour development. Among chemical carcinogens, MC (Homburger, 1972) appears to be a potent inducer, but unfortunately, as was the case for the MC-induced ovarian tumours, specific histological diagnoses were not given. Hiraki (1971) reported an 86% (12/14) incidence of uterine adenocarcinomas following prolonged treatment with *N,N'*-dimethylnitrosourea. Prenatal treatment with DES followed by postnatal treatment with DMBA appears to potentiate the effects of DMBA. DMBA alone induced three uterine polyps and six squamous cell papillomas of the vagina in 50 females, but following DES prenatal treatment, it produced 13 uterine polyps, 2 carcinosarcomas, 1 cervical squamous cell papilloma, 3 cervical polyps and 8 ovarian granulosa-theca-cell tumours in 19 females.

Vagina and clitoris

Among the different structures comprising the reproductive tract of the female hamster, the vagina is a target organ that responds most reliably and efficiently to the inductive effects of some chemical carcinogens. For example, Althoff *et al.* (1978) reported a 74% (67/90) incidence of squamous cell papilloma after treatment with *N*-nitroso-2,6-dimethylmorpholine. Likewise, an 89% (40/45) incidence of squamous cell papilloma was obtained following administration of *N*-nitroso-(2-hydroxypropyl)-(2-oxopropyl)amine (Pour *et al.*, 1979). Lower incidences of squamous cell papilloma have also been obtained after treatment with urethane (3.3%, 1/30) (Toth *et al.*, 1961), 1-oxopropylnitroso-propylamine (25%, 14/56) (Althoff *et al.*, 1977a), ethylurea plus sodium nitrite (22%, 8/36) (Rustia, 1974) and DMBA (12%, 6/50). A 26% (5/19) incidence of squamous cell papilloma has also been induced after prenatal treatment with DES followed by postnatal administration of DMBA (Rustia & Shubik, 1979). The application of DMBA on the uterine cervices of nine hamsters resulted in vaginal and perineal carcinomas in all treated animals (Chu & Malmgren, 1965).

There is only one report of tumour induction in the clitoral gland. Five solid and follicular-type adeno-mas (14%) were found in 36 females treated with ethylurea and sodium nitrite (Rustia, 1974).

PROGRESSION, METASTASIS, TRANSPLANTATION AND REGRESSION

Smooth muscle tumours in the hamster appear to be under hormonal influence. Tumour progression has been observed in the androgen/estrogen-induced leiomyosarcoma. Growth of early transplants *in vivo* requires hormone treatment of the host, but they become autonomous after serial passage. However, autonomous variants are still regarded as hormone-responsive, since their growth is retarded significantly in progesterone-treated hosts (Kirkman & Algard, 1970b). The occurrence of metastasis has been documented in one spontaneous leiomyosarcoma of the uterine cervix (Table 2) and in a cervical carcinoma from an estrogen-treated animal. Carcinosarcomas are usually multicentric in origin and have been found only in uterine horns. When metastasis occurs in *in vivo* transplantation of uterine neoplasms, the lungs are usually the site of metastases. Growth or regression of transplanted squamous cell carcinoma of the cervix is influenced by exposure to X-ray irradiation (Eddy, 1979).

PRENEOPLASTIC CHANGES

Treatment of female hamsters with sex hormones or a variety of non-specific carcinogens is often followed by precocious reproductive tract neoplasia as compared to untreated females (Toth, 1969, 1970; Toth & Shubik, 1969; Kirkman & Yau, 1972). However, little is known about constitutional factors in the host that may predispose to the development of spontaneous or induced neoplasms.

COMPARATIVE ASPECTS

The majority of human tumours of surface epithelium consist of either pure mucinous or pure serous cells. In the hamster, they are usually classified as potentially mucinous even though serous-like cells may also be present. The typical broad papillary structures present in human serous tumours have not been described in the hamster counterparts. Malignant surface ovarian tumours have not been reported in the hamster although in humans they are the commonest type.

Human thecomas contain estrogen but it is unknown if this occurs among the thecoma-fibroma group in the hamster. Although the incidence of stromal thecal cell tumours in the hamster is extremely low, it is possible that some of these tumours may be classified as either fibromas or fibrosarcomas. Thecomas are composed of steroid-producing cells and, at least by immunohistochemistry, they could be differentiated from other spindle cell tumours. Kirkman and Kempson (1982) favoured the diagnosis of diffuse stromal luteinization – a non-neoplastic process similar to the human pregnancy luteomas, for some of the reported stromal luteomas.

Hamsters have a high incidence of endometrial hyperplasia (Rakoff *et al.*, 1951; Ward & Moore, 1969; Van Hoosier *et al.*, 1971; Schmidt *et al.*, 1983), but spontaneous uterine cervical carcinomas are rare (Kirkman & Chesterman, 1972; Kirkman & Yau, 1969; Kirkman & Kempson, 1982). Squamous cell carcinoma of the cervix, the most common malignancy of the genital tract of American women and accounting for about 5% of all cancers in females (Cotran *et al.*, 1989), has been also reported in hamsters (Rustia, 1974; Rustia & Shubik, 1976, 1979); however, none were found in the Stanford colony (Kirkman & Kempson, 1982). Hamster endometrial adenocarcinomas vary in differentiation as the human counterparts do. Several carcinogens have been shown to induce endometrial neoplasms.

Spontaneous and induced smooth-muscle tumours, i.e., leiomyoma and leiomyosarcoma, are histologically similar to those of man and other animal species.

ACKNOWLEDGEMENTS

Acknowledgements are extended to Academic Press for permission to reproduce Figure 1 and to the *Journal of the National Cancer Institute* for permission to reproduce Figures 17, 25, 33 and 34. Figures 2–16, 18–24, 26–32 and Tables 1 and 2 are reproduced from the first edition of this volume (Kirkman & Kempson, 1982).

REFERENCES

Algard, F.T. (1965) Characteristics of an androgen/estrogen induced, dependent leiomyosarcoma of the ductus deferens of the Syrian hamster. II. In vitro. *Cancer Res.*, 25, 147–151

Althoff, J. (1974) Simultaneous tumors in the respiratory system and urinary bladder of Syrian golden hamsters. *Z. Krebsforsch.*, 82, 153–158

Althoff, J. & Grandjean, C. (1979) In vivo studies in Syrian golden hamsters: a transplacental bioassay of ten nitrosamines. *Natl. Cancer Inst. Monogr.*, 51, 251–255

Althoff, J. & Lijinsky, W. (1977) Urinary bladder neoplasms in Syrian hamsters after administration of N-nitroso-N-methyl-N-dodecylamine. *Z. Krebsforsch.*, 90, 227–231

Althoff, J., Kinzel, V., Mohr, U. & Wieser, O. (1969) Uber ein spontanes, transplantables Cystadenocarcinom des Syrischen Goldhamsters (*Mesocricetus auratus*). *Exp. Pathol.*, 3, 247–254

Althoff, J., Krueger, F.W. & Mohr, U. (1973) Carcinogenic effect of dipropylnitrosamine and compounds related by β-oxidation. *J. Natl Cancer Inst.*, 51, 287–288

Althoff, J., Wilson, R., Cardesa, A. & Pour, P. (1974) Comparative studies of neoplastic response to a single dose of nitroso compounds. III. The effect of N-nitrosopiperidine and N-nitrosomorpholine in Syrian golden hamsters. *Z. Krebsforsch.*, 81, 251–259

Althoff, J., Pour, P., Grandjean, C. & Eagen, M. (1976) Transplacental effects of nitrosamines in Syrian hamsters. I. Dibutylnitrosamine and nitrosohexamethyleneimine. *Z. Krebsforsch.*, 86, 69–75

Althoff, J., Grandjean, C., Gold, B. & Runge, R. (1977a) Carcinogenicity of 1-oxopropylpropylnitrosamine (N-nitroso-N-propylpropionamide) in Syrian hamsters. *Z. Krebsforsch.*, 90, 221–225

Althoff, J., Grandjean, C., Marsh, S., Pour, P. & Takahashi, M. (1977b) Transplacental effects of nitrosamines in Syrian hamsters. II. Nitrosopiperidine. *Z. Krebsforsch.*, 90, 71–77

Althoff, J., Grandjean, C., Russell, L. & Pour, P. (1977c) Vinylethylnitrosamine: a potent respiratory carcinogen in Syrian hamsters. *J. Natl Cancer Inst.*, 58, 439–442

Althoff, J., Pour, P., Grandjean, C. & Marsh, S. (1977d) Transplacental effects of nitrosamines in Syrian hamsters. III. Dimethyl and dipropylnitrosamine. *Z. Krebsforsch.*, 90, 79–86

Althoff, J., Grandjean, C. & Gold, B. (1978) Carcinogenic effect of subcutaneously administered N-nitroso-2,6-dimethylmorpholine in Syrian golden hamsters. *J. Natl Cancer Inst.*, 60, 197–199

Altman, P.L. & Katz, D.D. (1979) *Inbred and Genetically Defined Strains of Laboratory Animals. Part 2. Hamster, Guinea Pig, Rabbit and Chicken* (Handbook III), Bethesda, MD, Federation of American Societies for Experimental Biology

Bing, T.S. & Wynder, E.L. (1972) Induction of urinary bladder tumors in hamsters with 3,2'-dimethyl-4-amino-diphenyl. *Proc. Am. Ass. Cancer Res.*, 13, 6

Bivin, W.S., Olsen, G.A. & Murray, K.A. (1987) Morphophysiology. In: Van Hoosier, G.L., Jr & McPherson, C.W., eds, *Laboratory Hamsters*, New York, Academic Press, pp. 9–41

Brownstein, D.C. & Brook, A.L. (1980) Spontaneous endometrial neoplasms in aging Chinese hamsters. *J. Natl Cancer Inst.*, 64, 1209–1214

Cabral, J.R.P., Hall, R.K., Bronczyk, S.A. & Shubik, P. (1979) A carcinogenicity study of the pesticide dieldrin in hamsters. *Cancer Lett.*, 6, 241–246

Chesterman, F.C. (1972) Background pathology in a colony of golden hamsters. *Prog. Exp. Tumor Res.*, 16, 50–68

Christov, K. & Raichev, R. (1973) Proliferative and neoplastic changes in the ovaries of hamsters treated with 131-iodine and methylthiouracil. *Neoplasma*, 20, 511–516

Chu, E.W. & Malmgren, R.A. (1965) An inhibitory effect of vitamin A on the induction of tumors of forestomach and cervix in the Syrian hamster by carcinogenic polycyclic hydrocarbons. *Cancer Res.*, 25, 884–895

Chu, E.W., Herrold, K.M. & Wood, T.A., Jr (1962) Cytopathological changes of the uterine cervix of Syrian hamsters after painting with DMBA, benzo(a)pyrene, and tobacco tar. *Acta Cytol. (Balt.)*, 6, 376–384

Cotchin, E. (1964) Spontaneous uterine cancer in animals. *Br. J. Cancer*, 18, 209–227

Cotchin, E. & Marchant, J. (1977) *Animal Tumors of the Female Reproductive Tract*, New York, Springer-Verlag, pp. i–ix, 1–70

Cotran, R.S., Kumar, V. & Robbins, S.L. (1989) *Pathologic Basis of Disease*, 4th edition, Philadelphia, W.B. Saunders, p. 1141

Dontenwill, W., Mohr, U. & Bernhard, J. (1963) Die unterschiedliche Wirkung des Follikelhormons auf die Portio- und Vaginal-Schleimhaut bei parenteraler und lokaler Applikation. *Z. Krebsforsch.*, 65, 303–308

Dontenwill, W., Chevalier, H.-J., Harke, H.P., Lafrenz, U., Reckzeh, G. & Schneider, B. (1973a) Spontantumoren des syrischen Goldhamsters. *Z. Krebsforsch.*, 80, 127–158

Dontenwill, W., Chevalier, H.-J., Harke, H.P., Lafrenz, U., Reckzeh, G. & Schneider, B. (1973b) Investigations on the effects of chronic cigarette-smoke inhalation in Syrian golden hamsters. *J. Natl Cancer Inst.*, 51, 1781–1832

Eddy, H.A. (1979) Biological properties and radiation responses of the hamster uterine cervical squamous cell carcinoma. *Radiat. Res.*, 77, 561–576

Fabry, A. (1985) The incidence of neoplasms in Syrian hamsters with particular emphasis on intestinal neoplasia. *Arch. Toxicol.* [suppl.], 8, 124–127

Haemmerli, G., Schmid, W. & Lindemann, J. (1968) Cytogenetic and antigenetic properties of GW-127, a heterologously transplantable tumor. *Eur. J. Cancer*, 4, 279–285

Handler, A.H. (1951) Transplantation of heterospecific tumour tissue into the cheek pouch of the golden hamster. Doctoral dissertation, Boston University

Handler, A.H. (1965) Spontaneous lesions of the hamster. In: Ribelin, W.E. & McCoy, J.R., eds, *The Pathology of Laboratory Animals*, Springfield, IL, Thomas, pp. 210–240

Handler, A.H. (1976) Diseases of laboratory animals – neoplastic, transplantable tumors. In: Melby, E.C., Jr & Altman, N.H., eds, *CRC Handbook of Laboratory Animal Science*, Cleveland, OH, CRC Press, Vol. III, pp. 357–381

Hass, H., Mohr, U. & Krüger, F.W. (1973) Comparative studies with different doses of N-nitrosomorpholine, N-nitroso-piperidine, N-nitrosomethylurea, and dimethylnitrosamine in Syrian golden hamsters. *J. Natl Cancer Inst.*, 51, 1295–1301

Herrold, K.M. (1966) Carcinogenic effect of N-methyl-N-nitrosourea administered subcutaneously to Syrian hamsters. *J. Pathol. Bact.*, 92, 35–41

Hilfrich, J., Hecht, S.S. & Hoffmann, D. (1977) A study of tobacco carcinogenesis. XV. Effects of N'-nitrosonornicotine and N'-nitrosoanabasine in Syrian golden hamsters. *Cancer Lett.*, 2, 169–176

Hiraki, S. (1971) Carcingenic effect of N,N'-dimethylnitrosourea on Syrian hamsters. *Gann*, 62, 321–323

Homburger, F. (1968) The Syrian golden hamster in chemical carcinogenesis research. *Prog. Exp. Tumor Res.*, 10, 163–237

Homburger, F. (1969) Chemical carcinogenesis in the Syrian golden hamster: A review. *Cancer*, 23, 313–338

Homburger, F. (1972) Chemical carcinogenesis in Syrian hamster. *Prog. Exp. Tumor Res.*, 16, 152–175

Homburger, F. (1979) Chemical carcinogenesis in Syrian hamsters: A review (through 1976). *Prog. Exp. Tumor Res.*, 23, 100–179

Homburger, F., Hsueh, S.S., Kerr, C.S. & Russfield, A.B. (1972) Inherited susceptibility of inbred strains of Syrian hamsters to induction of subcutaneous sarcomas and mammary and gastro-intestinal carcinomas by subcutaneous and gastric administration of polynuclear hydrocarbons. *Cancer Res.* 32, 360–366

Kharkovskaya, N.A. (1979) Blastomogenic activity of 2-aminoacetophenone in Syrian hamsters [in Russian]. *Vopr. Onkol.*, 25, 81–84

Khrustalev, S.A. (1978) Comparative study of sensitivity of the animals of various species to the blastomogenic action of some metabolites [in Russian]. *Patol. Fiziol. Eksp. Ter.*, 4, 61–63

Kirkman, H. (1957) Steroid tumorigenesis. *Cancer*, 10, 757–764

Kirkman, H. (1959) Estrogen-induced tumors of the kidney. IV. Incidence in female Syrian hamsters. *Natl Cancer Inst. Monogr.*, 1, 59–91

Kirkman, H. (1972) Hormone-related tumors in Syrian hamsters. *Prog. Exp. Tumor Res.*, 16, 201–240

Kirkman, H. & Algard, F.T. (1965) Characteristics of an androgen/estrogen-induced, dependent leiomyosarcoma of the ductus deferens of the Syrian hamster. I. In vivo. *Cancer Res.*, 25, 141–146

Kirkman, H. & Algard, F.T. (1968) Spontaneous and nonviral-induced neoplasms. In: Hoffman, R.A., Robinson, P.E. & Magalhaes, H., eds, *The Golden Hamster, its Biology and Use in Medical Research*, Ames, Iowa State University Press, pp. 227–240

Kirkman, H. & Algard, F.T. (1970a) Autonomous variants of an androgen/estrogen-induced and dependent ductus deferens leiomyosarcoma of the Syrian hamster. *Cancer Res.*, 30, 35–40

Kirkman, H. & Algard, F.T. (1970b) Characteristics of an androgen/estrogen-induced uterine smooth muscle cell tumor of the Syrian hamster. *Cancer Res.*, 30, 794–800

Kirkman, H. & Bacon, R.L. (1958) Transplanted, estrogen-androgen induced tumors of the uterus and vas deferens in Syrian hamsters. *Proc. Am. Ass. Cancer Res.*, 2, 315

Kirkman, H. & Chesterman, F.C. (1972) Additional data on transplanted tumours of the golden hamster. *Prog. Exp. Tumor Res.*, 16, 580–621

Kirkman, H. & Kempson, R.L. (1982) Tumours of the female genitalia. In: Turusov, V.S., ed., *Pathology of Tumours in Laboratory Animals*, Vol. III, *Tumours of the Hamster*, (IARC Scientific Publications No. 34), Lyon, IARC, pp. 221–253

Kirkman, H. & Yau, P.K.S. (1969) Transplantable, Syrian hamster tumours, stored in liquid nitrogen. *Proc. Am. Ass. Cancer Res.*, 10, 46

Kirkman, H. & Yau, P.K.S. (1972) Longevity of male and female, intact and gonadectomized, untreated and hormone-treated, neoplastic and non-neoplastic Syrian hamsters. *Am. J. Anat.*, 135, 205–220

Kiseleva, N.S., Milievskaja, I.L. & Chaklin, A.V. (1977) Development of tumours in Syrian hamster during prolonged experimental exposure to nas. *Bull. World Health Org.*, 54, 597–605

Leavitt, W.W., Evans, R.W. & Hendry, W.J. (1981) Etiology of DES-induced uterine tumors in the Syrian hamster. *Adv. Exp. Med. Biol.*, 138, 63–86

Leiter, J., Abbott, B.J. & Schapartz, S.A. (1965) Screening data from the Cancer Chemotherapy National Service Center Screening Laboratories. XXII. *Cancer Res.*, 25 (Part 2), 1–195

Lindt, V.S. (1958) Uber krankheiten des syrischen Goldhamsters (Mesocricetus auratus). *Schweiz. Arch. Tierheilk.*, 100, 86–97

Milievskaya, I.L. & Kiseleva, N.S. (1977) Comparative study of the carcinogenic activities of nas and some chemical carcinogens when introduced into the buccal pouch of the Syrian hamster. *Bull. World Health Org.*, 54, 607–614

Mohr, U., Emura, M., Aufderheide, M.A., Riebe, M. & Ernst, H. (1987) Transplacental carcinogenesis, mouse, rat, hamster. In: Jones, T.C. & Hunt, R.D., eds, *Genital System*, Berlin, Springer-Verlag, pp. 148–157

Nicolov, I.G. & Chernozemsky, I.N. (1979) Tumors and hyperplastic lesions in Syrian hamsters following transplacental and neonatal treatment with cigarette smoke condensate. *J. Cancer Res. Clin. Oncol.*, 94, 249–256

Noble, R.L. (1964) Tumors and hormones. In: Pincus, G., Thimann, K.V. & Astwood, E.B., eds, *The Hormones*, New York, Academic Press, Vol. V, pp. 559–695

Poulsen, H.E., Taylor, C.W. & Sobin, L.H. (1975) *Histological Typing of Female Genital Tract Tumours* (International Histological Classification of Tumours, No. 13), Geneva, WHO

Pour, P., Krüger, F.W., Cardesa, A., Althoff, J. & Mohr, U. (1973) Carcinogenic effect of di-*N*-propylnitrosamine in Syrian golden hamsters. *J. Natl Cancer Inst.*, 51, 1019–1027

Pour, P., Krüger, F.W., Althoff, J., Cardesa, A. & Mohr, U. (1975) Effect of beta-oxidized nitrosamines on Syrian golden hamsters. III. 2,2-dihydroxy-di-n-propylnitrosamine. *J. Natl Cancer Inst.*, 54, 141–145

Pour, P., Althoff, J., Gingell, R., Kupper, R., Krüger, F.W. & Mohr, U. (1976a) A further pancreatic carcinogen in Syrian golden hamsters: N-nitroso-bis(2-acetooxypropyl)-amine. *Cancer Lett.*, 1, 197–202

Pour, P., Kmoch, N., Greiser, E., Mohr, U., Althoff, J. & Cardesa, A. (1976b) Spontaneous tumors and common diseases in two colonies of Syrian hamsters. I. Incidence and sites. *J. Natl Cancer Inst.*, 56, 931–935

Pour, P.M., Mohr, U., Althoff, J., Cardesa, A. & Kmoch, N. (1976c) Spontaneous tumors and common diseases in two colonies of Syrian hamsters. III. Urogenital system and endocrine glands. *J. Natl Cancer Inst.*, 56, 949–961

Pour, P.M., Althoff, J. & Nagel, D. (1977) Induction of epithelial neoplasms by local administration of N-nitrosobis (2-hydroxy-propyl)amine and N-nitrosobis (2-acetoxy-propyl) amine. *Cancer Lett.*, 3, 109–113

Pour, P.M., Salmasi, S.Z. & Runge, R.G. (1978) Selective induction of pancreatic ductular tumors by single doses of N-nitrosobis(2-oxopropyl)amine in Syrian golden hamsters. *Cancer Lett.*, 4, 317–323

Pour, P., Wallcave, L., Gingell, R., Nagel, D., Lawson, T., Salmasi, S. & Tines, S. (1979) Carcinogenic effect of N-nitroso-(2-hy-droxypropyl)(2-oxopropyl)amine, a postulated proximate pancreatic carcinogen in Syrian hamsters. *Cancer Res.*, 39, 3828–3833

Rakoff, A.E., Gross, M.L. & Wellenbach, B.L. (1951) Induction of cystic endometrial hyperplasia in the hamster with estradiol; prevention and treatment with progesterone. *J. Clin. Endocrinol.*, 11, 785–786

Rivière, M.R., Chouroulinkov, I. & Guérin, M. (1961) Actions hormonales expérimentales de longue durée chez le hamster du point de vue de leur effet cancérigène. I. Etude de la testostérone associée à un oestrogène. *Bull. Ass. franç. Cancer*, 48, 499–524

Rivière, M.R., Chouroulinkov, I. & Guérin, M. (1962a) Leiomyosarcomes de l'épididyme développés chez des hamsters dorés après un traitement simultané par la testostérone et un oestrogène. *C.R. Séanc. Soc. Biol. (Paris)*, 156, 1033–1035

Robinson, F.R. (1976) Hamsters. In: Melby, E.C., Jr & Altman, N.H., eds, *Handbook of Laboratory Animal Science*, Cleveland, OH, CRC Press, Vol. III, pp. 253–270

Russfield, A.B. (1966) *Tumors of Endocrine Glands and Secondary Sex Organs* (Public Health Service Publication No. 1332), Washington, DC, US Government Printing Office, pp. 1–148

Rustia, M. (1974) Multiple carcinogenic effects of the ethylnitrosourea precursors ethyl-urea and sodium nitrite in hamsters. *Cancer Res.*, 34, 3232-3244

Rustia, M. (1975) Inhibitory effect of sodium ascorbate on ethylurea and sodium nitrite carcinogenesis and negative findings in progeny after intestinal inoculation of precursors into pregnant hamsters. *J. Natl Cancer Inst.*, 55, 1389–1394

Rustia, M. (1976) The effect of gonadal ablation on transplacentally induced neurogenic tumors in hamsters. *Cancer Res.*, 36, 240–245

Rustia, M. (1979) Role of hormone imbalance in transplacental carcinogenesis induced in Syrian golden hamsters by sex hormones. *Natl Cancer Inst. Monogr.*, 51, 77–87

Rustia, M. & Schenken, J. (1976) Transplacental effects of ethylnitrosourea precursors ethyl-urea and sodium nitrite in hamsters. *Z. Krebsforsch.*, 85, 201–217

Rustia, M. & Shubik, P. (1973) Life-span carcinogenicity tests with 4-amino-N10-methylpteroylglutamic acid (methotrexate) in Swiss mice and Syrian golden hamsters. *Toxicol. Appl. Pharmacol.*, 26, 329–338

Rustia, M. & Shubik, P. (1976) Transplacental effects of diethylstilbestrol on the genital tract of hamster offspring. *Cancer Lett.*, 1, 139–146

Rustia, M. & Shubik, P. (1978) Thyroid tumours in rats and hepatomas in mice after griseofulvin treatment. *Br. J. Cancer*, 38, 237–249

Rustia, M. & Shubik, P. (1979) Effects of transplacental exposure to diethylstil-bestrol in carcinogenic susceptibility during postnatal life in hamster progeny. *Cancer Res.*, 39, 4636–4644

Saffiotti, U., Montesano, R., Sellakumar, A.R., Cefis, F. & Kaufman, D.G. (1972) Respiratory tract carcinogenesis in hamsters induced by different numbers of administrations of benzo[a]pyrene and ferric oxide. *Cancer Res.*, 32, 1073–1081

Schmidt, R.E., Eason, R.L., Hubbard, G.B., Young, J.T. & Eisenbrandt, D.L. (1983) *Pathology of Aging Syrian Hamsters*, Boca Raton, FL, CRC Press, pp. 219–225

Serov, S.F., Scully, R.E. & Sobin, L.H. (1973) *Histological Typing of Ovarian Tumours* (International Histological Classification of Tumours, No. 9), Geneva, World Health Organization

Shank, R.C. & Newberne, P.M. (1976) Dose-response study of the carcinogenicity of dietary sodium nitrite and morpholine in rats and hamsters. *Food Cosmet. Toxicol.*, 14, 1–8

Shimizu, H. & Toth, B. (1974) Effect of lifetime administration of 2-hydroxyethylhydrazine on tumorigenesis in hamsters and mice. *J. Natl Cancer Inst.*, 52, 903–906

Shubik, P. (1972) The use of the Syrian hamster in chronic toxicity testing. *Prog. Exp. Tumor Res.*, 16, 176–184

Shubik, P., Rustia, M. & Plesnicar, S. (1980) Modified carcinogenesis by contraceptive Enovid in hamster. *Proc. Am. Ass. Cancer Res.*, 21, 124

Squire, R.A., Goodman, D.G., Valerio, M.G., Fredrickson, T.N., Strandberg, J.D., Levitt, M.H., Lingenman, C.H., Harschbarger, J.C. & Dawe, C.J. (1978) Tumors. In: Benirschke, K., Garner, K.M. & Jones, T.C., ed., *Pathology of Laboratory Animals*, Berlin, Heidelberg, New York, Springer-Verlag, Vol. II, pp. 1051–1283

Stenback, F., Sellakumar, A. & Shubik, P. (1975) Magnesium oxide as carrier dust in benzo(a)pyrene-induced lung carcinogenesis in Syrian hamsters. *J. Natl Cancer Inst.*, 54, 861–867

Strandberg, J.D. (1987) Neoplastic diseases. In: Van Hoosier, Jr, G.L. & McPherson, C.W., eds, *Laboratory Hamsters*, Berlin, Heidelberg, New York, Academic Press, pp. 9–41, 157–168

Tomatis, L. & Cefis, F. (1967) The effects of multiple and single administration of dimethylnitrosamine to hamsters. *Tumori*, 53, 447–452

Toolan, H.W. (1967) Lack of oncogenic effect of the H-viruses for hamsters. *Nature*, 214, 1038

Toth, B. (1967) Studies in the incidence, morphology, transplantation, and cell-free filtration of malignant lymphomas in the Syrian golden hamster. *Cancer Res.*, 27, 1430–1442

Toth, B. (1969) The induction of malignant lymphomas and other tumors by 7,12-dimethylbenz[a]anthracene in the Syrian golden hamster. *Cancer Res.*, 29, 1476–1484

Toth, B. (1970) Tumor induction with single urethane injection in newborn and adult Syrian golden hamsters. A study of age influence. I. *Int. J. Cancer*, 6, 63–68

Toth, B. (1971) Tumor induction by repeated injections of urethane in newborn and adult hamsters: Age influences. II. *J. Natl Cancer Inst.*, 46, 81–93

Toth, B. (1972) Tumorigenesis studies with 1,2-dimethylhydrazine dihydrochloride, hydrazine sulfate, and isonicotinic acid in golden hamsters. *Cancer Res.*, 32, 804–807

Toth, B. & Boreisha, I. (1969) Tumorigenesis with isonicotinic acid hydrazide and urethane in the Syrian golden hamster. *Eur. J. Cancer*, 5, 165–172

Toth, B. & Shimizu, H. (1973) Methylhydrazine tumorigenesis in Syrian golden hamsters and the morphology of malignant histiocytomas. *Cancer Res.*, 33, 2744–2753

Toth, B. & Shubik, P. (1969) Lack of carcinogenic effects of isonicotinic acid hydrazide in the Syrian golden hamster. *Tumori*, 55, 127–135

Toth, B., Tomatis, L. & Shubik, P. (1961) Multipotential carcinogenesis with urethane in the Syrian golden hamster. *Cancer Res.*, 21, 1537–1541

Trentin, J.J. (1987) Experimental biology: use in oncological research. In: Van Hoosier, Jr, G.L. & McPherson, C.W., eds, *Laboratory Hamsters*, New York, Academic Press, pp. 201–214

Turusov, V.S., ed. (1982) *Pathology of Tumours in Laboratory Animals*. Vol. III, *Tumours of the Hamster* (IARC Scientific Publications No. 34), Lyon, IARC

Van Hoosier, G.L., Jr (1971) Comparative viral oncology-rodents and man. In: *Animal Models for Biomedical Research* IV, Washington, DC, National Academy of Sciences, pp. 1–10

Van Hoosier, G.L., Jr & Trentin, J.J. (1979) Naturally occurring tumors of the Syrian hamster. *Prog. Exp. Tumor Res.*, 23, 1–12

Van Hoosier, G.L., Jr, Spjut, H.J. & Trentin, J.J. (1971) Spontaneous tumors of the Syrian hamster: Observations in a closed breeding colony and a review of the literature. In: *Defining the Laboratory Animal*. Washington, DC, National Academy of Sciences, pp. 450–473

Vasilieva, N.N. & Milevskaja, I.L. (1977) *N*-Nitroso-*N*-methylurea-induced neurogenic tumors of the stomach in Syrian hamsters [in Russian]. *Arh. Pat.*, 39, 66–71

Ward, B.C. & Moore, W., Jr (1969) Spontaneous lesions in a colony of Chinese hamsters, Cricetulus griseus. *Lab. Anim. Care*, 19, 516–521

Yabe, Y., Kataoka, N. & Koyama, H. (1972) Spontaneous tumors in hamsters; incidence, morphology, transplantation and virus studies. *Gann*, 63, 329–336

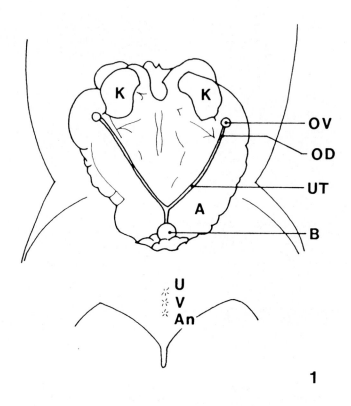

Figure 1. Diagrammatic representation of the female urogenital tract illustrating the relative positions of the kidney (K), bladder (B), ovary (OV), oviduct (OD), uterine horn (UT), adipose tissue (A), urethral opening (U), vaginal opening (V), and anus (An) (from Bivin *et al.*, 1987)

Figure 2. Ovarian mucinous cystadenoma. H & E; × 500 (from Kirkman, 1972)

Figure 3. Ovarian mucinous cystadenoma. H & E; × 50 (from Kirkman, 1972)

Figure 4. As for Figure 3. × 500 (from Kirkman, 1972)

Figure 5. Ovarian tubular clear cell (mesonephric) adenoma. Mallory-azan stain; × 200

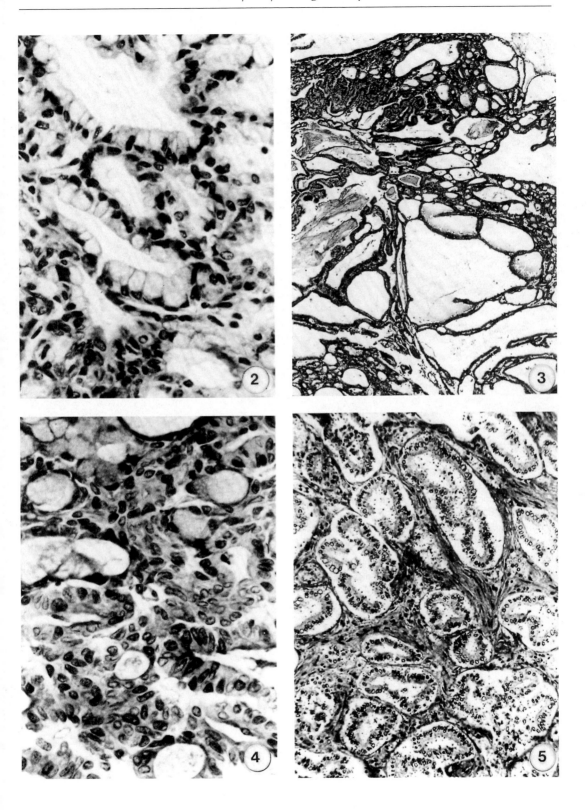

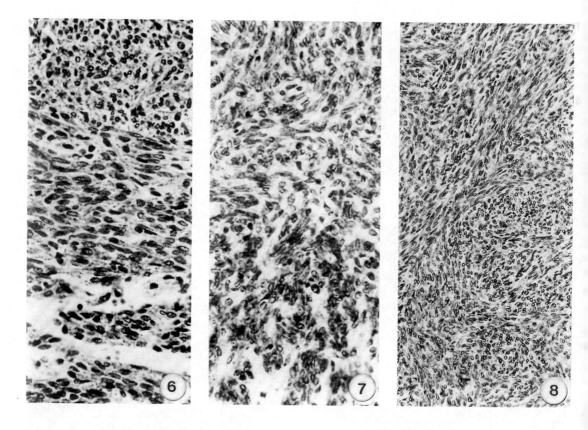

Figure 6. Ovarian fibrosarcoma. H & E; × 375

Figure 7. As for Figure 6

Figure 8. Ovarian fibrosarcoma. H & E; × 200

Figure 9. Pulmonary metastases from the 8th serial subpannicular passage of the ovarian fibrosarcoma shown in Figure 8. H & E; × 375

Figure 10. Ovarian thecoma–fibrosarcoma. Mallory-azan stain; × 200

Figure 11. The first serial subpannicular transplant of the tumour in Figure 10. H & E; × 375

Figure 12. Arrhenoblastoma. H & E; × 100 (from Kirkman, 1972)

Figure 13. Unilateral ovarian stromal luteinization, or possible stromal luteoma. H & E; × 50 (from Kirkman, 1972)

Figure 14. As for Figure 13. × 500 (from Kirkman, 1972)

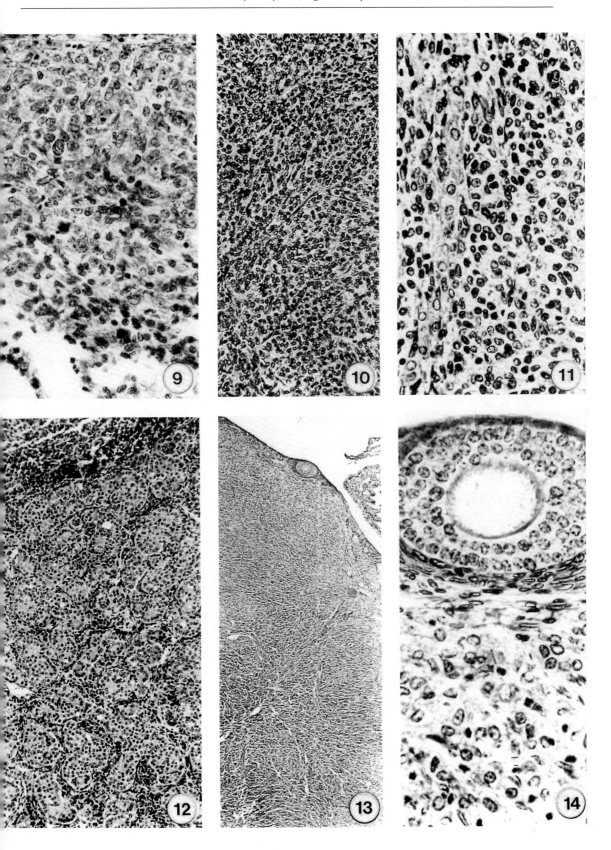

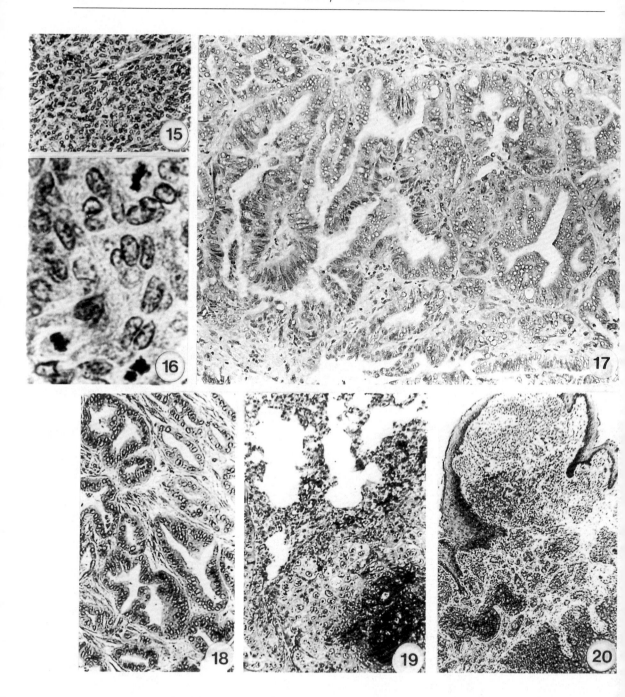

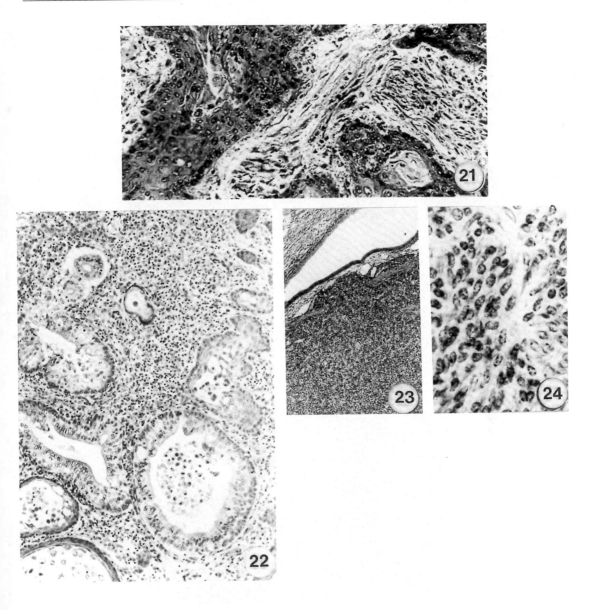

Figure 15. Benign theca-granulosa-cell tumour. H & E; × 200

Figure 16. Malignant theca-granulosa-cell tumour. H & E; × 460

Figure 17. Cervical adenocarcinoma with papillary formation and pleomorphic cells. H & E; × 100 (from Pour *et al.*, 1976c)

Figure 18. The 21st serial subpannicular passage of a uterine cervical adenocarcinoma. H & E; × 150

Figure 19. Pulmonary metastasis from the 23rd serial passage of the transplant shown in Figure 18. Mallory-azan stain; × 150

Figure 20. Primary uterine cervical adenocarcinoma. H & E; × 50

Figure 21. Primary uterine horn adenocarcinoma with squamous metaplasia. H & E; × 200

Figure 22. Endometrial squamous metaplasia. H & E; × 100 (from Kirkman, 1972)

Figure 23. Benign stromal nodule of the uterine horn. H & E; × 50 (from Kirkman, 1972)

Figure 24. As for Figure 23. × 500 (from Kirkman, 1972)

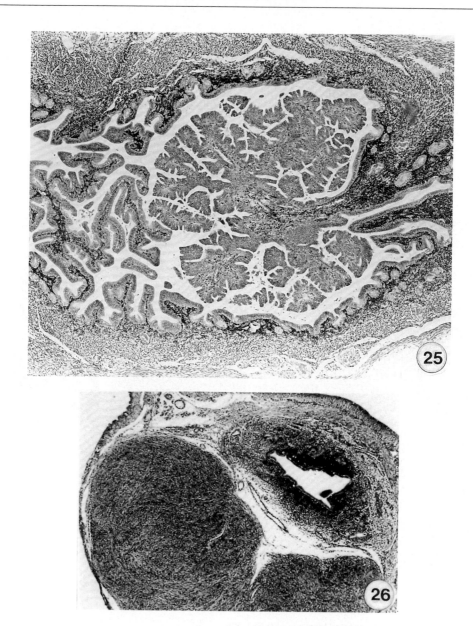

Figure 25. Papillary endometrial polyp with hyperplasia of adjacent endometrium. H & E; × 40 (from Pour *et al.*, 1976c)

Figure 26. Spontaneous leiomyoma of the uterine horn. Mallory-azan stain; × 50

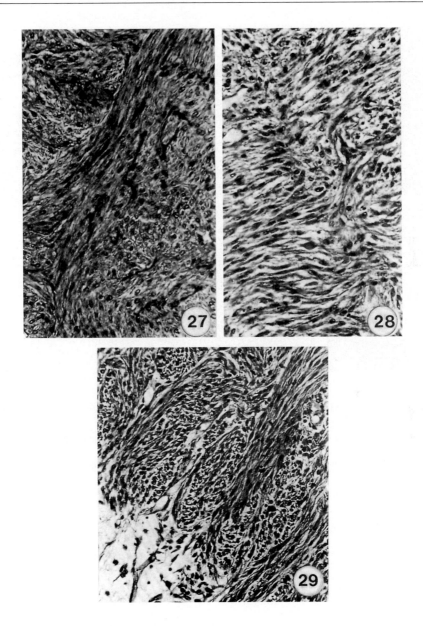

Figure 27. Spontaneous leiomyoma of the uterine cervix. H & E; × 200

Figure 28. Uterine horn leiomyosarcoma. H & E; × 200

Figure 29. Interlacing fasciculi at the growing margin of the 10th serial subpannicular passage of an autonomous variant of an originally DES/Tpr-induced-and-dependent uterine horn leiomyosarcoma. H & E; × 140 (from Kirkman & Algard, 1970b)

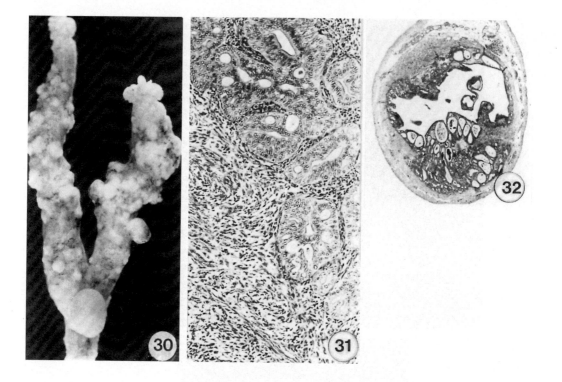

Figure 30. Multiple, DES/Tpr-induced-and-dependent bilateral uterine horn leiomyosarcoma. × 2 (from Kirkman, 1957)

Figure 31. Primary DES-induced-and-dependent, malignant mixed Müllerian tumour (carcinosarcoma). H & E; × 100 (from Kirkman, 1972)

Figure 32. Uterine horn showing typical DES-induced cystic glandular hyperplasia of the endometrium. H & E; × 12

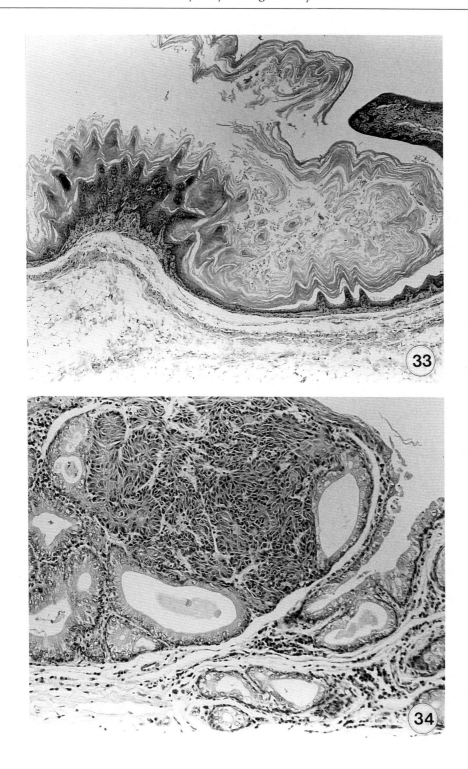

Figure 33. Squamous cell papilloma of vagina. H & E; × 40 (from Pour *et al.*, 1976c)

Figure 34. Inverted vaginal papilloma with simultaneous glandular proliferation. H & E; × 100 (from Pour *et al.*, 1976c)

Tumours of the endocrine glands

R.E. SCHMIDT AND G.B. HUBBARD

INTRODUCTION

This chapter is principally concerned with primary tumours of the endocrine glands of various strains of Syrian hamsters. Most of the literature documenting endocrine tumours concerns Syrian hamsters, although endocrine neoplasms in Chinese, European and Dzungarian hamsters have also been described (Ladiges, 1987; Mohr & Ernst, 1987; Cantrell & Padovan, 1987). Adenomas and adenocarcinomas are described in the pituitary, thyroid, parathyroid, adrenal glands and the islets of Langerhans.

PITUITARY GLAND

Tumours of the pituitary gland occur relatively infrequently, based on reviews and reports of large numbers of hamster necropsies (Fortner, 1957; Kirkman & Algard, 1968; Kirkman, 1972; Pour *et al.*, 1976b; Schmidt *et al.*, 1983; Strandberg, 1987). Reported tumours occur in the pars distalis and pars intermedia, with both adenomas and carcinomas described.

NORMAL STRUCTURE

The hamster pituitary is divided into pars distalis, intermedia, nervosa and tuberalis (Reiter & Hoffman, 1968). Cells of the pars distalis are arrayed in anastomotic cords and are classified as acidophils, basophils or chromophobes, depending on their stain affinity. Chromophobes are concentrated at the periphery as are acidophils, although the latter are also scattered throughout parenchyma of the pars distalis. Basophils form the largest cell of the pars distalis.

The pars intermedia and pars nervosa are closely associated. The pars nervosa is composed of well vascularized neural tissue including fibres of the hypothalamo-hypophyseal tract. The pars tuberalis forms the cover of the stalk of the pituitary.

MORPHOLOGY AND BIOLOGY OF TUMOURS

Pars intermedia tumours are usually histologically benign. They are composed of large cuboidal or columnar cells forming sheet-like structures often oriented around blood vessels. Reported tumours of the pars distalis include adenomas of eosinophilic, basophilic and chromophobic types, as well as adenocarcinomas. Tumours of mixed cell types are occasionally seen. Benign tumours are composed of enlarged polygonal cells forming nests, cords and glandular structures (Figures 1 and 2). Sinusoid dilation is variable. Carcinomas are composed of more pleomorphic, anaplastic cells with enlarged nuclei and less cytoplasmic granule differentiation. Nuclei may be multiple in cells. The cells usually form whorls and cords or alveolar patterns. These tumours invade surrounding structures (Figure 3).

INDUCTION OF TUMOURS

Estrogens have been used by several investigators to induce pituitary tumours in Syrian hamsters (Vasquez-Lopez, 1944; Koneff *et al.*, 1946; Horning & Whittick, 1954; Hamilton, 1975). Tumours of the pars intermedia and chromophobe adenomas of the distalis both have been induced by stilbestrol. Carcinomas of the pituitary were reported following radio-thyroidectomy (Russfield *et al.*, 1963). These tumours were easily transplanted and metastasized.

COMPARATIVE ASPECTS

Estrogen-induced pituitary tumours in hamsters are usually chromophobic, while in rats they are acidophilic (Lacour, 1950; Clifton & Meyer, 1956). In one study, steroid-induced tumours in rats and mice were found to contain prolactin, growth-hormone- and adenocorticotrophic-hormone-producing cells. In hamsters there were hyperplasia of prolactin-secreting cells and hyperplasia and neoplasia of pars intermedia cells producing melanocyte-stimulating hormone. In studies with native carrageenan, tumours of the pituitary were induced in rats, but not in hamsters (Rustia *et al.*, 1980).

THYROID GLAND

Several studies on hamster tumours have reported low incidences of thyroid neoplasia (Kirkman & Algard, 1968; Pour *et al.*, 1976b; Schmidt *et al.*, 1983). Tumours reported include follicular adenomas and carcinomas, as well as medullary (C-cell) tumours. The latter can be differentiated by immunohistochemistry that identifies the calcitonin content of the cells (DeLellies *et al.*, 1987). Some inbred strains of Syrian hamster have a higher incidence of thyroid tumours (Pour *et al.*, 1979).

NORMAL STRUCTURE

Follicular epithelial cells vary from cuboidal to columnar. Nuclei are basally located. Follicles in the central portion of the gland tend to be smaller than those in the periphery. Colloid is homogeneous and absorption vacuoles are seen adjacent to the apical portions of epithelial cells. Parafollicular cells, which secrete calcitonin, and fat cells are present between follicles. The interfollicular connective tissue is vascular (Reiter & Hoffman, 1968).

MORPHOLOGY AND BIOLOGY OF TUMOURS

Follicular adenomas are usually well circumscribed and composed of follicles lined by fairly well differentiated cuboidal epithelial cells. Some papillary variations are seen and adenomas may also contain solid nests. Basement membranes are intact and the cells are well oriented on the basement membranes (Figures 4–6). Carcinomas are composed of more anaplastic cells with loss of polarity and attachment to basement membrane (Figure 7). Invasion of stroma and capsule is present. Medullary tumours are composed of large cells with granular cytoplasms and vesicular nuclei. These cells form trabecular structures and solid sheets with isolation and destruction of follicles (Figure 8). Minimal stroma is present. Both adenomas and carcinomas are present with anaplasia and invasion of surrounding tissue as the primary criteria for malignancy. The more anaplastic cells often have spindle granular patterns (DeLellies *et al.*, 1987). Specific differentiation of solid medullary tumours may depend on histochemical demonstration of calcitonin (DeLellies *et al.*, 1987).

INDUCTION OF TUMOURS

Goitrogenic agents, iodine-deficient diets, radioactive iodine and carcinogenic agents have all produced thyroid tumours in hamsters (Fortner *et al.*, 1958, 1960; Christov & Raichev, 1972; Dontenwill & Mohr, 1962). When pregnant female hamsters were treated with *N*-nitroso-bis-(2-oxypropyl)amine (BOP), thyroid follicular adenomas were seen only in the F1 generation (Pour, 1986).

COMPARATIVE ASPECTS

Although C-cell hyperplasia has been observed in familial medullary carcinoma of rats and humans, none was seen in hamsters with proved medullary carcinoma (DeLellies *et al.*, 1987). Although adult rats treated with BOP developed follicular adenomas, only fetal (F1) hamsters from BOP-treated pregnant females developed similar tumours (Pour, 1986). In one study of experimentally induced follicular adenomas, no difference in morphology was detected between hamsters and rats (Christov, 1981).

PARATHYROID GLAND

The incidence of parathyroid tumours varies between several published studies (Van Hoosier & Trentin, 1979; Schmidt *et al.*, 1983; Pour, 1983). Pour (1983) indicated that there are strain variations in the incidence of parathyroid tumours. Most reported tumours are benign. Parathyroid nodules (including hyperplastic lesions) were the second most common proliferative lesion of endocrine glands other than the adrenal in one study (Schmidt *et al.*, 1983).

NORMAL STRUCTURE

Parenchymal cells have irregular borders and round to oval nuclei. Cytoplasm is darkly basophilic in principal cells. Large cells with clear cytoplasm are randomly distributed among the principal cells. Gland stroma is minimal and there is a thin connective tissue capsule (Reiter & Hoffman, 1968).

MORPHOLOGY AND BIOLOGY OF TUMOURS

Although usually unilateral, parathyroid tumours can be bilateral. Differentiating between hyperplasia and neoplasia can be difficult, with compression of adjacent tissue and capsule formation being the primary criteria for neoplasia (Figures 9 and 10). Cells making up adenomas are large and fairly uniform, with clear or granular cytoplasms and vesicular nuclei. Cell boundaries are often indistinct. Carcinomas are composed of more anaplastic cells, and invasion of adjacent tissue and occasional metastasis are seen (Figures 11 and 12).

INDUCTION OF TUMOURS

High-fat diets resulted in a higher incidence of parathyroid adenoma (Birt & Pour, 1985). Parathyroid adenomas were enhanced in both male and female hamsters injected with BOP and fed a low-protein diet after eight weeks of age (Pour & Birt, 1986).

COMPARATIVE ASPECTS

No specific information on this topic is present in the literature reviewed.

ADRENAL GLAND

Cortical and medullary tumours are both reported in the adrenal glands of hamsters. Tumours of the cortex comprise one of the most common types of spontaneous tumours in Syrian hamsters (Kirkman & Algard, 1968; Homburger & Russfield, 1970; Pour *et al.*, 1976b; Van Hoosier & Trentin, 1979; Schmidt *et al.*, 1983). The zona glomerulosa and zona fasciculata are both sites of tumour origin. Medullary tumours (phaeochromocytomas) have been reported less frequently.

NORMAL STRUCTURE

The hamster adrenal gland is histologically similar to that of other rodents (Reiter & Hoffman, 1968). The cortex is separated into the zona glomerulosa, fasciculata and reticularis. The zona fasciculata is the most prominent and is composed of columns of cells with round nuclei and abundant eosinophilic cytoplasm. The medulla consists of a central zone of dark cells arranged in cords and a peripheral area of clear cells in follicular structures. Sympathetic ganglion cells can be found in the medulla.

MORPHOLOGY AND BIOLOGY OF TUMOURS

Cortical tumours can be unilateral or bilateral (Figure 13). Histologically, the differentiation between hyperplasia and neoplasia may be arbitrary in some cases. Adenomas tend to be circumscribed and to compress adjacent cortex (Figure 14). Two morphological cell types are present in cortical tumours. Spindle-shaped cells have moderate amounts of cytoplasm and hyperchromatic nuclei, and more cuboidal cells have moderate to abundant cytoplasm and vesicular nuclei (Figure 15). Adenomas can be of a single cell type or a mixed cell type. Ultrastructurally, the spindle cells are anaplastic variants of the cuboidal cells with fewer mitochondria and secretory granules. Cortical carcinomas tend to be larger with variable amounts of cellular anaplasia. Occasional giant cells are seen. Metastasis of cortical carcinomas is rare (Anderson & Capen, 1978) (Figure 16).

Phaeochromocytomas are composed of large cuboidal or polygonal cells with abundant cytoplasm and vesicular nuclei. The cells are arranged in nests, cords or trabeculae with minimal amounts of stromal proliferation (Figure 17). The borders of the tumours are usually well defined. A ganglioneuroma is a tumour of ganglion cells of neuroectodermal origin. They are occasionally seen in hamster adrenal glands (Kirkman, 1972).

INDUCTION OF TUMOURS

Hyperplastic cortical nodules have been noted in gonadectomized hamsters (Agate, 1952). In another study, castrated males had a significantly higher incidence of cortical hyperplasia and adenoma formation than their controls (Fortner, 1961). Stilbestrol treatment also results in hyperplasia of the adrenal cortex (Horning & Whittick 1954; Franks & Chesterman, 1957).

Exposure to chemicals of several types including 3-methylcholanthrene, 4-dimethylaminoazobenzene, urethane and 3-indolylacrylic acid, has produced cortical neoplasms (Franks & Chesterman, 1957; Shubik *et al.*, 1962; Matsuyama & Suzuki, 1970; Khrustalev *et al.*, 1976). High-fat diets fed after eight weeks of age led to an elevated incidence of cortical adenomas in female hamsters (Birt & Pour, 1983). The incidence of adrenal hyperplasia increased in male hamsters fed high-fat and high-protein diets before or after eight weeks of age (Birt & Pour, 1985).

COMPARATIVE ASPECTS

The incidence of cortical tumours in hamsters is similar to that seen in rats and mice (Fabry, 1985). Levels of P-glyco-protein mRNA were measured to determine if there was a relationship between the levels and the occurrence of drug resistance during cancer therapy. No correlation was found; however, hamsters and rats have low levels in the adrenal gland, whereas in man they are high (Baas & Borst, 1988).

ISLETS OF LANGERHANS

Small numbers of islet cell tumours have been reported (Kirkman, 1972; Pour *et al.*, 1976a,b). Both adenomas and carcinomas are seen.

NORMAL STRUCTURE

The islets of Langerhans are compact masses of cells surrounded by a thin reticular layer that separates them from exocrine pancreas. Alpha and beta cells are found in a 1:4 ratio. Alpha cells have spherical basal nuclei and eosinophilic cytoplasmic granules. They are located near small blood vessels. Beta cells have large cytoplasmic granules and randomly distributed nuclei (Jewell & Charipper, 1951; Muller, 1959).

MORPHOLOGY AND BIOLOGY OF TUMOURS

Adenomas must be differentiated from hyperplasia. Pour *et al.* (1976a,b) classified adenomas as being larger than 1.0 mm diameter and consisting of one cell type. The cells are large cuboidal or columnar that form cords, nests and ribbons. Minimal stroma is present and cystic or follicular patterns are described (Figures 18 and 19). Carcinomas usually are more anaplastic and there is invasion of surrounding tissue. Metastases are seen in some cases.

INDUCTION OF TUMOURS

Hamsters treated with adrenal corticosteroids will develop slight islet cell hyperplasia. When chlorothiazide was added, a more severe hyperplasia was present (Frenkel, 1960). The formation of new islet cells was induced by lifetime weekly oral or subcutaneous administration of N-nitroso-bis-(2-hydroxypropyl)amine. No difference was noted due to the route of administration (Gariot *et al.*, 1983).

Mixed ductular–insular neoplasms were produced in hamsters by low single doses of N-nitroso-2-methoxy-2,6-dimethylmorpholine (Pour *et al.*, 1981).

COMPARATIVE ASPECTS

P19, a group of 19 000 molecular weight cytosolic proteins, has been identified in AtT20 mouse pituitary tumour cells, RIN-1122 rat insulinoma cells and hamster insulinoma cells (Pasmantier *et al.*, 1986). Somatostatin-28 receptors in hamster islet cell tumours differ from those of acinar membranes of guinea-pigs. Specific inhibitor proteins are involved (Cotroneo *et al.*, 1988).

ACKNOWLEDGEMENT

The authors wish to thank the authors of the corresponding chapters in the first edition for the use of Figures 1, 2, 4, 5, 6, 9, 11, 12 and 16.

REFERENCES

Agate, F.J., Jr (1952) Functional significance of adrenal change following gonadectomy in the hamster. *Anat. Rec.*, 112, 303–304

Anderson, M.P. & Capen, C.C. (1978) The endocrine system. In: Benirschke, K., Garner, F.M. & Jones T.C., eds, *Pathology of Laboratory Animals*, New York, Springer-Verlag, pp. 423–508

Baas, F. & Borst, P. (1988) The tissue dependent expression of hamster P-glycoprotein genes. *FEBS Lett.*, 229, 329–332

Birt, D.F. & Pour, P.M. (1983) Influence of dietary fat on spontaneous lesions of Syrian golden hamsters. *J. Natl Cancer Inst.*, 71, 401–406

Birt, D.F. & Pour P.M. (1985) Interaction of dietary fat and protein in spontaneous diseases of Syrian golden hamsters. *J. Natl Cancer Inst.*, 75, 127–133

Cantrell, C.A. & Padovan, D. (1987) Biology, care and use in research. In: Van Hoosier, G.L., Jr & McPherson, C.W., eds, *Laboratory Hamsters*, Chapter 21, Orlando, FL, Academic Press, pp. 369–387

Christov, K. (1981) Ultrastructure of thyroid tumors. I. Follicular adenomas and carcinomas in rats and hamsters. *Pathol. Res. Pract.*, 173, 30–44

Christov, K. & Raichev, R. (1972) Thyroid carcinogenesis in hamsters after treatment with 131-iodine and methylthiouracil. *Z. Krebsforsch. Klin. Onkol.*, 77, 171–179

Clifton, K.H. & Meyer, R.K. (1956) Mechanism of anterior pituitary tumour induction by estrogen. *Anat. Rec.*, 125, 65–81

Cotroneo, P., Marie, J.-C. & Rosselin, G. (1988) Characterization of covalently cross-linked somatostatin receptors in hamster beta cell insulinoma. *Eur. J. Biochem.*, 174, 219–224

DeLellies, R.A., Wolfe, H.J. & Mohr, U. (1987) Medullary thyroid carcinoma in the Syrian golden hamster: an immunohistochemical study. *Exp. Pathol.*, 31, 11–16

Dontenwill, W. & Mohr, U. (1962) Experimentelle Erzeugung metastasierender Strumen nach Behandlung von Goldhamstern mit Tabakrauchkondensaten. *Z. Krebsforsch.*, 65, 69–74

Fabry, A. (1985) The incidence of neoplasms in Syrian hamsters with particular emphasis on intestinal neoplasia. *Arch. Toxicol. Suppl.,* 8, 124–127

Fortner, J.G. (1957) Spontaneous tumors, including gastrointestinal neoplasms and malignant melanomas, in the Syrian hamster. *Cancer,* 10, 1153–1156

Fortner, J.G. (1961) The influence of castration on spontaneous tumorigenesis in the Syrian (golden) hamster. *Cancer Res.,* 21, 1491–1498

Fortner, J.G., George, P.A. & Sternberg, S.S. (1958) The development of thyroid cancer and other abnormalities in Syrian hamsters maintained on an iodine deficient diet. *Surg. Forum,* 9, 646–650

Fortner, J.G., George, P.A. & Sternberg, S.S. (1960) Induced and spontaneous thyroid cancer in the Syrian (golden) hamster. *Endocrinology,* 66, 364–376

Franks, L.M. & Chesterman, F.C. (1957) Adrenal degeneration and tumour formation in the golden hamster following treatment with stilbestrol and methyl-cholanthrene. *Br. J. Cancer,* 11, 105–111

Frenkel, J.K. (1960) Pancreatic islet cell hyperplasia in hamsters treated with cortisone and chlorothiazide (Diuril). *Fed. Proc.,* 19, 160

Gariot, P., Zbinden, G., Fluckiger, B. & Foliquet, B. (1983) Lesions pancréatiques précoces induites par le N-nitrosobis(2-hydroxypropyl)amine chez le Syrian golden hamster. *Toxicol. Eur. Res.,* 5, 265–271

Hamilton, J.M. (1975) Renal carcinogenesis. *Adv. Cancer Res.,* 22, 1–56

Homburger, F. & Russfield, A.B. (1970) An inbred line of Syrian hamsters with frequent spontaneous adrenal tumours. *Cancer Res.,* 30, 305–308

Horning, E.S. & Whittick, J.W. (1954) Histogenesis of stilboestrol-induced renal tumours in male golden hamster. *Br. J. Cancer,* 8, 451–457

Jewell, H.A. & Charipper, H.A. (1951) The morphology of the pancreas of the golden hamster Cricetus auratus, with special reference to the histology and cytology of the islets of Langerhans. *Anat. Rec.,* 111, 401–415

Khrustalev, S.A., Khar'kovskaya, N.A. & Vasil'eva, N.N. (1976) On blastomogenic activity of 3-indolylacrylic acid in experiments on Syrian hamsters [in Russian]. *Vopr. Onkol.,* 22, 52–57

Kirkman, H. (1972) Hormone-related tumors in Syrian hamsters. *Prog. Exp. Tumor Res.,* 16, 201–240

Kirkman, H. & Algard, F.T. (1968) Spontaneous and nonviral-induced neoplasms. In: Hoffman, R.A., Robinson, P.F. & Magalhaes, H., eds, *The Golden Hamster; Its Biology and Use in Medical Research,* Ames, Iowa State University Press, pp. 227–240

Koneff, A.A., Simpson, M.E. & Evans, H.M. (1946) Effects of chronic administration of diethylstibestrol on the pituitary and other endocrine organs of hamsters. *Anat. Rec.,* 94, 169–191

Lacour, P. (1950) Recherches sur la relation entre les cellules hypophysaires à granulations orangées (cellules de Romeis) et les phénomènes de lactation. *C.R. Séances Soc. Biol.,* 144, 248–249

Ladiges, W.C. (1987) Diseases. In: Van Hoosier, G.L., Jr & McPherson, C.W., eds, *Laboratory Hamsters,* Orlando, FL, Academic Press, pp. 321–328

Matsuyama, M. & Suzuki, H. (1970) Adrenal tumours and endocrine lesions induced in Syrian hamsters by urethane injected during suckling period. *Br. J. Cancer,* 24, 312–318

McMartin, D.N. (1979) Morphologic lesions in aging Syrian hamsters. *J. Gerontol.,* 34, 502–511

Mohr, U. & Ernst, H. (1987) Biology, care and use in research. In: Van Hoosier, G.L., Jr & McPherson, G.W., eds, *Laboratory Hamsters,* Orlando, FL, Academic Press, pp. 351–366

Muller, D. (1959) Investigation of the morphology of the islands of Langerhans and of Feyrter's duct of the pancreas of the Syrian golden hamster. *Anat. Anz.,* 106, 369–385

Pasmantier, R., Danoff, A., Fleischer, N. & Schubart, U.K. (1986) P19, a hormonally regulated phosphoprotein of peptide hormone-producing cells: secretagogue-induced phosphorylation in AtT-20 mouse pituitary tumor cells and in rat and hamster insulinoma cells. *Endocrinology,* 119, 1229–1238.

Pour, P.M. (1983) Adenoma carcinoma, parathyroid, hamster. In: Jones, T.C., Mohr, U. & Hunt, R.D., eds, *Endocrine System* (Monographs on Pathology of Laboratory Animals), Berlin, Heidelberg, New York, Springer-Verlag, pp. 275–281

Pour, P.M. (1986) Induction of exocrine pancreatic, bile duct, and thyroid gland tumors in offspring of Syrian hamsters treated with N-nitrosobis(2-oxypropyl)-amine during pregnancy. *Cancer Res.*, 46, 3663–3666

Pour, P.M. & Birt, D.F. (1986) Effect of dietary protein on N-nitrosobis-(2-oxypropyl)-amine-induced carcinogenesis and on spontaneous disease in Syrian golden hamsters. *J. Natl Cancer Inst.*, 76, 67–72

Pour, P., Kmoch, N., Greiser, E., Mohr, U., Althoff, J. & Cardesa, A. (1976a) Spontaneous tumors and common diseases in two colonies of Syrian hamsters. I. Incidence and sites. *J. Natl Cancer Inst.*, 56, 931–935

Pour, P., Mohr, U., Althoff, J., Cardesa, A. & Kmoch, N. (1976b) Spontaneous tumors and common diseases in two colonies of Syrian hamsters. III. Urogenital system and endocrine glands. *J. Natl Cancer Inst.*, 56, 949–961

Pour, P., Althoff, J., Salmasi, S.Z. & Stepan, K. (1979) Spontaneous tumors and common diseases in three types of hamsters. *J. Natl Cancer Inst.*, 63, 797–811

Pour, P.M., Wallcave, L. & Nagel, D. (1981) The effect of N-nitroso-2-methoxy-2,6-dimethylmorpholine on endocrine and exocrine pancreas of Syrian hamsters. *Cancer Lett.*, 13, 233–240

Reiter, R.J. & Hoffman, R.A. (1968) The endocrine system. In: Hoffman, R.A., Robinson, P.F. & Magalhaes, H., eds, *The Golden Hamster, its Biology and Use in Medical Research*, Ames, Iowa State University Press, pp. 139–155

Russfield, A.B., Friedler, G. & Frenkel, J.K. (1963) Biological characteristics of two transplantable pituitary tumors of Syrian hamsters. *Cancer Res.*, 23, 720–724 + plate

Rustia, M., Shubik, P. & Patil, K. (1980) Life-span carcinogenicity tests with native carrageenan in rats and hamsters. *Cancer Lett.*, 11, 1–10

Schmidt, R.E., Eason, R.L., Hubbard, G.B., Young, J.T. & Eisenbrandt, D.L. (1983) Endocrine glands. In: Schmidt, R.E. & Eason, R.L., eds, *Pathology of Aging Syrian Hamsters*, Boca Raton, FL, CRC Press, pp. 141–174

Shubik, P., Della Porta, G., Pietra, G., Tomatis, L., Rappaport, H., Saffiotti, U. & Toth, B. (1962) Factors determining the neoplastic response induced by carcinogen. In: Brennan, M.J. & Simpson, W.L., eds, *Biological Interactions in Normal and Neoplastic Growth; A Contribution to the Host-tumor Problem*, Boston, Little, Brown, pp. 285–297

Strandberg, J.D. (1987) Neoplastic diseases. In: Van Hoosier, G.L., Jr & McPherson, C.W., eds, *Laboratory Hamsters*, Orlando, FL, Academic Press, pp. 157–168

Van Hoosier, G.L., Jr & Trentin, J.J. (1979) Naturally occurring tumors of the Syrian hamster. *Prog. Exp. Tumor Res.*, 23, 1–12

Vasquez-Lopez, E. (1944) The reaction of the pituitary gland and related hypothalamic centres in the hamster to prolonged treatment with oestrogens. *J. Pathol. Bacteriol.*, 56, 1–13

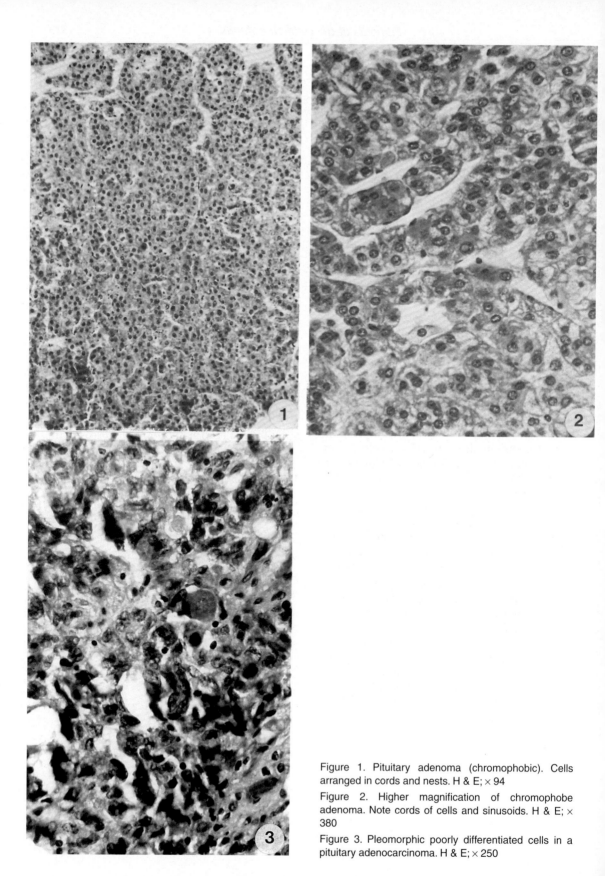

Figure 1. Pituitary adenoma (chromophobic). Cells arranged in cords and nests. H & E; × 94

Figure 2. Higher magnification of chromophobe adenoma. Note cords of cells and sinusoids. H & E; × 380

Figure 3. Pleomorphic poorly differentiated cells in a pituitary adenocarcinoma. H & E; × 250

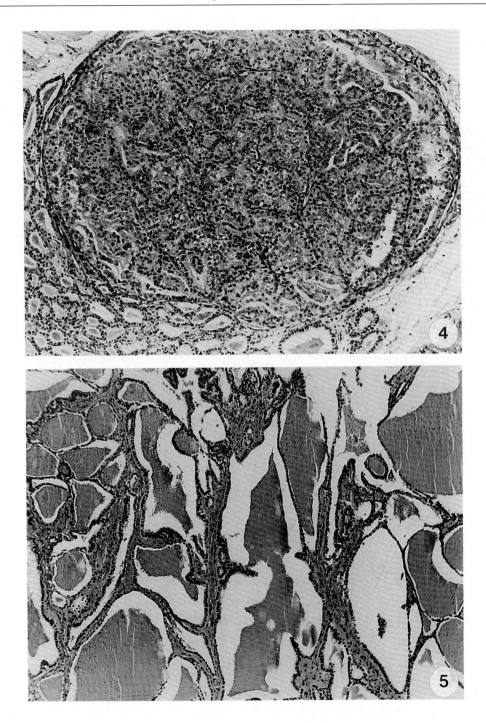

Figure 4. Papillary adenoma of thyroid gland. The tumour is well encapsulated. H & E; × 94

Figure 5. Macrofollicular adenoma with large colloid-filled follicles. H & E; × 94

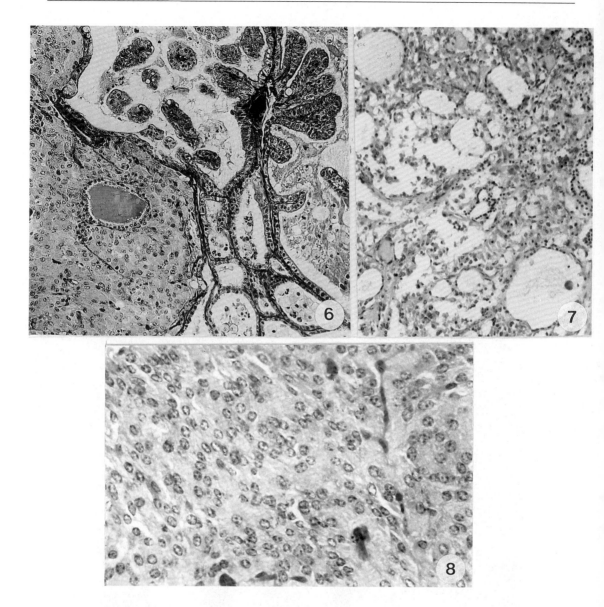

Figure 6. Thyroid adenoma with both papillary and solid foci. H & E; × 130

Figure 7. Follicular carcinoma of a thyroid gland. There is a loss of structural integrity and variation in follicular size and shape. H & E; ×100

Figure 8. Medullary tumour of the thyroid gland. Sheets of large cells have replaced normal thyroid tissue. H & E; × 400

Figure 9. Circumscribed parathyroid adenoma with compression of adjacent tissue. H & E; × 189

Figure 10. Boundary of parathyroid adenoma. Note compression of adjacent tissue but no capsule formation. H & E; × 400

Figure 11. Parathyroid carcinoma. Anaplastic cells forming poorly defined nests and sheets. H & E; × 473

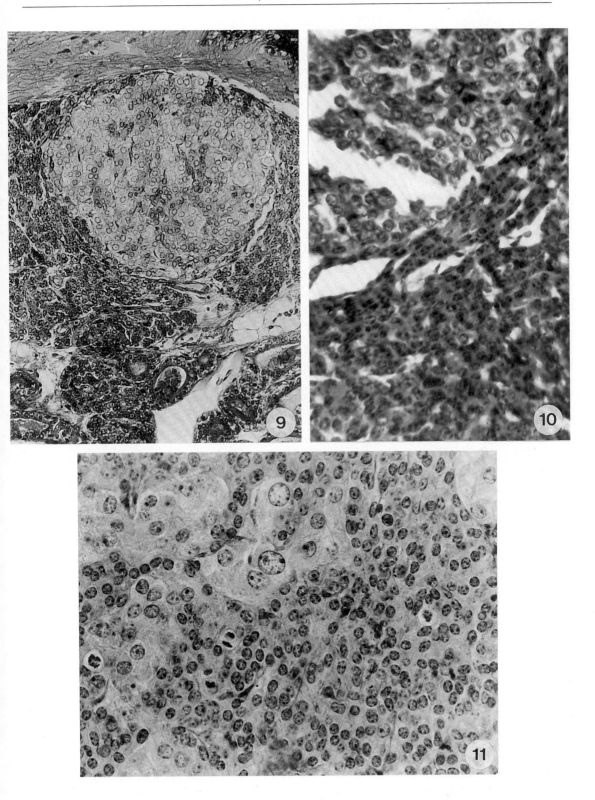

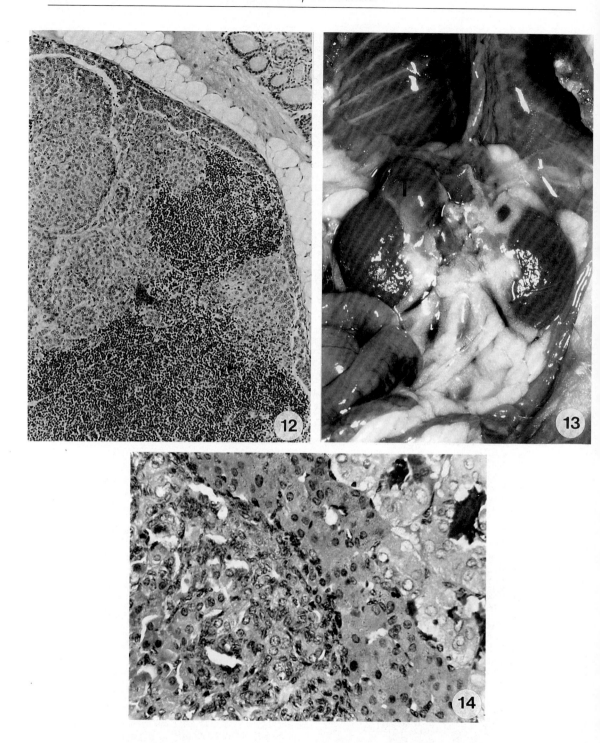

Figure 12. Parathyroid carcinoma metastatic to lymph node, with effacement of normal gland. H & E; × 94

Figure 13. Large unilateral adrenal cortical tumour (T) that is approximately half the size of the kidney.

Figure 14. Adrenal cortical adenoma compressing adjacent cortical epithelial cells. H & E; × 100

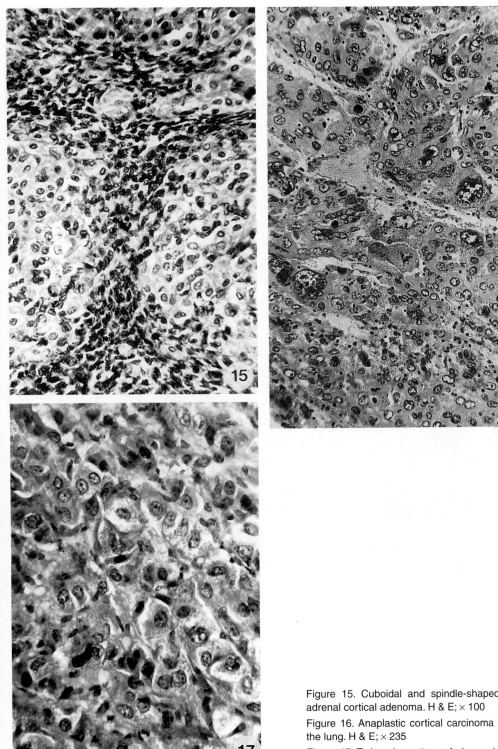

Figure 15. Cuboidal and spindle-shaped cells in an adrenal cortical adenoma. H & E; × 100

Figure 16. Anaplastic cortical carcinoma metastatic to the lung. H & E; × 235

Figure 17. Trabecular pattern of phaeo-chromocytoma. Minimal stroma is present. H & E; × 400

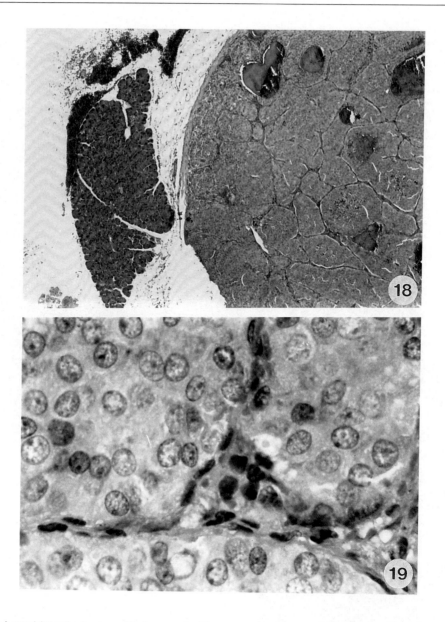

Figure 18. Large islet cell adenoma with circumscribed border compressing pancreatic tissue. H & E; × 40
Figure 19. Nests of large cuboidal cells in islet cell adenoma. H & E; × 400

Tumours of soft tissues

L.D. Berman

The term 'hamster' is used exclusively in reference to the Syrian (or golden) hamster (*Mesocricetus auratus*), since the vast majority of lesions have been described in this species.

The term 'soft tissue' is used here to refer to any of the generalized supporting mesenchymal tissues and includes the following: fibrous, adipose, peripheral, neural, vascular and muscular tissue. The skeletal, central nervous system, lymphoid, synovial and haematological tissues are covered elsewhere. The tumours arise not only in the muscular and subcutaneous tissues, but also in most of the visceral organs where supporting tissue is present. As in the preceding review (Berman *et al.*, 1982), the latter types of tumour are only briefly mentioned, since many of them are discussed in the chapters dealing with those visceral organ systems.

These tumours are of particular interest due to the unique susceptibility of the hamster to viral oncogenesis. Virtually all major varieties of known oncogenic viruses are tumorigenic in the hamster, and they induce some unique lesions that are not known in any other species. Since most of these tumours are soft-tissue lesions, the hamster provide a singular yardstick for morphological and biological comparison.

MORPHOLOGY AND BIOLOGY OF TUMOURS

In the preceding edition (Berman *et al.*, 1982), the difficulties in making precise histogenetic diagnoses were discussed. The main problem was the fact that most of the induced tumours and many of the spontaneous ones were so poorly differentiated that they defied standard histological diagnostic criteria. In some cases a single tumour can also have divergent histological appearances in different areas. It was, therefore, best to regard many of these tumours as primitive mesenchymal lesions with a limited potential to differentiate along one or several pathways. Since that time, however, a number of well defined entities have become firmly established in human soft-tissue tumour pathology. Many of the hamster tumours are either compatible with, or bear a close enough resemblance to these human lesions to be confidently classified by the same criteria.

Since most oncogenic viruses and parenteral carcinogens are administered subcutaneously, most of the tumours arise in this area. The site of spontaneous tumours is somewhat more variable, but many also grow in the subcutaneous area. Although locally invasive, they grow primarily in an expansile manner. Because of the loose, highly elastic integument, these tumours can grow to dimensions as great as the total size of the rest of the animal. The animals eventually die from inanition produced by this massive tumour burden. Yet, even in these cases, metastases usually do not occur; if they do, it is only when the tumours have grown to a large size.

321

This absence of metastasis raises the question of the basic malignant nature of these tumours. Many of these lesions can be characterized as malignant because they do fulfil most of the other criteria that are commonly accepted for malignancy, i.e. they are frequently locally invasive, they eventually kill their hosts, and they usually satisfy the commonly accepted histological and cytological criteria of malignancy, such as dysplastic features and the presence of numerous mitoses, many of which are abnormal.

The situation with spontaneous tumours is less clear. Although some of these are also locally invasive, others grow predominantly by purely expansile means. Although some appear to be high-grade malignancies, in others cellular pleomorphism may be mild, dysplastic features not very prominent, and mitoses not very conspicuous. Clearly these latter tumours are low-grade in character, and some are likely benign.

SPONTANEOUS TUMOURS

Spontaneous soft-tissue tumours make up a small proportion of all spontaneous tumours. In terms of incidence, Van Hoosier and Trentin (1979), tabulating 'malignant' tumours only, found 5.8% soft-tissue tumours among a total of 719. When uterine and other abdominal visceral tumours were excluded, the incidence was 3.4%. In the same publication Berman (1979), tabulating both benign and malignant tumours, found that 3.8% of 2672 spontaneous tumours were soft-tissue tumours. The incidence was only 1.7% when uterine and other abdominal visceral tumours were excluded.

By far the most common spontaneous mesenchymal tumours are the vascular tumours of the liver and spleen (Berman, 1979; Van Hoosier & Trentin 1979), which comprise at least 50% of these lesions. Most are benign. Other visceral lesions that have been reported at a much lower incidence, include leiomyoma/leiomyosarcoma/fibroma of the uterus, a leiomyoma of the prostate, a leiomyosarcoma of the bladder, a fibrosarcoma of the testis, and six intestinal tumours: four leiomyosarcomas, one angiosarcoma and one liposarcoma. Four osteo- or chondrosarcomas were recorded, and five cheek pouch tumours: four myxoid lesions and one haemangiopericytoma.

The remaining lesions which constitute the soft-tissue tumours of non-visceral organs are listed in Table 1 and discussed in more detail. Most of these are fibrosarcomatous spindle cell lesions having a greater or lesser degree of collagenization and growing for the most part in a fascicular 'herring-bone' or storiform pattern (Figure 1). The less collagenized lesions tend to have more cellular pleomorphism and moderate numbers of mitoses; however, abnormal mitotic figures are usually absent. They grow predominantly by expansion, and infiltration of surrounding tissues is not a striking feature. Prominent areas of geographic tumour necrosis can frequently be seen. In many areas patterns of differentiation can occur; the most common of these is an haemangiopericytomatous pattern featuring numerous irregular vascular channels surrounded by spindle cells (Figure 2) or an osteosarcomatous pattern, featuring areas of osteoid formation (Figure 3).

The more collagenized tumours are obvious low-grade fibrosarcomas characterized by absence of necrosis, a dense collagenous stroma and few mitoses (Figure 4). Occasional lesions have a myxosarcomatous pattern in which the cells permeate a loose watery collagenous matrix. This pattern may be focal (Figure 5).

Haemangiopericytomas also occur. These consist of fairly uniform spindle cells surrounding vascular channels, which may be irregular in contour (Figure 6), or small and slit-like in appearance. Foci with these characteristics may appear in areas which are otherwise poorly differentiated fibrosarcoma. Other tumours include the following.

Table 1. Spontaneous hamster soft tissue tumours: classification and incidence

Histological types of tumour	Numbers reported and/or verified
Tumours of fibrous tissue	
Fibroma	1
Fibrosarcoma	12
Tumours of vascular tissue	
Haemangioendothelioma	3
Haemangiopericytoma	5
Tumours of adipose tissue	
Liposarcoma	3
Tumours of nerve tissue	
Neurofibroma	1
Neurofibrosarcoma	5
Tumours of muscle tissue	
Leiomyosarcoma	4
Rhabdomyosarcoma	3
Other tumours	
Histiocytoid tumour (fibrous histiocytoma)	4
Undifferentiated (polymorphous, round-cell,	
spindle cell) sarcoma	11
TOTAL	52

This tabulation lists reported spontaneous tumours, including reported tumours that occurred in experimental animals in which any relationship to the original treatment was highly doubtful, and also unreported tumours reviewed by the authors. The diagnoses listed are those of the original sources of reference where material was not reviewed. In some cases the original diagnoses have been changed upon review of the material.

Fibrous histiocytoma (histiocytic variant). These tumours were originally characterized as 'periarticular giant cell' tumours by Ruffolo and Kirkman (1965). Histologically, they consist of predominantly small round cells or spindle cells with round or ovoid nuclei containing homogeneous chromatin of varying density. The distinctive feature of these lesions is the presence of sharply outlined round or polygonal Touton giant-cells with 6–30 small round nuclei marginating around the periphery of the cytoplasm in a circular or or horseshoe pattern (Figure 7). The giant cells seem to form from local nodular aggregations of the surrounding small tumour cells and their nuclear detail is similar to those cells. Mitoses are very rare. Although histologically benign, the lesions are transplantable.

Muscle tumours. Rhabdomyosarcomas and leiomyosarcomas have been observed (see Figure 8 and 9 in Berman *et al.*, 1982). The former contain irregular strap-and-ribbon cells in which cross-striations can be demonstrated. The latter are composed of interlacing uniform bundles of spindle cells with cigar-shaped nuclei.

Tumours of peripheral nerve and adipose tissue. Neurofibro- and liposarcomas have been described by Fortner *et al.* (1961) and others. The former are basically low-grade spindle cell lesions in which there was suggestive evidence of peripheral nerve tissue, such as fascicles resembling nerve fibres and palisading of nuclei. I have identified one lesion which had these features.

Liposarcomas consist of spindle cell lesions with areas of cells with vacuolated cytoplasm resembling lipoblasts. However, these lesions also contain prominent myxoid areas and varying numbers of vascular channels, suggesting that the cells are multipotential. Other low-grade liposarcomas have been described.

INDUCTION OF TUMOURS

Chemically induced tumours (Table 2)

The first chemically induced hamster sarcomas were reported in 1939 by Gye and Foulds, who observed tumours at the site of inoculation after administration of polycyclic aromatic hydrocarbons. A number of other investigators have obtained similar results and have reported that tumours can be observed after 8–10 weeks in up to 100% of animals if high enough doses of carcinogen are administered.

Tumours induced by benzo[a]pyrene, dimethylbenz[a]anthracene and 3-methyl cholanthrene (Homburger & Hsueh, 1970) were reviewed. They are essentially undifferentiated pleomorphic spindle cell sarcomas that histologically have a fascicular 'herring-bone' pattern (Figure 8) and are of the general histological category of malignant fibrous histiocytoma. The cells are oriented in parallel with little if any intercellular matrix. The cytoplasmic borders are indistinct and the cytoplasm is abundant, homogeneous and eosinophilic. The nuclei are fusiform with rounded ends and the chromatin has a vesicular bubbly character with prominent single or multiple nucleoli (Figure 9). Mitotic figures are plentiful, including frequent bizarre forms. Areas of round polygonal cells in the lesions may represent tumour cells cut transversely. These tumours grow aggressively and infiltrate through surrounding muscular and adipose tissues. Areas of geographic tumour necrosis are usually prominent.

A distinctive feature of these lesions is the characteristic tumour giant cells which are irregular in shape and 50–100 µm in size (Figure 10). The nuclei vary from one or two irregular distinct structures to a conglomerate mass in which the outlines

Table 2. Chemical and physical agents inducing soft tissue tumours in the hamster

Sarcomagenic agent [a]	Type of tumour
Definite	
Polycyclic aromatic hydrocarbons	
Benzo[a]pyrene (5)	Malignant fibrous histiocytoma (MFH)[b]
	Dimethylbenz[a]anthracene (7) (high-grade sarcoma)
	3-Methylcholanthrene (5)
Nitroso compounds	
	Nitrosomethylurea (2)MFH (dimorphic sarcoma) [b]
	Nitrosodimethylamine (1) [c]No histological report
	4-Nitroquinoline-1-oxide and derivatives (2) [c]Fibrosarcoma
Aromatic amines	
	N-Hydroxyacetyl-aminofluorene (1)Fibrosarcoma
Radiation	
	Thorium dioxide (1)MFH (polygonal cell sarcoma)[b]
Possible	
Cholesterol (1)	Leiomyosarcoma
Iron dextran complex (1)	Pleomorphic sarcoma
Polyethylene film (1)	Pleomorphic sarcoma and fibrosarcoma
Powdered steel (1)	Fibrosarcoma

The diagnoses are those of the original authors unless reviewed
[a] Numbers of reports by different authors are shown in parentheses
[b] Tumours reviewed

of individual forms cannot be easily discerned. The nuclear chromatin pattern has the same vesicular bubbly character present in most of the tumour cells. The cytoplasm has a fine, slightly granular, eosinophilic character and the cell boundaries are usually indistinct and occasionally tend to engulf neighbouring tumour cells.

With regard to tumours produced by carcinogens other than the polycyclic aromatic hydrocarbons, lesions produced by N-nitrosomethylurea (Haas *et al.*, 1973) and by thorium dioxide (Mori *et al.*, 1966) have been reviewed. The former were first described by Herrold (1966). The lesions reviewed also consisted of pleomorphic spindle cell sarcomas histologically resembling malignant fibrous histiocytomas. There were basically two types of cells with some intermediate forms: small cells with ovoid or rounded homogeneous nuclei having varying chromatin density and occasional nucleoli, and large cells with pale eosinophilic cytoplasm, indistinct borders, and rounded vesicular nuclei with frequent nucleoli (Figure 11). A variant of the latter population consisted of cells, usually in mitosis, with well demarcated abundant glassy pale cytoplasm and a small amount of dense chromatin material. In some areas abundant collagenous matrix was present suggesting fibrosarcoma. The boundaries of the tumours were for the most part sharply demarcated from the surrounding tissue, although residual muscle fibres were present in focal areas of the tumour. Sharply outlined areas of ischaemic-type necrosis sometimes occurred in the centre of a lesion.

One thorium dioxide-induced tumour was also reviewed. It consisted of a spindle cell/polygonal cell lesion with sharply outlined cellular borders and homogeneous cytoplasm, also falling into the category of malignant fibrous histiocytoma. Nuclei were irregularly rounded and vesicular, with prominent nucleoli. A characteristic feature was the presence of a single large central nucleolus (Figure 12). Mitotic figures were fairly frequent.

Miller *et al.* (1964) reported induction of fibrosarcomas by N-hydroxyacetylaminofluorene. These lesions could not be reviewed, and the one figure in their report is too poor to warrant any comment.

Other reported miscellaneous lesions include fibroangiomas of the pinnae, induced by estrogen in orchiectomized animals (Kirkman, 1962). There have also been isolated reports of lesions associated with cholesterol, iron dextran complex, polyethylene film and powdered steel. These latter cases are somewhat dubious, since the possibility that they were spontaneous lesions fortuitously associated with the experimental protocol cannot be excluded. None of these has been reviewed.

There are a number of reports of visceral mesenchymal tumours induced by chemical carcinogens, recent examples being reports of splenic and hepatic haemangiomas and haemangiosarcomas and urinary bladder sarcomas induced by various members of the alkylnitrosourea group of carcinogens (Lijinsky & Kovatch, 1988, 1989). Since splenic and hepatic tumours of this type occur spontaneously (Berman, 1979; Van Hoosier & Trentin, 1979), these results may be regarded as carcinogen-induced enhancement of spontaneous tumorigenesis, rather than a completely *de novo* carcinogenic event. Other examples of this phenomenon in the hamster have been previously reported (Berman *et al.*, 1973).

Viruses

The fundamental advances in the field of viral oncogenesis in the 1960s and 1970s owed much to the use of the hamster as a model system. The main reason for this is the fact that the neonatal hamster has exceptionally high susceptibility to tumorigenesis by most of the major classes of oncogenic viruses, both DNA and RNA (Table 3). In some cases the hamster is even more susceptible than the original host species of the virus (e.g., polyomavirus); in other cases the hamster is susceptible whereas the original host species appears to be entirely resistant (e.g., SV40 and adenoviruses). In addition, most of the classes of known oncogenic virus produce soft-tissue tumours (i.e., sarcomas) at the site of inoculation. Because of this, the hamster can serve as a useful yardstick to compare tumorigenesis by the different oncogenic viruses. Such comparisons show that the tumours induced by each major class of oncogenic virus have a characteristic and distinct histological appearance (Berman, 1967). Such information has proved useful in studying the effects of the different viral

oncogenes, especially when viruses of mixed or hybrid character are assayed (Huebner *et al.*, 1964), and to etiologically characterize tumours induced by inocula-containing possible contaminant oncogenic agents (Gaugas *et al.*, 1969).

Adenoviruses

The oncogenic adenoviruses were discovered by Trentin *et al.* (1962), who were searching for new oncogenic agents by systematically inoculating neonatal hamsters with known animal and human viruses. Originally a number of oncogenic human serotypes were discovered. Subsequently several additional simian serotypes, at least two bovine, two canine

Table 3. Viruses inducing soft tissue tumours in the hamster

Viral group	Virus	Histological type of tumour
DNA viruses		
Adenopapova viruses	Adenovirus (several human and simian serotypes: 2 bovine, 1 canine and 1 avian)	Typical small cell undifferentiated sarcoma. Bovine, canine and avian viruses also produce fibromas and fibrosarcomas.
	Simian virus 40 BK and JC viruses	Malignant fibrous histiocytomas with typical giant cells
	Polyoma virus	Malignant fibrous histiocytomas with varying histogenetic patterns
	Bovine papillomavirus	Dermal fibromas (low-grade fibrosarcomas)
Herpes viruses [a]	Human herpes simplex virus and human cytomegalovirus, guinea-pig and bovine herpes viruses	Fibrosarcomas with typical giant cells; 'adenocarcinomas' [b]
RNA viruses		
Retroviruses	Rous sarcoma virus (several strains)	Typical pleomorphic polygonal sarcomas (? malignant rhabdoid tumours) and fibrosarcomas
	Murine sarcomas virus (3 strains)	Histiocytoid tumours (fibrous histiocytomas) with Touton-type giant cells. Also pleomorphic sarcomas (? malignant rhabdoid tumours)

[a] Tumours have so far only been produced by transplantation of cells transformed *in vitro*.
[b] These have been reported but not reviewed.

(infectious canine hepatitis virus and respiratory-associated canine adenovirus), and an avian (chicken embryo lethal orphan) were added to this list. None of these agents has ever been implicated as oncogenic in the species of origin of the respective virus. The highly oncogenic human serotypes (types 12, 18, and 31) produce soft, translucent, dull pearly white lesions of almost gelatinous character after latent periods of 30–60 days in up to 100% of animals when high-dose inocula are used. Similar lesions are produced by the moderately oncogenic human (types 3, 7, 14 and 21), simian, bovine, canine and avian viruses with somewhat longer latent periods and lower percentages. Histologically these lesions are unique. They are typical small-cell tumours growing in sheets of uniform cells permeated by delicate stromal strands and small vessels (Figure 13). The cytoplasm is scant and indistinct and the nuclei are round to ovoid with a punctate ('salt and pepper') chromatin pattern. A focal organoid pattern is produced when the tumour cells form true rosettes around stromal strands or pseudorosettes around small blood vessels (Figures 13 and 14). Mitotic figures are numerous. Tumours induced by some of the simian and bovine serotypes tend to have somewhat more of a spindle cell pattern, in which the cells are larger and grow in fascicles. Occasionally round giant cells with four to six peripherally located nuclei resembling those of most of the surrounding tumour cells are found.

Necrosis is a very prominent feature of these lesions and characteristically occurs even in small tumours. There are two types: ischaemic and haemorrhagic. In the former, large areas of tumour cells become densely pyknotic, assuming an almost lymphoid character. In some cases the tumour cells around small blood vessels are spared, leaving islands of viable tumour surrounded by large areas of ischaemic necrosis. Haemorrhagic necrosis is associated with small vascular channels

that frequently appear to be lined directly by tumour cells. This may result in vascular instability. Occasional vessels are seen to be only partially lined by tumour cells, a defect is created and the surrounding tissue becomes haemorrhagic (Figure 14).

In bovine adenovirus-inoculated animals, firm rubbery lesions develop in addition to the more characteristic small-cell tumours, usually with a longer latent period (Darbyshire *et al.*, 1968). Histologically these are low-grade, non-transplantable, slowly growing, spindle cell lesions, that do not have the characteristic cytological features of the more usual small-cell tumours. They grow in loose fascicles, frequently with a collagenous matrix and thus can be characterized as low-grade fibrosarcomas. Cytoplasmic boundaries are indistinct, and mitoses are rare. The nuclei have irregularly tapered or blunted ends, and show a vesicular chromatin pattern with small nucleoli. In addition to these lesions, cystic endothelialized lesions also occur.

SV40 and the human polyomaviruses

These agents are indigenous primate viruses that induce sarcomas at the site of inoculation in neonatal hamsters with a 5–12 month latent period (Eddy *et al.*, 1961; Nase *et al.*, 1975; Shah *et al.*, 1975; Dougherty, 1976). Tumours induced by SV40 and the BK virus were reviewed. Grossly, the tumours are firm and rubbery. Microscopically, they are spindle-cell sarcomas, frequently growing in a fascicular ('herring-bone') pattern and generally classifiable as malignant fibrous histiocytomas. The tumour cells have a moderately well demarcated light granular cytoplasm. The nuclei are ovoid or cigar-shaped with a vesicular pattern, clumped chromatin and frequent prominent nucleoli (Figure 15). Mitoses are fairly abundant, and areas of ischaemic necrosis are common, especially in lesions over 5 mm in diameter. Occasionally some tumours show areas of intercellular collagenous matrix consistent with a fibrosarcomatous pattern.

A distinctive feature of these tumours is the presence of characteristic giant cells (Figure 16). These are 40–80 μm in size and have an irregular somewhat densely eosinophilic cytoplasm. The nuclei consist of either one to four distinct irregular forms or an indistinct aggregate of several nuclei. The nuclear appearance is either similar to the surrounding individual tumour cells, or more densely pyknotic.

Murine polyomavirus

The polyomavirus is distinctive in that the hamster is so sensitive to this agent that the tumours arise with an exceedingly short latent period (6–10 days), not only at the site of inoculation, but also in a variety of visceral organs. The latter most commonly include the kidneys and heart, but lesions have also been reported in the intestine, lungs, meninges and serosal surfaces (Chesterman & Negroni, 1960; Stanton & Otsuka, 1963; Berman, 1967). Microscopically, these malignant fibrous histiocytomas resemble the SV40 tumours, except for differences such as greater pleomorphism in both cytological and organizational detail. Thus, the fascicular pattern is frequently not so tight and the cells may be separated by a loose collagenous stroma. Cellular variability can be considerable, with some cells closely resembling the SV40 tumour cells, while others are smaller and more uniform in appearance, having a homogeneous chromatin pattern (Figure 17). Giant cells, when present, resemble the SV40 giant cells (Figure 18), but may not be as distinct or striking. Various differentiation patterns can be seen, especially in some of the visceral lesions, including fibro-, myxo-, neurofibro-, lipo- or angiosarcomatous patterns. In the cardiac lesions, foci of cartilage, osteoid and calcification can be found. The renal lesions are distinctive in that they can almost completely replace the medulla while sparing the cortex.

A unique lesion produced by the virus is the cystic angiosarcoma of the liver (Chesterman & Negroni, 1960; Stanton & Otsuka, 1963; Defendi & Lehman, 1964). These appear to involve the Kupffer cells which enlarge and become prominent (Figure 19). Their proliferation appears to destabilize the plates of hepatocytes which consequently break up, creating large blood-filled cystic spaces in which a few clusters of papillary tumour cells can be found. The cysts continue to enlarge and eventually may rupture through the liver capsule, resulting in massive haemoperitoneum and death.

Bovine papillomavirus

This member of the papillomavirus group produces warty tumours at the site of inoculation after a 1–2-month latent period (Boiron *et al.*, 1964). Histologically, however, rather than being typical epithelial papillomas, they are dermal fibromatous lesions that appear to be either fibromatoses or low-grade fibrosarcomas. The lesions cause marked dermal thickening, are indistinctly demarcated from adjacent uninvolved tissue, and penetrate into the subcutaneous fat (Figure 20). The lesions are composed of tightly compacted bland, ovoid to cigar-shaped spindle cells in a fibrous stroma growing in a storiform pattern (Figure 21). They are not very aggressive and mitoses are rare. One characteristic feature is the presence of small round dense nuclei (presumably lymphocytes) superimposed on some of the tumour cell nuclei (Figure 21). There are occasional areas of ischaemic necrosis. After some time, additional lesions appear on peripheral body areas, such as the extremities, scrotum and pinna (see Figure 29 of Berman *et al.*, 1982).

Rous sarcoma virus (RSV)

The tumorigenicity of Rous sarcoma virus in the hamster was first demonstrated by Ahlstrom and Forsby (1962), who observed tumours at the site of inoculation in neonatal animals after 30–60 days with the Schmidt–Ruppin strain. Subsequently, most of the other strains were also reported to induce tumours in hamsters. Histologically, these are extremely pleomorphic sarcomas. Some are tightly knit, poorly differentiated fibrosarcomatous lesions with cells growing in fascicles with abundant collagenous matrix, while others are predominantly polygonal cell lesions with no appreciable intercellular matrix. Frequently these diverse features can be found in different parts of the same tumour. In the polygonal and even in many of the spindle cell lesions, cellular outlines appear distinct. The cytoplasm varies from pale granular to a dense, dark, homogeneous glassy consistency. Nuclei are characteristically vesicular, often with a single large central nucleolus (Figure 22). Rhabdoid-type giant cells are frequently present, containing one to four nuclei similar to those in the surrounding tumour cells. Sometimes cytoplasmic concretions fill most of the cell, with the nuclei displaced eccentrically (Figure 23). Mitotic figures, particularly in slower-growing tumours induced by the Bryan strain may not be very numerous. A mixed inflammatory cell infiltrate frequently can be found at the periphery of the lesions and occasionally acute inflammatory cells (neutrophils) overlie necrotic tumour giant cells (see Figure 50 in Berman, 1967). Distinct areas of ischaemic necrosis are usually present, frequently occupying most of the tumour.

Murine sarcoma virus (MSV)

Hamster tumours have been induced by all three strains of murine sarcoma virus (Moloney, Harvey and Kirsten) at the site of inoculation (Chesterman *et al.*, 1966; Berman, 1967). The tumours are histologically of two types: fast-growing polygonal cell lesions closely resembling the Rous sarcomas (Figure 24), and slower-growing lesions having a number of distinctive features. Histologically, the slower-growing lesions are fibrous histiocytomas (histiocytic variant) with cells having endothelioid features. These neoplasms consist of small spindle cells in a loose matrix with indistinct cellular borders set in a loose matrix. The irregular ovoid nuclei have a pale homogeneous chromatin pattern with a few cells having nucleoli. Mitoses are few. The lesions are permeated by a focal infiltrate of plasma cells and mast cells. The most distinctive feature of these lesions is the formation of irregular angiomatoid spaces (Figure 25) and characteristic Touton-type giant cells with 15–40 nuclei, usually arranged in a circular or horseshoe-shaped configuration (Figure 26). Frequently the giant cells project into the angiomatoid spaces. The giant cell nuclei resemble those of the surrounding tumour cells and occasionally circular whorls of tumour cells are present (Figure 27), suggesting that the giant cells form by fusion of the cells in these masses.

Another distinctive feature of the MSV–hamster system is that inoculated animals (usually with primary tumours) frequently develop diffuse swelling of a paw or focal area of an extremity (see Figure 34 in Berman *et al.*, 1982). In these lesions, the entire soft-tissue structures between skin and bone may be replaced by sarcomatous growth.

Although herpes viruses have generally not been shown to be directly oncogenic in hamsters (see below), there is a more recent report (Hadjiolov *et al.*, 1993) which claims the induction of tumours in 10–15 months when a promoter (TPA) was applied to the skin for six months over the site of herpes simplex virus type 1 inoculation. The tumours, described as angiolipomas, chondromyxomas, a hibernoma and a Kaposi sarcoma-like tumour, have not been reviewed.

Transformation

The term transformation implies changes occurring in tissue-cultured cells of non-neoplastic origin, endowing them with the phenotypic properties associated with neoplasia, i.e. loss of anchorage dependence for cell growth, loss of contact inhibition, cytological changes and, most importantly, the ability to form tumours when transplanted to a syngenic recipient. Hamster cells have been very popular for transformation studies since most hamster tumours are transplantable, even in random outbred animals. In addition, the hamster cheek pouch offers an immunologically privileged site for transplantation.

Transformation may either occur spontaneously or be induced by chemical or viral carcinogenic agents. There seem to be basic differences between these two types of phenomenon. As regards spontaneous transformation, it is almost axiomatic that any normal hamster tissue explanted into culture will become spontaneously transformed if the cells are passaged long enough. Such cell lines are characterized by immortality and can be passaged indefinitely. Most of the cells, however, still maintain contact inhibition and anchorage dependence for cell growth. They will produce tumours when inoculated into adult animals. However, large numbers of cells (10^5–10^7) must be used. The best known of these spontaneous cell lines is the BHK-21 line developed by Stoker and MacPherson (1964) from subcultures of kidney cells derived from one-day-old animals. This and most other similar lines are probably derived from fibroblastoid cells. The tumours induced by BHK-21 cells are spindle-cell sarcomas growing in a fascicular pattern. The cells are small with pale indistinct cytoplasm and round to cigar-shaped nuclei with a vesicular or homogeneous chromatin pattern. Sometimes one or two small nucleoli are present and mitotic figures are sparse. The distinctive feature is the presence of numerous round cells with dense eosinophilic cytoplasm and one small vesicular or pyknotic nucleus (Figure 28). Although these cells resemble myoblastic cells, the tumours are basically fibrosarcomas. Tumours induced by at least one other spontaneous line of transformed cells were examined and found similar to the BHK-21 cell tumours.

Transformation studies with chemical and viral carcinogens have been complicated by the fact that sometimes the spontaneous lines have been used as a starting point. In such cases many of the tumours have resembled the BHK-21 tumours. Therefore only tumours produced by transformation of primary cells will be discussed.

With regard to chemical carcinogens, tumours have been reported to be induced by cells transformed by polycyclic aromatic hydrocarbons (Berwald & Sachs, 1963; Dipaolo & Donovan 1967), nitrosodimethylamine (Huberman *et al.*, 1968), and 4-nitroquinoline *N*-oxide (Kamahora & Kakunaga, 1967; Kuroki & Sato, 1968). Tumours induced by the polycyclic aromatic hydrocarbon transformed cells are similar to the primary carcinogen-induced tumours described above. The tumours induced by nitroquinoline-transformed cells were described as spindle-cell or round-cell sarcomas with no other distinguishing features and were not reviewed. Those from nitrosodimethylamine-transformed cells arose only after long-term serial tissue-culture passage. Therefore the possibility of spontaneous transformation cannot be excluded.

With regard to viruses, tumours induced by cells transformed by the oncogenic adenoviruses, polyoma and MSV all resemble the lesions induced by these viruses *in vivo*. In the case of SV40 this is also true in some cases where one can assume that the original transformed cells were of fibroblastoid origin (see below).

There are three cases, however, in which tumours originating from virally transformed cells have proven to be novel lesions.

The first of these concerns tumours induced by the adenovirus–SV40 hybrid viruses. These are adenoviruses in which some of the adenovirus genetic material has been replaced by early SV40 genes. Tumours induced by these viruses may have the histological appearance of adenovirus or SV40 tumours, or be intermediate in appearance (Huebner *et al.*, 1964; Black *et al.*, 1969). The latter occasionally has well demarcated contrasting areas of both adenovirus and SV histological types in a geographic configuration.

The second case involves tumours induced by SV40-transformed cells (see Figure 37 from Berman *et al.*, 1982). Although tumours induced by transformed cells (presumed fibroblastoid) resemble the tumours induced virally *in vivo* (as described above), tumours induced by SV40–transformed hamster kidney cells frequently contain an epithelial tubular-type pattern (see Figure 41 from Berman *et al.*, 1982) in addition to the usual malignant fibrous histiocytoma (Black *et al.*, 1966). Also, tumours induced with transformed hamster embryo cells occasionally show foci of epidermoid and small-cell carcinoma (Diamandopoulos & Enders, 1966; Diamandopoulos & Sanborn-Redmond, 1973). It thus appears that SV40 has the capacity to transform a variety of cell types, each of which subsequently imparts to the tumour some of its original histological features. However, fibroblastoid cells are either the most sensitive or the most virally exposed cells when the virus is administered *in vivo*. Fibroblastoid cells also comprise the majority of cells when hamster tissues are explanted into culture.

The third case concerns various members of the herpes virus group that are capable of inducing tumorigenic transformants in tissue culture, although they are unable to directly induce tumours *in vivo*. These viruses include the human

herpes simplex viruses (HSV) types 1 and 2 (Duff & Rapp, 1971, 1973), human cytomegalovirus (CMV) (Albrecht & Rapp, 1973), guinea-pig herpes virus (Michalski *et al.*, 1976) and the infectious bovine rhinotracheitis virus (Michalski & Hsiung, 1975). The HSV-transformed cell tumours are tight pleomorphic spindle cell lesions with a scant collagenous matrix and a vesicular punctate nuclear chromatin pattern. They appear to be poorly differentiated fibrosarcomas. Mitoses are moderate in number and there are characteristic irregular mostly mononuclear giant cells with dense cytoplasm (Figure 29). They differ from the BHK-21 giant cells in that they are more variable in size and some are much larger. The cellular outlines are also more irregular and the nuclei are larger with a more vesicular chromatin pattern. Similarly to SV40, HSV-transformed cells have also produced lesions reported as adenocarcinomas (Duff & Rapp, 1973). These tumours have not been reviewed. Two tumours from guinea-pig herpes virus-transformed cells were reviewed. One was a spindle cell lesion similar to the HSV-transformed cell tumours but without the giant cells. The other was an irregular pleomorphic round cell–polygonal cell lesion with abundant mitoses, in which there were discrete foci of small round, almost lymphoid-like tumour cells interspersed throughout the lesion.

HISTOGENESIS, TUMORIGENESIS AND COMPARATIVE ASPECTS

With regard to spontaneous tumours, the 'periarticular giant-cell tumours' do not necessarily arise in relation to joints and do not resemble the giant-cell tumours of bone and tendon sheath in humans, which are currently designated as nodular tenosynovitis. Since they appear to be benign and resemble some of the human fibrous histiocytomas, I prefer to designate them as fibrous histiocytomas or simply as benign histiocytoid tumours. In addition, giant cells formed by cell fusion are frequently histiocytic in cell type and some of the MSV tumours which these lesions resemble also appear to be of histiocytic cell origin (Hallowes *et al.*, 1973) (see below). Further studies on fresh material will be necessary to substantiate this, however.

The only study with chemical carcinogens is that of Nettleship and Smith (1950), who reported the early events after subcutaneous administration of 3-methylcholanthrene. They observed oedema and the accumulation of nodules of altered fibroblasts starting at 24 hours. At 2–2.5 months, invasive sarcomas arose from these foci. Histologically these lesions resemble malignant fibrous histiocytomas in humans (see below).

The adenovirus lesions have been studied by a number of investigators. Ogawa *et al.* (1966) concluded that these tumours are of neuroectodermal origin, since the earliest lesions were microproliferative foci that appeared always in relation to peripheral nerve fibres within 10 days after subcutaneous inoculation. Furthermore, they and others (Berman, 1967) have called attention to the characteristic formation of Homer–Wright rosettes and pseudorosettes around small vessels similar to those seen in human neuroblastic tumours. The only other serious histogenic consideration is that the tumours are haemangiopericytomas that may differentiate to leiomyosarcomas, a contention put forward by Levenbook and Strizhachenko (1971) and Levenbook *et al.* (1982) on the basis of ultrastructural and histochemical observations and their studies reporting the relation of tumour micronodules to small vessels. Although immunohistochemical stains for human neuroglial and neuroectodermal markers (GFAP, NSE, S-100 protein, NF and vimentin) have all been negative (Ogawa, 1989; L. Berman, unpublished observations) in hamster tumours, Kobayashi *et al.* (1985) and Kyritis *et al.* (1984) showed positive

NSE and S-100 staining in adenovirus-induced rat retinoblastoma, which are histologically similar. There are several lines of evidence that indicate that the characteristic features are a function of the adenovirus genome. Adenovirus-transformed BHK-21 cells produce tumours of characteristic adenovirus type (rather than BHK-21 type) when transplanted to hamsters (Strohl *et al.*, 1967), implying that the virus imparts the characteristic cellular appearance upon transformation, regardless of the original cell type transformed. In tissue-cultured adenovirus 12 tumour lines, a correlation was found between loss of the viral genome over time and reversion from the characteristic epithelioid to a fibroblastoid morphology. Furthermore, tumours induced by the latter cells were fibrosarcomas (Kuhlmann *et al.*, 1982). Rat kidney cells could be immortalized by transfection with the early region IA (EIA) gene of adenovirus type 5, but the cells retained a fibroblastoid appearance. The characteristic adenovirus-type cytology was obtained only after transfection with segments containing both the EIA and EIB genes, thus again indicating the direct effect of viral genetic material on morphological phenotypic expression (Houweling *et al.*, 1980). In addition, adenovirus-induced mouse and rat tumours also have the same histological appearance as the hamster tumours.

The development of tumours in animals inoculated with polyomavirus was studied by Chesterman (1961) and Stanton and Otsuka (1963). Within 24–48 hours, inflammatory infiltrates, oedema, focal necrosis and atypical cellular proliferation were found in the kidneys and heart. Tumours were clearly recognizable in the kidneys at three days and in the heart at five days. Tumours at the site of subcutaneous inoculation appeared later in animals not dying with the early renal, cardiac and hepatic lesions. The subcutaneous lesions had areas with differentiation towards haemangiomas, neurofibrosarcomas and liposarcomas. The cardiac lesions had areas of osteosarcoma, and the renal lesions and some of the subcutaneous tumours were essentially undifferentiated. In a more recent report, Combette *et al.* (1990) found desmin and actin (alpha smooth muscle isoform) present in the cardiac and renal tumours, suggesting some degree of muscular origin. All these results implied that polyomavirus affected a primitive mesenchymal cell which has the potential to undergo limited differentiation into a number of cell types (as lipoblasts, osteoblasts, myoblasts, etc.) or not at all.

In studies characterizing the tumorigenicity of the viral genes, transgenic mice with the polyoma middle T antigen gene developed only haemangiomata, while animals with only the polyoma large T antigen gene remained tumour-free over the same period (Bautch *et al.*, 1987). Tissue-culture experiments (similar to the adenovirus system) showed that the large T gene could immortalize primary cells to continuous growth; however, only the middle T gene could fix the transformed phenotype (Treisman *et al.*, 1981; Rassoulzadegan *et al.*, 1982). Why the middle T transgenic animals developed only haemangiomas, rather than the full spectrum of polyomavirus tumours, may possibly be related to the failure to activate other proto-oncogenes which are activated when the complete virus is administered *in vivo*. The spectrum of tumours produced also varies with the viral strain (Dawe *et al.*, 1987; Freund *et al.*, 1987, 1988) and may depend on duplications or point mutations in the viral genome. These in turn may also trigger the activation of secondary oncogenes (or anti-oncogenes).

The SV40 virus tumours were characterized as leiomyosarcomas by Levenbook (1975) on the basis of ultrastructural study. Histologically, they resemble the malignant fibrous histiocytomas observed in humans (see below). The large T antigen gene appears to be the primary and only oncogene; linking this gene to heterogeneous promoters in transgenic mice caused a variety of tumours (Ornity *et al.*, 1985; Suda *et al.*, 1987). In a somewhat anomalous result, however, Carbone *et al.* (1989) showed that SV40 small t antigen deletion mutants induced histiocytic lymphomas of the abdominal cavity in addition to the usual sarcomas, suggesting that the small t antigen may have some direct influence on the oncogenic process.

In the retrovirus systems, Hallowes *et al.* (1973), studying MSV, observed proliferation of histiocytic-type cells at the site of inoculation and in draining lymph nodes, with cyst formation in the lymph nodes as the earliest histological changes two weeks after administration of the virus. Tumours developed in these areas from three to six weeks. They concluded that the tumours were most likely of histiocytic origin. Perk and Hod (1971) characterized the hamster tumours as undifferentiated sarcomas with myoblastic features. The histogenesis of these mouse tumours has been quite controversial; the lesions have been variously described as undifferentiated sarcomas (Berman & Allison, 1969; Siegler 1970), rhabdomyosarcomas (Moloney, 1966), or even non-neoplastic granulomatous lesions (Stanton *et al.*, 1968). The RSV hamster tumours have been classified as rhabdomyosarcomas by Levenbook *et al.* (1974, 1982).

The extreme histological pleomorphism of these lesions and especially the character of the giant cells are strongly reminiscent of a more recently described entity in human soft-tissue tumour pathology—malignant rhabdoid tumour (Tsuneyoshi *et al.*, 1985; Schmidt *et al.* 1989). In this neoplasm, although the lesions are strongly suggestive of myoblastic origin, the cells are negative for myoglobin, frequently negative for desmin, and frequently positive for epithelial antigens (cytokeratin and epithelial membrane antigen).

The entity of malignant fibrous histiocytoma, first described by O'Brien and Stout (1964) and later extensively studied in a large series by Weiss and Enziger (1978), has become firmly established in human soft-tissue tumour pathology. These lesions appear to be derived from primitive mesenchymal cells having the capacity to differentiate along fibroblastic and histiocytic cell lines. In their variability they have many of the features described above for some of the chemically and virus-induced tumours. These include the extreme pleomorphic character of SV40, RSV and MSV-induced tumours, the tumour giant cells of the SV40, polyoma and polycyclic aromatic hydrocarbon induced lesions, the xanthoma-type giant cells of the RSV- and MSV-induced tumours, the fascicular and storiform growth patterns of many of these lesions, and the angiomatoid and myxoid patterns of growth. If the obviously malignant SV40, polyomavirus, RSV- and MSV-induced tumours represent lesions consistent with malignant fibrous histiocytoma, the benign spontaneous histiocytoid, and MSV giant cell lesions could represent their more benign counterparts.

In summary, a number of conclusions can be drawn from these studies:

1. All of the tumorigenetic studies cited above support the multistage theory of carcinogenesis. They have all demonstrated an initial non-specific preneoplastic proliferative reaction, frequently similar in nature to a response to some form of injury, followed subsequently by neoplastic growth.

2. All of the genetic studies support the concept that the DNA tumour viruses contain one or two potent oncogenes that are indispensable for inciting unrestricted growth and fixing the characteristic phenotypic morphological alteration.

3. Attempts to attach histogenetic diagnoses to some of the induced tumours are inconclusive. This is due to the lack of definitive markers, the fact that many of the lesions show considerable variability from one area to the next and that exact counterparts do not exist in humans. Nevertheless, many of these lesions do have enough similarity to well characterized human soft-tissue tumours that reasonable assumptions can be made regarding their histogenetic origin.

4. All of the systems of induced tumours have some unique features which are useful to characterize and identify them. This uniqueness includes the histological features of the characteristic sarcomatous soft-tissue lesions produced by the major classes of oncogenic viruses and carcinogens.

ACKNOWLEDGEMENTS

Acknowledgement is given for the use of histological material kindly provided by the following: Drs R.M. Dougherty, H. Haas, F. Homburger, L.S. Kaplow, H. Kirkman, A.M. Lewis, R. Mantyjarvi, R. McGandy, T. Mori, C. Olson, J.D. Strandberg, I. Wodinsky and Y. Yabe. I am also indebted to Dr Sharon Weiss for review of the histological material along with helpful suggestions and discussion.

REFERENCES

Ahlstrom, C.G. & Forsby, N. (1962) Sarcomas in hamsters after injection with Rous chicken tumor material. *J. Exp. Med.*, 115, 839–852

Albrecht, T. & Rapp, F. (1973) Malignant transformation of hamster embryo fibroblasts following exposure to ultraviolet-irradiated human cytomegalovirus. *Virology*, 55, 53–61

Bautch, V.L., Toda, S., Hassell, J.A. & Hanahan, D. (1987) Endothelial cell tumors develop in transgenic mice carrying polyoma virus middle T oncogene. *Cell*, 51, 529–538

Berman, L.D. (1967) Comparative morphologic study of the virus induced solid tumors of Syrian hamsters. *J. Natl Cancer Inst.*, 39, 847–901

Berman, L.D. (1979) Naturally occurring tumors: Hamster. In: Altman, P.L. & Katz, D.D., eds, *Biological Handbooks* III. *Inbred and Genetically Defined Strains of Laboratory Animals*. Part 2. *Hamster, Guinea Pig, Rabbit, and Chicken*, Bethesda, MD, Federation of American Societies for Experimental Biology, pp. 493–495

Berman, L.D. & Allison, A.C. (1969) Studies on murine sarcoma virus; A morphological comparison of tumorigenesis by the Harvey and Moloney strains in mice, and the establishment of tumor cell lines. *Int. J. Cancer*, 4, 820–836

Berman, L.D., Hayes, J.A. & Sibay, T.M. (1973) Effect of streptozotocin in the Chinese hamster (*Cricetulus griseus*). *J. Natl Cancer Inst.*, 51, 1287–1294

Berman, L.D., Soto, E. & Chesterman, F.C. (1982) Tumors of the soft tissues. In Turusov, V.S., ed., *Pathology of Tumours in Laboratory Animals*. Vol. III, *Tumours of the Hamster* (IARC Scientific Publications No. 34), Lyon, IARC, pp. 293–324

Berwald, Y. & Sachs, L. (1963) *In vitro* cell transformation with chemical carcinogen. *Nature*, 200, 1182–1184

Black, P.H., Berman, L.D. & Dixon, C.B. (1969) In vitro transformation of adenovirus simian virus 40 hybrid viruses. IV. Properties of clones isolated from cell lines transformed by adenovirus 2-simian virus 40 and adenovirus 12-simian virus 40 transcapsidant viruses. *J. Virol.*, 4, 694–703

Boiron, M., Levy, J.P., Thomas, M., Friedmann, J.C. & Bernard, J. (1964) Some properties of the bovine papilloma virus. *Nature*, 201, 423–424

Carbone, M., Lewis, A.M., Jr., Matthews, B.J., Levine, A.S. & Dixon, K. (1989) Characterization of hamster tumors induced by simian virus 40 small t deletion mutants as true histiocytic lymphomas. *Cancer Res.*, 49, 1565–1571

Chesterman, F.C. (1961) The pathological effects of the Mill Hill polyoma virus (MHP). *Med. Press*, 245, 350–355

Chesterman, F.C. & Negroni, G. (1960) Tumours and other lesions induced in golden hamsters by a polyoma virus (Mill Hill strain): induction time and dose response. *Br. J. Cancer*, 14, 790–797

Chesterman, F.C., Harvey, J.J., Dourmashkin, R.R. & Salaman, M.H. (1966) The pathology of tumors and other lesions induced in rodents by virus derived from a rat with Moloney leukemia. *Cancer Res.*, 26, 1759–1768

Cheville, N.F. (1966) Studies on connective tissue tumors in the hamster produced by bovine papilloma virus. *Cancer Res.*, 26, 2334–2339

Combette, J.M., Sappino, A.P. & Turler, H. (1990) Heterogeneity of polyoma tumors in hamsters: analysis of cytoskeletal proteins and viral gene expression. *Int. J. Cancer*, 45, 521–528

Darbyshire, J.H., Berman, L.D., Chesterman, F.C. & Pereira, H.G. (1968) Studies on the oncogenicity of bovine adenovirus type 3. *Int. J. Cancer*, 3, 546–557

Dawe, C.J., Freund, R., Mandel, G., Ballmer-Hofer, K., Talmage, D.A. & Benjamin, T.L. (1987) Variations in polyoma virus genotype in relation to tumor induction in mice. *Am. J. Pathol.*, 127, 243–261

Defendi, V. & Lehman, J. (1964) Nature of the hemorrhagic lesions induced by polyoma virus in hamsters. *Cancer Res.*, 24, 329–343

Diamandopoulos, G.T. & Enders, J.F. (1966) Comparison of the cytomorphologic characteristics of *in vitro* transformed hamster embryo cells with the histologic features of the neoplasms they induce in the homologous host. *Am. J. Pathol.*, 49, 397–417

Diamandopoulos, G.T. & Sanborn-Redmond, S. (1973) Adenovirus-like transformation of hamster embryo cells mediated by simian virus 40. *Am. J. Pathol.*, 71, 81–92

Dipaolo, J.A. & Donovan, P.J. (1967) Properties of Syrian hamster cells transformed in the presence of carcinogenic hydrocarbons. *Exp. Cell Res.*, 48, 361–377

Dougherty, R.M. (1976) Induction of tumors in Syrian hamsters by a human renal papovavirus RF strain. *J. Natl Cancer Inst.*, 57, 395–400

Duff, R. & Rapp, F. (1971) Properties of hamster embryo fibroblasts transformed *in vitro* after exposure to ultraviolet irradiated herpes simplex virus type 2. *J. Virol.*, 8, 469–477

Duff, R. & Rapp, F. (1973) Oncogenic transformation of hamster embryo cells after exposure to inactivated herpes simplex virus type 1. *J. Virol.*, 12, 209–217

Eddy, B.E., Borman, G.S., Berkeley, W.H. & Young, R.D. (1961) Tumors induced in hamsters by injection of rhesus monkey kidney cell extracts. *Proc. Soc. Exp. Biol. (N.Y.)*, 107, 191–197

Fortner, J.G., Mahy, A.C. & Cotran, R.S. (1961) Transplantable tumors of the Syrian (golden) hamster. Part II. Tumors of the hematopoietic tissues, genitourinary organs, mammary glands and sarcomas. *Cancer Res.*, 21 (part 2), 199–229

Freund, R., Mandel, G., Carmichael, G.G., Barncastle, J.P., Dawe, C.J. & Benjamin, T.L. (1987) Polyomavirus tumor induction in mice – influences of viral coding and noncoding sequences on tumor profiles. *J. Virol.*, 61, 2232–2239

Freund, R., Dawe, C.J. & Benjamin, T.L. (1988) Duplication of noncoding sequences in polyomavirus specifically augments the development of thymic tumors in mice. *J. Virol.*, 62, 3896–3899

Gaugas, J.M., Chesterman, F.C., Hirsch, M.S., Rays, R.J.W., Harvey, J.J. & Gilchrist, C. (1969) Unexpected high incidence of tumours in thymectomized mice treated with anti-lymphocytic globulin and Mycobacterium leprae. *Nature*, 221, 1033–1036

Gye, W.W. & Foulds, L. (1939) A note on the production of sarcomas in hamsters by 3:4-benzpyrene. *Am. J. Cancer*, 35, 108

Haas, H., Mohr, U. & Kruger, F.W. (1973) Comparative studies with different doses of N-nitrosomorpholine, N-nitrosopiperidine, N-nitrosomethylurea and dimethylnitrosamine in Syrian golden hamsters. *J. Natl Cancer Inst.*, 51, 1295–1301

Hadjiolov, D., Hadjiolov, N. & Zur Hausen, H. (1993) The soft tissue tumors induced in Syrian hamsters by herpes simplex virus type 1 and a chemical promoter. *J. Cancer Res.. Clin. Oncol.*, 119, 309–311

Hallowes, R.C., Chesterman, F.C. & West, D.G. (1973) The histogenesis of tumors induced in golden hamsters by murine sarcoma virus-Harvey (MSVH). *Int. J. Cancer*, 12, 705–721

Herrold, K. McD. (1966) Carcinogenic effect of N-methyl-N-nitrosourea administered subcutaneously to Syrian hamsters. *J. Pathol. Bact.*, 92, 35–41

Homburger, F. & Hsueh, S.S. (1970) Rapid induction of fibrosarcomas by 7,12-dimethylbenzanthracene in an inbred line of Syrian hamster. *Cancer Res.*, 30, 1449–1452

Houweling, A., Van den Elsen, P.J. & Van der Eb, A.J. (1980) Partial transformation of primary rat cells by the leftmost 4.5% fragment of adenovirus 5 DNA. *Virology*, 105, 537–550

Huberman, E., Salzberg, S. & Sachs, L. (1968) The in vitro induction of an increase in cell multiplication and cellular life span by the water soluble carcinogen dimethylnitrosamine. *Proc. Natl Acad. Sci. USA*, 59, 77–82

Huebner, R.J., Channock, R.M., Rubin, B.A. & Casey, M.J. (1964) Induction by adenovirus type 7 of tumors in hamsters having the antigenic characteristics of SV 40 virus. *Proc. Natl Acad. Sci. USA*, 52, 1333–1340

Kamahora, J. & Kakunaga, T. (1967) Malignant transformation of hamster embryonic cells in vitro by 4-nitroquinoline-1-oxide. *Biken J.*, 10, 219–242

Kirkman, H. (1962) A preliminary report concerning tumors observed in Syrian hamsters. *Stanford Med. Bull.*, 20, 163–166

Kirschstein, R. & Gerber, P. (1962) Ependymomas produced after intracerebral inoculation of SV 40 into newborn hamsters. *Nature*, 195, 299–300

Kobayashi, M., Sawada, T. & Mukai, N. (1985) Immunochemical evidence of neuron specific enolase (NSE) in human adenovirus 12-induced retinoblastoma-like tumor cells *in vitro*. *Acta Histochem. Cytochem.*, 18, 551–556

Kuhlmann, I., Achten, S., Rudolph, R. & Doerfler, W. (1982) Tumor induction by human adenovirus type 12 in hamsters: loss of the viral genome from adenovirus type 12-induced tumor cells is compatible with tumor formation. *EMBO J.*, 1, 79–86

Kuroki, T. & Sato, H. (1968) Transformation and neoplastic development in vitro of hamster embryonic cells by 4-nitroquinoline-1-oxide and its derivatives. *J. Natl Cancer Inst.*, 41, 53–71

Kyritis, A.P., Tsokos, M., Triche, T.S. & Chader, G.L. (1984) Retinoblastoma-origin from primitive neuroectodermal cell? *Nature*, 307, 471–473

Levenbook, I.S. (1975) The role of the virus in the tumor morphology [in Russian]. *Vop. Virus*, 4, 397–402

Levenbook, I.S. & Strizhachenko, N.M. (1971) Morphology of tumors induced in hamster soft tissues by bovine adenovirus type 3. *Int. J. Cancer*, 8, 531–540

Levenbook, I.S., Kolomietz, O., Polukhina-Nikolaeva, M. & Tsetlin, E. (1974) Rhabdomyosarcomas induced by Rous sarcoma virus in golden hamsters. *Fol. biol. (Praha)*, 20, 238–243

Levenbook, I.S., Kolomiyetz, O.L. & Nikolayeva, M.A. (1982) Ultrastructural and histochemical studies on soft tissue tumours and tumorigenesis induced by oncogenic adenoviruses and Rous sarcoma virus in hamsters. In: Turusov, V.S., ed., *Pathology of Tumours in Laboratory Animals*. Vol. III, *Tumours of the Hamster* (IARC Scientific Publications No. 34), Lyon, IARC, pp. 325–342

Lijinsky, W. & Kovatch, R.M. (1988) Comparative carcinogenesis by nitrosomethylalkylamines in Syrian hamsters. *Cancer Res.*, 48, 6648–6652

Lijinsky, W. & Kovatch, R.M. (1989) The uniform carcinogenic action of alkylnitrosoureas in Syrian hamsters. *Biomed. Environ. Sci.*, 2, 167–173

Michalski, F. & Hsiung, G.D. (1975) Malignant transformation of hamster cells following infection with a bovine herpesvirus (infectious bovine rhinotracheitis virus). *Proc. Soc. Exp. Biol. (N.Y.)*, 148, 891–896

Michalski, F.J., Fond, C.K.Y., Hsiung, G.D., Schneider, R.D. & Kaplow, L.S. (1976) Induction of angioid sarcoma and fibrosarcoma by a guinea-pig herpes virus-transformed hamster cell line. *Bibl. haemat.*, 43, 400–402

Miller, E.C., Miller, J.A. & Enomoto, M. (1964) The comparative carcinogenicities of 2-acetylaminofluorene and its *N*-hydroxy metabolite in mice, hamsters and guinea-pigs. *Cancer Res.*, 24, 2018–2026

Moloney, J.B. (1966) A virus induced rhabdomyosarcoma of mice. *Natl Cancer Inst. Monogr.*, 22, 139–142

Mori, T., Sakai, T., Okamoto, T., Tamura, N., Nozue, Y., Ishida, T & Umeda, M. (1966) Preliminary report on a spindle-cell sarcoma in the Syrian hamster produced by Thorotrast. *Gann*, 57, 431–433

Nase, L.M., Karkkairen, M. & Mantyjarvi, R.A. (1975) Transplantable hamster tumors induced with the BK virus. *Acta pathol. microbiol. scand.*, B83, 347–352

Nettleship, A. & Smith, A.G. (1950) Studies on the early phase of induced fibrosarcoma in the hamster. *Proc. Soc. Exp. Biol. (N.Y.)*, 74, 800–802

O'Brien, J.E. & Stout, A.P. (1964) Malignant fibrous xanthomas. *Cancer*, 17, 1445–1458

Ogawa, K. (1989) Embryonal neuroepithelial tumors induced by human adenovirus type 12 in rodents. I. Tumour induction in the peripheral nervous system. *Acta Neuropathol.*, 77, 244–253

Ogawa, K., Tsutsumi, A., Iwata, K., Fujii, Y., Ohmori, M., Taguchi, K. & Yabe, Y. (1966) Histogenesis of malignant neoplasm induced by adenovirus type 12. *Gann*, 57, 43–52

Ornity, D.M., Palmiter, R.D., Messing, A., Hammer, R.D., Pinkert, C.A. & Brinster, R.L. (1985) Elastase I promotor directs expression of human growth hormone and SV40 T antigen genes to pancreatic acinar cells in transgenic mice. *Cold Spring Harbor Symp. Quant. Biol.*, 50, 399–409

Perk, K. & Hod, I. (1971) Comparative pathology and ultrastructure of rodent sarcomas induced by the murine sarcoma virus (Moloney). *J. Comp. Pathol.*, 81, 173–182

Rassoulzadegan, M., Cowie, A., Carr, A., Glaichenhaus, N., Kamen, R. & Cuzin, F. (1982) The roles of individual polyoma virus early proteins in oncogenic transformation. *Nature*, 300, 713–718

Ruffolo, P.R. & Kirkman, H. (1965) Malignant, transplantable giant cell tumors of periarticular connective tissues in Syrian golden hamsters (*Mesocricetus auratus*). *Br. J. Cancer*, 19, 573–580

Schmidt, D., Leuschner, I., Harms, D., Sprenger, E. & Schafer, H.-J. (1989) Malignant rhabdoid tumor. A morphological and flow cytometric study. *Pathol. Res. Pract.*, 184, 202–210

Shah, K.V., Daniel, R.W. & Strandberg, V.O. (1975) Sarcoma in a hamster with BK virus, a human papova virus. *J. Natl Cancer Inst.*, 54, 945–950

Siegler, R. (1970) Pathogenesis of virus induced murine sarcoma. I. Light microscopy. *J. Natl Cancer Inst.*, 45, 135–137

Stanton, M.F. & Otsuka, H. (1963) Morphology of the oncogenic response of hamsters to polyoma virus infection. *J. Natl Cancer Inst.*, 31, 365–409

Stanton, M.F., Law, L.W. & Ting, R.C. (1968) Some biologic, immunologic and morphologic effects in mice after infection with a murine sarcoma virus. II. Morphological studies. *J. Natl Cancer Inst.*, 40, 1113–1129

Stoker, M. & MacPherson, I. (1964) Syrian hamster fibroblast cell line BHK21 and its derivatives. *Nature*, 203, 1355–1357

Strohl, W.A., Rabson, A.S. & Rouse, H. (1967) Adenovirus tumorigenesis: Role of the viral genome in determining tumor morphology. *Science*, 156, 1631–1633

Suda, Y., Aizawa, S., Hirai, S-I., Inoue, T., Furuta, Y., Suzuki, M., Hirohashi, S. & Ikawa, Y. (1987) Driven by the same Ig enhancer and SV40 T promoter ras induced lung adenomatous tumors, myc induced pre-B cell lymphomas and SV40 large T gene a variety of tumors in transgenic mice. *EMBO J.*, 6, 4055–4065

Treisman, R., Novak, U., Favaloro, J. & Kamen, R. (1981) Transformation of rat cells by an altered polyoma virus genome expressing only the middle T protein. *Nature*, 292, 595–600

Trentin, J.J., Yabe, Y. & Taylor, G. (1962) The quest for human tumor viruses. *Science*, 137, 835–841

Tsuneyoshi, M., Daimaru, Y., Hashimoto, H. & Enjoji, M. (1985) Malignant soft tissue neoplasms with the histologic features of renal rhabdoid tumors: an ultrastructural and immunohistochemical study. *Human Pathol.*, 16, 1235–1242

Van Hoosier, G.L., Jr & Trentin, J.J. (1979) Spontaneous tumor development: hamster. In: Altman, P.L. & Katz, D.D., eds, *Biological Handbooks*, III. *Inbred and Genetically Defined Strains of Laboratory Animals*. Part 2, *Hamster, Guinea Pig, Rabbit and Chicken*, Bethesda, MD, Federation of American Societies for Experimental Bio-logy, pp. 480–484

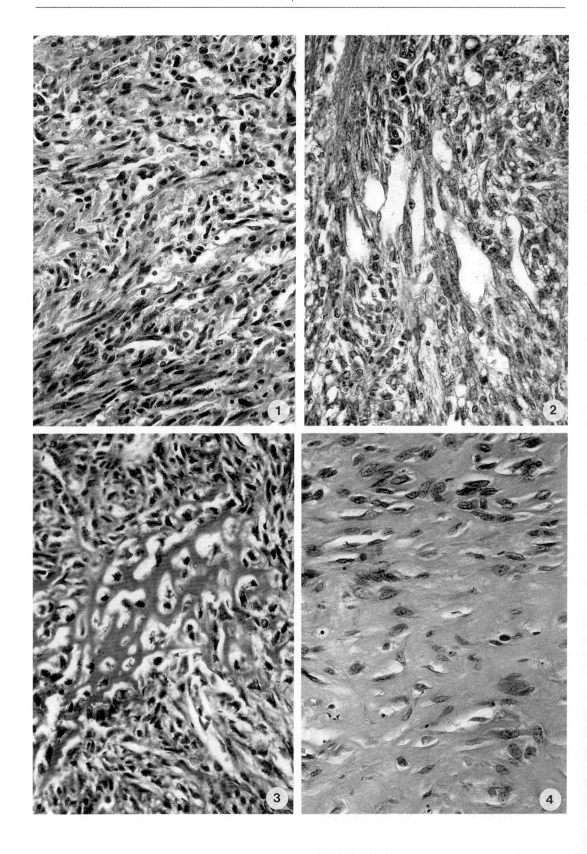

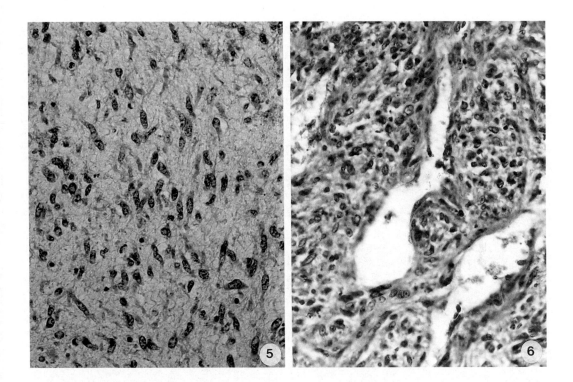

Figure 1. Spontaneous pleomorphic high-grade fibrosarcoma. H & E; × 250

Figure 2. Spontaneous fibrosarcoma with a local haemangiopericytomatous pattern. H & E; × 250

Figure 3. Spontaneous fibrosarcoma with a focal osteogenic pattern.H & E; × 250

Figure 4. Spontaneous low-grade collagenized fibrosarcoma. H & E; × 250

Figure 5. Spontaneous fibrosarcoma with a myxoid pattern. H & E; × 250

Figure 6. Spontaneous haemangiopericytoma. H & E; × 250

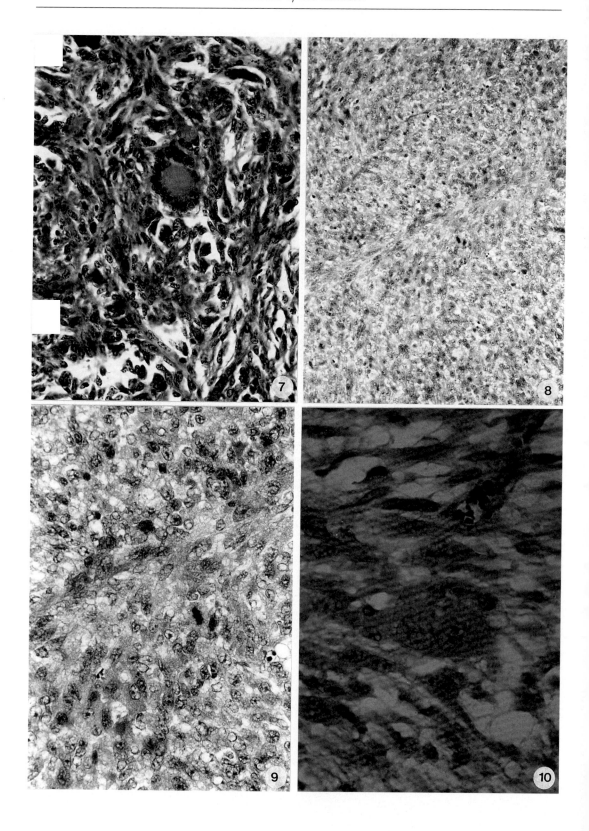

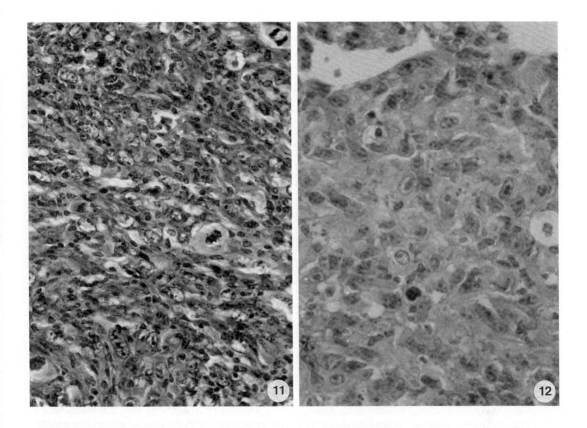

Figure 7. Spontaneous fibrous histiocytoma with characteristic Touton giant cell. H & E; × 250

Figure 8. Benzo[*a*]pyrene-induced tumour. Malignant fibrous histiocytoma with a fascicular pattern. H & E; × 100

Figure 9. Higher magnification of tumour in Figure 8, showing bubbly vesicular nuclei with mitoses. H & E; × 250

Figure 10. Methylcholanthrene-induced tumour. Characteristic giant cell with bubbly nuclei and indistinct borders. H & E; × 400

Figure 11. Nitrosourea-induced tumour. Dimorphic sarcoma (malignant fibrous histiocytoma). Large and small cells with larger rounded cells in mitoses. H & E; × 400

Figure 12. Thorotrast-induced tumour. Pleomorphic polygonal sarcoma (malignant fibrous histiocytoma). Prominent single macronucleoli. H & E; × 400

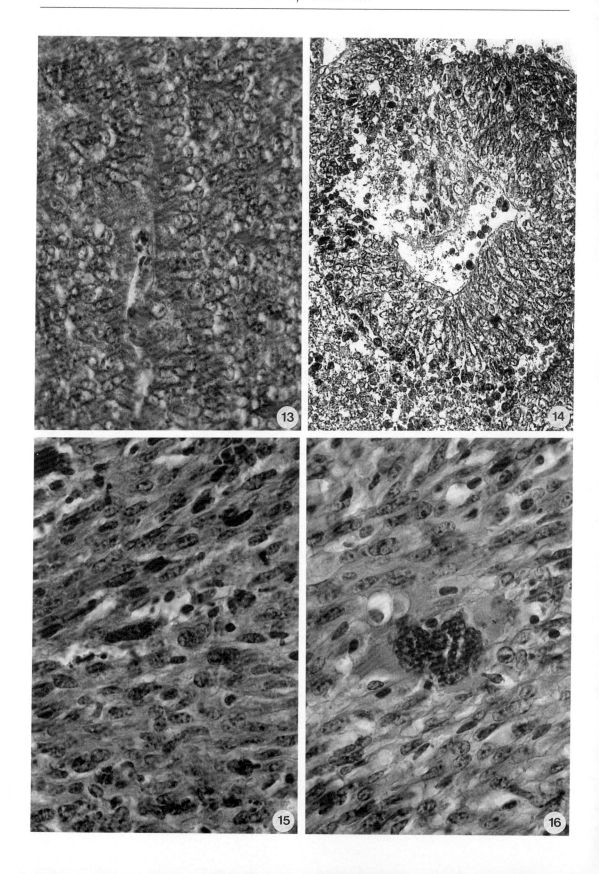

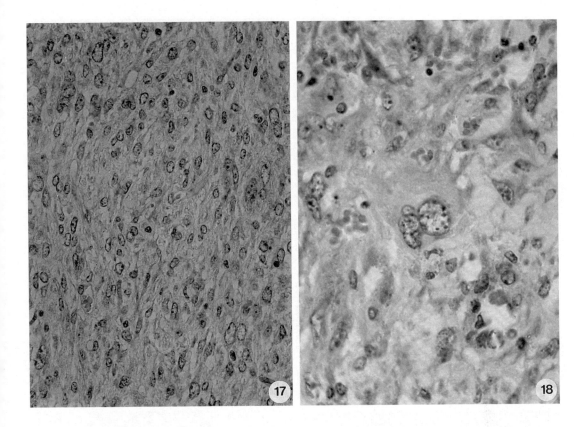

Figure 13. Human adenovirus type 3 tumour. Sheets of small undifferentiated small cells with 'salt and pepper' nuclei. Cells are palisading around a small vascular channel. H & E; × 400

Figure 14. Human adenovirus type 3 tumour. Tumour cells rosetting around a small vessel. On one side the vascular wall is disrupted. H & E; × 250

Figure 15. SV40 virus tumour. Pleomorphic malignant fibrous histiocytoma. H & E; × 400

Figure 16. SV40 virus tumour. Characteristic giant cell with fused pyknotic nuclear structure. H & E; × 400

Figure 17. Polyomavirus tumour. Pleomorphic malignant fibrous histiocytoma. H & E; × 250

Figure 18. Polyomavirus tumour. Characteristic giant cell with four vesicular nuclei. H & E; × 400

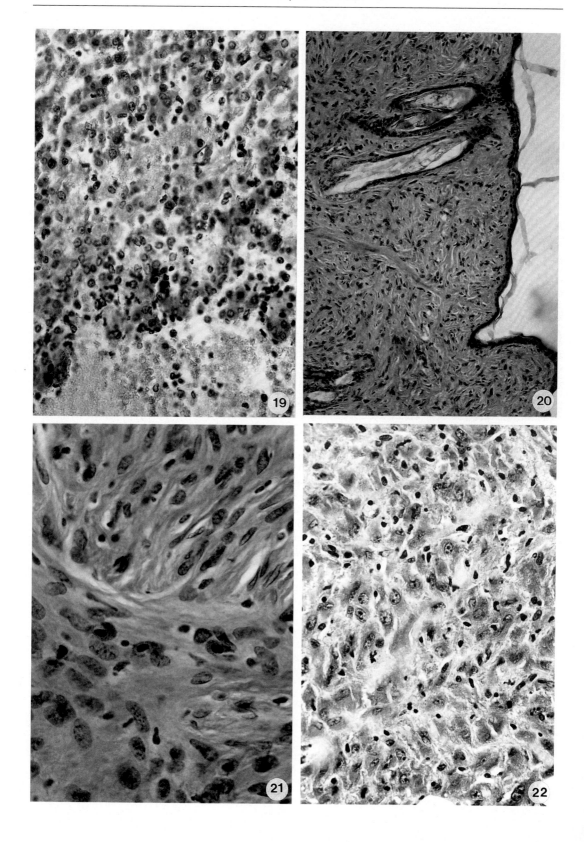

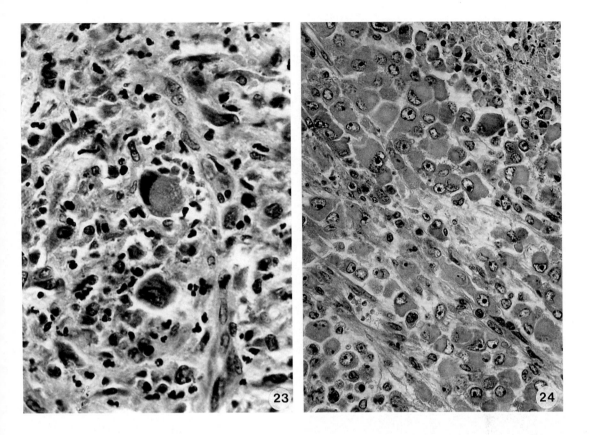

Figure 19. Polyomavirus. Liver lesion. Haemorrhagic cavity (bottom) being formed by disruption of liver cell cords. H & E; × 250

Figure 20. Bovine papillomavirus tumour. Marked dermal thickening with infiltration of bland fibroblastoid cells surrounding adnexal structures. Atrophy of overlying epidermis. H & E; × 100

Figure 21. Bovine papillomavirus tumour. Fibroblastoid cells growing in a storiform pattern. Small dark nuclei superimposed on larger tumour cell nuclei. H & E; × 400

Figure 22. Rous sarcoma virus (Schmidt–Ruppin) tumour. Pleomorphic sarcoma with scattered inflammatory cells. H & E; × 250

Figure 23. Rous sarcoma virus (Schmidt–Ruppin) tumour. Round giant cell with central nodular cytoplasmic concretion. A scattered acute inflammatory infiltrate is apparent. H & E; × 400

Figure 24. Murine sarcoma virus (Moloney) tumour. Pleomorphic round cell sarcoma. Many cells with a single macronucleolus. H & E; × 250

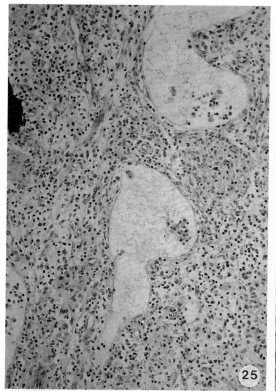

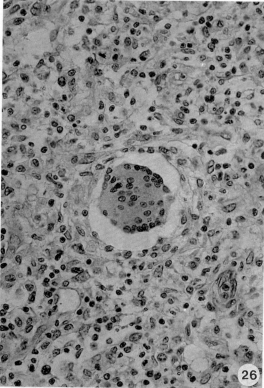

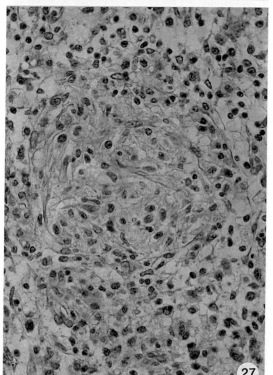

Figure 25. Murine sarcoma virus (Moloney) tumour. Fibrous histiocytoma with angiomatous formations. H & E; × 100

Figure 26. Murine sarcoma virus (Moloney) tumour. Fibrous histiocytoma with typical Touton-type giant cell projecting into an angiomatous space. H & E; × 400

Figure 27. Murine sarcoma virus (Moloney) tumour. Whorled nodule of tumour cells. H & E; × 250

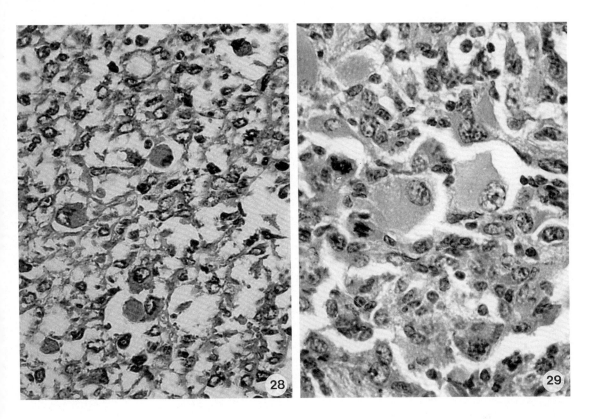

Figure 28. BHK 21/C13. Spontaneously transformed cell tumour. Pleomorphic fibrosarcoma with characteristic cell rounding. H & E; × 400

Figure 29. Tumour induced by herpes simplex virus-transformed cells. Pleomorphic spindle cell sarcoma with characteristic mononuclear giant cells. H & E; × 400

Ultrastructure of virus-induced soft-tissue tumours

I.S. LEVENBOOK AND O.L. KOLOMIYETS

Only a small number of studies on the ultrastructural characteristics of the soft-tissue tumours of hamsters have been reported. They deal mainly with virus-induced tumours. No new studies have appeared since the publication of the first edition. In this revision, we have elected to delete studies of histochemistry, as the later studies of immunohistochemistry are covered in other chapters.

TUMOURS INDUCED BY ADENOVIRUSES OF MAMMALS

The ultrastructure of tumours induced by human adenovirus type 12 was described by Ogawa et al. (1966) and Chino et al. (1967). Ogawa et al. (1966) reported that these tumours were of neuroectodermal nature and, specifically, noted the presence of desmosomes and digitiform recesses in the contact zones of the tumour cells. They stressed that similar structures have been observed in human schwannomas. Chino et al. (1967) observed viral particles in the cytoplasm of local mesenchymal cells as early as two hours after subcutaneous injection. Some of these cells were subsequently transformed into tumour cells. They described the tumours as consisting of poorly differentiated cells with multiple processes and numerous pinocytotic vesicles located along their plasma membrane. In contrast to the findings of Ogawa et al. (1966), they did not find any desmosomes

in the zones of cellular contact. No basal lamina was noted around the cells, but electron-dense material was present in the narrow intercellular spaces. It was concluded that mesenchymal cells were the target cells for this oncogenic virus.

The ultrastructure of tumours induced by simian adenovirus 30 was described by Merkow et al. (1968). These tumours consisted of large, poorly differentiated cells capable of synthesizing collagenous fibres and were likely of mesenchymal origin. Annulate lamellae and virus-like particles were found in both the nucleus and the cytoplasm of these cells. Ohmori et al. (1972), studying transplanted tumours initially induced by bovine adenovirus type 3, noted the presence of cilia and desmosomes in the contact zones of the tumour cells, which they considered indicative of an epithelial origin for these tumours. Our findings (Levenbook, 1972), based on the use of a variety of special stains, led us to believe that tumours induced by simian adeno-viruses constitute poorly differentiated malignant haemangiopericytomas tending to differentiate into leio- (angioleio-) myosarcomas (Figures 1 and 2).

Most of the tumours induced by bovine adenovirus type 3 (BA3) were also, in our opinion, poorly differentiated haemangiopericytomas with leiomyo-sarcomatous areas (Figure 3) (Levenbook & Strizhachenko, 1971). In many of these tumours, the cytoplasm of many cells was vacuolated, but had little stainable poly-saccharide content, and almost no stainable fat. The extensively distributed capillaries of these tumours were always lined with only one layer of rather typical endothelial cells corresponding to the original description by Stout and Murray (1942).

The tumours induced by simian adenovirus SA7 (C8) and by BA3, diag-nosed by us as haemangiopericytomas, were ultrastructurally similar. We also found typical capillaries which were sur-rounded by basal lamina. Maculae occlu-dentes were identified in the contact zones of usually normal cells. Not infrequently, however, the basal laminae surrounding the capillaries were loosened (Figure 4) and in a number of endothelial cells the cytoplasmic matrix and mitochondria were swollen. Fine fibrillar material coated the surface of many tumour cells.

During the early stages of growth, the tumours consisted of poorly differentiated round or polygonal cells with large nuclei with dispersed fine chromatin. The cells had a scanty cytoplasm, numerous free ribosomes, centrioles, a poorly developed Golgi complex and mitochondria with a greatly swollen matrix and contracted intermembranous space (Figure 5). With further growth, the tumours were com-posed predominantly of poorly dif-ferentiated elongated cells (Figure 6). Fibroblast-like cells were also present and had a highly developed granular endo-plasmic reticulum and bundles of fila-ments 3–7 nm in diameter, located mostly in the cytoplasmic processes. In some cells, these bundles were associated with dark bodies, either suspended in the cytoplasm or associated with the plasma membrane (Figure 7). Pinocytotic vesicles were sometimes seen along the plasma membrane.

Individual cells similar to smooth-muscle cells were observed, especially in more slowly growing tumours induced by

the large-plaque variant (Altstein *et al.*, 1969) of SA7 (C8) virus. Their cytoplasm contained bundles of short thin (4–8 nm in diameter) and thick (12–16 nm in diameter) filaments sometimes associated with dark bodies (Figure 8), numerous free ribosomes, a poorly developed Golgi complex, and rough endoplasmic reti-culum. Pinocytotic vesicles were located along the plasma membranes. Some of these cells were partially surrounded by a basal lamina which was fragmented and poorly defined in some areas. Cells of transitional type, intermediate between fibroblasts and smooth-muscle cells, were also encountered. Such cells have been described in some leiomyomas of humans (Apatenko *et al.*, 1974).

After prolonged cultivation *in vitro* (more than 50 passages) of a BA3-induced haemangiopericytoma, Graevskaja *et al.* (1972) established a permanent cell line (HTC). These cells, when inoculated sub-cutaneously in hamsters, produced tu-mours that, by light microscopy, had features typical of a leiomyosarcoma (Figure 9). From this it was inferred that a haemangiopericytoma can precede smooth-muscle tumour development. This assumption conforms to the quite wide-spread opinion that it is possible for pericytes to differentiate into smooth-muscle cells, both in normal and patho-logical conditions, including those of tumour growth (Stout, 1956; Movat & Fernando, 1964; Kuhn & Rosai, 1969; Hahn *et al.*, 1973).

The ultrastructural cell types of the HTC tumours included some smooth-muscle-type cells with bundles of thin filaments and individual thick filaments in their cytoplasm. Bundles of such filaments were associated with dark bodies (Figure 10). In the contact zones of these cells, local densities were observed in the cyto-plasmic areas adjoining the plasma membrane. Between plasma membranes, there was single- or multi-layered electron-dense material, and an intermittent basal lamina surrounded the cells. Some areas consisted of round cells, with cytoplasmic free ribosomes, individual mitochondria, and bundles of filaments 8–10 nm in diameter. In their contact zones, adhesion of opposing plasma membranes was observed.

In all the tumours described above, many cells had cytoplasmic myelin-like structures (Figure 11), annulate lamellae (Figure 12), pentalamellar formations, and cilia with bundles of densely packed filaments 7–8 nm in diameter (Figure 13). Kalnins *et al.* (1967) and Stich and John (1969) described such filaments in the cells of tumours induced in hamsters by human and simian adenoviruses. Since these filaments were also found in cultures of transformed cells, and in cells acutely infected by adenoviruses, and because they reacted with ferritin-labelled antibodies to adenovirus T antigen, the authors concluded that these filaments could be regarded as a manifestation of viral infection. Cilia (Welsh & Meyer, 1969; Ferenczy *et al.*, 1971) and myelin-like formations (Apatenko *et al.*, 1974) have been observed in some human tumours of smooth-muscle origin. Cilia also were described by Sorokin (1962) in embryonal smooth-muscle cells cultivated *in vitro*.

TUMOURS INDUCED BY ROUS SARCOMA VIRUS

The ultrastructure of tumours induced by Rous sarcoma virus (RSV) in hamsters was described by Lindberg (1969). Two types of cells were identified as the basic elements of these lesions. Cells of the A type, ultrastructurally indistinguishable from fibroblasts, had large round or oval nuclei. The cytoplasmic elements of these cells included a well developed granular endoplasmic reticulum, a moderately developed Golgi complex, and fibrillae. Cells of the C type contained oval or round nuclei, and scanty cytoplasm. The author designated these lesions as

fusiform-cellular sarcomas and suggested that the A-type cells were purely neoplastic, whereas the C cells might be stromal cells occurring in the tumour during the course of its growth. He did not, however, rule out the possibility of interconversion between them.

By light microscopy, these tumours were identified by us as rhabdomyosarcomas, predominantly of the embryonal type (Levenbook *et al.*, 1974) (Figures 14 and 15). The cytoplasm of some of the fusiform cells stained red with azan after Heidenhain, similar to the sarcoplasmal staining of muscle cells. In PAS-stained sections, granular and pulverized PAS-positive material was observed, which disappeared after pretreatment of the sections with amylase. Silver impregnation according to Gomori demonstrated argyrophile 'cuffs' surrounding the individual cells.

In electron micrographs, we observed cells of different types, with large fusiform cells predominant. Thick bundles of collagenous fibres were present in the intercellular spaces. Most of the cells had elongated nuclei with uneven contours and, sometimes, deep invaginations (Figure 16). The copious cytoplasm was characterized by a highly developed rough endoplasmic reticulum resembling that seen in fibroblasts. In some cells, the canaliculi of the rough endoplasmic reticulum paralleled the long axis of the cell. Mitochondria were not numerous and most of them had a markedly swollen matrix with contracted intermembranous space. Bundles of densely packed filaments, 3–5 nm in diameter, running parallel to each other and to the long axis of the cell, were seen in proximity to the plasma membrane (Figure 17). Identical filaments were described by Auber (1969) in developing skeletal muscles of rats at early stages of embryogenesis, and designated as initial myofilaments with immature Z lines. The same structures were also described by Dalton (1966) in mouse tumours induced by Moloney strain of murine sarcoma virus.

We also found parallel bundles of more loosely arranged filaments (5–7 nm in diameter), corresponding to the diameter of actin, in the large fusiform cells. Electron-dense Z-like lines occurred along the length of these filaments (Figure 18). Individual filaments of greater thickness (12–13 nm in diameter), corresponding to myosin, were also identified in these filaments. Since few filaments were found, no formation of I and A discs, produced by the alternate arrangements of thin and thick myofilaments, was observed. This can explain the difficulty in detecting transverse striations by light microscopy.

In some large fusiform cells there were convoluting bundles of filaments 8–11 nm in diameter (the so-called "100 Å filaments" of Ishikawa *et al.* (1968)) (Figure 19). Such filaments have been described also in experimental (Cencov, 1961; Dalton, 1966; Levy *et al.*, 1969) and human (Raihlin, 1973) rhabdomyosarcomas by many investigators.

Areas consisting of poorly differentiated cells arranged in tandem were often found, as well as some tumours composed mostly of large round cells with some giant multinucleated (5–6 nuclei) cells. No fibrillar structures or cytoplasmic filaments were found in any of these multinuclear giant cells. Filaments of diameter 8–11 nm, irregularly scattered in the cytoplasm, were, however, identified in large mononuclear cells, and were considered features of cytodifferentiation and initial stages of myofibrillogenesis.

REFERENCES

Altstein, A.D., Dodonova, N.N., Tsetlin, E.M., Babakova, S.V. & Levenbook, I.S. (1969) Large- and small-plaque variants of oncogenic simian adenovirus SA7 (C8). *Int. J. Cancer*, 4, 446–454

Apatenko, A.K., Vtjurin, B.V. & Sarkisov, D.S. (1974) On some peculiar features of the ultrastructure of skin leiomyomas [in Russian]. *Arkh. Patol.*, 36, 16–23

Auber, J. (1969) La myofibrillogenèse du muscle strié. 2. Vertèbres. *Microscopie,* 8, 367–390

Cencov, Ju. S. (1961) Some peculiarities of the ultrastructure of experimental tumour cells [in Russian]. *Z. Obshch. Biol.*, 22, 383–387

Chino, F., Tsuruhara, T. & Egashira, G. (1967) Pathological studies on the oncogenesis of adenovirus type 12 in hamsters. *Jap. J. Med. Sci. Biol.*, 20, 483–500

Dalton, A.S. (1966) An electron microscopic study of a virus-induced murine sarcoma (Moloney). *Nat. Cancer Inst. Monogr.*, 22, 143–168

Ferenczy, A., Richan, R. M. & Okagaki, T. (1971) A comparative ultrastructural study of leiomyosarcoma, cellular leiomyoma, and leiomyoma of the uterus. *Cancer*, 28, 1004–1018

Graevskaja, N.A., Strizacenko, N.M., Karmyseva, V.Ja., Gumina, I.I. & Tjufanov, A.V. (1972) Cell lines derived from tumours induced in hamsters by bovine adenovirus type 3 [in Russian]. *Vopr. Onkol.*, 18, 79–83

Hahn, M.D., Dawson, R., Esterly, G.A. & Joseph, D.J. (1973) Hemangiopericytoma: an ultrastructural study. *Cancer*, 31, 255–261

Ishikawa, H., Bischoff, R. & Holtzer, H. (1968) Mitosis and intermediate-sized filaments in developing skeletal muscle. *J. Cell Biol.*, 38, 538–555

Kalnins, V.I., Stich, H.F., Gregory, G. & John, D.I. (1967) Localization of tumor antigens in adenovirus-12-induced tumor cells and in adenovirus-12-infected human and hamster cells by ferritin-labeled antibodies. *Cancer Res.*, 27, 1874–1886

Kuhn, C. & Rosai, J. (1969) Tumors arising from pericytes. Ultrastructure and organ culture. *Arch. Pathol.*, 88, 653–663

Levenbook, I.S. (1972) Induction of angiogenic sarcomas by certain adenoviruses of mammals [in Russian]. *Bjull. Eksp. Biol. Med.*, 10, 71–75

Levenbook, I.S. & Strizhachenko, N.M. (1971) Morphology of tumors induced in hamster soft tissues by bovine adenovirus type 3. *Int. J. Cancer*, 8, 531–540

Levenbook, I.S., Kolomietz, O.L., Polukhina-Nikolaeva, M. & Tsetlin, E. (1974) Rhabdomyosarcomas induced by Rous sarcoma virus in golden hamsters. *Folia biol., Praha,* 20, 238–243

Levy, B.M., Taylor, A.C., Hampton, S. & Thoma, G.W. (1969) Tumors of the marmoset produced by Rous sarcoma virus. *Cancer Res.,* 29, 2237–2248

Lindberg, L.G. (1969) Comparative electron microscopic study of Rous sarcoma in Syrian hamster and rat. *Acta Pathol. Microbiol. Scand.,* 76, 539–566

Merkow, L., Slifkin, M., Pardo, M. & Rapoza, N.P. (1968) The histopathology and ultrastructure of tumors induced by simian adenovirus 30. *Cancer Res.,* 28, 1180–1190

Movat, H.Z. & Fernando, N.V.P. (1964) The fine structure of the terminal vascular bed. IV. The venules and their perivascular cells (pericytes, adventitial cells). *Exp. Molec. Pathol.,* 3, 98–114

Ogawa, K., Tsutsumi, A., Iwata, K., Fujii, J., Ohmori, M., Taguchi, K. & Jabe, J. (1966) Histogenesis of malignant neoplasm induced by adenovirus type 12. *Gann,* 57, 43–52

Ohmori, M., Otsuki, Y. & Ogawa, K. (1972) Brief note. Some characteristic fine structures in the bovine adenovirus-induced tumors. *Acta Med. Okayama,* 26, 75–79

Raihlin, N. T. (1973) Ultrastructural organ-specificity and polymorphism of the cancer cells. *Neoplasma,* 20, 567–568

Sorokin, S. (1962) Centrioles and formation of rudimentary cilia by fibroblasts and smooth muscle cells. *J. Cell Biol.,* 15, 363–377

Stich, H. F. & John, D.J. (1969) Submicroscopic fibrous complexes in adenovirus infected and transformed cells. *Proc. Am. Assoc. Cancer Res.,* 10, 88

Stout, A.P. (1956) Tumors featuring pericytes, glomus tumor and hemangiopericytoma. *Lab. Invest.,* 5, 217–223

Stout, A.P. & Murray, M.R. (1942) Hemangiopericytoma. *Ann. Surg.,* 116, 26–33

Welsh, R.A. & Meyer, A.T. (1969) Ultrastructure of gastric leiomyoma. *Arch. Pathol.,* 87, 71–82

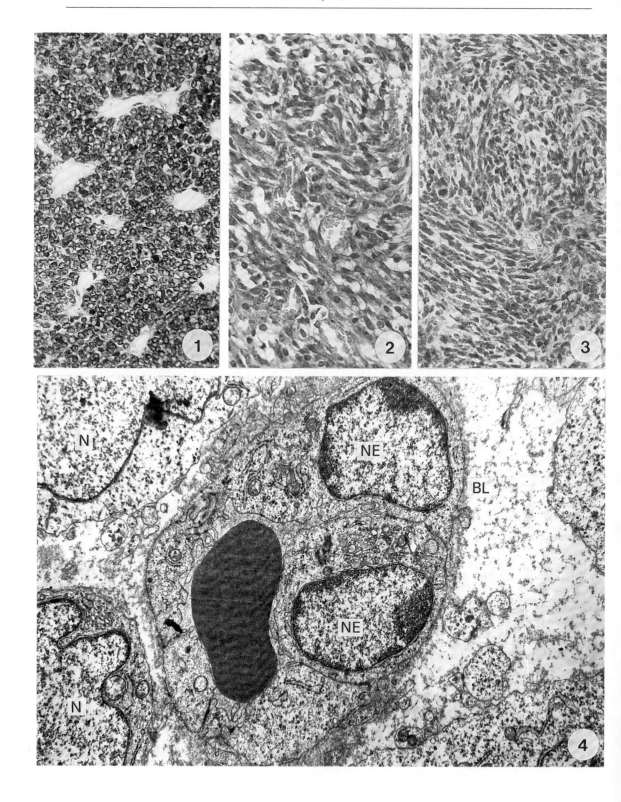

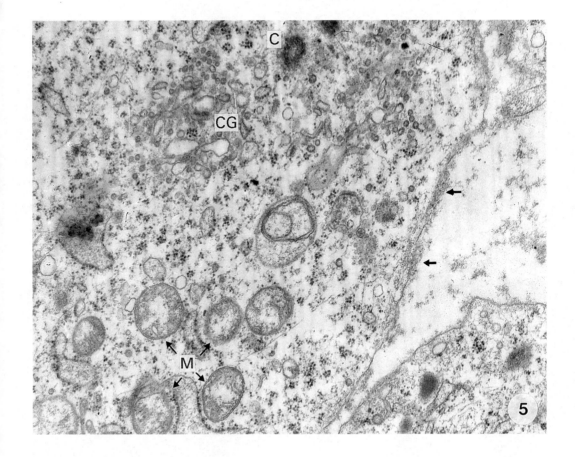

Figures 1–3. Tumours induced by SA7 (C8) and BA3.

Figure 1. SA7 (C8)-induced haemangiopericytoma. Sinusoidal vessels are surrounded by rather monomorphous round cells. H & E; × 345

Figure 2. An area of the same tumour with an angioleiomyosarcomatous structure. Fusiform tumour cells are arranged around vessels (arrows) in whirling bundles. H & E; × 345

Figure 3. Leiomyosarcomatous area of BA3-induced tumour. H & E; × 345

Figures 4–8. Ultrastructure of haemangiopericytomas induced by SA7 (C8)

Figure 4. Pericapillary arrangement of round tumour cells. (NE = nucleus of an endothelial cell; N = nucleus of a tumour cell.) Basal lamina (BL) surrounding the capillary is loosened. Material identical to basal lamina is present in the broad intercellular spaces. × 5200

Figure 5. A cell of the same nodule. Thin fibrillar material (arrows) similar to the basal lamina surrounds the surface of the cell. (CG = Golgi complex; M = mitochondria with swollen matrix and condensed intermembrane space; C = centriole.) × 22 500

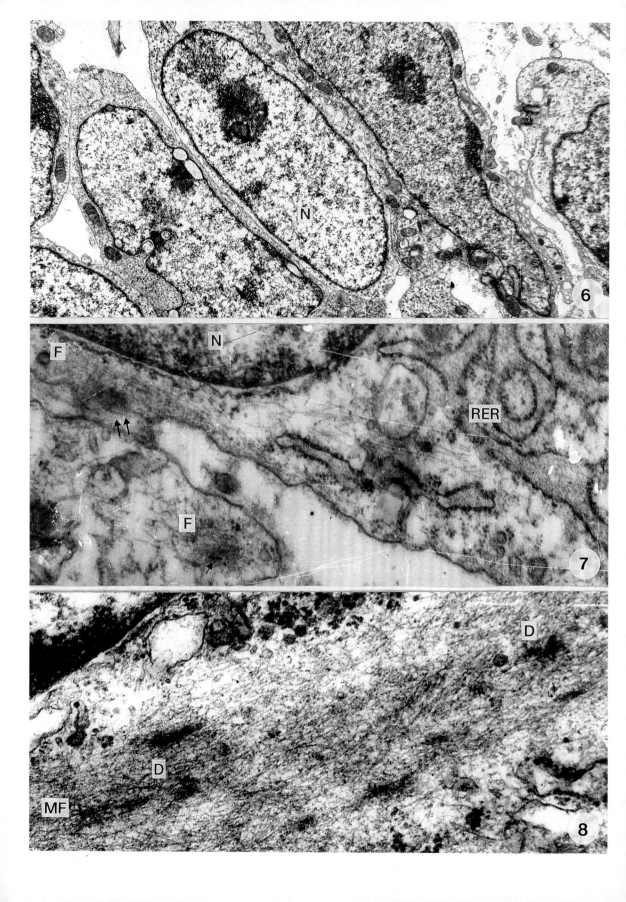

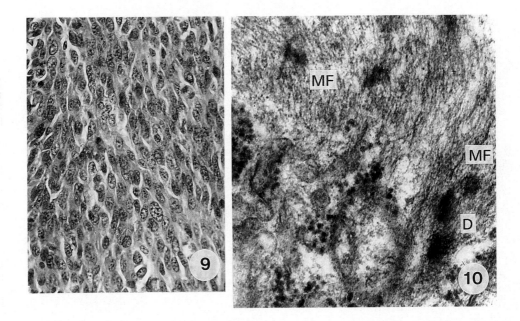

Figure 6. Elongated tumour cells. (N = nucleus.) × 3200

Figure 7. Fibroblast-like cells. (N = nucleus.) Bundles of filaments (F) are associated with dark bodies suspended in the cytoplasm (arrow) or associated with the plasma membrane (two arrows). (RER = rough endoplasmic reticulum.) × 3000

Figure 7. Bundle of myofilaments (MF) associated with dark bodies (D). × 78 000

Figure 9. Leiomyosarcoma induced by inoculation of HTC cells. H & E; × 345

Figures 10–13. Ultrastructure of leiomyosarcomas produced by inoculation of HTC cells

Figure 10. Bundle of myofilaments in a tumour cell. (MF = myofilaments; D = dark bodies.) × 80 400

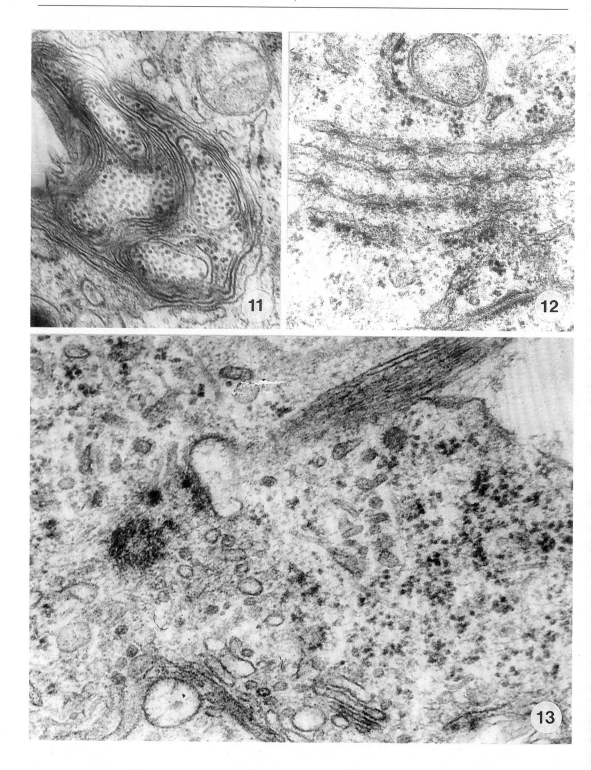

Figure 11. Myelin-like structures in the tumour-cell cytoplasm. × 40 300
Figure 12. Annulate lamellae in the tumour-cell cytoplasm. × 52 500
Figure 13. Cilia containing filaments in the tumour-cell cytoplasm. × 58 500

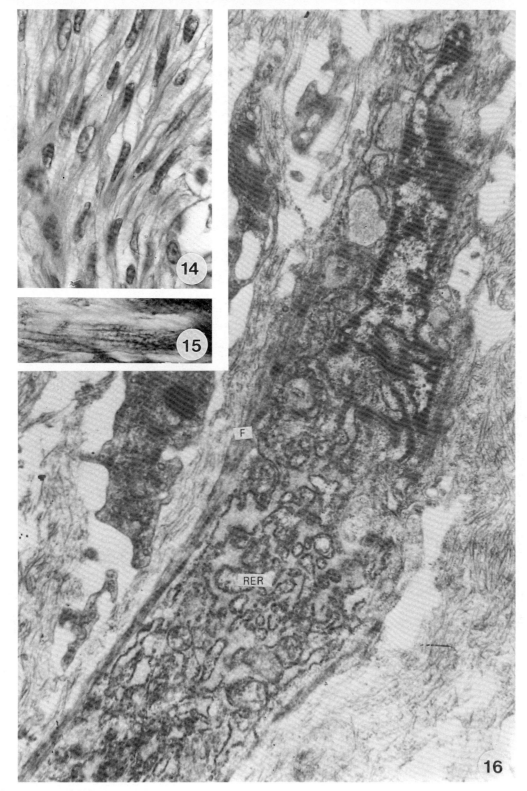

Figures 14–15. RSV-induced tumours

Figure 14. Syncytium of fusiform tumour cells showing rod-shaped nuclei and longitudinal fibrillarity in the cytoplasm. Iron haematoxylin (Heidenhain); × 880

Figure 15. Cross-striated myofibrils in a fusiform cell. Iron haematoxylin (Heidenhain); × 880

Figures 16–20. Ultrastructure of RSV-induced tumours

Figure 16. Fibroblast like cell. (F = filaments; RER = rough endoplasmic reticulum). × 9000

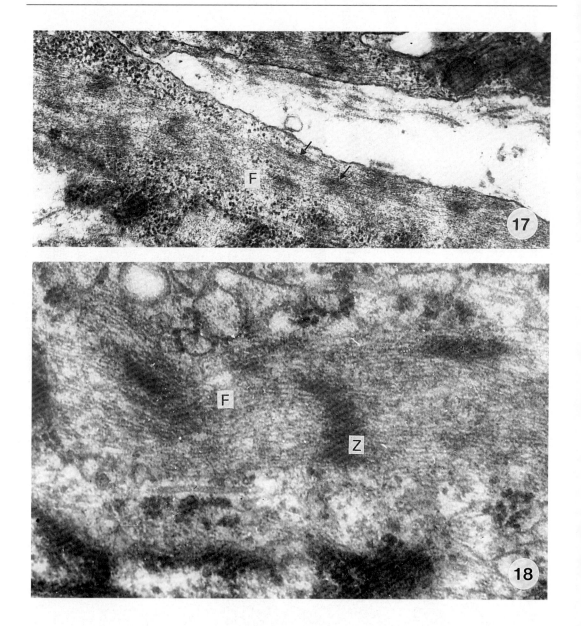

Figure 17. Bundle of filaments (F) 3–7 nm in diameter with electron-dense zones periodically located along the bundle (arrows) × 30 000

Figure 18. Bundle of filaments (F) 5–7 nm in diameter with immature Z lines (Z). × 62 000

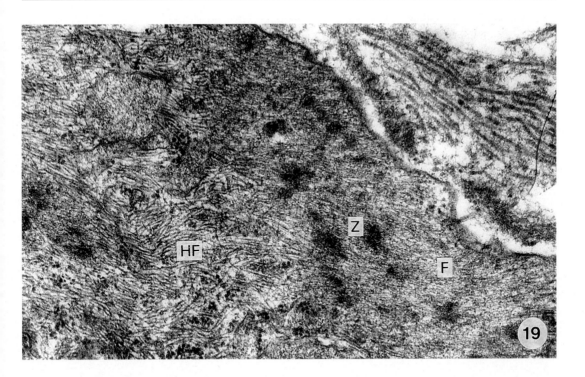

Figure 19. Irregularly oriented bundles of "100 Å filaments" (HF) near the bundles of other filaments (F) 5–7 nm in diameter and Z-like zones (Z). × 35 700

Tumours of the haematopoietic system

S.W. Barthold

Tumours of the haematopoietic system are an important group of tumours in the hamster from a number of perspectives. Tumours of lymphoreticular origin are among the most common spontaneous tumours in aged hamsters and appear to be the most frequent malignant neoplasm. Lymphoreticular tumours have also been induced experimentally by a number of means, including X-irradiation, chemical carcinogens, viruses and tissue extracts. Their relatively high rate of occurrence in untreated hamsters has often obscured the significance of their induction by experimental means. These tumours often contain a number of virus-like particles of unknown biological significance. A virus of clear significance is hamster papovavirus, which can cause epizootics or enzootics of transmissible lymphoma. It has confounded a number of hamster experiments, including ones investigating its own pathogenesis.

NORMAL STRUCTURE AND FUNCTION

During early mammalian embryonic development, mesenchymal stem cells form blood islands in the yolk sac. Cells from these sites enter the embryonic plasma and colonize the liver, then spleen, lymph nodes and bone marrow. These pleuripotential stem cells give rise to two lineages of stem cells: multipotential myeloid stem cells and lymphoid-committed stem cells. Multipotential myeloid stem cells differentiate into progenitor committed cells for erythrocytic and myeloid lines. Recent evidence has suggested that neutrophilic granulocytes and monocytes arise from a common granuloid progenitor cell, which is separate from eosinophilic and megakary-ocytic progenitor cells. Monocytes circulate in the blood, enter tissues and become the activated macrophages of alveoli, liver (Kupffer's cells), spleen and other sites (Bell, 1987). This is an important consideration in classification of haemolymphatic tumours, which reflect aberrations of these developmental sequences.

The developmental sequence of progenitor to functional cells has been deduced from functional studies *in vitro*. Standard morphological criteria are not useful, since progenitor cells are not recognizable in bone marrow smears. They resemble early lymphoid series cells with fine chromatin, nucleoli and scant blue, non-granulated cytoplasm. Haematopoiesis takes place in the extravascular space, with migration of mature cells through sinusoidal endothelium, regardless of tissue site (Bell, 1987).

Hamster bone marrow resembles that of other rodents. In pups less than one week old, bone marrow is predominantly erythroid, but the myeloid:erythroid ratio shifts to 8–10:1 in adults. In adults, marrow of long bones become inactive (fatty). Hamster haemolymphatic cells are not notably unique, except for a large number of ring- or doughnut-shaped nuclei in immature granulocytes. Neutrophils possess finely granulated, acidophilic

365

cytoplasm, which must be differentiated from eosinophils. Extramedullary haematopoiesis is active in the splenic red pulp of newborn hamsters, as well as modest activity in liver. Haematopoietic activity is usually absent from livers by weaning age and decreases in spleen, but foci of activity may remain in adult spleens (Desai, 1968; Tomson & Wardrop, 1987).

Haematology of hamsters has been thoroughly reviewed elsewhere, and normal values are available in these references for Syrian hamsters (Desai, 1968; Tomson & Wardrop, 1987) as well as European hamsters (Mohr & Ernst, 1987). At birth, Syrian hamsters are relatively anaemic, but normal values are attained by 8–9 weeks of age. Adult peripheral blood leukocytes range around 7–8000/ml, with lymphocytes representing approximately 70% of the relative count and neutrophils up to 30%, with only approximately 1–2% eosinophils and monocytes. Basophils are extremely rare.

The lymphoreticular system of hamsters is anatomically similar to that of other rodents. At birth, the lymphoreticular system is functionally and morphologically immature. Cortical and medullary differentiation in the thymus does not begin until three days of age and normal morphology is not attained until nine days. Lymphocytic population of spleen and lymph nodes is minimal at birth. The immunological response of neonatal hamsters is, not surprisingly, immature and does not attain full competence until well after weaning (Streilein, 1987).

MORPHOLOGY AND BIOLOGY OF TUMOURS

Haemolymphatic tumours have been subjected to a number of classification schemes, and debate over classification and terminology continues. In the past, classification schemes have relied on morphology, but current terminology with cytochemical markers is revealing the

inaccuracy of morphological criteria. For example, so-called histiocytic tumours (based on morphology) are usually of lymphoid lineage. In more extensively studied species such as the mouse, older morphological classification schemes have merged with contemporary immunohistochemical classification schemes to allow an accurate and unified immunomorphological classification scheme (Table 1) that also attempts to correlate mouse tumour types with equally well studied human lymphomas and leukaemias (Frith *et al.*, 1985). Such a system for hamster tumours would be desirable, but at present remains impossible. Attempts to merge morphological criteria alone from the hamster literature into the murine or human immunomorphological scheme would only create inaccuracy. Cytochemical markers have not been generally applied to hamster tumours, although T and B cell markers have been defined on epizootic lymphomas in hamsters (Coggin *et al.*, 1983). Complex morphological classification is useful with human tumours, where accurate correlation with clinical course is known and important, but imposition of these criteria on hamster tumours is inappropriate. Until better methods and data are available, hamster tumours can only be classified in as simple a scheme as possible. Furthermore, grouping of tumour types under a simplified scheme allows better analysis of the past literature, which often lacks detailed description.

Although not perfect, the WHO classification of haematopoietic and lymphoid tissue neoplasia seems the most suitable for hamster oncology (Jarrett & Mackey, 1974). This system is based solely on morphology and allows classification of tumours between species, using common terminology (Table 2). Cytochemical classification of tumours should be used whenever possible, but is likely to be independent of this classification scheme. Lymphoid neoplasia is represented in the hamster as lymphosarcoma, lymphoid leukaemia, tumours of immunoglobulin-forming cells and thymoma. A few cases of myeloid neoplasia and myelosclerosis have been reported. Only entities that have been found in hamsters will be defined in this chapter. Details of these categories of neoplasia are readily available elsewhere (Jarrett & Mackey, 1974; Jones & Hunt, 1983; Moulton & Dungworth, 1978). In spite of this classification scheme, terms will be used interchangeably in this chapter to reflect various authors' terminology.

Lymphosarcoma is generally applied to animal neoplasms, and is synonymous with malignant lymphoma in humans. The term lymphosarcoma was once used in humans to designate a specific pattern of lymphoma, and thus unfortunately has not been universally applied as a general term in human lymphoid neoplasia. Lymphosarcomas are solid masses of fleshy, uniform-textured tumours in lymph nodes, spleen, thymus, bone marrow and

Table 1. Immunomorphologic classification of haemolymphatic tumours of mice (after Frith *et al.*, 1985)

Lymphoid neoplasms

   B-cell lymphoma
      Small lymphocyte
      Lymphoblastic
      Follicular centre cell
         Small
         Large
         Mixed (small and large)
      Plasma cell
      Immunoblastic
   T-cell lymphoma
      Lymphoblastic
   Non-T, non-B-cell lymphoma
      Lymphoblastic

Granulocytic leukaemia

Mast cell tumours

Thymoma

Metastatic neoplasms

Table 2. Histological classification and nomenclature of haemolymphatic tumours (after Jarrett & Mackey, 1974)

Lymphoid neoplasms	*Myeloid neoplasms*
*A. Lymphosarcoma	*A. Myeloid leukaemia
1. Poorly differentiated	1. Poorly differentiated
2. Lymphoblastic	2. Well differentiated
3. Lymphocytic and prolymphocytic	a. neutrophilic
4. Histiocytic, histioblastic, and histiolymphocytic	b. eosinophilic
*B. Lymphoid leukaemia	B. Erythroleukaemia
C. Nodular lymphoid hyperplasia of the canine spleen	C. Acute erythraemia (di Guglielmo)
*D. Tumours of immunoglobulin-forming cells	D. Polycythaemia vera
1. Solitary plasmacytoma	E. Megakaryocytoid leukaemia
2. Myeloma	F. Panmyelosis
3. Primary macroglobulinaemia (Waldenstrom)	*G. Myelosclerosis
*E. Thymoma	H. Myeloproliferative disease
1. Predominantly epithelial	I. Monocytic (monocytoid) leukaemia
2. Predominantly lymphocytic	
	Mast cell neoplasms
	A. Mastocytoma
	B. Malignant mastocytosis

* Groups represented in hamsters (see text)

other organs. They are usually multicentric, but there can be alimentary, thymic or other forms. They represent neoplasia of lymphoid cells, and thus are subclassified morphologically by cell type: poorly differentiated, lymphoblastic, lymphocytic (Figure 1) or histiocytic (Figure 2), although they are often mixed and may change as the course of disease progresses. Histiocytic lymphosarcomas were formerly designated reticulum cell sarcomas. This type of tumour displays considerable cellular pleomorphism. Cells usually possess large vesicular nuclei with prominent nucleoli and varying amounts of acidophilic or amphophilic cytoplasm. Reticulum fibres and phagocytosis can be present, but not consistently. The volume of cytoplasm, size and number of nuclei and nucleoli can be quite variable, with giant cells sometimes formed. Pleomorphism gives rise to Reed–Sternberg-like cells, which are commonly seen in Hodgkin's disease in humans. Since similar cells arise in hamster lymphosarcomas, the term 'Hodgkin's-like' has been used, but should be avoided, since the term refers to a specific clinical entity in humans. Histiocytic lymphosarcomas are probably heterogeneous with regard to cell of origin, and most represent transformed lymphocytes or immunoblasts, rather than true histiocytes. The term should thus be viewed as expedient, rather than functionally accurate.

Lymphoid leukaemia refers to primary neoplasia of bone marrow involving lymphoid cells, with haematogenous (leukaemic) growth (Figure 3). Cell types should be classified morphologically, as in lymphosarcomas. This may be an arbitrary distinction, since involvement of bone marrow and blood can take place in multicentric lymphosarcoma.

Tumours of immunoglobulin-forming cells are composed of lymphoid cells that have sufficient differentiation to produce immunoglobulins. The cells thus morphologically resemble plasma cells, with eccentric dark nuclei with coarsely clumped chromatin and variable staining affinity of the cytoplasm (Figure 4). In poorly differentiated tumours, only a few of the cells may resemble plasma cells. Solitary plasmacytomas are apparently benign and localized to lymph nodes. In contrast, myelomas are less well differentiated and multicentric, usually involving bone marrow and other sites.

Thymomas are benign, localized tumours which arise from epithelial or lymphocytic components of the thymus, and often possess both cell types. Lymphosarcoma involving the thymus is more common, and can be distinguished by its malignant growth characteristics.

Myeloid neoplasms will not be described in detail. These tumours involve cells of the granulocyte, monocyte, erythrocyte and megakaryocyte series. They thus arise in bone marrow (myeloid) and circulate in peripheral blood (leukaemia). They are classified morphologically on discernable cell type. Myelofibrosis is an obscure entity, in which some forms of leukaemia may be accompanied by fibrosis of the bone marrow. This lesion is sometimes viewed as 'preleukaemia'.

SPONTANEOUS TUMOURS

Lymphoid tumours are among the most common spontaneously occurring tumours in Syrian hamsters and represent the most frequent malignancy. Actual prevalence rates are difficult to state because of marked variation between hamster populations studied. The single most important variable appears to be age, since these tumours generally arise in animals one year of age or older. The first published report on spontaneous tumours in Syrian hamsters (Ashbel, 1945) described a 'polymorph sarcoma' involving lymphoid organs and other tissues in the original hamster colony in Israel. Although this is not convincing evidence of lymphoid origin, lymphoid tumours have been noted with regularity in Syrian hamsters ever since. There are numerous published reports on their occurrence and prevalence rates (reviewed by Kirkman & Algard, 1968; Schmidt *et al.*, 1983; Sträuli & Mettler, 1982; Van Hoosier & Trentin, 1979). Detailed descriptions of these tumours are often lacking and the terminology used for them has been diverse and frequently anthropomorphic, making accurate retrospective analysis of tumour or cell types difficult. Nevertheless, lymphosarcomas clearly emerge as the most frequent life-limiting spontaneous neoplasm of ageing hamsters. Plasma cell tumours are considerably less common and other forms of haemolymphatic neoplasia appear to be very rare in Syrian hamsters.

Lymphosarcomas, lymphomas, lymphomatosis and reticulum cell sarcomas have been noted among hamsters by different authors, with cell types interpreted as histiocytic, epithelioid, lymphocytic, lymphoblastic, undifferentiated and mixed (Kirkman & Algard, 1968). Few reports have provided substantive supportive detail, but it can be assumed that most represented lymphosarcomas, using the classification discussed above. Furthermore, interpretation of cell types by different authors is vague and should not be taken too literally. It is clear, however, that histiocytic lymphosarcomas (which include reticulum cell sarcomas) are frequent. Organ distribution has likewise been poorly defined or lacking, but several reports have suggested that spontaneous lymphosarcomas can be localized or multicentric. Local sites of involvement included skin (Figure 5) (McMartin, 1979; Brindley & Banfield, 1961), cervical lymph node (Coggin *et al.*, 1983; Finkel *et al.*, 1968; Fortner, 1961; McMartin, 1979; Pour *et al.*, 1979), renal lymph node (McMartin, 1979), inguinal lymph node (Pour *et al.*, 1976, 1979), mesenteric lymph node (Pour *et al.*, 1976, 1979; McMartin, 1979), spleen (McMartin, 1979), retroperitoneal tissue (Greene & Harvey, 1960; Handler, 1965), and liver, mesentery, thigh or cheek pouch (Sträuli & Haemmerli, 1960; Sträuli, 1962). Most were multicentric, involving thymus, thoracic lymph node, mediastinal lymph node, liver and spleen (Finkel *et al.*, 1968), superficial lymph nodes, liver, kidney and sternal bone marrow (Lee *et al.*, 1964), mesenteric lymph nodes, gut, spleen, mediastinum and pancreas (McMartin, 1979), generalized (Pour *et al.*, 1976, 1979), lymph nodes, skin, spleen, kidney, liver and occasionally bone marrow (Toth, 1967, 1969), superficial lymph nodes, skin, spleen and liver (Yabe *et al.*, 1972), liver, mesentery, kidneys, spleen and intestine (Sträuli & Haemmerli, 1960; Sträuli, 1962). In most of these reports, involvement of tissues other than lymph nodes and skin was not grossly visible, but was found upon microscopic examination.

Spontaneous lymphoid leukaemia has only rarely been reported, and has not been well described. It appears to arise as a result of multicentric lymphosarcoma, rather than primary bone marrow disease (Dontenwill *et al.*, 1973; Fortner, 1965; Kirkman, 1962; Lindt, 1958).

Spontaneous tumours of immunoglobulin-forming cells have been relatively rare and usually represented solitary (localized) plasmacytomas. The site of tumour growth was not specified by some authors (Dontenwill *et al.*, 1973; Kirkman, 1962; Fortner, 1961; Kirkman & Algard, 1968; Dunham & Herrold, 1962). Others have reported these tumours in cervical lymph node (Finkel *et al.*, 1968; Fortner, 1961; Garcia *et al.*, 1961; Pour *et al.*, 1976, 1979), inguinal lymph node (Pour *et al.*, 1976, 1979), and mesenteric lymph node (Fortner, 1961). Pour *et al.* (1976, 1979) noted a generalized plasmacytic lymphoma and bone marrow plasma cell tumour in another hamster. Plasma cell tumours, like spontaneous lymphosarcomas, arise in aged hamsters (one year of age or older).

Spontaneous thymomas or myeloid leukaemias have not been reported in Syrian hamsters, with the exception of two cases of myeloid leukaemia reported by Dontenwill *et al.* (1973) without further detail.

Information on haemolymphatic neoplasia in other types of hamster is considerably less documented. Benjamin and Brooks (1977) noted a high frequency of bone marrow granulocytic hyperplasia and three cases of myelogenous leukaemia among 157 ageing Chinese hamsters (*Cricetulus griseus*). The hamsters with leukaemia had splenomegaly and diffuse bone marrow neoplasia, with leukaemic infiltration of liver, kidney, brain and spinal cord. Two of these hamsters had myelofibrosis. Although Djungarian hamsters (*Phodopus sungorus*) develop a high prevalence of neoplasia with ageing, no haemolymphatic tumours have been documented (Pogosianz, 1975). Ghadially and Illman (1965) examined five aged European hamsters (*Cricetus cricetus*) that were wild-trapped in Germany. Two of these hamsters had thymomas. Tumours were composed of two cell types: lymphocytic and large, pale reticular cells with epithelial characteristics, including tonofilaments. They were localized to the thymus and adjacent tissues. Others (Mohr & Ernst, 1987) have noted a spontaneous tumour incidence of 70% in European hamsters greater than two years of age, with lymphatic tumours the most common.

INDUCTION OF TUMOURS

Haemolymphatic tumours, especially lymphoid tumours, have been experimentally induced in Syrian hamsters with X-irradiation, chemical carcinogens, viruses and tumour extracts. Hamsters are also subject to natural infection with hamster papovavirus, which can cause epizootics or enzootics of lymphosarcoma. Hamster haemolymphatic tumours, whether spontaneous or induced, often contain various virus-like particles. These agents are incidental findings and do not appear to have oncogenic significance.

X-irradiation

The hamster is remarkably radio-resistant compared to mice (Stenbäck *et al.*, 1979). Rivière *et al.* (1960) induced lymphosarcoma in nine of 80 hamsters given whole-body 300–600 R X-irradiation in single or fractionated doses. Lymphoblastic tumours arose at 8–10 months, involving lymph nodes, spleen, liver, lungs and kidneys. Stenbäck *et al.* (1979) induced a 7% rate of lymphosarcomas (reticulum cell sarcomas and undifferentiated lymphoreticular tumours) among 200 hamsters treated with weekly fractionated doses of X-irradiation totalling 200–3000 R. Most tumours arose in spleen and liver. In an earlier study, Stenbäck *et al.* (1969) induced a single lymphoma among 29 weanling hamsters given four doses of 240 R at seven-day intervals.

Chemical carcinogens

Haemolymphatic tumours have occurred in Syrian hamsters following treatment with a number of chemical carcinogens. In several cases, cause and effect have been obscured by the high background rate of lymphosarcomas among control hamsters relative to the low prevalence of tumours in treated groups. Toth (1969) treated adult Syrian hamsters intravenously with single and multiple weekly injections of 7,12-dimethylbenz[a]anthracene, resulting in 25–30% lymphomas in hamsters receiving a single injection and 7–18% lymphomas in hamsters receiving multiple injections, compared to 2–7% among controls. Among the 25 lymphomas induced, six were composed of stem cells (undifferentiated), eight were lymphocytic and 11 were histiocytic, involving lymph nodes, spleen, liver, kidney and occasionally bone marrow.

Hamsters treated with oral 3-methylcholanthrene (Della Porta, 1961), urethane (Toth *et al.*, 1961), subcutaneous injections of 7,12-dimethylbenz[*a*]anthracene (Lee *et al.*, 1964), cheek pouch implants of betel quid (Dunham & Herrold, 1962) and a number of other chemicals (Toth, 1967) have developed a few lymphoid neoplasms, but their appearance cannot be attributed to carcinogen treatment. A single male Syrian hamster developed an extremely rare eosinophilic leukaemia at 92 weeks in a lifetime lung-carcinogenesis bioassay using benzo[*a*]pyrene–haematite. The number of animals treated was not specified. The hamster had extensive pulmonary involvement, as well as heart, kidney, liver, intestine and bone marrow (Port & Richter, 1977). This was the only report of a tumour of this type in hamsters.

European hamsters are susceptible to carcinogenesis with a variety of chemicals, but haemolymphatic neoplasia is not readily induced (Mohr & Ernst, 1987). European hamsters treated with subcutaneous and intragastric *N*-nitroso-2,6-dimethylmorpholine (Althoff *et al.*, 1985), subcutaneous *N*-nitrosodimethylamine (Richter-Reichhelm *et al.*, 1978) and subcutaneous 1,1-dimethylhydrazine (Ernst *et al.*, 1987) developed a low incidence of lymphomas, but within control rates.

Oncogenic viruses

In addition to the hamster papovavirus (discussed in the next section), the papovavirus SV40, several human adenoviruses and selected murine retroviruses have been shown to experimentally induce haemolymphatic neoplasia in Syrian hamsters. When SV40 was inoculated by subcutaneous, intracerebral, intraperitoneal or intrathoracic routes into newborn hamsters, it induced sarcomas at the site of inoculation. Older hamsters tended to be resistant to SV40

oncogenesis (Allison *et al.*, 1967), except when the virus was given intravenously. Following intravenous inoculation of weanling hamsters, 85–95% developed neoplasia within 3–6 months, of which 72–78% had 'reticulum-cell sarcomas', 3–4% had lymphosarcomas and 1% had lymphocytic leukaemia. The reticulum cell sarcomas primarily involved mediastinal and mesenteric lymph nodes, with secondary infiltration of liver, spleen, intestine and Peyer's patches. The lymphosarcomas involved superficial lymph nodes, with less involvement of liver and spleen. These were poorly differentiated to lymphoblastic in morphology. The thymus was never involved in these hamsters (Diamandopoulos, 1972, 1973).

The initial observation of human adenovirus 12 oncogenicity in newborn hamsters (Trentin *et al.*, 1962) was followed by other reports of human adenovirus oncogenicity in hamsters, including adenovirus 12 and 18 (Huebner *et al.*, 1962), adenovirus 7, 12 and 18 (Girardi *et al.*, 1964), adenovirus 7 (Larson *et al.*, 1965), and adenovirus 12 (Pereira & McCallum, 1964; Larson *et al.*, 1965). Later, 30 human adenovirus types were tested, and types 1, 7, 8, 12, 14, 18, 21 and 24 were confirmed to be oncogenic when inoculated intraperitoneally or subcutaneously into newborn hamsters. Tumour type, prevalence and latent period varied with adenovirus type, isolate and dose. Tumour prevalence ranged from 62% (with a short latent period) with highly oncogenic adenovirus 12 to 4% (with a latent period greater than one year) with weakly oncogenic adenovirus 7 (Trentin *et al.*, 1968). Highly oncogenic adenovirus types 12 and 18 appeared to induce undifferentiated mesenchymal neoplasms with epithelioid characteristics at the site of subcutaneous inoculation (Trentin *et al.*, 1962; Huebner *et al.*, 1962; Girardi *et al.*, 1964), but Pereira and McCallum (1964) noted the induction of lymphosarcomas by adenovirus 12 and Trentin *et al.* (1968) likewise noted lymphoma-like features in adenovirus 18-induced tumours. These may represent interpretive differences, since lymphoid tumours clearly arise with other adenoviruses. Larson *et al.* (1965) noted 'undifferentiated sarcomas, undifferentiated sarcomas resembling malignant lymphoma, malignant lymphomas and lymphosarcomas' (denoting local invasiveness) at the site of subcutaneous inocu-lation with adeno-virus 7 in 7–21% of hamsters following a long latent period (155–405 days). The predominant tumour type induced by adenovirus types 1, 7, 8, 14, 21 and 24 following intra-peritoneal inoculation of newborn hamsters was noted to be 'lymphoma, lymphosarcoma or reticulum cell sarcoma' (Trentin *et al.,* 1968). Mesenteric lymph nodes were a common site of origin. In summary, lymphoid tumours, regardless of ter-minology, are frequently induced by adenoviruses in hamsters.

Lymphoid tumours have also been induced in hamsters with murine retro-viruses. Gerber and Brown (1972) inocu-lated 300 newborn Syrian hamsters intraperitoneally with cell-free leukaemia extracts from mice infected with murine leukaemia virus GC. A single hamster developed a reticulum cell sarcoma after 18 months. The tumour lacked infectious GC virus, but contained the virus genome, murine retrovirus gs antigen and co-cultivation of hamster tumour cells with susceptible murine cells generated infectious GC virus. The GLOH- retrovirus, which is a Gross M-MSV/hamster retro-virus pseudotype, also induces lymphomas in hamsters after long latent periods (Huebner, cited by Okabe *et al.,* 1974).

Hamster papovavirus (transmissible lymphoma)

Hamster papovavirus (HaPV) is a highly transmissible, naturally occurring virus that has infected several Syrian hamster colonies in Europe and the United States. It can manifest itself in a number of ways, including silent infections, epizootics of lymphoma, cutaneous trichoepitheliomas (also referred to as epitheliomas and papil-lomas), and possibly other disease syn-dromes (Barthold *et al.,* 1987; Ambrose & Coggin, 1975; Bottger *et al.,* 1971; Coggin *et al.,* 1978, 1981, 1983, 1985; Delmas *et al.,* 1985; Graffi *et al.,* 1967, 1968a,b, 1969a,b; Horn & Siewert, 1968; Leinbach *et al.,* 1987; Scherneck *et al.,* 1979, 1984, 1987, 1988; Vogel *et al.,* 1986; Zimmerman *et al.,* 1984).

There are several features of HaPV and its disease complex that have made incrimination of HaPV as the cause of transmissible lymphoma difficult. During natural epizootics, in which previously unexposed hamsters are exposed to HaPV, lymphomas can arise at devastatingly high rates. In contrast, when the virus is enzootic within a colony, lymphoma rates are markedly less, so that infection is nearly silent. Hamsters in infected colo-nies also develop a low prevalence of cutaneous trichoepitheliomas (less than 5%), but they do not correlate with development of lymphoma in individual animals. HaPV-induced lymphoid tumours do not contain detectable HaPV, but may contain C-type virus particles. Exami-nation of trichoepitheliomas reveals HaPV replication in nuclei of keratinizing epithelial cells (Ambrose & Coggin, 1975; Coggin *et al.,* 1978, 1981, 1983, 1985; Graffi *et al.,* 1967, 1968a,b, 1969a,b, 1972). When HaPV is inoculated into naive hamsters, it readily induces lymphomas (Barthold *et al.,* 1987; Graffi *et al.,* 1968a,b, 1969a,b). However, when HaPV is inocu-lated into hamsters from enzootically infected colonies, lymphomas are not, but trichoepitheliomas are, induced (Graffi *et al.,* 1968, 1969a,b).

Because of these features, the history of HaPV pathogenesis investigation has been circuitous. Graffi *et al.* (1967, 1968a,b, 1969a,b) originally discovered HaPV in embryo tissue cultures and epitheliomas from Syrian hamsters in Germany, maintained in a colony at their institute, without an obvious problem with lymphosarcoma. HaPV or its DNA induced lymphomas in hamsters from an un-infected colony, but hamsters from the enzootically-infected colony developed only epitheliomas. DNA infectivity was abrogated by DNase, but not RNase or pronase. Electron microscopic examination of epitheliomas revealed HaPV, but lymphomas contained only C-type virus particles. Although they did not establish oncogenicity of the C-type particles, they concluded that HaPV or its DNA was activating a latent retrovirus, rather than acting as a primary oncogen. Their hypothesis was reinforced when they showed that extracts from several human tumours were also oncogenic in their hamsters. In retrospect, the highly contagious nature of HaPV between treatment groups probably accounted for the oncogenicity of the human tumour extracts. Subsequent studies have unequivocally demonstrated the presence of HaPV DNA, but not HaPV virions, in lymphomas induced with the Graffi isolate of HaPV (Mothes, 1973; Scherneck et al., 1987,1988), and the non-oncogenic nature of hamster C-type virus (McCormick & Trentin, 1979).

Repeated epizootics of transmissible lymphoma were investigated in a University of Tennessee facility in the United States by Ambrose & Coggin (1975), Coggin et al. (1978, 1981, 1983, 1985) and Manci et al. (1984). Newborn to three-week old hamsters brought into the contaminated facility developed lymphomas at an average rate of 53%, with a range between 28% and 96% among different groups. Lymphomas developed within 4–30 weeks of exposure. A small percentage (3%) of introduced hamsters, as well as hamsters in the infected colony, developed epitheliomas. Electron microscopy of epitheliomas revealed HaPV, but lymphomas contained no discernable virus. When hamsters of different ages

from their colony were inoculated with extracts of epitheliomas containing HaPV or its DNA by different routes, epitheliomas but not lymphomas developed. Lymphomas were induced in one-day-old but not 10-day-old hamsters with protamine sulfate buffered extracts of primary and low-passaged lymphomas. The oncogenic extract was filterable, showed variable sensitivity to DNase, was inactivated by phenol and potassium hydroxide, and was resistant to RNase. Since no virus particles were visualized, these workers concluded that the agent of transmissible lymphoma was a naked DNA viroid-like agent (Coggin et al., 1981), and emphasized the lack of association of HaPV with lymphomas, since HaPV did not induce lymphomas (Coggin et al., 1985). They found that hamsters from the infected colony resisted experimental induction of lymphoma, as Graffi's group showed in their work. Barthold et al. (1987) obtained naturally infected University of Tennessee hamsters from Ambrose and isolated HaPV from a skin tumour. Taking precautions to preclude natural contamination of experimental groups with HaPV, they demonstrated that skin tumour homogenates or HaPV grown in embryo culture were highly lymphomagenic in naive newborn and weaning age hamsters. Finally, Leinbach et al. (1987) demonstrated HaPV DNA in primary and transplanted lymphomas from the Tennessee hamsters.

HaPV is a papovavirus of the polyomavirus subgroup which is related to, but distinct from other polyomaviruses (Bottger et al., 1971; Delmas et al., 1985; Scherneck et al., 1979, 1984, 1987, 1988; Vogel et al., 1986; Zimmerman et al., 1984). Its biology closely resembles that of polyoma virus of mice (Barthold et al., 1987). HaPV replicates in various tissues, including kidney (Graffi et al., 19691b; Bottger et al., 1971; Leinback et al., 1987). Neoplasia is unessential to polyomavirus epizootiology, but when neonatal mice are

inoculated parenterally with polyomavirus, they develop multiple tumours,
which contain viral DNA, but not repli-
cating virus. An exception is that a few
mice can develop cutaneous trichoepitheliomas, which allow replication of
virus. HaPV is therefore quite similar,
except that hamsters of all ages are susceptible to oncogenesis and tumour induction does not require experimental,
parenteral inoculation (Barthold *et al.*,
1987).

Horn and Siewert (1968) were the first
to describe HaPV lymphoid neoplasia in
35 hamsters aged 2–7 months, as well as
two hamsters with cutaneous papillomas.
Most had lymphosarcomas arising from
mesentery, which is typical of the HaPV
syndrome (Figures 6 and 7), with invasion
of abdominal organs, although a few cases
involved only axillary and cervical lymph
nodes. This was the colony in which Graffi
et al. (1967, 1968a) described virus-
associated skin tumours and later showed
that HaPV induced 30–40% leukoses when
inoculated into naive hamsters. Induced
tumours arose in liver (Figure 8), with
extension into the abdominal cavity, and
also infiltrated kidney and thymus, but
not spleen. Tumours were usually lymphatic, but erythroblastic, reticulosarco-
matous and myeloid types were seen
occasionally. Stunzi *et al.* (1977) reported
another epizootic in Germany among
inbred Syrian hamsters aged 5–14 months,
in which over 70% developed lymphosarcoma. Most tumours were localized to
the intestinal wall and mesentery, but
liver, kidney, axillary lymph nodes and
cervical lymph nodes were also often
affected. Cells were lymphocytic, with
variable differentiation, including occasional plasmacytoid features. In the
repeated epizootics of lymphoma at the
University of Tennessee, most lymphomas
arose in the intestinal wall and mesenteric
lymph node, with the liver being the
second most frequent site. Involvement of
kidney, thymus, superficial lymph nodes

and other sites was less common. Tumours
varied cytologically. Most were composed
of monotonous populations of immature
lymphoid cells, but some displayed
cellular pleomorphism. Occasional plasmacytomas were seen (Ambrose & Coggin,
1975; Coggin *et al.*, 1978, 1983, 1985).
Lymphomas of the abdomen contained
cells with B-cell markers, while those of
thymus possessed T-cell characteristics
(Coggin *et al.*, 1983).

Because of its variable presentation and
frequent lack of recognition, it is unclear
how prevalent HaPV is among hamster
colonies. Several colonies in Europe have
been infected. Coggin *et al.* (1985) cited
three geographically separate outbreaks in
the USA, but one of these, which involved
experimental studies in HaPV-infected
hamsters from Coggin's facility (Barthold
et al., 1987) was not an outbreak. Other
possible epizootics included clusters of
reticulum cell sarcomas, lymphosarcomas
and plasma cell tumours among young
Syrian hamsters in Switzerland, involving
liver, mesentery and other sites (Sträuli &
Haemmerli, 1960; Sträuli, 1962). It is of
interest that an HaPV-like agent has also
been described in European (*Cricetus
cricetus*) hamsters in Europe (Hannoun *et
al.*, 1974). Clearly, much remains to be
discovered about the source of HaPV and
its prevalence among hamster colonies. It
has had devastating consequences,
resulting in loss of unique inbred hamster
lines (Streilein, 1987), has significantly
obscured spontaneous and experimental
hamster tumour biology and is the most
clinically significant viral agent of Syrian
hamsters.

Non-oncogenic tumour-associated
viruses

A number of virus-like particles with
unknown biological significance have
been observed ultrastructurally in hamster tissues, cultured cells and tumours,
including spontaneous tumours and
those induced by irradiation, viruses and

chemicals. These particles include R-type particles, A-type particles and C-type particles, and have been reviewed elsewhere (McCormick & Trentin, 1979). R-type particles are approximately 100 nm in diameter with spoked structures radiating from a 50 nm nucleoid. They arise in the endoplasmic reticulum. They have also been termed H (hamster)-type particles and Bernhard particles. A-type particles occur in the cytoplasm, often in clusters. They are approximately 80 nm in diameter with an electron-lucent core of 56 nm. C-type particles measure 99 nm, with a nucleoid of approximately 54 nm and are often found budding into the endoplasmic reticulum. All three virus-like particles have been found in lymphoid tumours of hamsters, including radiation-induced lymphomas, spontaneous lymphomas, transplantable tumours and adenovirus-induced tumours (Stenbäck *et al.*, 1966, 1968, 1969). C-type virus particles have also been observed in hamster papovavirus-induced lymphomas (Graffi, 1972; Graffi *et al.*, 1968; 1970).

Oncogenicity of human and animal tissue extracts

The newborn hamster has been used to seek potentially oncogenic agents in human and animal tumours. Most studies have been equivocal, with induction of lymphoid tumours at rates equivalent to those in the control population. Nastac *et al.* (1973) induced a single lymphosarcoma among 14 hamsters injected with human leukaemic spleen and lymph node. Hamsters injected with human osteosarcoma extracts developed osteosarcomas and a low prevalence of lymphoid tumours, which were considered within the normal range (Finkel *et al.*, 1968). Lussier and Pavilanis (1969) injected hamsters with bovine leukaemia extract and noted a wasting syndrome and malignant lymphomas in 16% of inoculated hamsters. Lymphomas arose in the peritoneal cavity after 8–9 months. Graffi

et al. (1969) induced lymphomas in neonatal hamsters with cell-free filtrates of human gastric carcinomas, pancreatic carcinoma, ovarian tumours, lung carcinoma and mammary carcinoma. However, there is a very strong probability that these results were due to contamination of treatment groups with hamster papovavirus (Coggin *et al.*, 1985). Karpas and Samso (1972) induced lymphosarcomas in single hamsters from each of two litters at 8 and 22 months after inoculation as newborns with primary hamster embryo cell cultures infected with equine herpesvirus 3. Virus alone had no effect. Ultracentrifuged extracts of the original tumours induced a 20% rate of lymphomas when inoculated intraperitoneally into newborn hamsters.

TRANSPLANTATION

Lymphoreticular tumours, in addition to a variety of other tumours and tissues, are readily transplantable in Syrian hamsters. This is not surprising, when the high degree of genetic homozygosity among Syrian hamsters is considered (Streilein, 1987). Syrian hamsters readily accept intra-strain, as well as interstrain skin grafts (Handler, 1968). Numerous investigators have demonstrated transplantability of spontaneous and induced lymphosarcomas and plasma cell tumours. These studies have been thoroughly reviewed elsewhere (Handler, 1968; Strauli & Mettler, 1982; Toth, 1967). It is of interest to note that lymphoreticular tumours of hamsters have been shown to be so transplantable that they can be contagious by contact and by arthropod among hamsters (Banfield *et al.*, 1966; Brindley & Banfield, 1961).

COMPARATIVE ASPECTS

Haemolymphatic tumours represent a significant life-limiting disease in hamsters, as they do in many other species. Their morphology resembles that in other species, including humans, but direct correlations are never possible. Cyto-chemical classification techniques are required to accurately define cell of origin in hamster tumours, especially for 'histio-cytic' lymphosarcomas. The hamster is unique in several ways. Its high degree of genetic homozygosity, even among different strains, allows transplantation of tumours, even by contact. Lymphoid tumours can be readily induced in hamsters with a number of viruses, but unlike other laboratory rodents, retro-viruses are not directly involved in oncogenesis, if at all. The hamster is resistant to both radiation and chemical induction of haemolymphatic tumours. The hamster is unquestionably unique in its natural susceptibility to transmissible papovavirus lymphoma. This is a double-edged sword, since it offers important information on non-retrovirus onco-genesis, but also threatens the validity of cancer data derived from enzootically infected hamsters. Methodology for detecting hamster papovavirus in hamster colonies is needed for precluding this agent as a variable in cancer research.

ACKNOWLEDGEMENTS

Preparation of this manuscript was supported in part by grant number RR00393 from the Division of Research Resources, National Institutes of Health, U.S. Public Health Service.

REFERENCES

Allison, A.C., Chesterman, F.C. & Baron, S. (1967) Induction of tumours in adult hamsters with simian virus 40. *J. Natl Cancer Inst.*, 38, 567–572

Althoff, J., Mohr, U. & Lijinsky, W. (1985) Comparative study on the carcinogenicity of N-nitroso-2,6-dimethylmorpholine in the European hamster. *J. Cancer Res. Clin. Oncol.*, 109, 183–187

Ambrose, K.R. & Coggin, J.H., Jr. (1975) An epizootic in hamsters of lymphomas of undetermined origin and mode of transmission. *J. Natl Cancer Inst.*, 54, 877–880

Ashbel, R. (1945) Spontaneous transmissible tumours in the Syrian hamster. *Nature*, 155, 607

Banfield, W.G., Woke, P.A. & Mackay, C.M. (1966) Mosquito transmission of lymphoma. *Cancer*, 19, 1333–1336

Barthold, S.W., Bhatt, P.N. & Johnson, E.A. (1987) Further evidence for papovavirus as the probable etiology of transmissible lymphoma of Syrian hamsters. *Lab. Animal Sci.*, 37, 283–288

Bell, A. (1987) Haematopoeisis. In: Pittiglio, D.H. & Sacher, R.A. eds, *Clinical Haematology and Fundamentals of Haemostasis*. Philadelphia, F.A. Davis, pp. 1–14

Benjamin, S.A. & Brooks, A.L. (1977) Spontaneous lesions in Chinese hamsters. *Vet. Pathol.*, 14, 449–462

Bottger, M., Bierwolf, D., Wunderlich, V. & Graffi, A. (1971) New calibration correlations for molecular weights of circular DNA: the molecular weight of the DNA of an oncogenic papova virus of the Syrian hamster. *Biochem. Biophys. Acta*, 232, 21–31

Brindley, D.C. & Banfield, W.G. (1961) A contagious tumour of the hamster. *J. Natl Cancer Inst.*, 26, 949–957

Coggin, J.H. Jr, Vassa-Thomas, K., Huebner, R. (1978) Horizontally transmitted lymphomas of Syrian hamsters. *Fed. Proc.*, 37, 2086–2088

Coggin, J.H. Jr, Oakes, J.E., Huebner, R.J. & Gilden, R. (1981) Unusual filterable oncogenic agent isolated from horizontally transmitted Syrian hamster lymphomas. *Nature*, 290, 336–338

Coggin, J.H. Jr, Bellomy, B.B., Vassa-Thomas, K. & Pollock, W.J. (1983) B-cell and T-cell lymphomas and other associated diseases induced by an infectious DNA viroid-like agent in hamsters (*Mesocricetus auratus*). *Am. J. Pathol.*, 110, 254–266

Coggin, J.H. Jr, Hyde, B.M., Heath, L.S., Leinbach, S.S., Fowler, E. & Stadmore, L.S. (1985) Papovavirus in epitheliomas appearing on lymphoma-bearing hamsters: lack of association with horizontally transmitted lymphomas in Syrian hamsters. *J. Natl Cancer Inst.*, 75, 91–97

Della Porta, G. (1961) Induction of intestinal, mammary, and ovarian tumours in hamsters with oral administration of 20'-methylcholanthrene. *Cancer Res.*, 21, 575–579

Delmas, V., Bastien, C., Scherneck, S. & Feunteun, J. (1985) A new member of the polyomavirus family: the hamster papovavirus. Complete nucleotide sequence and transformation properties. *EMBO J.*, 4, 1279–1286

Desai, R.G. (1968) Haematology and microcirculation. In: Hoffman, R.A., Robinson, P.F. & Magalhaes, H., eds, *The Golden Hamster: its Biology and Use in Medical Research*, Ames, Iowa State University Press, pp. 185–194

Diamandopoulos, G.T. (1972) Leukaemia, lymphoma, and osteosarcoma induced in the Syrian golden hamster by simian virus 40, *Science*, 176, 173–175

Diamandopoulos, G.T. (1973) Induction of lymphocytic leukaemia, lymphosarcoma, reticulum cell sarcoma, and osteogenic sarcoma in the Syrian golden hamsters by oncogenic DNA simian virus 40. *J. Natl Cancer Inst.*, 50, 1347–1365

Dontenwill, W., Chevalier, H.-J., Harke, H.-P., Lafrenz, U., Reckzeh, G. & Schneider, B. (1973) Spontantumouren des syrischen Goldhamsters. *Z. Krebsforsch.*, 80, 127–158

Dunham, L.J. & Herrold, K.M. (1962) Failure to produce tumours in the hamster cheek pouch by exposure to ingredients of betel quid: histopathological changes in the pouch and other organs by exposure to known carcinogens. *J. Natl Cancer Inst.*, 29, 1047–1067

Ernst, H., Rittinghausen, S., Wahnschaffe, U. & Mohr, U. (1987) Induction of malignant peripheral nerve sheath tumours in European hamsters with 1,1-dimethylhydrazine (UDMH). *Cancer Lett.*, 35, 303–311

Finkel, M.P., Biskis, B.O. & Farrel, C. (1968) Osteosarcomas appearing in Syrian hamsters after treatment with extracts of human osteosarcomas. *Proc. Natl Acad. Sci. USA*, 60, 1223–1230

Fortner, J.G. (1961) The influence of castration on spontaneous tumorigenesis in the Syrian (golden) hamster. *Cancer Res.*, 21, 1491–1498

Jarrett, W.F.H. & Mackey, L.J. (1974) Neoplastic diseases of the haematopoietic and lymphoid tissues. In: *International Histological Classification of Tumours of Domestic Animals. Bull. W.H.O.*, 50, 21–34

Jones, T.C. & Hunt, R.D. (1983) *Veterinary Pathology,* 5th edition, Philadelphia, Lea & Febiger

Karpas, A. & Samso, A. (1972) A new malignant lymphoma induced in the Syrian hamster. *Eur. J. Cancer*, 8, 231–237

Kirkman, H. (1962) A preliminary report concerning tumours observed in hamsters. *Stanford Med. Bull.*, 20, 163–166

Kirkman, H. & Algard, F.T. (1968) Spontaneous and non-viral induced neoplasms. In: Hoffman, R.A., Robinson, P.F. & Magalhaes, H., eds, *The Golden Hamster: its Biology and Use in Medical Research*, Ames, Iowa State University Press, pp. 227–240

Larson, V.M., Girardi, A.J., Hilleman, M.R. & Zwickey, R.E. (1965) Studies of oncogenicity of adenovirus type 7 viruses in hamsters. *Proc. Soc. Exp. Biol. Med.*, 118, 15–24

Lee, K.Y., Toth, B. & Shubik, P. (1964) Carcinogenic response of the Syrian golden hamster treated with 7,12-dimethylbenz(a)anthracene. *Proc. Soc. Exp. Biol. Med.*, 114, 579–582

Leinbach, S.S., Fowler, E., Heath, L.S., Hyde, B. & Coggin, J.H., Jr (1987) Complete, circular papovavirus genome in the cells of hamsters exposed to a horizontally transmitted lymphomagenic agent. *J. Natl Cancer Inst.*, 79, 273–279

Lindt, V.S. (1958) Über Krankheiten des Syrischen Goldhamsters. *Schweiz. Arch. Tierheilkd.*, 100, 86–97

Lussier, G. & Pavilanis, V. (1969) Malignant lymphomas in hamsters following a wasting disease produced by bovine leukaemic extract – a preliminary report. *Can. J. Comp. Med.*, 33, 81–82

Manci, E.A., Heath, L.S., Leinbach, S.S. & Coggin, J.H., Jr (1984) Lymphoma-associated ulcerative bowel disease in the hamster (*Mesocricetus auratus*) induced by an unusual agent. *Am. J. Pathol.*, 116, 1–8

McCormick, K.J. & Trentin, J.J. (1979) Tumour-associated viruses of the Syrian hamster: relation to neoplasia. *Prog. Exp. Tumour Res.*, 23, 13–55

McMartin, D.N. (1979) Morphologic lesions in aging Syrian hamsters. *J. Gerontol.*, 34, 502–511

Mohr, U. & Ernst, H. (1987) The European hamster. Biology, care, and use in research. In: Van Hoosier, G.L., Jr & McPherson, C.W., eds, *Laboratory Hamsters,* New York, Academic Press, pp. 351–366

Mothes, E. (1973) Untersuchungen über Sequenzhomologien zwischen DNS aus Normal- und Tumourgewebe des Golden-hamsters und Papovavirus-DNS mittels DNS × DNS-hybridisierung. *Acta Biol. Med. Germ.,* 30, 341–351

Moulton, J.E. & Dungworth, D.L. (1978) Tumours of the lymphoid and haema-topoietic tissues. In: Moulton, J.E., ed., *Tumours in Domestic Animals,* 2nd edition, Berkeley, University of California Press, pp. 150–204

Nastac, E., Ionescu, T., Athanasiu, P., Demetrescu, R., Velciu, V. & Ursea, N. (1973) Hamster lymphosarcomatosis and sarcomas induced by human leukaemic material. I. The action of leukaemic human spleen and lymph nodes suspension on Syrian hamster. *Neoplasma,* 20, 655–663

Okabe, H., Gilden, R.V. & Hatanaka, M. (1974) Specificity of the DNA product of RNA-dependent DNA polymerase in type C viruses: III. Analysis of viruses derived from Syrian hamsters. *Proc. Natl Acad. Sci. USA,* 71, 3278–3282

Pereira, M.S. & McCallum, F.O. (1964) Infection with adenovirus type 12. *Lancet,* I, 198–199

Pogosianz, H.E. (1975) Djungarian hamster – a suitable tool for cancer research and cytogenetic studies. *J. Natl Cancer Inst.,* 54, 659–664

Port, C.D. & Richter, W.R. (1977) Eosinophilic leukaemia in a Syrian hamster. *Vet. Pathol.,* 14, 283–286

Pour, P., Mohr, U., Althoff, J., Cardesa, A. & Kmoch, N. (1976) Spontaneous tumours and common diseases in two colonies of Syrian hamsters. IV. Vascular and lymphatic systems and lesions of other sites. *J. Natl Cancer Inst.,* 56, 963–974

Pour, P., Althoff, J., Salmasi, S. & Stepan, K. (1979) Spontaneous tumours and common diseases in three types of hamsters. *J. Natl. Cancer Inst.,* 63, 797–811

Richter-Reichelm, H.-B., Green, U., Ketkar, M.B. & Mohr, U. (1978) The carcinogenic effect of dimethylnitrosamine in laboratory-bred European hamsters (*Cricetus cricetus*). *Cancer Lett.,* 4, 1–4

Rivière, M.R., Chouroulinkov, I. & Guerin, M. (1960) Tumeurs observées chez le hamster après irradiation générale au moyen des rayons X. *Bull. Ass. Etude Cancer,* 47, 542–557

Rowe, W.P. & Lane, W.T. (1962) Oncogenic effects in hamsters of human adenovirus type 12 and 18. *Proc. Natl Acad. Sci. USA,* 48, 2051–2058

Scherneck, S., Bottger, M. & Feunteun, J. (1979) Studies on the DNA of an oncogenic papovavirus of the Syrian hamster. *Virology,* 96, 100–107

Scherneck, S., Vogel, F., Nguyen, H.L. & Feunteun, J. (1984) Sequence homology between polyoma virus, simian virus 40 and a papilloma-producing virus from a Syrian hamster: evidence for highly conserved sequences. *Virology,* 137, 41–48

Scherneck, S., Delmas, V., Vogel, F. & Feunteun, J. (1987) Induction of lymphomas by the hamster papovavirus correlates with massive replication of nonrandomly deleted extrachromosomal viral genomes. *J. Virol.,* 61, 3992–3998

Scherneck, S., Vogel, F., Arnold, W., Horn, K.H., Mothes, E., Rudolf, M., Delmas, V. & Feunteun, J. (1988) Analysis of hamster lymphomas for the presence of hamster papovavirus DNA. *Acta Virol.,* 32, 97–103

Schmidt, R.E., Eason, R.L., Hubbard, G.B., Young, J.T. & Eisenbrandt, D.L. (1983) *Pathology of Aging Hamsters,* Boca Raton, CRC press

Stenbäck, W.A., Van Hoosier, G.L., Jr & Trentin, J.J. (1966) Virus particles in hamster tumours as revealed by electron micro-scopy. *Proc. Soc. Exp. Biol. Med.,* 122, 1219–1223

Stenbäck, W.A., Van Hoosier, G.L., Jr & Trentin, J.J. (1968) Biophysical, biological, and cytochemical features of a virus associated with transplantable hamster tumours. *J. Virol.,* 2, 1115–1121

Stenbäck, W.A., Van Hoosier, G.L., Jr, Ferguson, D.B. & Trentin, J.J. (1969) Significance of virus particles observed in spontaneous and in-duced tumours of the Syrian hamster. *Comp. Leukaemia Res., Bibl. Haematol.,* 36, 559–565

Stenbäck, W.A., Bryan, M.E. & Trentin, J.J. (1979) Radiation carcinogenesis in the Syrian hamster. *Prog. Exp. Tumour Res.*, 23, 89–99

Sträuli, P. (1962) Morphogenetische untersuchungen an einem lymphoreticulocytaren Sarkom des Goldhamsters. *Pathol. Microbiol.*, 25, 301–305

Sträuli, P. & Haemmerli, G. (1960) Über ein spontanes, transplantables lymphoreticulocytares Sarkom des Goldhamsters. *Z. Krebsforsch.*, 63, 503–520

Sträuli, P. & Mettler, J. (1982) Tumours of the haematopoeitic system. In: Turusov, V.S., ed., *Pathology of Tumours in Laboratory Animals*, Vol. III, *Tumours of the Hamster*, Lyon, IARC, pp. 343–369

Streilein, J.W. (1987) Experimental biology: use in immunobiology. In: Van Hoosier, G.L., Jr & McPherson, C.W., eds, *Laboratory Hamsters*, New York, Academic Press, pp. 215–225

Stunzi, H., Dossenbach, P. & Mettler, F. (1977) Ein übertragbares Lymphosarkom beim Goldhamster. *Dtsch. tierarztl. Wschr.*, 84, 111–113

Tomson, F.N. & Wardrop, K.J. (1987) Clinical chemistry and haematology. In: Van Hoosier, G.L. Jr & McPherson, C.W., eds, *Laboratory Hamsters*, New York, Academic Press, pp. 43–59

Toth, B. (1967) Studies on the incidence, morphology, transplantation, and cell-free filtration of malignant lymphomas in the Syrian golden hamster. *Cancer Res.*, 27, 1430–1442

Toth, B. (1969) The induction of malignant lymphomas and other tumors by 7,12-dimethylbenz(a)anthracene in the Syrian golden hamster. *Cancer Res.*, 29, 1476–1484

Toth, B. Tomatis, L. & Shubik, P. (1961) Multipotential carcinogenesis with urethan in the Syrian golden hamster. *Cancer Res.*, 21, 1537–1541

Trentin, J.J., Van Hoosier, G.L., Jr & Samper, L. (1968) The oncogenicity of human adenoviruses in hamsters. *Proc. Soc. Exp. Biol. Med.*, 127, 683–689

Trentin, J.J., Yabe, Y. & Taylor, G. (1962) The quest for human cancer viruses. A new approach to an old problem reveals cancer induction in hamsters by human adenovirus. *Science*, 137, 835–841

Van Hoosier, G.L, Jr & Trentin, J.J. (1979) Naturally occurring tumours of the Syrian hamster. *Prog. Exp. Tumour Res.*, 23, 1–12

Vogel, F., Rhode, K., Scherneck, S., Bastien, C., Delmas, V. & Feunteun, J. (1986) The hamster papovavirus: evolutionary relationships with other polyomaviruses. *Virology*, 154, 335–343

Yabe, Y., Kataoka, N. & Koyama, H. (1972) Spontaneous tumours in hamsters: incidence, morphology, transplantation and virus studies. *Gann*, 63, 329–336

Zimmerman, W., Krause, H., Scherneck, S., Feunteun, J. & Geissler, E. (1984) Molecular cloning of the hamster papovavirus genome in *Escherichia coli* plasmid vector pBR322. *Gene*, 29, 243–246

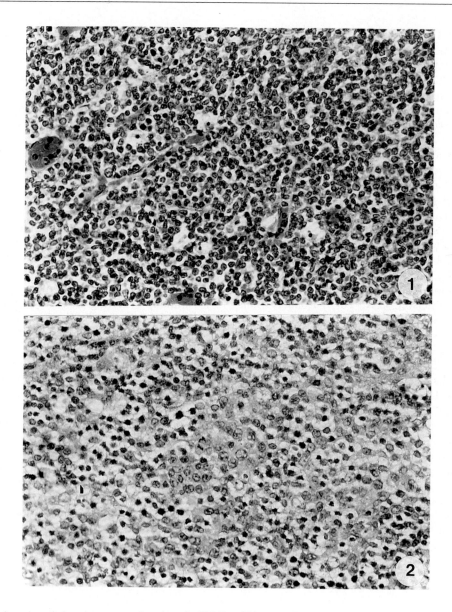

Figure 1. Lymphocytic lymphosarcoma, lymph node. H & E; × 200
Figure 2. Histiocytic lymphosarcoma, lymph node. H & E; × 200

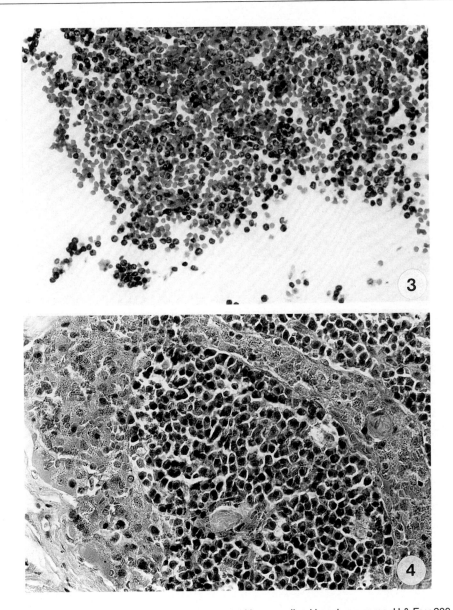

Figure 3. Lymphocytic leukaemia, heart blood, in a hamster with generalized lymphosarcoma. H & E; × 200

Figure 4. Plasmacytoma, lymph node. Adjacent, non-neoplastic histiocytes contain abundant eosinophilic cytoplasmic granules, presumably secretory product from neoplastic plasma cells. H & E; × 200

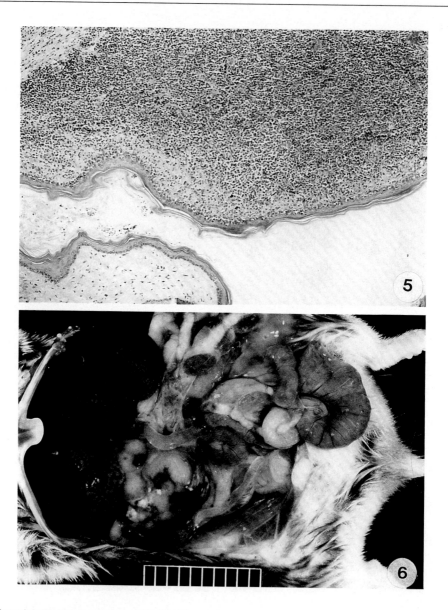

Figure 5. Lymphocytic lymphosarcoma, skin. H & E; × 50

Figure 6. Hamster papovavirus-induced lymphosarcoma (transmissible lymphoma). A 3 cm neoplasm is present in the mesentery adjacent to the liver. The liver has an accentuated lobular pattern due to neoplastic infiltration.

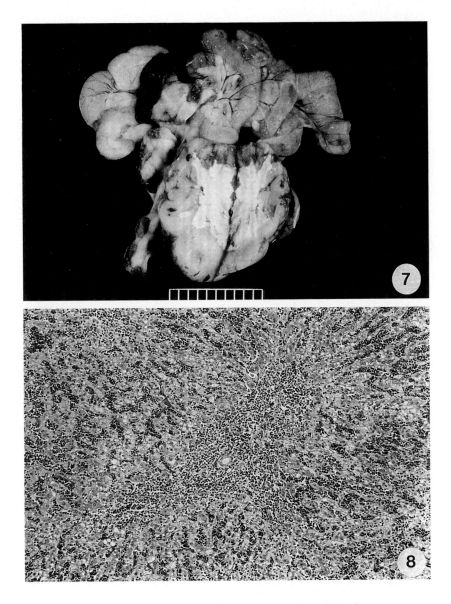

Figure 7. Mesenteric mass depicted in Figure 6. Cross-section, revealing necrotic interior.

Figure 8. Liver from hamster depicted in Figure 6. Neoplastic infiltration of sinusoids and portal connective tissue. H & E; × 50

Tumours of the bone

P.M. POUR

The Syrian golden hamster (*Cricetus auratus*) has not been used extensively for studies of experimental induction of bone tumours. Therefore, in comparison with other laboratory rodents, less is known of the development, anatomy and spontaneous diseases of its skeleton. However, this species provides a suitable model for comparative studies, of not only skeletal but also odontogenic diseases, because some spontaneous and induced lesions of the bone, supporting tissues and dental structures resemble morphologically those occurring in humans (Kirkman, 1962; Ruffolo & Kirkman, 1965; Herrold, 1968; Soehner & Dmochowski, 1969; Fujinaga *et al.*, 1970; Dmochowski *et al.*, 1972; Yabe *et al.*, 1972; Diamandopoulos, 1972, 1973; Baer & Kilham, 1974). The etiology of bone tumours (including dental neoplasms) in humans is unknown and a practical experimental model could provide information about the factors involved in the pathogenesis of skeletal and dental neoplasms.

NORMAL STRUCTURE

The Syrian golden hamster has a 16-day gestation period and the first centres of ossification begin on the 12th day of gestation; bone development occurs 'explosively' within four days before birth (Beatty & Hillemann, 1950; Boyer, 1968). During this period the greater portion of the entire skeleton is represented by ossification centres and, in many cases, the characteristic shape of the definitive bone structure may be seen. At birth, the vertebrae (formula: C-7, T-13, L-6, S-4, Cd-13/14) (Salih & Kent, 1964), all bones of the pelvic and pectoral girdles, the sternum (except for the last two sternebrae, which ossify on the first post-natal day) and the long bones of the fore and hind legs, are well developed. However, the epiphyseal centres do not begin to ossify until the sixth and seventh post-natal days. At the end of the seventh post-natal day, the skull bones have greatly expanded and sutures are established. The developmental stages have been reported as follows: development of Meckel's cartilage (Friant, 1957, 1958a,b); osteogenesis of other portions of the hamster skeleton (Kerschner *et al.*, 1957; Boyer, 1968); palatogenesis (Shah & Chaudhry, 1972; Chaudhry & Shah, 1973); the ossicles of the semilunar cartilages (Pedersen, 1949) and abnormalities in bone development (Beatty & Hillemann, 1950; Shklar, 1972).

The joints of hamsters differ structurally from those of humans and these differences can influence the comparative pattern of articular disease. In adult hamsters, the epiphysis of the fibia remains open, but the capital epiphysis of the femur does not (Sokoloff, 1958). Another special feature is ossification of the knee menisci. The ossicles, completely surrounded by cartilage, may be found in joints having no alterations of disease.

Spontaneous degenerative changes in the hamster bony skeletal system occur frequently in aged animals. Progressive fibrillation may be seen, as well as erosion of the articular knee cartilage, followed by sclerosis of the underlying bone, fibrillation of the cruciate ligaments, fibrosis of the synovial membranes and occasional posterior subluxation of the femur or tibia (Sokoloff, 1958). Similar alterations, particularly involving the intervertebral cartilage, were observed, especially in several strains of untreated hamsters from the Eppley Institute, kept for their lifetime (Table 1). The luxation of the vertebral plates and the separation and dislocation of altered cartilage sometimes resulted in progressive paralysis, due to spinal cord damage (Figures 1–4). Genetic factors seem to influence this process, but nutritional and endocrine elements might also be involved (Sokoloff & Jay, 1956).

The alteration of epiphyseal cartilage in desalivated hamsters has been described (Chauncey *et al.,* 1963); pathological skeletal growth after viral infection (Ferm & Kilham, 1965; Heggie, 1971; Heggie & Stjernholm, 1973), (Kilham & Margolis, 1971); dental structures and their diseases (Keyes, 1968; Coleman *et al.* 1971, Jordan & Van Houte, 1972; Shklar, 1972); pathology of tooth movement (Gisondi & Kronman, 1972; Deemys & Kronman, 1973); and disturbances in odontogenesis (Herrold, 1968; Baer & Kilham, 1964).

MORPHOLOGY AND BIOLOGY OF TUMOURS

Spontaneous tumours of the hamster skeleton are rare. Moreover, clinical observations are scanty and induced bone tumours have only recently been described. The difficulties of classifying the relatively few known tumours are also complicated by the fact that these neoplasms often have great variations in tissue composition within a single tumour and, hence, present mixed osteogenic, chondrogenic, angiomatous, sclerosing, and myxomatous areas (Soehner & Dmochowski, 1969; Fujinaga *et al.,* 1970). However, tumours of soft tissues which involve bone may have reactive bone formation which resembles osteoclastoma (Chesterman *et al.,* 1972). Differentiation between a primary bone tumour and secondary involvement is often difficult and even ultrastructural features do not provide clear-cut morphological guidelines (Fujinaga *et al.,* 1970; Kay, 1971). Accordingly, information available for the histological typing of bone neoplasms in hamsters is scanty. The present classification of skeletal tumours (including tumours of the supporting tissue and dental structures) is based on the predominant malformation and the differentiation of cell types in spontaneous and induced neoplasms provided by

Table 1. Spontaneous degeneration of the intervertebral cartilage in Syrian hamsters from different sources and strains

Strain	Source	Incidence (%) of lesions		Average age (weeks)	
		F	M	F	M
Golden	Eppley colony	10	29	94 (67–114)	95 (52–129)
Golden	Hanover colony	81	83	71 (32–152)	98 (33–137)
Yellow	Eppley colony	84	97	61 (25–113)	70 (22–114)
White	Eppley colony	32	65	92 (66–124)	110 (65–138)
Albino	Eppley colony	89	34	77 (55–101)	108 (92–126)

selected laboratories or observed in our hamster colony. An attempt was also made to follow a classification method which could apply to such neoplasms in other species, and to those in humans (Spjut *et al.*, 1971; Schajowicz *et al.*, 1972). Some of the lesions included in the general classification may not be neoplastic, but in many instances it is difficult to decide whether a lesion represents malformation, dysplasia, metaplasia, preneoplasia, or neoplasia.

Histological types of tumour

Tumours and tumour-like lesions of chondroblastic origin

    Chondroma

    Chondromatosis

    Chondrosarcoma

Tumours and tumour-like lesions of osteoblastic origin

    Osteogenic exostosis

    Osteochondroma

    Osteosarcoma

Tumours of unknown origin

    Giant-cell tumour

Tumours or tumour-like lesions of odontogenic origin

    Malassez' epithelial rests

    Ectodermal odontogenic cysts

    Denticles

    Cementicles

    Periodontal cartilaginous dysplasia

    Periodontal hyperostosis

    Ameloblastoma

    Ameloblastic fibroma

    Odontoma (complex or compound)

Miscellaneous

    Osteopathia fibrosa generalisata (von Recklinghausen's disease, brown tumour of the bone)

    Tumoral calcinosis

Tumours and tumour-like lesions of chondroblastic cell origin

Tumours arising from cartilage cells appear to be exceptionally rare in Syrian golden hamsters.

Chondroma. Only one spontaneous chondroma (Kirkman, 1962) has been reported, but details of its size, topography and morphology are not available.

Chondromatosis. Cartilaginous metaplasia of periarticular connective tissue is common in older hamsters, particularly in the vertebral region of Syrian golden hamsters and in the maxillomandibular joints of albino hamsters. The metaplastic changes of the vertebrae, apparently originating at the intervertebral cartilage, sometimes have wide peripheral extensions simulating neoplasia (Figures 5 and 6). Osteocartilaginous tissue may develop in surrounding fibromuscular connective tissue, and may detach and float free in the spinal canal (Figure 7). Osteoblastic activities with reactive hyperostosis or osteoclasia may be encountered (Figures 8 and 9). The proliferated mature and immature cartilaginous tissues have great variations in growth patterns, as well as the mixture of both hyaline and fibrous cartilage (Figures 10 and 12). Cartilaginous metaplasia of the maxillomandibular joints is often indistinguishable from periarticular chondroma (Figures 10–12). Sometimes the metaplastic tissue extends widely into the surrounding tissues and protrudes into the lumen of large blood vessels. These features, in association with focal nuclear abnormalities, have been incorrectly interpreted as neoplasia. However, the non-neoplastic nature of these lesions is indicated by progressive dysplasia in the periphery of the lesion. Nodular proliferation of fibrocartilage and elastic cartilage of the pinnae, sometimes reminiscent of well differentiated chondrosarcoma, has been observed in Syrian golden hamsters treated with estriol and estrone (Ruffolo & Kirkman, 1966).

Chondrosarcoma. Apart from the above-mentioned chondrosarcoma-like lesions of the hamster's external ear, only one spontaneously occurring chondrosarcoma has been described. The neoplasm, 4 cm in diameter, weighed 29 g and appeared to originate from a rib, and protruded into the abdominal cavity. Microscopically, the almost completely encapsulated tumour was composed of immature hyaline cartilage with pleomorphic chondroblasts and chondrocytes and was lobulated by thin connective tissue septa, which projected from the surrounding capsule; focal calcification was noted. Metastases were not found.

Tumours and tumour-like lesions of osteoblastic cell origin

Osteogenic exostosis. Two small osteogenic exostoses were observed in hamsters of the Eppley colony. One lesion was located in the distal portion of a tibia and the other in the distal metaphysis of a femur (Figures 13 and 14). Both were composed of lamellar osseous structures, probably of periosteal origin. Both of these lesions were externally covered by cartilaginous-like tissue. They may be interpreted as the result of metaplastic processes or they might have resulted from the growth of aberrant cartilaginous tissue at the surface of the bone.

Osteochondroma.   Osteochondromas were found in two untreated Eppley colony hamsters; both lesions were in the lumbar spine. The larger tumour was 4 × 2 × 2 mm and compressed the spinal cord (Figure 15). Microscopically, the tumours were composed primarily of immature cartilaginous tissue, which surrounded small islets of lamellar bone spicules and osteoid (Figures 16–18). In some areas, formation of new bone was prominent. These tumour-bearing hamsters simultaneously had chondrosis of the vertebral cartilage with both degenerative and regenerative lesions. A correlation may exist between these lesions in the cartilage

and the development of a tumour at the same site.

Osteosarcoma (osteogenic sarcoma). Osteosarcomas are probably the most frequently encountered malignant bone tumours in hamsters. The principal locations of these neoplasms, both spontaneously occurring and induced, are the bones of the hind limbs, followed by the ribs and bones of the forelegs. A few tumours have also developed in the sternum and scapulae. The neoplasms vary in size and may be up to 9 cm in diameter, are firm, mostly encapsulated and can be prominently lobulated (Figures 19 and 20). These neoplasms usually grow expansively and invade surrounding tissue. Osteosarcomas arising from the ribs tend to protrude into the pleural or abdominal cavities (Figure 21). Osteosarcomas have variable amounts of cartilaginous, fibrous and osseous tissues. The gross appearance of the tumours is variable, depending upon the predominance of one or another of these three tissues. Neoplasms consisting primarily of either fibrous or cartilaginous tissues are grey-white and glistening on cut surface. Those neoplasms composed mainly of boney components are hard. Necrotic and haemorrhagic areas are present in many osteosarcomas (Figure 21).

Bone tumours can be detected radiographically at an early stage as areas of increased density or irregular radio-paque masses (Figure 22a–d). Localized thickening in long bones, primarily in the proximal metaphysis of the humerus or tibia and distal metaphysis of the femur, can be followed by endosteal hyperostosis with extensive invasion of the marrow spaces (Figure 22e). In some animals early lesions are identifiable as osteoblastic or osteolytic areas (Figure 22f–i); these lesions seem to grow very slowly and perforate the cortex shortly before death. Growth of the peripheral portions of the tumour can be rapid shortly before death (Figure 22 j–m).

The histological patterns of osteosarcomas vary greatly. Even within the same tumour, the morphological features differ considerably from section to section. In some neoplasms, a sarcomatous cellular pattern predominates, and osteoid, material histologically indistinguishable from osteoid, and bone occur as small foci (Lichtenstein, 1965; Dahlin, 1970). In other tumours, or in a portion of the same neoplasm, osteoid, chondroid, fibromatous, myxomatous or angiomatous tissue patterns can be dominant. These malignant neoplasms can be histologically subclassified as is done with those of humans (Dahlin, 1970) as osteoblastic, chondroblastic and fibroblastic. The osteoblastic type of osteosarcoma can have a framework of uncalcified and calcified osteoid, branching or densely sclerotic structures intermingled with osteoid or osteoblastic and osteoclastic cell activity (Figures 23–26). The irregular bone spicules can coalesce to form a solid tumour mass within the cellular matrix (Figure 23). These atypical boney trabeculae must be distinguished from Codman's reactive bone formation of the regular cortical bone by invasion of various mesenchymal tumours. The intertrabecular spaces of these osteosarcomas can be filled with loose connective tissue having scattered cells resembling osteoblasts or osteoclasts (Figures 27–29), or have numerous multinucleated giant cells. These latter tumours sometimes resemble a giant-cell tumour of bone. In some areas, the cellular pattern can lack bone or osteoid. In other areas, focal calcification can occur along with osteoid, fibrillary interlacing processes, or hyalin-like bands or filigree patterns of calcified, fibrous matrices with intervening nests of malignant osteoblasts (Figures 27–32). Highly cellular, poorly differentiated areas resemble neoplasms of humans diagnosed as osteoblastoma. Chondroblastic cellular areas are not identified in most osteosarcomas and are primarily found as small foci, mainly at the periphery of encapsulated tumours (Figures 33 and 34). These foci usually contain large, atypical cells within areas of calcification or osseous transformation. Chondroblast-like cells, similar to those found in chondroblastomas in humans, occur in some hamster lesions.

The fibroblastic osteosarcoma is the most common type and the histological patterns vary, even in the same tumour. These neoplasms sometimes have interlacing, compact bundles, streams or whorls of spindle-shaped cells (Figures 35–37), and a conical plug of tumour tissue within the medullary cavity (Figure 38). They might not have any obvious foci of calcification. In some areas the tumour attenuates the cortex or breaks through the cortex and protrudes into the surrounding tissues, causing Codman's reactive zones in some cases (Figures 39 and 40). Bizarre multinucleated cells, sometimes with large intracytoplasmic vacuoles, can be found in different regions of the same tumour (Figures 41 and 42). These resemble areas seen in non-osteogenic fibroma described in humans (Lichtenstein, 1965). However, focal osteoid trabeculae and islets of malignant cartilage or bone spicules are often found within these tumours (Figures 43–45), allowing a diagnosis of osteosarcoma. In other neoplasms, the malignant cells form clefts and sinusoid-like spaces bordered by compact spindle or multinucleated cells, which sometimes form papillary projections, and such neoplasms resemble synovial sarcoma (Figures 46–48). Areas similar to chondromyxoid fibroma described in humans can be found in some osteosarcomas. These have prominent vascular patterns with intervening spindle-shaped cells arranged in waves (Figures 49 and 50) or clusters of epithelioid cells (Figure 51). Tumour patterns can also imitate epithelial tumours (Figures 45 and 51).

In electron micrographs, some induced osteosarcomas have, in certain areas, a fully calcified boney matrix. The osteo-cytes have a well developed granular endoplasmic reticulum and other ultra-structural features typical of osteoblasts. The round or oval chondrocytes in lacunae of uncalcified matrix can have numerous cell processes that extend into the lacunar space (Figure 52), a well developed granular endoplasmic reticu-lum and Golgi apparatus, and glycogen granules. Nuclei of the multi-nucleated giant cells are usually distributed ran-domly throughout the cytoplasm, which contains filamentous granular endoplas-mic reticulum, abundant free ribosomes, round or oval mitochondria and Golgi apparatuses near to the nuclei (Figure 53). Sometimes multiple centrioles can be seen within individual giant cells (Figure 54). Anaplastic and fibroblastic cells vary in shape, size, electron density, and develop-ment of cell organelles (Figure 55).

Type-C virus particles have been found in virus-induced osteosarcomas (Fujinaga *et al.*, 1970). They were mature particles with electron-dense nucleoids surrounded by an outer membrane. Immature and budding viral particles with an outer double-layered membrane, an interme-diate and an inner, more electron-dense, membrane were also observed (Figure 56). In some osteosarcomas, particles resem-bling type H virus were seen (Figure 57). The particles were located within cisternae of endoplasmic reticulum or in cyto-plasmic vacuoles. The electron micro-scopic characteristics of osteosarcomas have been described (Fujinaga *et al.*,1970; Chesterman *et al.*, 1972).

The different cellular patterns of osteo-sarcomas appear not related to the bio-logical behaviour, as each of the described tumour types can metastasize (Figures 58–65). The most common sites for metastases are the lungs. The metastatic lesions are usually multiple and of various sizes; they sometimes coalesce and form a large solid mass in the mediastinum (Figure 62). In a few hamsters, metastases have been found

in the kidneys (Figures 64 and 65), but lymph-node metastases have not been reported.

Tumours of uncertain cellular origin

Giant cell tumours develop within bones and apparently arise from the mesenchymal cells of the connective tissue framework (Spjut *et al.*, 1971). These are extremely rare in rodents. In Syrian golden hamsters, only two neoplasms have been reported and these arose spon-taneously from connective tissue around the metacarpal joints (Kirkman, 1962; Ruffolo & Kirkman, 1965). Microscopi-cally, both tumours were composed main-ly of two cell types. The cells were pre-dominantly spherical or spindle-shaped with dense or vesicular nuclei, sometimes resembling epithelioid cells (Figure 66). They were usually arranged as clusters, cords, streams or whorls, often with rosettes (Figure 67). When arranged as palisades around necrotic areas, such neo-plasms or areas of neoplasms resemble epithelioid cell granulomas (Figure 68) and can have scattered eosinophilic leuko-cytes in such areas. The next most prominent cell was the giant cell, with various shapes and containing 20 or more, usually peripherally arranged, hyper-chromatic nuclei. These giant cells had neither stainable pigment nor foreign materials and frequently appeared in clusters and, occasionally, in a concentric arrangement (Figures 69 and 70). The intracellular matrix of the tumour was finely fibrillar, and focally dense or hy-alinized. In reticulum fibre-stained sec-tions, the neoplastic cells were sur-rounded both individually and in small clusters by reticulum fibres. The two giant-cell tumours had metastasized to the lungs and kidneys and both were trans-plantable.

Tumours or tumour-like lesions of odontogenic origin

Tumour-like lesions. In most cases, odontogenic lesions in rodents are not neoplasms but rather are malformations or dysplastic lesions probably associated with chronic periodontitis. A variety of lesions have been reported in several species (Orr, 1936; Ratcliffe, 1940; Zegarelli, 1944). However, little information is available for such lesions in Syrian golden hamsters.

Malassez' epithelial rests are considered a part of normal periodontium; however, they can occur in large epithelial clusters, forming cords or glandular patterns similar to those of ameloblastoma (Figures 71–73) and, thus, give rise to problems in differential diagnosis. Ameloblastomas have not been observed in untreated hamsters.

Ectodermal odontogenic cysts associated with an osteoblastic reaction of the periodontal membrane of the lower jaw, are lined by non-cornified epithelium. They have occurred under certain experimental conditions (Herrold, 1968). It is not known whether these lesions are the origin of the rare squamous cell type of ameloblastoma.

Abnormal dentin production *(denticles)* may be found occasionally within the pulp or in the periodontal membrane of the upper incisors (Figures 74 and 75). Islets of cementum (cementicles) (Figures 76–78) and cartilage *(periodontal cartilaginous dysplasia)* can also occur (Figure 79) in the same area. The presence of chronic inflammation and fibrosis suggests that these lesions, found sometimes in both treated and untreated Eppley colony hamsters, represent a dysplastic alteration, rather than neoplasia. Excessive new bone formation (periodontal hyperostosis) of the alveolar bone, reminiscent of osteogenic tumours, might also occur as a result of periodontitis (Figures 81 and 82).

Ameloblastomas, which have been observed only under experimental conditions, have characteristic features including interlacing strands and epithelial-cell islands embedded in a connective tissue stroma. The epithelial aggregates characteristically have palisading of cells at the periphery of the aggregates and, occasionally, keratinization in the central portion. They can be locally invasive and destructive; however, distant metastases have not been observed (Herrold, 1968). The keratinizing ameloblastoma can be confused with epidermoid carcinoma of the gingiva (Figures 82 and 83), which sometimes occurs in untreated hamsters (Pour, unpublished data). The presence of ameloblasts in a portion of the tumour is required for a diagnosis of ameloblastoma. Ameloblastomas can have various stages of differentiation.

Ameloblastic fibromas are characterized by neoplastic proliferation of both ameloblastic epithelium and connective tissue. Microscopically, they are composed of ramifying islands and nests of cuboidal epithelial cells embedded in loose connective tissue stroma.

Ameloblastic odontoma (odontoameloblastoma) are composed of proliferating ameloblastic and odontoblastic epithelium which retains its capacity to produce irregular dentin and preenamel, so toothlike structures are characteristic of these neoplasms.

Odontoma (complex or compound). Most odontomas (hamartomas) have been experimentally induced (Herrold, 1968; Baer & Kilham, 1974) and are composed of calcified dental tissue. Complex odontomas lack ameloblastic tissue corresponding to a later stage of tooth development. These tumours consist of disorderly mixtures of dentin, enamel, cementum and fibrous connective tissue. Compound odontomas are often agglomerations of large numbers of small and deformed teeth (Figure 84) varying in shape and size.

Miscellaneous lesions

Lesions simulating generalized fibrous osteopathy (von Recklinghausen's disease) may occur in hamsters with parathyroid gland alterations. However, many lesions in bone have been found in the course of severe, generalized calcinosis in hamsters treated with various carcinogenic and non-carcinogenic compounds (Pour, un-published data); the parathyroid glands had, in many (but not all) cases, hyper-plasia or benign neoplasia. The most commonly affected sites are the calvaria and bones of the nasal cavity and jaws. The small lesions usually seen in the bones of the maxillae and mandibulae are characterized by mottling and subperi-osteal scalloping with rarification, de-mineralization, bone resorption and replacement fibrosis (Figures 81, 85 and 86). In the calvaria, the lesions are more severe and have different stages of development (Figure 88).

Costochondral hyperplasia and pre-cancerous lesions of the palate have been observed in male Syrian hamsters treated with N-nitroso-N-diethylamine and ex-posed to cigarette smoke (Harada *et al.,* 1987).

Occasionally, nodular calcinosis of tissues, particularly of the lungs, was found in hamsters of the Eppley colony, and resembled the tumoral calcinosis described in humans (Spjut *et al,* 1971) with regard to histological appearance, but not location. However, these lesions have a different etiology in hamsters as compared to humans, such as aspiration of severely degenerated tracheal cartilages (tracheomalacia), which is not infrequent in older hamsters, or perhaps results from calcium deposits in the lungs by hyper-calcinosis. These foci of calcinosis may be the precursors of the ossicles commonly found in the lungs of hamsters.

SPONTANEOUS TUMOURS

Spontaneous neoplasms arising from the skeletal system and supporting tissues of Syrian golden hamsters have rarely been reported, but might be more numerous because their generally microscopic size or unusual locations allow them to be overlooked at necropsy. When the skeletal system of hamsters of various strains (golden, yellow, white, albino) kept for their lifetime was examined systema-tically, some benign tumours and tumour-like lesions were detected only at microscopic examination. This indicates that benign lesions have either long latencies or slow growth rates, in contrast to malignant tumours, which have an apparently greater incidence and a more rapid growth rate. Nevertheless, osteo-sarcomas have also been found in the *in situ* stage (Diamandopoulos, 1973).

Among the benign spontaneous tumours, a chondroma has been reported in one of 7200 Stanford colony hamsters (Kirkman, 1962). The skeletal system of 65 Syrian golden and 113 Syrian white hamsters (of the Eppley colony) were examined and two osteochondromas found, both located in the lumbar spine (Figure 15), one in a 115-week-old and the other in a 112-week-old male hamster. In addition, extra-osseous exostosis was detected in two white hamsters, in one case originating in the distal femur (female, 94 weeks) and in the other in the distal tibia (female, 81 weeks) (Figures 13 and 14).

Chondromatosis of the periarticular connective tissue of vertebral joints, sometimes indistinguishable from true neoplasms, was also a relatively frequent finding (golden, yellow, white and albino hamsters). These lesions were always asso-ciated with chondrosis and degeneration of intervertebral cartilage, as were the two osteochondromas. These observations indicate a relationship between de-generative, dysplastic and benign neo-plastic changes of the skeletal system in hamsters, in contrast to malignant lesions, which are of different tissue origins and apparently also of different etiology. A high incidence of chondromatosis in the periarticular region of the jaws (Figure 10) was observed in albino hamsters from our breeding colony. This alteration occurred in 16.7% of the females and 3.4% of males. Since similar lesions were not observed in other hamster strains, genetic influences should be considered primary.

Spontaneous malignant neoplasms of cartilage and bone occur sporadically in some hamster colonies. Chondrosarcomas are extremely rare (Graubmann, 1967), whereas osteosarcoma occurs in incidences up to 0.5% (Fortner *et al.*, 1961; Dunham & Herrold, 1962; Cox *et al.*, 1972; Yabe *et al.*, 1972; Dontenwill *et al.*, 1973). Osteosarcoma was found in 0.3–1.8% of Syrian golden hamsters of our colony treated with various carcinogenic and non-carcinogenic substances and the tumour incidence was not related to compound administration. The greater numbers of tumours in treated hamsters is probably due to the generally larger number of experimental animals as compared to controls. In the Eppley colony, the incidence of spontaneous osteosarcomas in albino hamsters was about 0.5%.

Spontaneous malignant neoplasms of periarticular tissue and tendon sheaths are extremely rare, as are neoplasms arising in cartilage. Malignant giant-cell tumours originating in connective tissue around metacarpal joints have been reported in two (0.17%) untreated, 575-day-old male hamsters (Kirkman, 1962; Ruffolo & Kirkman, 1965). A chondrosarcoma of the mandible and one of the falx cerebri have been reported in two Chinese hamsters (Ninomiya *et al.*, 1988). Ernst *et al.* (1989) recorded four neoplasms of bone and one odontogenic neoplasm in 285 European hamsters ranging in age between one and five years. Three of the bone neoplasms were osteosarcomas arising in mandible, external ear and femur. The other bone neoplasm was a chondroma located in the external ear. The odontogenic neoplasm was an unusual invasive cementoblastoma located in the maxilla.

Lesions of odontogenic origin, such as Malassez' epithelial rests (which sometimes resemble ameloblastomas), cementicles, denticles, periodontal chondroid dysplasia and hyperostosis, have occasionally been observed in untreated hamsters. The possible relationship between these lesions and periodontitis has already been mentioned. However, neoplasia, incorrectly described as odontoma, might also occur (Dontenwill *et al.*, 1973).

Lesions similar to tumorous carcinosis in humans were observed in a few Eppley colony hamsters, but spontaneous neoplasms originating from bone-marrow elements were not seen. Bone lesions have been reported in cardiomyopathic hamsters (Togari *et al.*, 1989).

INDUCTION OF TUMOURS

Viruses

The induction of bone tumours in Syrian golden hamsters was initially derived from an observation that FBJ-virus, isolated from a spontaneous murine bone tumour, induced osteosarcoma when injected into newborn mice (Finkel *et al.*, 1966 a, b). In the search for a similar agent responsible for malignant bone tumours in humans, it was found that intraperitoneal injections of extracts of human osteosarcomas into newborn hamsters produced localized, calcium-containing lesions in the abdominal wall at the injection site in 70% of the animals within a few days after injection. In addition, many of the hamsters developed multiple bone fractures, mainly of the ribs, fibulae, zygomatic arch and ulna, 1–3 weeks later (Finkel *et al.*, 1967). Inflammatory reactions observed microscopically included numerous giant cells and abundant intercellular calcium deposits. Virus-like particles were demonstrated in both the tumour extracts and lesions at injection sites. Later, between 427 and 559 days after injection, six of the 461 treated hamsters (1.3%) developed osteosarcomas arising from the proximal tibiae (two neoplasms), distal femora, proximal humeri, distal radii, fibulae and scapulae (Finkel *et al.*, 1968). An extraosseous sarcoma appeared in the right inguinal region at the inoculation site (Finkel *et al.*, 1969). Type-C particles were found in five of these neoplasms. Also, the muscle extract removed from the primary tumour in a patient induced osteosarcoma in a hamster. In addition, extracts from induced osteosarcomas in hamsters, one and two passages removed from patients, produced similar tumours, but with shorter latencies. The shorter latencies could have been related to the enhancement of tumorigenesis by passage through hamsters (Finkel *et al.*, 1968). In electron micrographs of these neoplasms, virus particles of two types, H and C, were observed.

In serial radiographs of the treated hamsters, it was observed that tumour development preceded such skeletal abnormalities as fracture of non-weight-bearing bones, thickening of cortices in long bones (primarily in the proximal metaphysis of the humeri or tibiae and the distal metaphysis of the femora), and endosteal hyperostosis with invasion of the marrow spaces (Finkel *et al.*, 1969). Osteosarcomas in hamsters, like those observed in mice, rats and humans, may be one component of a generalized disease in all these species, with osseous lesions of inflammation, degeneration and proliferation to malignancy (L. Dmochowski, personal communication).

Soehner and Dmochowski (1969) and Soehner *et al.* (1970) reported that cell-free extracts from bone tumours induced in New Zealand black (NB) rats by murine sarcoma virus-Moloney (MSV-M) and murine sarcoma virus-Harvey (MSV-H), when injected intraperitoneally, induced various types of mesenchymal neoplasms in eight of 14 hamsters. Four of these eight animals developed osteosarcomas after about 87 days. MSV-H inoculation did not induce osteosarcomas, but an unclassified neoplasm. However, an extract of this tumour induced osteosarcoma in 82 days in one of four inoculated hamsters (Soehner & Dmochowski, 1969). The osteogenic tumours induced by both viruses were located in the sternum, ribs, scapulae and bone of limbs, and had often remarkable variations in histological

pattern, being composed of cells of osteogenic, chondrogenic, fibrous, myxomatous, angiosarcomatous, histiocytic (including giant cells) and anaplastic types.

Type-C virus particles in different stages of development were found in all cells and tissues examined (Soehner & Dmochowski, 1969; Fujinaga *et al.*, 1970). Osteosarcomas were also induced by serial passages of Soehner-Dmochowski-adapted virus (SD-MSV-M) in rats and hamsters (Soehner *et al.*, 1970). However, the tumorigenicity of SD-MSV-M for the hamster was lost after passage in mouse or rat embryo cells, though retained after passage in rat and hamster embryos and 3T3 cells (Dmochowski *et al.*, 1972). These results were considered reflections of the influence of a 'helper' virus (Stenback *et al.*, 1966), of either murine or hamster origin.

After subcutaneous inoculation of MSV-H virus in the interscapular region of weanling hamsters, the induced neoplasms were mostly mesenchymal and developed mainly in the peripheral portions of the limbs, sometimes involving all four (Chesterman *et al.*, 1972). In radiographs, some limb tumours had either very little bone involvement, apart from some periosteal new bone formation, or had extensive destruction resulting in pathological fractures. Microscopically, the majority of bone tumours were composed of giant cells resembling osteoclasts, the tumours resembling osteoclastomas. These extensively invaded the medullary cavity. It was, therefore, suggested that the bone lesions were the results of an osteolytic response to tumour invasion, rather than an osteosarcoma. However, in a few cases new bone formation was sufficient to suggest a tentative diagnosis of osteosarcoma (Chesterman *et al.*, 1972). In contrast, Berman (1967) and Chesterman et al. (1972) reported the induction by MSV-M virus of tumours with histological features suggestive of myoblastic origin. The same virus may induce all types of lesions ranging from inflammatory, necrotizing and degenerative alterations to proliferative and, indeed, neoplastic changes, some of which derive, depending upon the reactive and responsive tissues, from soft tissues and others from osseous tissue. Because MSV-M virus also induced osteosarcoma in some strains of rats (Tanaka *et al.*, 1972, 1974), a common phenomenon appears to exist in the induction of bone tumours by a virus that originally induced leukaemia and, sometimes, rhabdomyo-sarcomas (Moloney, 1966)

Diamandopoulos (1972, 1973) reported that DNA viruses also will induce osteosarcomas in hamsters. The intravenous inoculation of male weanling hamsters (21–22 days old) with SV40 virus induced within 3–6 months various mesenchymal and lymphoid tumours in 85–95% of the inoculated hamsters and multicentric osteosarcomas in 50%. Of the 137 hamsters with bone tumours, two thirds of the larger primary neoplasms were in the bones of the posterior limbs, usually on the same side as the intravenous inoculation. Additional primary, but smaller, bone tumours originated from one or more of the ribs on either the same or the contralateral sides of the thorax. The bones of the anterior limbs were involved in only 10% of the hamsters. The sites of origin of the larger tumours were difficult to determine, because the neoplasms had invaded the surrounding tissues. The smaller bone tumours, however, arose from the periosteum and/or endosteum. Many of the rib tumours, which were multicentric, were at the *in situ* stage, being either within the bone medulla or subperiosteally located without local invasion. In this experiment, the osteosarcomas had various histological patterns (Diamandopoulos, 1973). In a later study, Diamandopoulos and McLane (1975) observed tumours in 3-week-old to 12-month-old male Syrian hamsters inoculated intravenously with $10^{8.5}$

median tissue culture infective dose of SV40 virus. The tumour incidence and latency were directly dependent on the age of the animals at the time of exposure to virus and the dose of the virus. However, this age–dose dependence was weaker than that usually observed in hamsters inoculated subcutaneously or intramuscularly with SV40 virus. Moreover, the spectrum of neoplasms induced (lymphosarcomas, osteosarcomas) by intravenous inoculation contrasted sharply with the anaplastic and spindle-cell sarcomas, which were the only types of malignant tumours produced when other routes were used. In a similar experiment with three inbred hamster strains (LSH/SsLak, LHC/Lak, MHA/SsLak) and one outbred stock (LVG/Lak), Diamandopoulos (1978) found that, although the incidence and latency of induced tumours (lymphocytic leukaemia, osteosarcoma) were similar in the three inbred strains, hamsters of the outbred stock were almost completely resistant to tumour induction. When SV40-virus-induced tumours were serially passaged, osteosarcoma cells lost their differentiated phenotype and their capacity to form osteoid during, but not before, their serial passage in culture. Lymphosarcoma cells remained differentiated and retained production of immunoglobulin after many *in vitro* passages (Diamandopoulos *et al.*, 1976). Singh *et al.* (1977) induced osteosarcoma in antilymphocyte-treated hamsters when TE-85 human osteosarcoma cells (maintained in tissue culture) infected with MSV-M (RD-114) virus were injected adjacent to the femur or the scapula. Tumours were palpable 10 to 14 days after the cells were injected and all hamsters had pulmonary metastases. Neither the subcutaneous sarcomas nor their metastases had either bone or osteoid; however, sarcomas adjacent to the femur and scapula had osteoid and calcified bone.

Several biological products, which included live and inactive viral vaccines (measles, smallpox, yellow fever, rabies, poliovirus, poliomyelitis, mumps), were not oncogenic when administered to newborn hamsters (Cox *et al.*, 1972). A small number of osteosarcomas developed in the test animals (8 of 7643 = 0.10%) and the incidence was within the range of spontaneously occurring malignant bone tumours in that colony of Syrian hamsters (Cox *et al.*, 1972).

Significant numbers of osteosarcomas have been induced in hamsters until recently only by viruses; the presence of virus-like particles in the majority of these neoplasms suggests a viral etiology for these tumours. However, the virus particles could be ubiquitous, since particles have been observed in various normal hamster tissues (Stenback *et al.*, 1966). Also, the possibility exists that X-radiation exposure during the taking of radiographs could have contributed to the induction of osteosarcomas. However, Finkel *et al.* (1969) considered it doubtful that 360 rads given in 12 fractions during the course of a year would induce bone tumours in a population of only a few thousand hamsters; furthermore, as discussed below, hamsters seem less sensitive than mice to the induction of bone tumours by radiation. Also, control hamsters subjected to the same radiographic procedures did not have bone tumours (Finkel *et al.*, 1969). Polyoncogenic prototype human papovavirus BKV (Gardner's strain), two small-plaque isolates (WT-500 and WT-502), and a large-plaque forming isolate (WT-501) induced brain tumours and a few osteosarcomas in hamsters (Watanabe *et al.*, 1982).

The possible viral etiology of osteosarcomas in hamsters, as well as in other species, is supported by immunological evidence and by the identification of SV40 virus T antigen and antibody against SV40 virus T antigen in the serum of adult hamsters which had received transplants of different tumours (Pope & Rowe, 1964; Diamandopoulos & McLane, 1972).

Furuno and Yogo (1983) analysed 10 clones from cell line OS-513 (which originated from a BK virus-induced osteosarcoma in hamsters) for viral DNA and found that all the clones had both monomeric and polymeric viral DNA. They suggested that the basic form of free viral DNA in the transformed cells is stably inherited by the progeny cells during cell growth.

Osteosarcomas were also induced in newborn Syrian hamsters by injecting productively infected TE-85 cells (cultured human osteosarcoma cells) adjacent to the femur. All of the hamsters had tumours and pulmonary metastases. Invasion of the marrow spaces and adjacent skeletal muscles by the malignant osteoblasts, anaplastic sarcoma cells and multi-nucleated giant cells was frequently observed. The tumour was transplantable and TE-85 cell surface antigens were demonstrable on the surface of the tumour cells (Singh *et al.*, 1979). Osteosarcomas of the ribs and mandibula were induced in weanling hamsters by intravenous inoculation of highly concentrated human papovavirus BK, propagated in human embryonic kidney cells. The sera of the tumour-bearing animals were positive for BK T-antigen and successfully transplanted tumour cells were positive for intranuclear T-antigen. Morphologically, these tumours had various areas of differentiation from mature sarcoma and angiomatous sarcoma to well-differentiated osteosarcoma (Yamaguchi *et al.*, 1980). BK virus induced ependymoma, carcinoma of the pancreatic islets, osteosarcomas and a variety of other tumours (Corallini *et al.*, 1978). A cell line was established from an osteosarcoma that occurred in a hamster inoculated at birth with an extract of a CF N01 mouse FBJ-osteosarcoma (Levy *et al.*, 1978). The transformed cell line contained the FBJ-MUSV genome, which could be 'rescued'. This 'rescued' genome induced osteosarcomas typical of those induced by FBJ-MUSV.

While it is generally agreed that some viruses are oncogenic to mesenchymal tissues, different opinions exist, chiefly in interpretations of the nature of induced bone tumours. Berman (1967) and Chesterman *et al.* (1972) suggested that the majority of bone lesions are due to secondary involvement by tumours arising from soft tissue or from undifferentiated cells of the marrow. Nevertheless, the direct formation of tumour osteoid, the presence of material microscopically indistinguishable from it, or of small foci of bone (demonstrated in the majority of the experimental tumours) identifies osteosarcoma (Lichtenstein, 1965; Dahlin, 1970). The concomitant presence of various malignant cells in induced (and also in spontaneously occurring) osteosarcomas may reflect the neoplastic response of either different mesenchymal elements or primitive cells in various stages of differentiation. Such could explain the morphological variety of 'virus-induced' neoplasms.

A few odontogenic lesions can also be induced by viruses. The intracranial and intraperitoneal inoculation of weanling hamsters with rat virus and with minute virus of mice (MVM) resulted in cementomas and odontomas within the mandibulae and about the apical portion of the mandibular incisors (Baer & Kilham, 1964, 1974). In addition, lesions such as thickening of the first molar roots by a large number of concentric layers of osteocementum, shortening and thickening of the roots of the second molars and severe loss of alveolar bone of the third molars were observed (Baer & Kilham, 1964). Odontogenic lesions and malformations preceded the development of odontogenic neoplasms.

Giant-cell tumours resembling those in humans have been observed in virus-induced bone tumours, particularly in hamsters inoculated with MSV-H and MSV-M. Murine sarcoma virus-Kirsten (MSV-Ki) produced, among other sar-comas, giant-cell tumours involving the femur (Chesterman *et al.*, 1972). Type-C particles have been found in both osteosarcoma and giant-cell tumours of humans (Dmochowski, 1971), suggesting that bone and giant-cell tumours of mice, rats and hamsters and some neoplasms in humans may conceivably be of viral etiology. The giant-cell tumours are distinguishable from giant-cell reactions of bone in osteopathia fibrosa by their different morphologies and distribution.

Radiation

In contrast to mice and rats, tumours have not been induced in hamsters by radiation. A dose of 2.0 mCi of ^{90}Sr/g body weight, which is highly oncogenic for the mouse skeleton (Finkel *et al.*, 1968), did not produce bone tumours in a group of 34 Syrian hamsters (Finkel *et al.*, 1969). However, the very severe radiation damage produced in treated hamsters may indicate that the dose was too large, and the failure to induce tumours was, therefore, not due to the lower sensitivity of the hamster skeleton (compared to that of the mouse) to oncogenesis by radiation. In fact, because of the difference in bone sizes between hamsters and mice and the range of the beta rays from the ^{90}Y daughter of ^{90}Sr, the energy absorbed by the hamster skeleton would exceed that absorbed by the mouse skeleton, for the same injected dose (M.P. Finkel, personal communication).

Chemicals

No chemical carcinogen is known to be organotropic for bone and supporting tissues in hamsters. The few osteosarcomas observed in the Eppley colony hamsters could not be attributed to the chemical compounds used.

In contrast to osseous tissue, odontogenic tissues are responsive to chemical carcinogens. A variety of odontogenic tumours were induced at incidences of 6/14 and 6/9, respectively, by *N*-methyl-*N*-nitrosourea injected intravenously or intragastrically into four-week-old Syrian golden hamsters (Herrold, 1968). Amelo-blastic fibromas and ameloblastic odon-tomas were the predominant types found at death in these animals (average age 8.5 months). Acanthomatous ameloblasto-mas (two tumours) and a compound odontoma (one tumour) developed only in hamsters treated intragastrically, whereas one complex odontoma devel-oped in an intravenously injected hamster. Most tumours originated in the mandi-bular incisors and only a few in the maxillary incisor area. In this experiment, as in the study on MVM-induced lesions (Baer & Kilham, 1974), odontogenic le-sions and malformations preceded development of odontogenic neoplasms in many animals.

Lesions similar to generalized fibrous osteopathy (von Recklinghausen's disease) associated with hyperparathyroidism were found in two Eppley colony hamsters receiving single injections of nitroso-hexamethyleneimine and nitrosopiperi-dine (Althoff *et al.*, 1974). It was not clear whether the development of fibrous osteo-pathy was attributable to the treatment, since spontaneous parathyroid gland adenomas were relatively frequent in this colony (2% of males and 7% of females). However, no bone lesions were found in hamsters with parathyroid gland adeno-mas. In hamsters of the Eppley colony exposed to various carcinogenic and noncarcinogenic compounds, marked fibrous osteopathy was observed in several hamsters which had lesions of severe generalized calcinosis. Since hyperplasia and neoplasia of the parathyroid glands were not found in all animals, the lesions in bone seem to reflect a primary dis-turbance of calcium metabolism of un-determined etiology and alterations of the parathyroid glands were secondary.

Hormones

Hyperplasia of fibrocartilage and chon-drosarcomas have been induced by prolonged administration of estrone and estriol in orchidectomized Syrian ham-sters (Ruffolo & Kirkman, 1966). No such lesions were seen in hamsters treated similarly with other steroids, namely ethinylestradiol, estradiol, diethylstilbes-trol, testosterone, cortisone, and deoxy-corticosterone acetate.

COMPARATIVE ASPECTS

The anatomy, histology and phy-siology of the hamster skeleton differ from that of humans, and this influences the comparison of skeletal diseases. However, some neoplasms and tumour-like lesions, which develop spontaneously or under experimental conditions, have morpho-logical similarities to skeletal lesions occurring in humans. Benign neoplasms of bones and supporting tissues are relatively rare in both humans and ham-sters. Osteosarcomas, as in humans, are also the most common malignant bone tumour in hamsters. The distribution of osteosarcomas and their histological features and biological behaviour in ham-sters are similar to observations made of these neoplasms in humans. Cellular pat-terns which resembled those of various bone neoplasms of humans, such as chon-droblastomas, osteoblastomas, non-osteo-genic and chondromyxoid fibromas, and giant-cell tumours, were observed in some areas of osteosarcomas in hamsters. This may indicate a similar tissue response in both species. However, a variety of pat-terns can be produced in hamsters that do not necessarily duplicate patterns found in bone lesions of humans. Most osteo-sarcomas in hamster are poorly differen-tiated and large areas of some tumours resembled fibrosarcoma. Multiple osteo-sarcomas, induced in hamsters, also develop in a few human patients. In this regard, the successful induction of osteo-sarcoma in hamsters by viruses is of some interest, since a viral etiology of human osteosarcomas has been suggested by several investigators (Dmochowski, 1970; Latarjet, 1971; Pritchard *et al.*, 1971; Reilly *et al.*, 1972). Lesions similar to osteopathia fibrosa generalisata (von Reckling-hausen's disease) can occur in Syrian golden hamsters, whereas the skeletons of many other species apparently do not respond to hyperparathyroidism in the same manner. The same is true for odontogenic structures, as the most common types of odontogenic neoplasms in humans have been reproduced in the hamster by viruses and certain chemicals.

The results on induction of skeletal tumours demonstrate the value of the hamster as a model system in studies of the origin of human skeletal tumours and of antiviral treatment of tumours. Antiviral drugs might evolve as a possible treatment for bone tumours, supplementary to surgery, radiotherapy and chemotherapy.

ACKNOWLEDGEMENTS

The author thanks Dr P.N. Baer, Dr G.T. Diamandopoulos, Dr L. Dmochowski, Dr M.P. Finkel, Dr H. Kirkman and Dr Y. Yabe for providing material for this chapter.

REFERENCES

Althoff, J., Wilson, R., Cardesa, A. & Pour, P. (1974) Comparative studies of neoplastic response to a single dose of nitroso compounds. 3. The effect of *N*-nitrosopiperidine and *N*-nitrosomorpholine in Syrian golden hamsters. *Z. Krebsforsch.*, 81, 251–259

Baer, P.N. & Kilham, L. (1964) Rat virus and periodontal disease. IV. The aged hamster. *Oral Surg.*, 18, 803–811

Baer, P.N. & Kilham, L. (1974) Dental defects in hamsters infected with minute virus of mice. *Oral Surg.*, 37, 385–389

Beatty, M.D. & Hillemann, H.H. (1950) Osteogenesis in the golden hamster. *J. Mammal.*, 31, 121–134

Berman, L.D. (1967) Comparative morphologic study of the virus-induced solid tumors of Syrian hamsters. *J. Natl. Cancer Inst.*, 39, 847–901

Boyer, C.C. (1968) Embryology. In: Hoffman, R.H., Robinson, P.F. & Magalhaes, H., eds, *The Golden Hamster: Its Biology and Use in Medical Research*, Ames, Iowa State University Press, pp. 227–240

Brown, P., Henderson, J., Hilton, T. J. & Parren, J. (1993) Chondroma of the foreleg in a Syrian hamster. *Lab. Anim.*, 27, 391–392

Chaudhry, A.P. & Shah, R.M. (1973) Palatogenesis in hamster. II. Ultrastructural observations on the closure of palate. *J. Morphol.*, 139, 329–350

Chauncey, H.H., Kronman, J.H., Spinale, J.J. & Shklar, F. (1963) Effect of partial desalivation and parotin administration on hamster epiphyseal plate. *J. Dent. Res.*, 24, 894

Chesterman, F.C., Harvey, J.J., Branca, M., Phillips, D.E.H., Hallowes, R.C. & Bassin, R.H. (1972) Tumors and other lesions induced by murine sarcoma viruses. *Prog. Exp. Tumor Res.* (Basel), 16, 426–453

Coleman, E.J., Gaffar, A. & Marcussen, H.W. (1971) The influence of inoculation of human cariogenic bacteria upon periodontal bone resorption in the golden hamster. *Arch. Oral Biol.*, 16, 1371–1376

Corallini, A., Altavilla, G., Cecchetti, M.G., Fabris, G., Grossi, M.P., Balboni, P.G., Lanza, G., & Barbanti-Brodano, G. (1978) Ependymomas, malignant tumors of pancreatic islets, and osteosarcomas induced in hamsters by BK virus, a human papovavirus. *J. Natl. Cancer Inst.*, 61, 875–883

Cox, C.B., Landon, J., Valerio, M.G., Palmer, A., Kirschstein, R.L. & Singer, S.H. (1972) Lack of significant oncogenicity of biological products in hamsters. *Appl. Micro-biol.*, 23, 675–678

Dahlin, D.C. (1970) *Bone Tumors, General Aspects and Data on 3,987 Cases*, 2nd ed., Springfield, IL, Charles C. Thomas

Deemys, G. & Kronman, J.H. (1973) Sequential tissue response and recovery after orthodontic tooth movement in hamsters. *Am. J. Orthodont.*, 63, 56–66

Diamandopoulos, G.T. (1972) Leukemia, lymphoma, and osteosarcoma induced in the Syrian golden hamster by simian virus 40. *Science*, 176, 173–175

Diamandopoulos, G.T. (1973) Induction of lymphocytic leukemia, lymphosarcoma, reticulum cell sarcoma, and osteogenic sarcoma in the Syrian golden hamster by oncogenic DNA simian virus 40. *J. Natl. Cancer Inst.*, 50, 1347–1365

Diamandopoulos, G.T. (1978) Incidence, latency, and morphologic types of neoplasms induced by Simian virus 40 inoculated intravenously into hamsters of three inbred strains and one outbred stock. *J. Natl. Cancer Inst.*, 60, 445–449

Diamandopoulos, G.T. & McLane, M.F. (1972) The tumor imprint technique for demonstrating SV40 T antigen by immunofluorescence (36716). *Proc. Soc. Exp. Biol. (N.Y.)*, 141, 62–66

Diamandopoulos, G.T. & McLane, M.F. (1975) Effect of host age, virus dose, and route of ino-culation on tumor incidence, latency, and morphology in Syrian hamsters inoculated intravenously with oncogenic DNA simian virus 40. *J. Natl. Cancer Inst.*, 55, 479–482

Diamandopoulos, G.T., Miller, M.H., McLane, M.F. & Evans, P.G. (1976) Loss persistence of the differentiated state of simian virus 40-induced hamster tumor cells before and after serial passage in culture. *Cancer Res.*, 36, 3171–3177

Dmochowski, L. (1970) Current status of the relationship of viruses to leukemia, lymphoma and solid tumors. In: *Proceedings of the 14th Annual Clinical Conference on Leukemia-Lymphoma, Houston, Texas,* Chicago, Year Book Medical Publishers, pp. 32–57

Dmochowski, L. (1971) Studies on the relationship of viruses to leukemia and solid tumours in man. In: *Proceedings of the Xth International Cancer Congress, Houston, Texas,* May 22–29, Chicago, Year Book Medical Publishers, pp. 134–145

Dmochowski, L., East, J.L., Bowen, J.M., Lewis, M.L. & Shigematsu, T. (1972) Studies on tumorigenicity of rat bone tumor virus (SD-MSV-M) in mice, rats and hamsters. *Tex. Rep. Biol. Med.*, 30, 301–312

Dontenwill, W., Chevalier, H.J., Harke, H.P., Lafrenz, U. & Reckzeh, G. (1973) Spontantumoren des syrischen Goldhamsters. *Z. Krebsforsch.*, 80, 127–158

Dunham, L.J. & Herrold, K.M. (1962) Failure to produce tumors in the hamster cheek pouch by exposure to ingredients of betel quid; histopathologic changes in the pouch and other organs by exposure to known carcinogens. *J. Natl. Cancer Inst.*, 29, 1047-1067

Ernst, H., Kunstyr, I., Rittinghausen, S.J. & Mohr, U. (1989) Spontaneous tumors of the European hamster (*Cricetus cricetus L.*). *Z. Versuchstierkd.*, 32, 38–96

Ferm, V.H. & Kilham, L. (1965) Skeletal studies of virus-induced dwarfism. *Growth*, 29, 7-16

Finkel, M.P., Biskis, B.O. & Jinkins, P.B. (1966a) Virus induction of osteosarcomas in mice. *Science*, 151, 698–701

Finkel, M.P., Jinkins, P.B., Tolle, J. & Biskis, B.O. (1966b) Serial radiography of virus-induced osteosarcomas in mice. *Radiology*, 87, 333–339

Finkel, M.P., Biskis, B.O. & Farrell, C. (1967) Pathogenic effects of extracts of human osteosarcomas. *Arch Pathol.*, 84, 425–428

Finkel, M.P., Biskis, B.O. & Farrell, C. (1968) Osteosarcomas appearing in Syrian hamsters after treatment with extracts of human osteosarcomas. *Proc. Natl. Acad. Sci. USA*, 60, 1223–1230

Finkel, M.P., Biskis, B.O. & Farrell, C. (1969) Nonmalignant and malignant changes in hamsters inoculated with extracts of human osteosarcomas. *Radiology*, 92, 1546–1552

Fortner, J.G. (1961) The influence of castration on spontaneous tumorigenesis in the Syrian (golden) hamster. *Cancer Res.*, 21, 1491–1498

Fortner, J.G., Mahy, A.G. & Schrodt, G.R. (1961) Transplantable tumors of the Syrian (golden) hamster. I. Tumors of the alimentary tract, endocrine glands and melanomas. *Cancer Res.*, 21, 161–198

Friant, M. (1957) Le début de l'ossification du cartilage de Meckel. *C.R. Acad. Sci. (Paris)*, 244, 1071–1073

Friant, M. (1958a) Sur les premiers stades d'ossification du cartilage de Meckel. *Acta Anat.*, 32, 100–114

Friant, M. (1958b) Sur l'évolution du cartilage de Meckel. *Acta Anat.*, 34, 292–297

Fujinaga, S., Poel, W.E. & Dmochowski, L. (1970) Light and electron microscopic studies of osteosarcomas induced in rats and hamsters by Harvey and Moloney sarcoma viruses. *Cancer Res.*, 30, 1698–1708

Furuno, A. & Yogo, Y. (1983) Free viral DNA present in BKV hamster osteosarcoma (OS-513) cell clones. *Jpn. J. Med. Sci. Biol.*, 36, 105–108

Gisondi, J.G. & Kronman, J.H. (1972) Thyroid influence on bone histology during tooth movement in hamsters. *Angle Ortho.*, 42, 310–318

Graubmann, H.D. von (1967) Spontanes Chondrosarkom beim syrischen Goldhamster. *Z. Versuchstierkd.*, 9, 216–220

Harada, T., Enomoto, A., Kitazawa, T., Maita, K. & Shirasu, Y. (1987) Oral leukoplakia and costochondral hyperplasia induced by diethylnitrosamine in hamsters exposed to cigarette smoke with or without dietary vitamin C. *Vet. Pathol.*, 24, 257–264

Heggie, A.D. (1971) Pathogenesis of H-1 virus infection of embryonic hamster bone in organ culture. *J. Exp. Med.*, 133, 506–519

Heggie, A.D. & Stjernholm, R.L. (1973) Altered mucopolysaccharide metabolism in organ cultures of fetal hamster bones infected by the H-1 strain of parvovirus. *Teratology*, 8, 147–152

Herrold, K.M. (1968) Odontogenic tumors and epidermoid carcinomas of the oral cavity. An experimental study in Syrian hamsters. *Oral Surg.*, 25, 262–272

Jordan, H.V. & Van Houte, J. (1972) The hamster as an experimental model for odontopathic infections. *Prog. Exp. Tumor Res.* (Basel), 16, 539–556

Kay, S. (1971) Ultrastructure of an osteoid type of osteogenic sarcoma. *Cancer*, 28, 437–445

Kerschner, A., Riehl, T. & Magalhaes, H. (1957) Osteogenesis in different strains of the golden hamster, *Mesocricetus auratus. Anat. Rec.*, 128, 575–576

Keyes, P.H. (1968) Odontopathic infection. In: Hoffman, R.H., Robinson, P.F. & Magalhaes, H., eds, *The Golden Hamster: Its Biology and Use in Medical Research*, Ames, Iowa State University Press, pp. 253–282

Kilham, L. & Margolis, G. (1971) Fetal infections of hamsters, rats, and mice induced with the minute virus of mice (MVM) *Teratology*, 4, 43–62

Kirkman, H. (1962) A preliminary report concerning tumors observed in Syrian hamsters. *Stanford Med. Bull.*, 20, 163–166

Latarjet, R. (1971) Sur l'étiologie virale de certains ostéoscomes ostéogènes. *Revue critique. Bull. Cancer*, 58, 277–286

Levy, J.A., Kazan, P.L., Reilly, C.A. & Finkel, M.P. (1978) FBJ osteosarcoma virus in tissue culture. III. Isolation and characterization of non-virus-producing FBJ-transformed cells. *J. Virol.*, 26, 11–15

Lichtenstein, L. (1965) *Bone Tumors*, 3rd ed., St. Louis, Mosby

Moloney, J.B. (1966) A virus-induced rhabdomyosarcoma of mice. *Natl Cancer Inst. Monogr.*, 22, 139–142

Ninomiya, H., Nakamura, T. & Yamazaki, K.V. (1988) Chondrosarcoma of the mandible and falx cerebri in a Chinese hamster (*Cricetulus griceus*): report of a case. *Jikken-Dobutsu*, 37, 317–320

Orr, J.W. (1936) Adamantinoma of the jaw in a rabbit. *J. Pathol. Bacteriol.*, 42, 703–704

Pedersen, H.E. (1949) The ossicles of the semilunar cartilages of rodents. *Anat. Rec.*, 105, 1–9

Pope, J.H. & Rowe, W.P. (1964) Detection of specific antigen in SV40-transformed cells by immunofluorescence. *J. Exp. Med.*, 120, 121–128

Pritchard, D.J., Reilly, C.A. & Finkel, M.P. (1971) Evidence for a human osteosarcoma virus. *Nature*, 234, 126–127

Ratcliffe, H.L. (1940) Spontaneous tumors in two colonies of rats of the Wistar Institute of Anatomy and Biology. *Am. J. Pathol.*, 16, 237–254

Reilly, C.A., Pritchard, D.J., Biskis, B.O. & Finkel, M.P. (1972) Immunologic evidence suggesting a viral etiology of human osteosarcoma. *Cancer*, 30, 603–609

Ruffolo, P.R. & Kirkman, H. (1965) Malignant, transplantable, giant cell tumors of periarticular connective tissues in Syrian golden hamsters (*Mesocricetus auratus*). *Br. J. Cancer*, 19, 573–580

Ruffolo, P.R. & Kirkman, H. (1966) Estriol- and estrone-induced hyperplasia and neoplasia of external ear elastic cartilage in the Syrian hamster. *Anat. Rec.*, 154, 573–580

Salih, M.S. & Kent, G.C., Jr (1964) The epaxial muscles of the golden hamster. *Anat. Rec.*, 150, 319–334

Schajowicz, F., Ackerman, L.V., Sissons, H.A., Sobin, L.H. & Torloni, H. (1972) *Histological Typing of Bone Tumours* (International Histological Classification of Tumours, No. 6), Geneva, World Health Organization

Shah, R.M. & Chaudhry, A.P. (1972) Palato-genesis in hamster. I. Light microscopic and cytochemical observations on the closure of the hard and soft palates. *J. Morphol.*, 139, 329–350

Shklar, G. (1972) Experimental oral pathology in the Syrian hamster. *Prog. Exp. Tumor Res.* 16, 518–538

Singh, I., Hatheway, J.M., Tsang, K.Y., Blakemore, W.S. & McAllister, R.M. (1977) An animal model for human osteosarcoma. *Surgery*, 81, 168–175

Singh, I., Tsang, K.Y. & Blakemore, W.S. (1979) A model for human osteosarcoma. *Clin. Orthop.*, 144, 305–310

Soehner, R.L. & Dmochowski, L. (1969) Induction of bone tumours in rats and hamsters with murine sarcoma virus and their cell-free transmission. *Nature,* 224, 191–192

Soehner, R.L., Fujinaga, S. & Dmochowski, L. (1970) Neoplastic bone lesions induced in rats and hamsters by Moloney and Harvey murine sarcoma viruses. *Bibl. Haematol.* (Basel), 36, 593–599

Sokoloff, L. (1958) Joint diseases of laboratory animals. *J. Natl. Cancer Inst.*, 20, 965–977

Sokoloff, L. & Jay, G.E., Jr (1956) Natural history of degenerative joint disease in small laboratory animals. I. Pathologic anatomy of degenerative joint disease in mice. *Arch. Pathol.*, 62, 118–142

Spjut, H.J., Dorfman, H.D., Fechner, R.E. & Ackerman, L.V. (1971) Tumors of bone and cartilage. In: *Atlas of Tumor Pathology,* Washington, D.C., Armed Forces Institute of Pathology, second series, fascicle 5

Stenback, W.A., Van Hoosier, G.L., Jr & Trentin, J.J. (1966) Virus particles in hamster tumors as revealed by electron microscopy. *Proc. Soc. Exp. Biol.* (N.Y.), 122, 1219–1223

Tanaka, K.K., Yoshida, T.O., Tanaka, T., Kojima, K. & Hanaichi, T. (1972) Different neoplastic response of mice and rats to infection by murine sarcoma virus (Moloney). *Gann*, 63, 445–457

Tanaka, K.K., Tanaka, T. & Ikemoto, K. (1974) Osteosarcoma induced in rats by murine sarcoma virus-Moloney. *Proc. Japan. Acad.*, 50, 641–644

Togari, A., Arai, M., Matsumoto, S., Tarumoto, Y. & Takahashi, H. (1989) Bone disorder in cardiomyopathic hamsters. *Bone Miner.*, 7, 127–136

Watanabe, S., Kotake, S., Nozawa, A., Muto, T., Uchida, S. (1982) Tumorigenicity of human BK papovirus plaque isolates, wild type and plaque morphology mutant, in hamsters. *Int. J. Cancer*, 29, 583–586

Yabe, Y., Kataoka, N. & Koyama, H. (1972) Spontaneous tumors in hamsters: incidence, morphology, transplantation and virus studies. *Gann*, 63, 329–336

Yamaguchi, K., Sata, S. & Aoyama, Y. (1980) Characteristics of osteogenic sarcoma of hamster induced BK virus. *Gann,* 71, 131–137

Zegarelli, E. V. (1944) Adamantoblastomas in the Slye stock of mice. *Am. J. Pathol.*, 20, 23–30

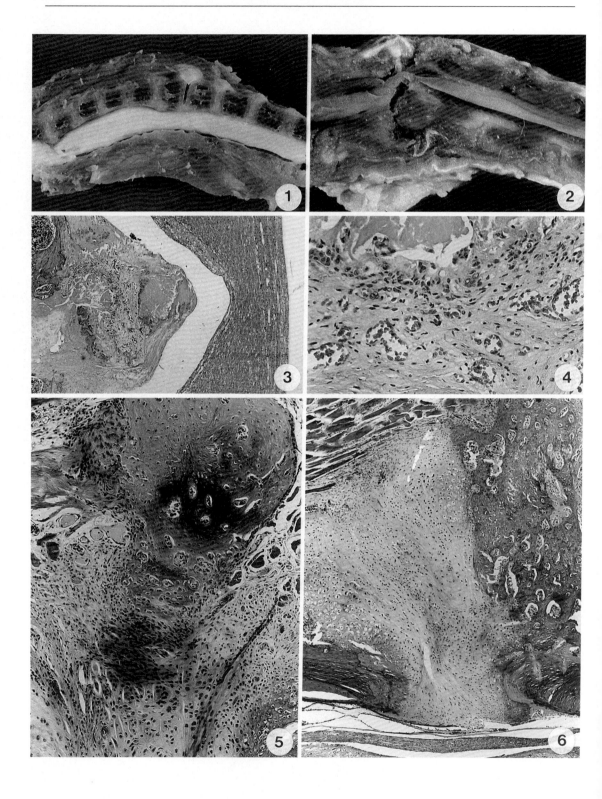

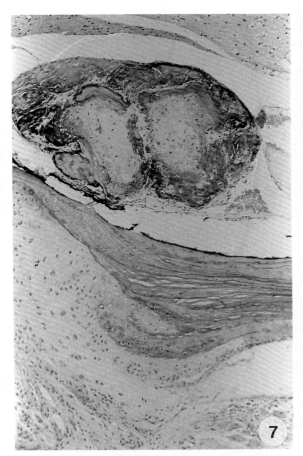
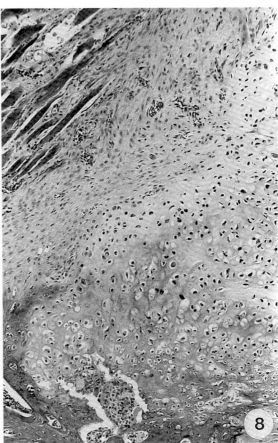

Figure 1. Chondrosis of vertebrae with focal compression of spinal cord. Excess extra-articular cartilage formation with dissection of vertebral joints and marked osteoporosis are also seen. Untreated male Syrian golden hamster (SGH), 118 weeks. × 4

Figure 2. Chondrosis with luxation of vertebral joint and severe spinal cord damage. Untreated male SGH, 115 weeks. × 5

Figure 3. Excess cartilage formation with focal degeneration and regeneration of intervertebral cartilaginous discs. Marked compression and atrophy of spinal cord is seen at right. Untreated male SGH, 120 weeks. H & E; × 40

Figure 4. Area of lesion of Figure 3, with fibrous regeneration of degenerated cartilage (top). H & E; × 250

Figure 5. Spontaneous chondromatosis of vertebral periarticular tissues characterized by hyperostosis (top), fibrosis (upper left-hand corner) and extended cartilaginous metaplasia of fibromuscular tissue. H & E; × 40

Figure 6. Another area of the chondromatosis of Figure 5, with hyperostosis (right) of vertebral bone and protrusion of lesion into spinal canal (bottom). H & E; × 40

Figure 7. Chondromatosis (bottom) of vertebrae with formation of calcified loose body in vertebral canal and compression of spinal cord (top). Untreated SGH, 98 weeks. H & E; × 50

Figure 8. Spontaneous, extensive periarticular chondromatosis of vertebral region. Remnant of atrophic muscle fibres is seen in lower left-hand corner. Female SGH, 45 weeks. H & E; ×100

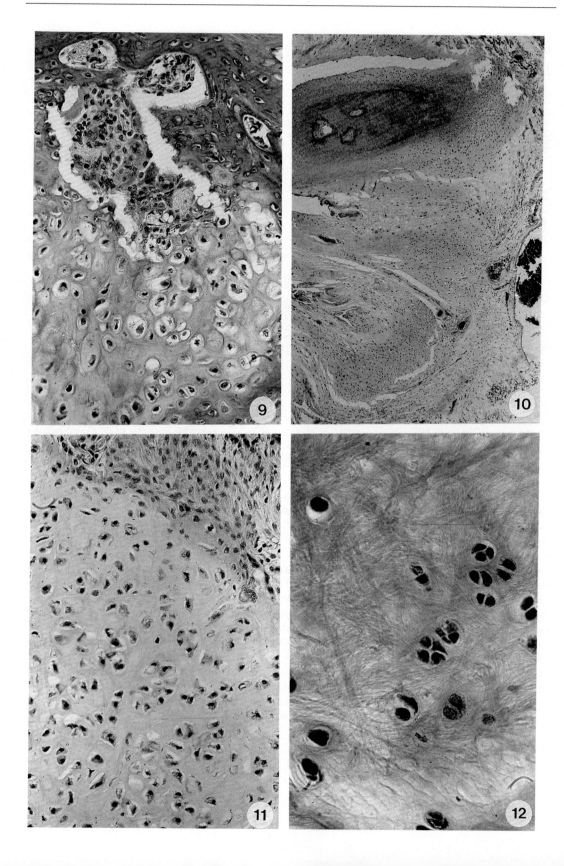

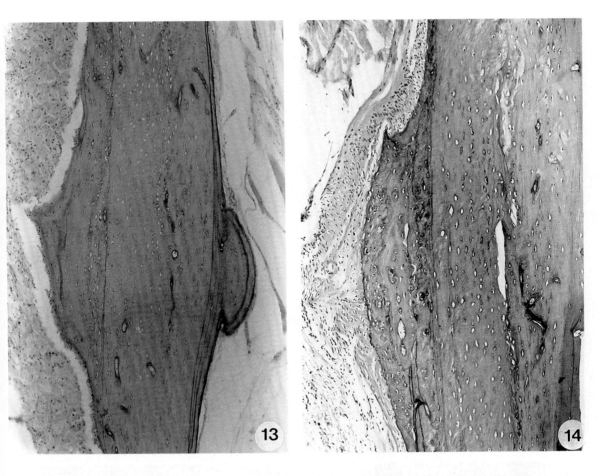

Figure 9. Area of lesion of Figure 8, with osteoclastic and chondroplastic activity in vertebral bone. H & E; × 250

Figure 10. Extensive chondromatosis around maxillomandibular joint in an untreated albino hamster (76 weeks). Part of metaplastic mandibular bone is seen in upper portion. H & E; × 100

Figure 11. Metaplastic cartilaginous tissue (left) extending into adjacent connective tissue (right). Maxillomandibular region of an untreated female albino hamster, 76 weeks. H & E; × 250

Figure 12. Area of chondromatosis in an untreated female albino hamster (76 weeks), has a mixture of collagenous bundles and cartilaginous tissue. The cells often showed bun-like nuclear structures. H & E; × 250

Figure 13. Spontaneous exostosis (osteoma) in the distal tibia of a female SGH (96 weeks), with lamellar structure on the outer layer, as also seen in subperiosteal bone region. H & E; × 30

Figure 14. Osteogenic exostosis in the distal femur of a female white hamster (81 weeks). The hyper-plastic and markedly vascularized bone tissue is demarcated from the femoral shaft by periosteal lines. The presence of collagenous fibres on the outer surface of the exostosis may indicate that the lesion is a result of physiological compensation. H & E; × 100

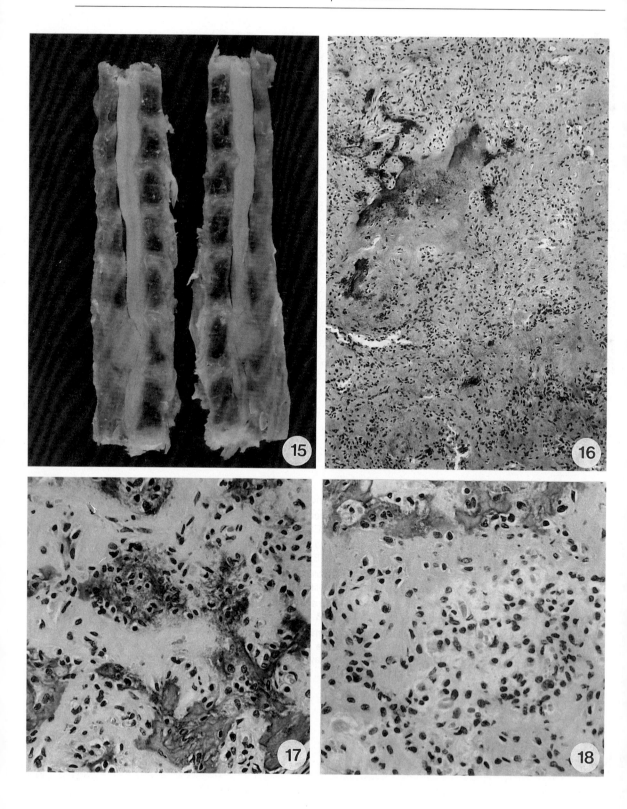

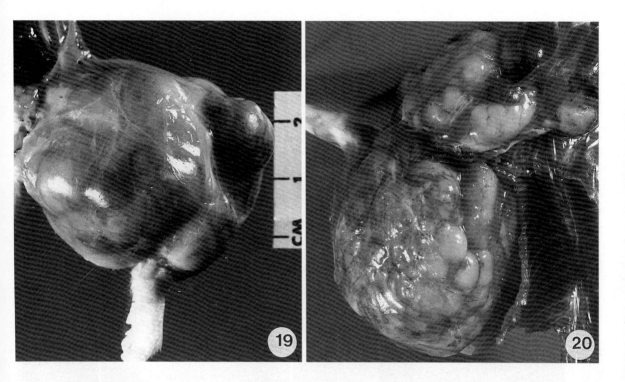

Figure 15. Spontaneous osteochondroma in longitudinal section of vertebrae (lower part), with marked compression and atrophy of lumbar spinal cord. Chondrosis of intervertebral cartilage is also seen (upper portion). Representative histological areas of osteochondroma are illustrated in Figures 16–18. × 6

Figure 16. Osteochondroma composed of irregular osteoid formations and calcium deposits surrounded by immature cartilage. H & E; × 100

Figure 17. Irregular bone spicules in osteochondroma. The uniformity of the cells indicates the benign character of the lesion. H & E; × 250

Figure 18. Irregular arrangement of cartilage cells surrounding newly formed bone trabeculae. H & E; × 250

Figure 19. Osteosarcoma originating in the left hind leg of a male SGH (76 weeks) whose dam was treated during pregnancy with a single dose of nitrosopiperidine.

Figure 20. Osteosarcoma (4×5×6 cm in diameter) which originated from the right foreleg and invaded shoulder and

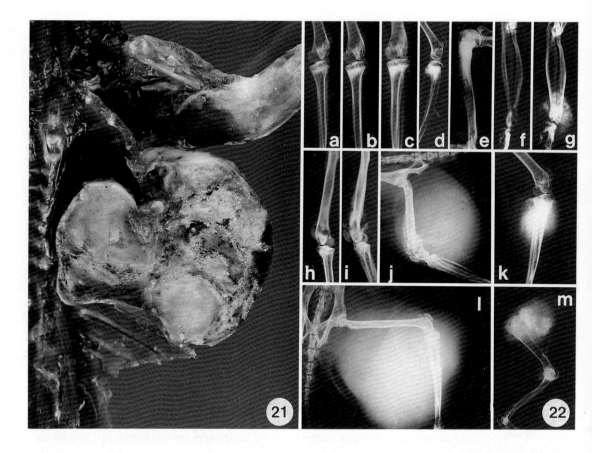

Figure 21. Osteosarcoma (4 cm in diameter) of ribs, protruding into the pleural cavity. The mediastinal organs were displaced and vertebrae had scoliosis. This female SGH (64 weeks) had received sodium cyclamate in drinking-water for its lifetime.

Figure 22. Radiographs of osteosarcomas of SGH inoculated with extracts of human osteosarcoma. a–d: Serial radiographs of enlarging osteosarcoma of proximal metaphysis of left tibia. Slow progression from a small area of increased density 421 days after inoculation (a), to a larger lesion at 504 (b) and 527 (c) days, with perforation of cortex by 575 days (d). e: Small sclerotic tumour of right humerus showing early extension through the cortex 544 days after inoculation. f and g: Osteosarcoma arising in distal metaphysis of the left radius 460 days after inoculation (f) has both osteolytic and osteoblastic processes; by 477 days, the osteoblastic activity was predominant (g). h–j: Osteosarcoma arising in distal metaphysis of the right femur. At 326 days after inoculation the small lesion (h) progressed to a large neoplasm having osteoblastic activity and by 385 days, to perforation of the cortex throughout the distal half of the bone (i). At 409 days there was a large, soft tissue component and a pathological fracture (j). k: Dense tumour of left tibia 559 days after inoculation. l: Large, invasive osteosarcoma of the left tibia 427 days after inoculation. m: Osteoblastic osteosarcoma of the left scapula 352 days after inoculation. From Finkel *et al.* (1968, 1969) by courtesy of Dr M.P. Finkel.

Figure 23. Sclerosing osteosarcoma with formation of excessive bone trabeculae, which are mature and lamellar. Tumour cells have little pleomorphism. Fibrous intertrabecular connective tissue lacks any activity. H & E; × 100

Figure 24. Osteosarcoma composed of massive bone trabeculae and hypercellular connective stroma. H & E; × 100

Figure 25. Area of tumour of Figure 24 illustrating pleomorphic osteoclastic cells. H & E; × 250

Figure 26. Osteosarcoma has large amounts of osteoid surrounded by pleomorphic cells. H & E: × 300. By courtesy of Dr G.T. Diamandopoulos.

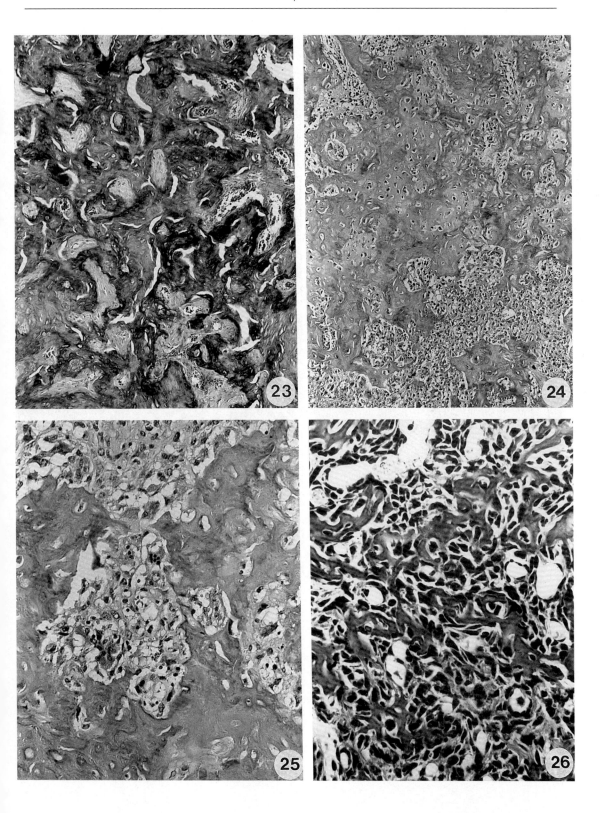

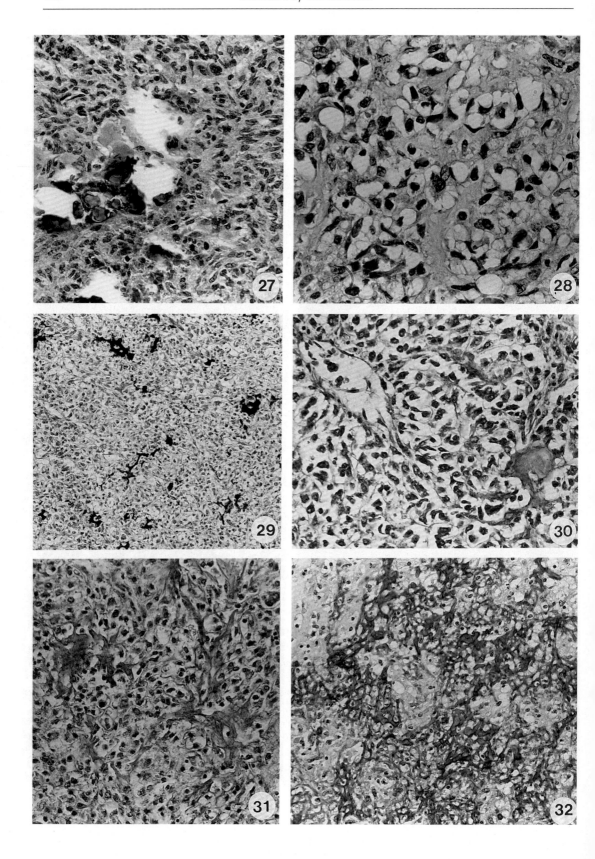

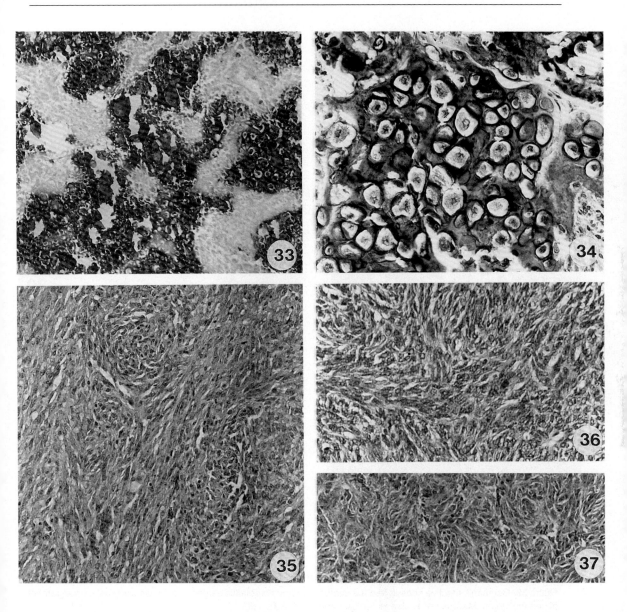

Figure 27. Calcium deposits in centre of an osteosarcoma, mainly composed of cellular patterns. H & E; × 250

Figure 28. Hyalin-like bands of fibrous matrix in osteosarcoma with intervening malignant osteoblasts. H & E; ×500

Figure 29. Filiform calcium deposits in osteosarcoma between tumour cells resembling immature osteoblasts. H & E; × 100

Figure 30. Another area of osteosarcoma in Figure 29, demonstrating radial arrangement of malignant osteoblasts around a blood vessel and focal mineralization. H & E; × 250

Figure 31. Osteoblastic osteosarcoma with formation of fibrillary mineralized stroma. H & E; × 250

Figure 32. Filigree patterns of osteosarcoma illustrating interlacing, net-like collagen fibres which have undergone calcification and osteoid conversion. H & E; × 250

Figure 33. Chondroblastic area of osteosarcoma, has calcification and necrosis of cartilaginous tissue. H & E; × 125

Figure 34. Calcification of matrix of cartilage in part of osteosarcoma. H & E; × 50

Figure 35–37. Fibroblastic osteosarcoma illustrating streams and whorls of anaplastic cells resembling fibrosarcoma. H & E; × 250

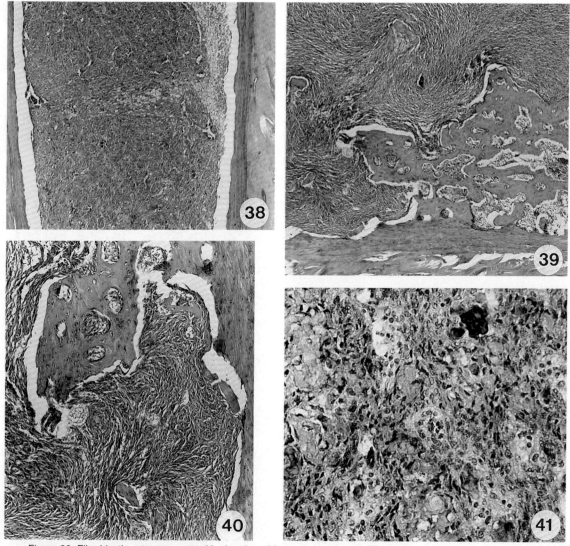

Figure 38. Fibroblastic osteosarcoma with plugging of femoral medulla. H & E; × 250

Figure 39. Codman's reactive zone in femoral shaft caused by fibroblastic osteosarcoma. Characteristic arrangement of non-malignant osseous trabeculae in vertical direction. H & E; × 50

Figure 40. Higher magnification of the lesion of Figure 39, illustrating coating of reactive bone trabeculae by malignant cells. H & E; × 100

Figure 41. Fibroblastic osteosarcoma composed of densely packed, malignant fibroblasts with interspersed calcified areas. H & E; × 250

Figure 42. Area of osteosarcoma of Figure 41 illustrating numerous multinucleated giant cells with large, intracytoplasmic vacuoles. H & E; × 400

Figure 43. Focal calcification of matrix in a fibroblastic osteosarcoma. Numerous giant cells and epithelioid cell nidus (lower left-hand corner) are present. H & E; × 250

Figure 44. Small foci of osteoid and osseous formation in osteosarcoma, composed largely of malignant fibroblasts. H & E; × 400

Figure 45. Area of fibroblastic osteosarcoma with osteoid formation and varied degrees of mineralization. The closely packed intervening cells are reminiscent of epithelial neoplasm. H & E; × 250

Figure 46. Angiomatous patterns in fibroblastic osteosarcoma. H & E; × 250

Figure 47. Sinusoid structures in osteosarcoma. Some sinusoids contain giant cells. H & E; × 250

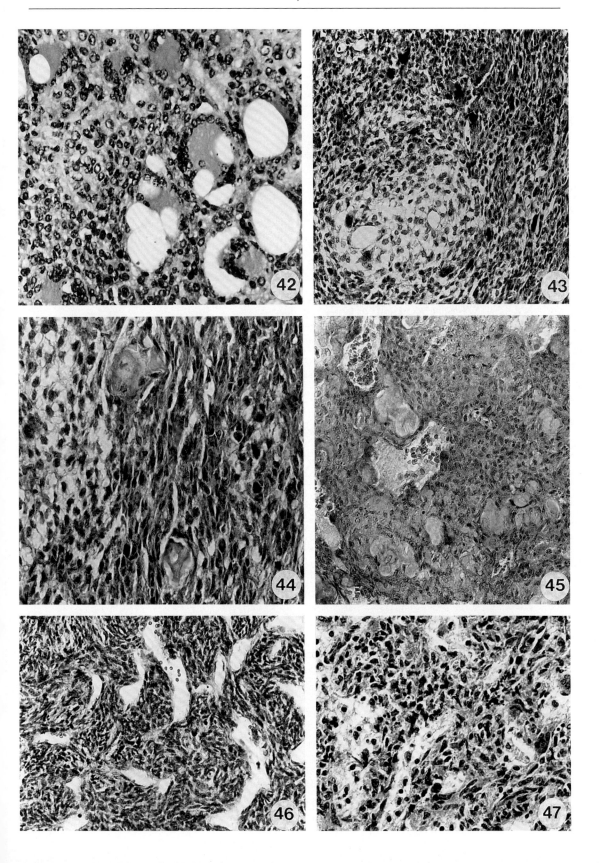

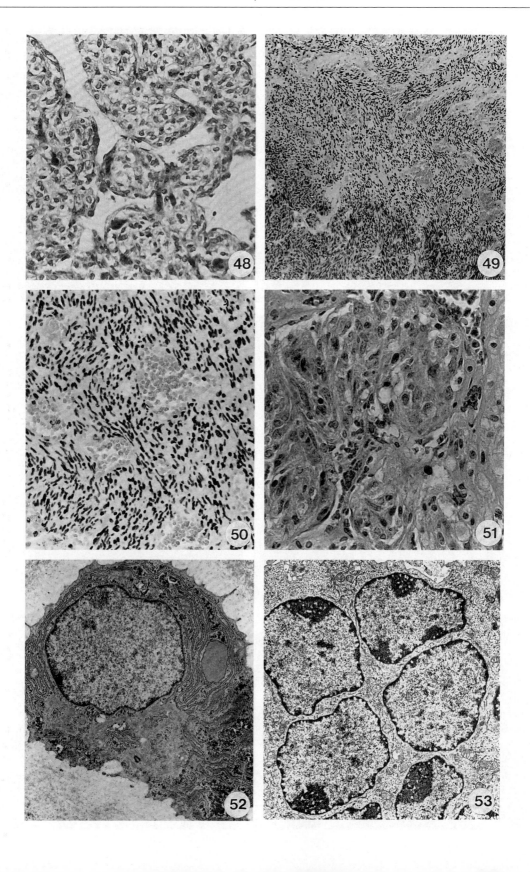

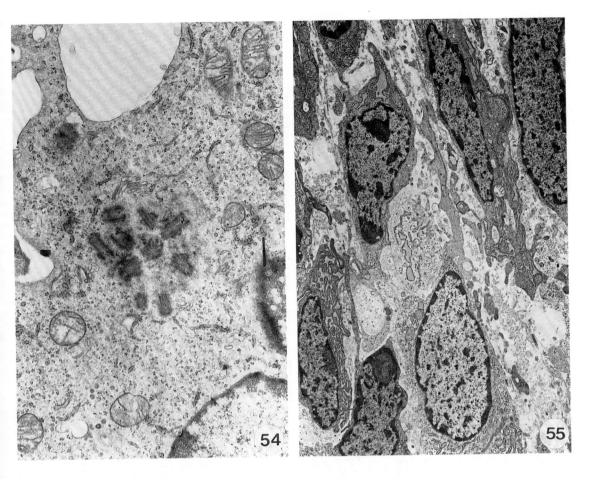

Figure 48. Vascular formation in osteosarcoma by malignant fibroblasts with interspersed, grotesque giant cells. H & E; × 250. By courtesy of Dr Y. Yabe.

Figure 49. Angiosarcomatous patterns of the osteosarcoma of Figure 46. H & E; × 100

Figure 50. Higher magnification of Figure 49 illustrating vascular spaces with intervening malignant spindle-shaped cells arranged in streams. H & E; × 250

Figure 51. Epithelioid structure in osteosarcoma. Lipid-filled cells seen at right-hand corner resemble features in non-osteogenic fibroma in man. H & E; × 400

Figure 52. Chondrocyte in uncalcified cartilage matrix in MSV-M-induced hamster osteosarcoma. The chondrocyte has many cell processes, well developed granular endoplasmic reticulum and Golgi apparatus and glycogen granules. × 5000

Figure 53–57. Electron microscopic findings in osteosarcomas. By courtesy of Dr L. Dmochowski.

Figure 53. Part of osteoclastic giant cell in an MSV-H-induced osteosarcoma. Mitochondria, granular endoplasmic reticulum and free ribosomes are scattered throughout the cytoplasm. × 6000

Figure 54. Multiple centrioles in an osteoblastic giant cell. × 12 000

Figure 55. Tumour cell in MSV-H-induced hamster osteosarcoma. Cells of low and high electron density with well developed granular endoplasmic reticulum are seen, as well as collagen fibres in intercellular spaces. × 6000

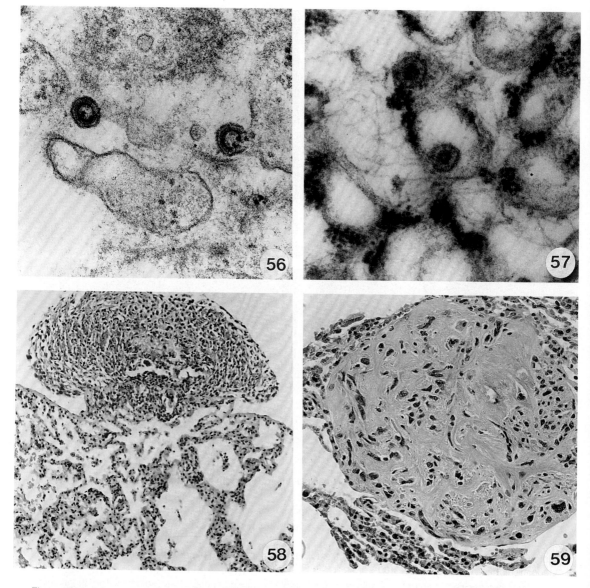

Figure 56. Immature and budding type-C virus particles in MSV-M-induced hamster osteosarcoma. × 90 000

Figure 57. Type-H virus particles in cisternae of endoplasmic reticulum of tissue culture cell in same tissue culture as Figure 59. × 70 000

Figure 58–65. Different patterns of metastases of osteosarcomas.

Figure 58. Lung metastases of the osteosarcoma of Figure 38. H & E; × 100

Figure 59. Lung metastases of the osteosarcoma of Figure 28. H & E; × 250

Figure 60. Lung metastases of the osteosarcoma of Figure 40. H & E; × 20

Figure 61. Lung metastases of the osteosarcoma of Figure 26. H & E; × 400

Figure 62. Mediastinal metastases of the osteosarcoma of Figure 46, illustrating invasion of the tracheal wall. H & E; × 50

Figure 63. Higher magnification of Figure 62 illustrating osteoid foci and mineralized matrix. H & E; × 250

Figure 64. Renal metastases of the osteosarcoma of Figure 43. H & E; × 250

Figure 65. Renal metastases of the osteosarcoma of Figure 24. H & E; × 250

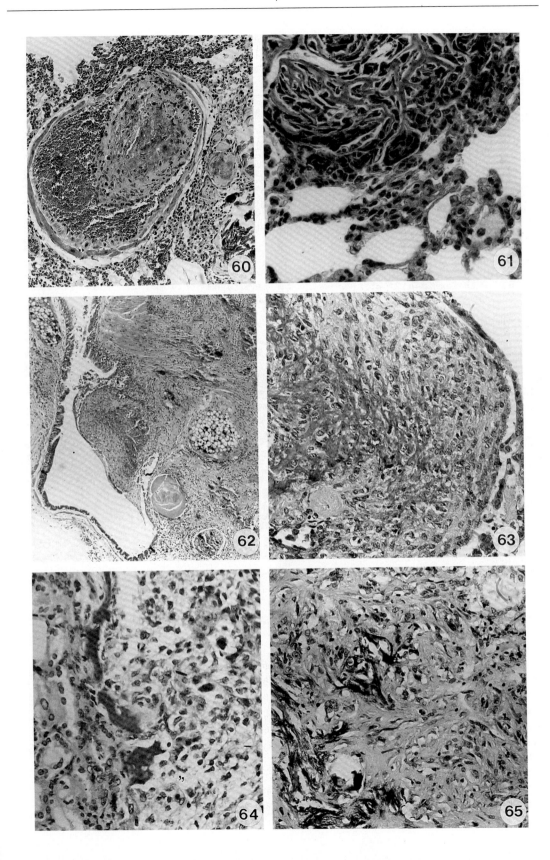

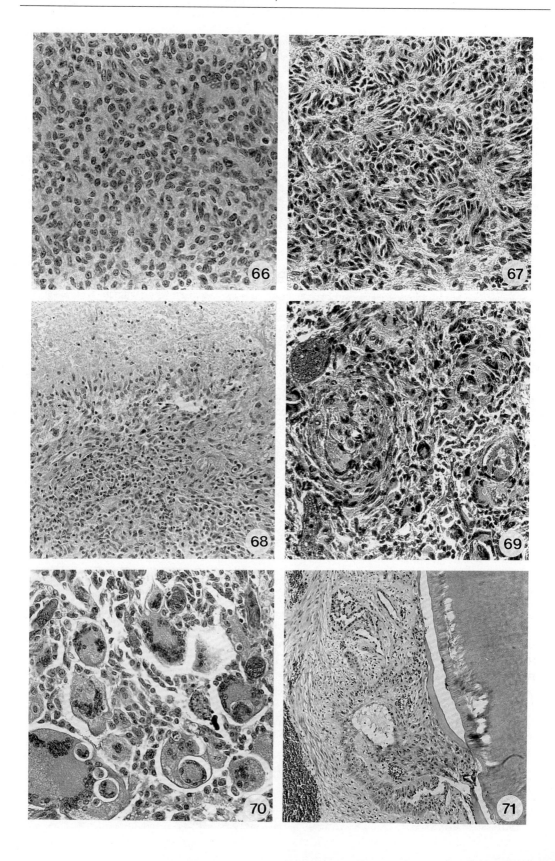

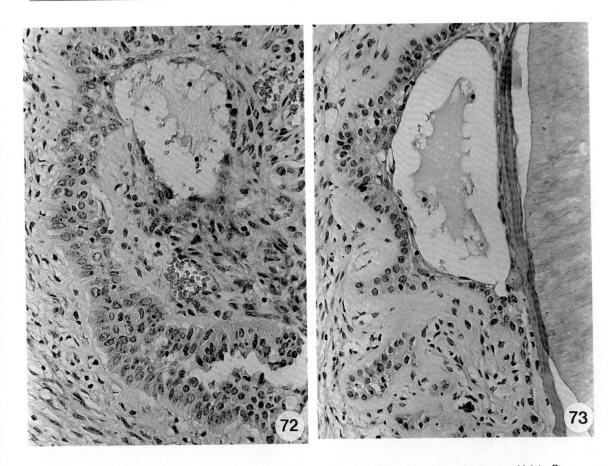

Figure 66–70. Different patterns of a giant cell tumour of peri-articular connective tissue around metacarpal joints. By courtesy of Dr H. Kirkman.

Figure 66. Area of tumour composed largely of epithelioid cells, some typical spindle-shaped cells, and cells with 'waisted' nuclei (upper left-hand corner). H & E; × 250

Figure 67. Another region of the same lesion illustrating rosette formations. H & E; × 250

Figure 68. Palisading of epithelioid cells around necrotic areas. Many eosinophilic leukocytes and lymphocytes are present in this region. H & E; × 250

Figure 69. Epithelioid and giant cells in focal concentric arrangements (left middle field). Numerous eosinophilic leukocytes and lymphocytes are present in right middle portion. H & E; × 250

Figure 70. Multinucleated giant cells with intervening epithelioid and lipid loaded cells (lower right-hand corner). Some giant cells contain smaller multinucleated cells (phagocytosis?). H & E; × 400

Figure 71. Malassez' epithelial rests in periodontium of the upper incisors teeth having glandular and cystis patterns. H & E; × 100

Figure 72. Higher magnification of the lesion of Figure 72, demonstrating epithelial cluster with tendency towards glandular or cyst formations. H & E; × 250

Figure 73. Cystic pattern of Malassez' epithelial rests in the lesion of Figure 72. H & E; × 250

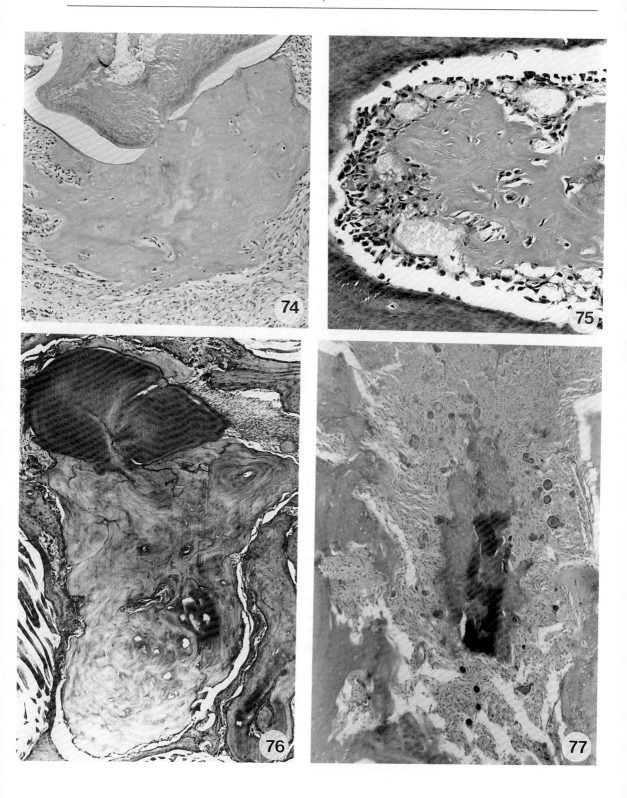

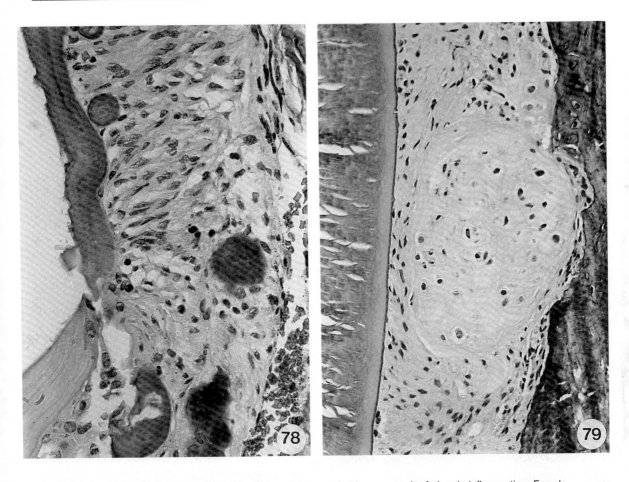

Figure 74. Periodontal denticle surrounded by fibrous tissue, probably as a result of chronic inflammation. Female untreated SGH, 95 weeks. H & E; × 100

Figure 75. Spontaneous denticle within the pulp of an upper incisor tooth of a 78-week-old male SGH. H & E; × 150

Figure 76. Cementicles about mandibular central incisor tooth in SGH infected with minute virus of mice. H & E; × 75. By courtesy of Dr P.N. Baer.

Figure 77. Spontaneous cementicles in the periodontium of an upper incisor tooth. Note the marked fibrosis. Male SGH, 104 weeks. H & E; × 65

Figure 78. Cement deposits in fibrosed periodontium. Disruption of alveolar bone (left) to which a foreign body is attached. Female SGH, 95 weeks. H & E; ×500

Figure 79. Periodontal cartilaginous dysplasia. The cartilaginous nidus, surrounded by dense fibrotic tissue, has cavitated the alveolar bone. H & E; × 400

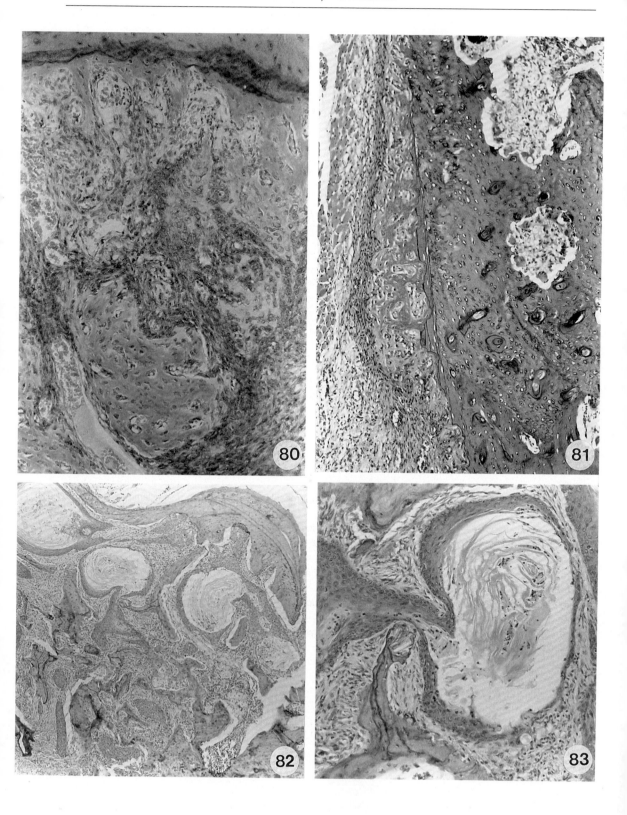

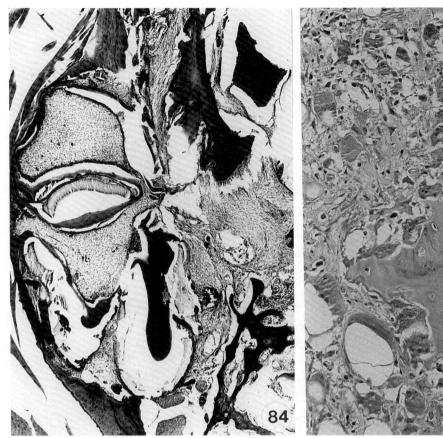

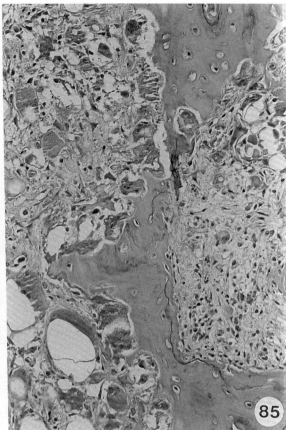

Figure 80. Periodontal hyperostosis in male SGH, 82 weeks of age. Islets of bone formations with intervening hypercellular matrix. H & E; × 100

Figure 81. Periodontal hyperostosis. Vertical arrangement of oppositional osteoid and bone trabeculae on alveolar bone, resembling Codman's reactive bone formation. H & E; ×200

Figure 82. Spontaneous, invading, gingival squamous cell carcinoma with focal cyst formations. Part of upper incisor tooth is seen in left-hand corner. H & E; × 25.

Figure 83. Higher magnification of lesion of Figure 83. Cystic spaces are filled with keratin lamellae. H & E; × 130

Figure 84. Odontoma composed of several teeth, enamel matrix, dentin and cementum fragments. Eighteen-month-old SGH infected with minute virus of mice at 5 days of age H & E; × 25. By courtesy of Dr P. N. Baer.

Figure 85. Generalized osteofibrosis with marked osteoclastic reaction in a female SGH, 36 weeks of age, treated with a single injection of nitrosodiisobutylamine at 8 weeks of age. This hamster had a parathyroid adenoma.

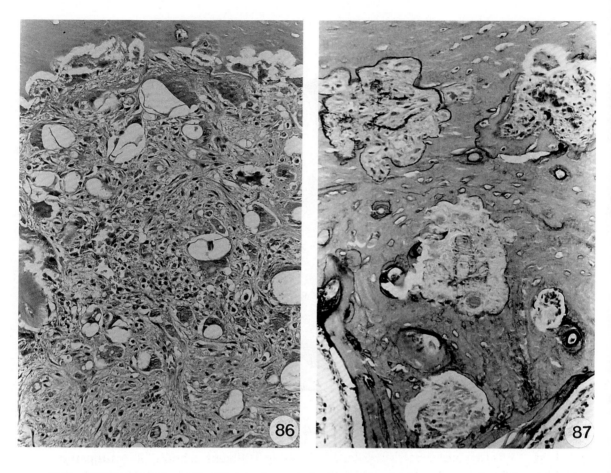

Figure 86. Osteofibrosis in maxillary bone, having marked osteoclastic containing numerous giant cells activity and fibrosis of bone marrow. H & E; × 65

Figure 87. Different stages of development of osteofibrosis in the calvarium of the animal of Figure 86. H & E; × 50

Tumours of the nervous system

A. Cardesa, G.M. ZuRhein, F.F. Cruz-Sanchez and V.S. Turusov

Advances in viral and chemical carcinogenesis have led to the development of new experimental approaches, resulting in the induction of a wide range of tumours of the nervous system. The intracerebral injection of oncogenic viruses into newborn animals (Rabson & Kirschstein, 1960) and the transplacental administration of resorptive chemical carcinogens capable of crossing both the placental and haematoencephalic barriers (Ivankovic & Druckrey, 1968) resulted in the induction of the first types of neurogenic tumours in hamsters. The considerable variety of tumours of nervous origin that have since been produced in the hamster, in contrast to the almost complete absence of spontaneous tumours, makes this animal species a useful biological system for studying the etiology, pathogenesis, morphology, biological behaviour and treatment of tumours of the central and peripheral nervous system. This is of interest since primary tumours of the central nervous system account for approximately 9% of all primary neoplasms in humans (Rubinstein, 1972a).

Since the first edition of this chapter was compiled (Cardesa *et al.*, 1982) the following new types of tumours of the nervous system have been experimentally induced in the hamster and are therefore described below: pinealocytoma, gliomatosis cerebri, medullo-epi-thelioma, ependymoblastoma, primitive polar spongioblastoma, neuroblastoma (central and peripheral), ganglioneuroblastoma, plexiform neurofibroma, esthesioneuroblastoma and retinoblastoma.

MORPHOLOGY AND BIOLOGY OF TUMOURS

The classification and terminology of tumours of the nervous system have been the subject of a great deal of controversy among different schools of neuropathology, and some aspects remain open to debate. Neurogenic tumours of the hamster are divided here mainly into tumours of the central nervous system (CNS) and tumours of the peripheral nervous system (PNS). In the CNS, tumours are classified according to their histogenesis, then subdivided according to their differentiation and cytological characteristics. Tumours originating in the PNS are classified according to cytological and textural features. Tumours of the sympathetic ganglia and tumours of the non-chromaffin paraganglia are listed separately. Tumours originating in the olfactory region and in the retina are also placed in separate groups. Tumours of paraganglionic chromaffin cells and tumours of the pituitary are omitted, since they are described in the chapter on endocrine tumours.

427

Histological types of tumour

Tumours of the central nervous system

Neuroepithelial tumours

Differentiated

    Astrocytoma
    Mixed glioma
    Ependymoma
    Choroid plexus papilloma
    Ganglioglioma
    Pinealocytoma

Poorly differentiated and embryonal

    Glioblastoma multiforme
    Undifferentiated tumours
    Medulloblastoma
    Medulloepithelioma
    Ependymoblastoma
    Primitive polar spongioblastoma
    Gliomatosis cerebri
    Neuroblastoma (central)

Mesodermal tumours

    Sarcomas
    Angiomatous lesions

Dysontogenetic tumours

    Teratomas and hamartomas

Tumours of the peripheral nervous system

    Neurinoma
    Neurofibroma
    Plexiform neurofibroma
    Neurofibrosarcoma
    Granular cell tumour

Tumours of the sympathetic ganglia

    Ganglioneuroma
    Ganglioneuroblastoma
    Neuroblastoma

Tumours of the non-chromaffin paraganglia

    Paraganglioma

Tumours of the olfactory region

    Esthesioneuroepithelioma
    Esthesioneuroblastoma

Tumours of the retina

    Retinoblastoma

Tumours of the central nervous system

Differentiated neuroepithelial tumours

These tumours are composed of differentiated neuroepithelial cellular elements showing a variable degree of maturation and differentiation. However, some of them may focally blend with areas lacking differentiation. According to the degree of differentiation and of phenotypic cellular expression, these tumours are classified in distinct categories.

Astrocytomas, first reported in hamster by Rabotti and Raine (1964), are tumours formed by neoplastic proliferation of astrocytes (Figures 1 and 2). Microscopically, astrocytes can be recognized by their characteristic shape. The nuclei are vesicular and present a fine chromatin network with centrally located nucleoli. Their cytoplasm possesses ramifications and varies from stellate to fusiform in shape, depending upon the degree of maturation (Figure 3). They mainly originate in the white matter of the brain, favouring the region of the subependymal plate, and have a tendency to grow diffusely by infiltrating the surrounding structures. Two different morphological patterns, namely the protoplasmic and pilocytic types, were seen after transplantation of primary intracerebral tumours in hamsters to the cheek pouch and subcutaneous tissue of this animal (Figures 4 and 5) (B.M.A. Davies and F.C. Chesterman, personal communication).

One of the criteria for evaluating the degree of malignancy of astrocytomas is the presence of mitoses. Many of these tumours induced in hamsters show a rich cellularity, numerous mitotic figures and varying degrees of cellular polymorphism; however, the astrocytic character of the cells is still recognizable (Figures 6 and 7). The term 'malignant astrocytoma' has been used for this kind of neoplasm (Bucciarelli *et al.*, 1967). Another feature of the malignant astrocytoma is the presence of numerous blood vessels with mild to moderate hyperplasia of endothelial and perivascular cells. Occasionally, the astrocytes may be arranged around the blood vessels, forming so-called vascular pseudorosettes or gliovascular formations. This type of pseudo-rosette must be differentiated from those seen in the cellular ependymomas. Foci of tissue degeneration, necrosis and haemorrhage and the formation of cystic spaces are features of rapidly growing astrocytomas. A careful search among numerous tissue sections may reveal some foci with anaplastic cellular features.

Mixed gliomas. When tumours are formed by the simultaneous proliferation of various cellular elements of glial origin, they are called mixed gliomas (Ivankovic & Druckrey, 1968). Grossly, they have an ill-defined nodular appearance with haemorrhagic areas (Figures 8 and 9). Microscopically, they are formed by the concomitant proliferation of astrocytes and oligodendroglia and contain areas in which either astrocytes or oligodendroglia predominate; when astrocytes predominate, they are classified as astrocytomas (Figure 10). The oligodendroglial cells are smaller than the astrocytes and have a lymphocyte-like nucleus surrounded by a clear, non-staining halo in the cytoplasm and a definite cell membrane. Round, pearl-like calcium deposits in the vicinity of areas populated by oligodendrocytes are occasionally seen (Figure 11). In some instances, particularly after transplacental exposure to ethylnitrosourea (ENU), these tumours may be almost entirely composed of oligodendrocytes, being therefore very closely related to oligodendrogliomas.

Ependymomas are well circumscribed exophytic tumours that usually protrude into the ventricular cavities and in some cases may obliterate their lumen (Figure 12). They originate from the ependymal epithelium lining the ventricles and interventricular channels of the CNS. Occasionally, obliterated ependymal streaks within the white matter can also give rise to these neoplasms.

Microscopically, three different patterns can be observed, but most of the tumours show a mixture of these patterns. When the ependymal cells show a predominantly papillary arrangement, the tumours are classified as papillary ependymomas (Figure 13) and must be distinguished from choroid plexus papillomas, which they closely resemble. Papillary ependymomas have been reported by Kirschstein and Gerber (1962), Eddy (1962), Gerber and Kirschstein (1962), Berman (1967) and ZuRhein *et al.* (1974). Tumours forming gland-like spaces called 'luminal rosettes', lined by ependymal cells differentiated towards their cylindrical epithelial aspect, which may even show cilia and blepharoplasts, correspond to the epithelial type. Ependymomas of cellular type are those neoplasms in which the cellular elements have a tendency to form elongated tail-like cytoplasmic appendages that are arranged around capillary blood vessels. These formations are called 'gliovascular processes' or 'vascular pseudo-rosettes'. Ependymomas with some of these last features have been reported by Mancini *et al.* (1969) and by Levenbook *et al.* (1968) in a malignant variant of ependymoma. More recent reports include those of Costa *et al.* (1976), Uchida *et al.* (1976), Corallini *et al.* (1978, 1982) and Altavilla *et al.* (1983).

Choroid plexus papillomas are formed by the epithelium that lines the choroid plexus of the ventricles and passages of the CNS. Grossly, they have a cauliflower-like appearance, growing within the ventricles and occupying their lumen, thereby presenting a close similarity to the exophytic growth pattern of ependymoma.

Microscopically, the tumours consist of fine papillary structures formed by a single layer of cuboidal or prismatic epithelial cells supported by delicate vascular connective tissue stroma (Rabotti *et al.*, 1965; Greenlee *et al.*, 1977; Uchida *et al.*,

1979; ZuRhein, 1983, 1987; Nagashima, 1986) (Figure 14). Differential diagnostic problems and discrepancies in interpretation may arise in distinguishing such tumours from papillary forms of ependymomas (Duffell *et al.*, 1964). The choroid plexus epithelium has its origin in the primitive medullary epithelium, being embryologically related to the ependymal cells. However, there are some histological differences that distinguish these tumour entities. In choroid plexus papillomas, the covering epithelium consists of a single layer of prismatic or cuboidal epithelium supported by vascular connective tissue. In papillary ependymoma, the epithelial cells may have a multilayered arrangement and are supported by a neuroglial stroma (Rubinstein, 1972a).

Malignant forms of choroid plexus papillomas can be recognized by the presence of anaplastic features in the epithelial cells and by the atypical histostructure of the tumours (Levenbook *et al.*, 1968).

Gangliogliomas are composed of the combined growth of neoplastic nerve cells and astrocytes; they have also been called neuroastrocytomas. The participation of the two cell types may vary considerably from case to case and also within different areas of the same tumour; it may therefore be difficult to decide which cellular type is predominant. To our knowledge, pure nerve-cell tumours or gangliocytomas of the CNS have not been reported in hamsters; however, pure astrocytomas were observed in the same set of experiments by Hosobuchi and Ishii (1967) in which gangliogliomas were induced (Figures 15 and 16). The histological criteria for the diagnosis of gangliogliomas require the identification of abnormal neurons, occasionally of binucleated type, and the concomitant proliferation of neoplastic astrocytes. The observation of mononucleated, well differentiated nerve cells within a field of

atypical proliferated astrocytes is rather indicative of invasive astrocytoma.

Pinealocytomas are tumours formed by the neoplastic proliferation of pinealocytes, which are derived from and composed of relatively mature cells of the pineal parenchyma. The first induction of such a tumour in any species was reported for the Syrian hamster by ZuRhein and Varakis (1975) and by Varakis and ZuRhein (1976). In subsequent experiments with JC viral strains, great variations in the yield of pinealocytomas were noted (Padgett *et al.*, 1977; ZuRhein, 1983, 1987) with a range from 0% to 45%. It is clear that the molecular structure of the JC viral genome is of particular importance for the induction of this type of tumour. Uchida *et al.* (1979) reported that another human papovavirus, BK virus, can induce pinealocytomas.

Grossly such tumours are located in the midline between the cerebral hemispheres and are superimposed on the quadrigeminal plate. They are encapsulated, greyish-white in colour, and can measure up to 9 mm in diameter (Figure 17). On sections they are solid and show neither haemorrhage nor necrosis.

On light microscopy, most of the tumours have a lobular architecture, the lobules having central nests of tumour cells and being bordered by non-collagenous, reticular connective tissue supporting thin-walled blood vessels (Figure 18). The cells are of small to medium size and of rounded to elongated shape. They have indistinct borders. The cytoplasm is pale eosinophilic, of moderate amount and contains infrequent small vacuoles. A majority of nuclei are spherical or oblong with rather pale nucleoplasm and distinct coarse chromatic clumps (Figure 19). Ultrastructural features include cell processes with microtubules and with bulbous endings filled with clear or dense core vesicles (Figure 20). Apical cell extensions contain cilia and aggregates of mitochondria, all these features pointing towards a photo-receptor differentiation. Quay *et al.* (1977) have found in homogenates of these tumours various levels of hydroxyindole-O-methyl-transferase, which is required for the synthesis of the hormone melatonin.

Poorly differentiated and embryonal neuroepi-thelial tumours

Grossly, the tumours are grey-white and semitransparent, often haemorrhagic or necrotic. Histologically, they are highly cellular and composed of either pleo-morphic small spindle or polygonal cells. According to their degree of limited differentiation, the characteristics of the cells and the predominance of some of their types, different tumour categories have been recognized. These categories are: glioblastoma multiforme, undif-ferentiated tumours not otherwise speci-fied (N.O.S.), medulloblastoma, medullo-epithelioma, ependymoblastoma, primi-tive polar spongioblastoma, gliomatosis cerebri and neuroblastoma (central).

Glioblastoma multiforme has been observed in the hamster in viral onco-genesis studies (Rapp *et al.*, 1969; Shein, 1970; Walker *et al.*, 1973; ZuRhein *et al.*, 1974; ZuRhein 1983, 1987). This neoplasm represents the most dedifferentiated glioma of astrocytic origin. The tumour cells show a marked degree of cellular pleomorphism, often adopting bizarre forms, with multinucleation and an increased number of atypical mitoses (Figure 21). In many areas within the tumour, necrotic foci can be found which are often surrounded by a palisade arrangement of the glial cells. The blood vessels have usually undergone marked proliferation, and show hyperplasia of the endothelial and perivascular cells. Alter-nating with zones of marked cellular polymorphism and poor differentiation, in which the glial origin of the cells is not recognizable, there are other regions in which the cells still contain some features that make their astrocytic origin obvious

(Figure 22). A common feature of astro-cytomas and glioblastomas is the presence of different amounts of glial fibres and the absence or scarcity of reticulum fibre formation, in contrast to the abundance of the reticulum network observed in sarcomas. Two cases of glioblastoma multi-forme were reported by Rapp *et al.* (1969) in which reticulum fibres were seen in some areas of the tumour, but were absent in others. This combined pattern was considered suggestive of the con-comitant occurrence of glioblastoma and fibro-sarcoma.

Undifferentiated tumours of the hamster CNS were reported by Merkow *et al.* (1968). These tumours are frequently located over the medulla oblongata and involve, by compression, the vermis of the cerebellum. They are occasionally ob-served as an area of haemorrhage on the surface of one cerebral hemisphere. Microscopically, the tumours are com-posed of cells with hyperchromatic, oval to round nuclei and semi-clear basophilic cytoplasm. In some areas the neoplastic cells are characterized by enlarged poly-gonal nuclei showing a monotonous undifferentiated pattern. Giant cells are frequently present, being either multi-nucleated with the nuclei arranged peripherally or megalonucleated with larger hyperchromatic bizarre nuclei. When glial fibrils are seen within the neoplasm, they are located in areas adjacent to compressed cortical tissue. Ogawa *et al.* (1969) reported the obser-vation of undifferentiated neuroecto-dermal tumours associated with the occurrence of medulloblastomas in the same experiment.

Medulloblastomas induced by various viruses have been reported (Rapp *et al.*, 1969; Ogawa *et al.*, 1969; ZuRhein & Varakis, 1979; Nagashima *et al.*, 1984, Nagashima *et al.*, 1986; Matsuda *et al.*, 1987). They are highly cellular and undifferentiated neoplasms, often multicentric in origin, which arise from the internal granular layer of the cerebellum (Figure 23) following JC virus inoculation or from the ventricular shorelines (adenovirus 12). By filling the 4th ventricle or extending into the cerebello-pontine angle, the tumours may produce hydrocephalus and herniation of brain tissue through the foramen magnum.

The tumours are composed of cells with ill-defined, scanty cytoplasm and small, round to oval, rather hyperchromatic and pleomorphic nuclei (Rapp *et al.*, 1969) (Figures 24 and 25). The mitotic activity is markedly variable. In some areas mitoses are numerous with many atypical figures. Ultrastructural analysis showed poorly differentiated cells with few cytoplasmic organelles but many ribosomes (ZuRhein, 1987; Ogawa, 1989b). An intercellular fibrillary support is often present within the tumour. Carrot-like cells, arranged in pseudo-rosette formation around fibrillary material, may be characteristic and suggestive of differentiation towards nerve cells (Figure 26). The presence of pseudo-rosette formation characterized by empty round spaces is a relatively common feature (Figure 27). Spindle-shaped cells arranged in palisades or whorled formations, and also pseudo-palisades around necrotic foci, may be seen. Perivascular pseudo-rosettes can also be observed, although a capillary vascular stroma is seldom seen. No reticulum, or very little, is produced by this kind of tumour. This property may help in distinguishing medulloblastomas from sarcomas in the brain, since the latter usually have an abundant reticulin network. The line of demarcation between the medulloblastoma and the brain is usually fairly sharp in cerebellar tumours.

Medulloepithelioma is very rare and is composed of cylindrical, medium or tall neuroepithelial cells showing darkly stained, elongated oval nuclei, with distinct granular chromatin. These cells are arranged in several layers or in rosettes of medulloepithelial type. Numerous mitoses are often observed near the lumen of rosettes. These cells characteristically show an internal limiting membrane mimicking the developing neural tube in the embryo (Ogawa, 1989b).

Ependymoblastoma is a form of phenotypic expression of some embryonal poorly differentiated neuroepithelial tumours in which characteristic 'ependymoblastic rosettes' are found. These rosettes are formed by multilayers of small or medium-sized oval cells, with numerous mitoses, positioned around a central lumen. Ultrastructurally, ependymoblastic rosettes show long and short junctional complexes, a few microvilli and sometimes basal bodies but no well developed cilia or filaments. (Ogawa, 1989b).

Primitive polar spongioblastomas are also very rare and arise from the subependymal plate. They feature the fascicular arrangement of slightly elongated spindle-shaped cells which occasionally form rhythmic parallel rows or palisading of small bipolar cells known as spongioblasts (Ogawa, 1989b).

Gliomatosis cerebri is a neoplastic process that was first described in the human by Nevin (1938) and consists of a proliferation of poorly differentiated glial elements infiltrating diffusely the white and grey matter without damaging the normal tissue. ZuRhein (1983, 1987), Nagashima *et al.* (1984, 1986) and Ogawa (1989b) described foci of gliomatosis cerebri in the thalamus, piriform lobe and brain stem of hamsters. The same neoplastic process was also noted in the spinal cord (Figure 28). Several glial elements with different cytological features are observed. Some of them are well differentiated glial elements such as astrocytes or oligodendrocytes, but most of them are less differentiated elements composed of small cells with hyperchromatic carrot-shaped nuclei and scanty eosinophilic cytoplasm. Unipolar and bipolar cells with elongated nuclei forming fascicular arrangements of elongated cells can be also found. These cells infiltrate the neuropil and the white matter. Myelinated fibres are separated by the proliferated glial cells but damage of the normal tissue is not observed.

Central neuroblastoma. Among the embryonal neuroepithelial tumours induced in the CNS of hamsters by human adenovirus type 12, Ogawa (1989b) reported the presence of neuroblastic rosettes of the Homer–Wright type which are characteristic of neuroblastoma. Homer–Wright rosettes consist of oval, unipolar cells radially arranged with or without neurofibrillary production in their centre. Ultrastructurally, these rosettes are composed of irregularly arranged, immature tumour cells loosely attached to each other, often with small slits in the centre. Microtubules or neurofilaments are not commonly present, but may be found.

Mesodermal tumours

Sarcomas in the CNS have similar histological features to those originating elsewhere (Rabson & Kirschstein, 1960; Romanul *et al.*, 1961; Girardi *et al.*, 1962; de Estable *et al.*, 1965; Harvey & East; 1971; Robl *et al.*, 1972; ZuRhein, 1987). Grossly, they are whitish nodular lesions generally located in the leptomeninges, but they have also been reported intracerebrally. Meningeal sarcomas may be composed of elongated cells arranged in interlacing bundles, whereas in other areas they may be disposed around the blood vessels (Figure 29). The nuclei are pleomorphic, hyperchromatic and show numerous atypical mitoses (Figure 30). Production of collagen fibres has also been found (Robl *et al.*, 1972). These tumours have a tendency to extend from the leptomeninges, infiltrating into the underlying brain tissue (Figures 31 and 32). Intracerebral sarcomas originate from the elements of the vascular walls (Harvey

& East, 1971). Reticulum fibres are particularly prominent in sarcomas and their presence is a considerable help in distinguishing these tumours from anaplastic astrocytomas and medulloblastomas (Bullon-Ramirez, 1962).

Angiomatous lesions. Conglomerates of capillary-type dilated vessels with increased numbers of endothelial cells and a gross appearance of a haemorrhagic focus have been observed in the brain and Gasserian ganglia of JC virus-inoculated hamsters (ZuRhein, 1983, 1987).

Dysontogenetic tumours

Teratoma and hamartoma. The induction of teratomas and hamartomas of the CNS has been reported by Hosobuchi and Ishii (1967). Teratomas are composed of ectodermal and/or mesodermal elements, such as skin, skin appendages, skeletal muscles, cartilage, bone and bone marrow. Histologically, hamartomas consists of fully differentiated brain tissue showing a disorderly architectural arrangement of the cellular components.

Tumours of the peripheral nervous system

Neurinomas are tumours of the PNS characterized by the exclusive proliferation of Schwann cells and are also called schwannomas or neurilemomas. Neurinomas in hamsters have been reported to occur in the root of the trigeminal nerve and in the peripheral nerves (Ivankovic & Druckrey, 1968; Levenbook & Strizhachenko, 1971; Mennel & Zülch, 1972; Rustia & Shubik, 1974; Rustia, 1974).

Grossly, neurinomas are well circumscribed, usually encapsulated nodules causing compression of the nerve (Figure 33). Frequently, they show cystic degeneration and a tendency to haemorrhage (Figure 34). Microscopically, the Schwann cells may have a round to spindle-shaped appearance, areas of dense cellularity alternating with others of scarce cellular population, among which there are abundant deposits of amorphous material (Figures 35 and 36). When the Schwann cells are numerous and arranged in rhythmic structures sometimes forming Verocay bodies, the neurinomas are classi-fied as Antoni type A (Figure 37). When the Schwann cells are arranged in a reticular pattern the tumour is considered Antoni type B (Figures 38 and 39). Both patterns have been described in hamsters by Levenbook and Strizhachenko (1971), Mennel and Zülch (1972) and Rustia (1974). The tendency to myxoid degeneration, cyst formation, and necrosis, or regression with hyalinosis and lymphoid-plasmocyte-like infiltration in these tumours has also been emphasized by these authors (Figure 40). In neurinomas originating either in the gasserian ganglion or in the spinal ganglia, the Schwann cells are seen to proliferate in between the apparently well preserved ganglion cells (Figure 41).

Neurofibromas are benign tumours of the PNS characterized by combined proliferation of all the cellular elements of a peripheral nerve: Schwann cells, perineurial cells and fibroblasts causing splitting of neurites. Grossly, neurofibromas are non-encapsulated neoplasms, which in some cases appear to be relatively well circumscribed. In other instances they form ill-defined swollen masses whose limits are impossible to define. They may measure up to several centimetres in diameter. The cut surface is usually greyish-white, translucent, smooth and glistening. Cystic and haemorrhagic changes are more common features in neurinomas than in neurofibromas.

Neurofibromas arise in cranial nerves, mainly from branches of the trigeminal nerves as well as in spinal nerve roots and in the cauda equina. Tumours arising in the spinal roots grow in the early stage as fusiform or nodular, sometimes inconspicuous enlargements of the roots. In more advanced tumours, the neoplastic growth infiltrates diffusely through the intervertebral disc and the paravertebral soft tissue. When neurofibromas involve the subcutaneous tissue, they may ulcerate the cutaneous surface.

Microscopically, the tumours are composed mainly of Schwann cells and are characterized by the concomitant presence of perineurial cells, fibroblasts and collagen bundles, all of them on occasions surrounding well preserved nerve fascicles. The Schwann cells are arranged in a texture of fusiform and twisted elements, often compactly arranged or alternating with other areas in which the cells may have a stellate shape and appear separated by considerable amounts of an amorphous matrix. Mast cells, often with enlarged nuclei, may be observed within these areas of loose texture. In subcutaneous tumours, the presence of cellular arrangements resembling tactoid-like or lamellar formations is a characteristic finding (Figure 42). Although in some instances the differential diagnosis between neurinoma and neurofibroma may be difficult, and in certain cases features of both lesions coexist, this does not justify combining the two categories. Neurofibromas have been observed in hamsters by Zülch and Mennel (1973), Rustia and Shubik (1974), Nakamura *et al.* (1989) and Cardesa and Mohr (unpublished data).

Plexiform neurofibroma. When bundles of distorted and sometimes bizarre nerves are entrapped within neurofibromatous textures, the tumours are classified as plexiform neurofibromas. In other words, besides Schwann cells, fibroblasts and perineurial cells which are distributed in a disorderly manner, these tumours show groups of convoluted nerve bundles with an increased endoneurial matrix. Grossly, no differences have been reported between plexiform and non-plexiform neurofibromas in hamsters.

Microscopically, plexiform neurofibromas show different degrees of differentiation. In the well differentiated plexiform neurofibromas, the plexiform pattern is characterized by sharply circumcribed and obviously thickened bundles of nerves. In the more aggressive PNS tumours, the plexiform pattern appears as poorly defined twisted conglomerates of convoluted nerve fascicles. Histologically, two types of plexiform structure are found, the first characterized by a pre-dominantly intraneural growth and the second by the presence of a more or less even distribution of both intraneural and extraneural components. The main basis for identification of the plexiform pattern, and hence of plexiform neurofibromas, is the recognition of a prominent intraneural growth of peripheral nerve sheath cells, which proliferate within bundles and trunks of nerves and give rise to irregularly distorted fascicles.

The histological features of plexiform neurofibromas were illustrated in the first edition of this book (Figures 43 and 44) from experiments performed by Rustia and Shubik (1974). Recently, Nakamura *et al.* (1989) have reported the induction of plexiform neurofibromas in the hamster, and considered this to correspond to an animal model for von Recklinghausen's neurofibromatosis. Plexiform neurofibromas induced in the hamster by Cardesa and Mohr (unpublished data) were morphologically similar to those reported in the rat (Cardesa *et al.*, 1989, 1990).

Neurofibrosarcoma. The malignant forms of PNS tumours are called neurofibrosarcoma, neurosarcoma, malignant schwannoma, malignant neurinoma or malignant neurilemoma. Histologically, these neoplasms show similar patterns to those previously described for neurinomas and neurofibromas; however, the Schwann cells in neurofibrosarcomas show a more marked degree of anaplasia (Figure 45). The neoplasms often consist of fusiform elements closely packed in interlacing bundles. Reticulin fibrils that extend in parallel rows among the spindle cells can be demonstrated ˙(Figure 46). Tumours with densely populated fusiform cells may show a general uniformity, but

there are frequently areas of pleomorphism with mononuclear or multinucleated giant cells and mitoses. Frequently, in the more loosely textured, myxoid tumours, the cells show a range of shapes, varying from relatively large elements with pale cytoplasm to small round or stellate cells with subtle elongated processes. In the myxoid neoplasms, Wagner–Meissner-like tactile corpuscles and arrangements of pseudorosette forms can be found.

Diffusely growing neurofibrosarcomas widely invade the neighbouring structures, dissecting and separating them. This happens most frequently to the skeletal muscle. Besides invasion, structural disorganization and cellular anaplasia, the main morphological criteria of malignancy are necrosis and particularly the presence of mitotic figures. The occurrence of these tumours in hamsters has been reported by Ivankovic and Druckrey (1968), Matsuyama and Suzuki (1971), Mennel and Zülch (1972), Althoff *et al.* (1973), Rustia and Shubik (1974) and Nakamura *et al.* (1989). Virus-induced malignant schwannomas have been reported by Levenbook and Strizhachenko (1971), Ohashi *et al.* (1978), ZuRhein (1983, 1987) and Nagashima *et al.* (1986). The latter were located either para-vertebrally or intraorbitally (Figure 47).

Granular cell tumour. This tumour represents a controversial entity about which there has been a great deal of discussion as to its histogenesis. Two cases were reported by Pour *et al.* (1973) in white hamsters, supporting the most widely accepted point of view that these tumours originate from Schwann cells rather than from muscle cells. The neoplasm is composed of nests and interlacing cords of large granular cells, often growing between nerve fibres. The cells are irregular in form and shape and contain uniform dense nuclei which are occasionally centrally located in the cytoplasm. The small intracytoplasmic granules are eosinophilic (Figure 48). These cells strongly immunoreact with protein S-100 antibody, which further supports their origin from Schwann cells.

Tumours of the sympathetic ganglia

Ganglioneuromas are benign neuroectodermal tumours composed of comparatively mature ganglion cells, Schwann cell elements and nerve fibres. These tumours originate from sympathetic ganglia retroperitoneally and/or retropleurally, apparently in the autonomic nervous system. Grossly, the tumours appear as firm, whitish masses of 1–2 cm in diameter, delineated by an incomplete capsule. Microscopically, they consist mainly of Schwann cell elements loosely arranged in the fibrillary matrix. The characteristic and comparatively mature ganglion cells are distributed in an irregular pattern within the tumour, but occasionally show tendency to form clusters. They contain abundant, pink, somewhat granular cytoplasm showing tigroid granulation and with usually one prominent vesicular nucleus and one or two eccentrically positioned nucleoli. Capsular satellite cells surrounding the ganglioneurons may or may not be present. Nerve fibres, frequently in a degenerate state, can be identified by special techniques (Figures 49 and 50). One case of ganglioneuroma, probably originating in the hamster coeliac plexus, has been reported by Della Porta (1961). Three of these tumours have been observed by Rustia and Cardesa (1975). Six additional cases have been documented by Beniashvili (1990).

Ganglioneuroblastoma is a tumour that differs from ganglioneuroma by the presence of immature ganglion cells alternating with mature ganglioneuroma areas. Beniashvili (1990) has reported two ganglioneuroblastomas in hamsters. In terms of histological structure, they also differ from ganglioneuromas by a greater number of cells and their cellular pleomorphism. Nuclear hyperchromatism and the presence of mitoses were frequently seen. Tigroid granulation was generally absent. Distorted, sometimes gigantic ganglion cells were present.

Neuroblastomas are immature tumours of the sympathetic nervous system which consist of small, round or oval cells containing markedly hyperchromatic nuclei and scarce cytoplasm. Tumour cells are generally closely attached to one another and tend to form rosettes. These neuroblastic rosettes, also known as Homer–Wright rosettes, are conspicuous within extremely cellular neoplastic tissue. Peripheral neuroblastomas induced by JC virus (Varakis *et al.*, 1978) or by human adenovirus type 12 (Ogawa, 1989a) consist of nodular, extensively necrotic and haemorrhagic tumours occurring mainly in the abdominal cavity, pelvis, mediastinum and neck region. In one tumour, an origin from the adrenal gland was demonstrated (Varakis *et al.*, 1978) (Figures 51 and 52), which strongly supports sympathetic derivation. Beniashvili (1990) has reported neuroblastomas after exposure to methylnitrosourea and ethylnitrosourea.

Tumours of the non-chromaffin paraganglia

Paragangliomas originate in chemoreceptor tissue and are also called chemodectomas. They consist of nests of polyhedral epithelioid cells with hyperchromatic oval nuclei, surrounded by a rich capillary network. The spontaneous occurrence of this tumour in hamsters has been observed by Kirkman (unpublished).

Tumours of the olfactory region

Esthesioneuroepithelioma. Tumours that have been termed esthesioneuroepithelioma originate from the olfactory region and are supposed to arise by the concomitant proliferation of epithelial cells and neurogenic elements that are the precursors of the sensory cells of the olfactory mucosa. These neoplasms have an expansive pattern of growth, breaking through the ethmoidal bone and invading the brain. Microscopically, the presence of 'true rosettes' is the most striking feature (Figure 53). These rosettes are formed by the arrangement of columnar cells, which resemble the sustentacular cells of the olfactory mucosa, around empty spaces. Frequently, wide areas of poorly differentiated small cells are identified which represent either reserve cells of the olfactory mucosa or neuroblasts. Identification of neuroblasts and neurofibrils is the requirement for establishing the diagnosis of this entity. Induction of such tumours in hamsters has been reported by Herrold (1964, 1967), Montesano and Saffiotti (1968) and Stenback (1973). Rosette formation in tumours arising from the olfactory epithelium was shown not to be conclusive of neurogenic origin; some of these tumours have therefore been considered as carcinomas (Pour *et al.*, 1974).

Esthesioneuroblastoma. Tumours located in the olfactory-frontal region (including olfactory bulbs) and resembling embryonal neuroepithelial tumours are termed esthesioneuroblastoma (Padgett *et al.*, 1977; ZuRhein, 1983, 1987). They consist essentially of masses of small cells with scanty cytoplasm and hyperchromatic nuclei showing neuroblastic rosettes of the Homer-Wright type (Figure 54).

Tumours of the retina

Retinoblastoma. The incidence of these tumours is low. They have arisen after intraocular injection of JC virus in newborn hamsters (Ohashi *et al.*, 1978; ZuRhein, 1983, 1987). Histologically, the cells are carrot-shaped or oval; they appear distributed diffusely or focally arranged in Homer–Wright rosettes but not in Flexner–Wintersteiner rosettes, as seen in man. The tumours are extremely cellular with numerous mitoses. Most of these tumours are poorly differentiated retinoblastomas (Figure 55).

SPONTANEOUS TUMOURS

The Syrian hamster is basically free of CNS tumours. Only one random neuro-ectodermal tumour was reported for the hamster species according to Luginbühl (1962). Two astrocytomas (Solleveld *et al.*, 1986) and a spontaneous giant cell glioblastoma in the brain of a six-month-old male Syrian hamster (Ernst *et al.*, 1991) have been reported. In other series, no spontaneous tumours of the CNS were seen (Luginbühl *et al.*, 1968; Pour *et al.*, 1976). In a series of ageing hamsters, only one metastatic lymphoma to the brain was recorded (Schmidt *et al.*, 1983). Only a few spontaneous tumours of the PNS have been reported in hamsters. They include neurofibromas (Fortner, 1958a,b; Kirkman, 1962), neurogenic sarcomas (Fortner & Gale, 1958; Kirkman, unpublished data), neurinomas (Garcia *et al.*, 1961), ganglioneuroma of the adrenal cortex (Kirkman, 1962), non-chromaffin paragangliomas (Kirkman, unpublished data) and granular cell tumour (Pour *et al.*, 1973).

INDUCTION OF TUMOURS

In the hamster, viruses and chemical compounds have proved to be effective agents in the induction of the wide spectrum of neurogenic tumours described above.

Viruses

Tumours of the CNS are induced by oncogenic viruses mainly after intracerebral (i.c.) injection into newborn hamsters. The viruses successfully employed for experimentation with hamsters in neurooncogenesis, of animal and human origin, are listed in Table 1 (Fenner, 1976).

Meningeal and intracerebral fibrosarcomas have been induced by inoculation of murine polyomavirus into the brain of 1–12-day-old hamsters (Rabson & Kirschstein, 1960; Romanul *et al.*, 1961; de Estable *et al.*, 1965). Bovine papillomavirus (BPV) (Lasneret *et al.*, 1965; Cheville, 1966; Robl *et al.*, 1972) and murine sarcoma virus (MSV) (Harvey & East, 1971) also produce sarcomas of leptomeningeal and intracerebral origin after i.c.

inoculation into hamster from newborn to weanling age. True neuroepithelial tumours, namely ependymomas, were induced by i.c. injection of SV40 into newborn hamsters (Kirschstein & Gerber, 1962; Eddy, 1962; Gerber & Kirschstein, 1962). Subsequently Duffell *et al.* (1964) reported the development of choroid plexus papillomas under similar conditions.

Table 1. Animal and human viruses neuro-oncogenic to the hamster

Animal viruses	Human viruses
DNA viruses	
(a) Papovaviruses	
Polyomavirus (murine)	JC polyomavirus
Simian virus 40 (SV40)	BK polyomavirus
Bovine papillomavirus	
(b) Adenoviruses	
Simian adenovirus 7 and 20	Adenovirus 12
Bovine adenovirus 3	Adenovirus 31
Avian adenovirus	
RNA viruses	
Avian sarcoma virus (Rous)	
Murine sarcoma virus	

Rous sarcoma virus after i.c. inoculation induces astrocytomas of the cerebral hemispheres (Rabotti & Raine, 1964; Bucciarelli *et al.*, 1967) and choroid plexus papillomas (Rabotti *et al.*, 1965). Burger *et al.* (1973), using three-day-old inbred (albino) hamsters, reported the induction of astrocytomas and spindle cell sarcomas.

A two-stage induction method was reported by Shein (1968, 1970), the first stage of which was the neoplastic transformation by SV40 and polyomavirus of cultured hamster astrocytes and choroid plexus cells. In the second stage, intracerebral or subcutaneous inoculation of the transformed cells into newborn hamsters resulted in the production of astrocytomas and choroid plexus tumours. In the same set

of experiments the inoculation of cloned transformed astrocytes resulted in the production of multiform glioblastomas. A similar approach has been used by Walsh *et al.* (1986).

Human and simian adenoviruses produced medulloblastoma and undifferentiated neoplasms of the brain (Ogawa *et al.*, 1969; Rapp *et al.*, 1969). Simian adenovirus type 7 also caused multiform glioblastomas and sarcomas (Rapp *et al.*, 1969) as well as ependymomas and choroid plexus papillomas of malignant type (Levenbook *et al.*, 1968). Simian adenovirus type 20 induced undifferentiated tumours (Merkow *et al.*, 1968). Bovine adenovirus type 3 gave rise to malignant schwannomas after subcutaneous injection (Levenbook & Strizhachenko, 1971). Motoi and Ogawa (1985) induced choroid plexus papilloma and glioblastoma multiforme using a pool of bovine adenovirus type 3. Avian adenovirus results in ependymomas (Mancini *et al.*, 1969). The intracerebral inoculation of the human adenovirus 12 induces CNS tumours of neuroectodermal origin (Ogawa *et al.*, 1969; Mukai, 1976; Ogawa, 1989a,b). These tumours are preferentially located along the ventricular shoreline arising from the subependymal matrix cells. Histologically they are embryonal neuroepithelial tumours showing a spectrum of tumour types: medulloblastomas, medulloepitheliomas, ependymoblastomas, primitive polar spongioblastomas and neuroblastomas (Ogawa, 1989b). Similar types of tumours were also induced after the intracranial inoculation of another human adenovirus, type 31 (Mizobuchi *et al.*, 1984).

The oncogenicity of JC virus has been repeatedly tested in Syrian hamsters (Walker *et al.*, 1973; Padgett *et al.*, 1977; Varakis *et al.*, 1978; ZuRhein & Varakis, 1979; Nagashima *et al.*, 1986; reviewed by ZuRhein, 1983, 1987). Tumours appeared clinically at three months after inoculation of newborns and at 7.5 months after inoculation of adults. The incidence was highest in hamsters that had been inoculated i.c. as newborns and lowest in animals which had been inoculated parenterally or intraocularly. Different tumour categories have been described after JC virus inoculation: medulloblastomas (Walker *et al.*, 1973; Padgett *et al.*, 1977; ZuRhein & Varakis, 1979; Nagashima *et al.*, 1984; Takakura *et al.*, 1987); primitive neuroectodermal tumours, malignant astrocytomas, glioblastoma multiforme and gliomatosis cerebri (Walker *et al.*, 1973; ZuRhein *et al.*, 1974; ZuRhein & Varakis, 1975), esthesioneuroblastomas (Padgett *et al.*, 1977), ependymomas and choroid plexus papillomas (Walker *et al.*, 1973; ZuRhein *et al.*, 1974; ZuRhein & Varakis, 1975), pinealocytomas (ZuRhein & Varakis, 1975; Varakis & ZuRhein, 1976), peripheral neuroblastomas (Varakis *et al.*, 1978), retinoblastomas (Ohashi *et al.*, 1978) and malignant schwannomas (Ohashi *et al.*, 1978).

The BK virus, another human DNA virus, induces several CNS tumour types, including ependymomas (Costa *et al.*, 1976; Uchida *et al.*, 1976; Corallini *et al.*, 1978), choroid plexus papillomas (Greenlee *et al.*, 1977; Altavilla *et al.*, 1983) and olfactory-frontal neuroblastomas and pinealocytomas (Uchida *et al.*, 1979). They mainly developed after i.c. inoculation into newborn hamsters and the latency period was 5–6 months (Costa *et al.*, 1976).

The role of immune response in the induction of CNS tumours by BK virus in the hamster has been studied (Greenlee *et al.*, 1977; Altavilla *et al.*, 1983). Immunosuppression did not enhance the tumour incidence, nor influence the latency period. However, neoplastic growth appeared to be more rapid and with more aggressive behaviour in immunosuppressed animals. De Micco *et al.* (1986) suggested that the blood–brain barrier allows immunocompetent effector cells to penetrate inside the CNS and prevented the locally elicited cell-mediated immune response from diffusing outside the CNS.

They concluded that the ability of the brain to develop a local immune response and the partial lack of circulation of immuno-competent cells across the blood–brain barrier could be largely responsible for the special immune status of the CNS and would greatly interfere with the establishment of an efficient immune response towards brain tumours. These concepts relate to adult hamsters but not to animals within a few days after birth, when the blood–brain barrier is still immature.

Chemicals

Chemical neurocarcinogens of the group of nitrosoureas produce tumours of the central and peripheral nervous system mainly after transplacental administration and crossing of the placental and haematoencephalic barriers.

Administration by intragastric tube of 60 mg/kg b.w. ENU to hamsters on the 11th day of pregnancy induced mixed gliomas of the cerebral hemispheres and spinal cord, as well as neurinomas and neurosarcomas in the offspring (Ivankovic & Druckrey, 1968).

Intravenous injection of 30 mg/kg b.w. ENU to hamsters on the 15th day of pregnancy (Mennel & Zülch, 1972) caused neurinomas and neurosarcomas of the trigeminal nerve and of the peripheral nerves in the progeny. No CNS tumours were seen.

The offspring of pregnant hamsters treated with 100 mg/kg of ethylurea and 50 mg/kg of sodium nitrite administered simultaneously by intragastric intubation from the 12th until the 15th day of pregnancy, and the offspring of hamsters similarly receiving a single dose of 200 mg/kg ethylurea and 100 mg/kg of sodium nitrite on the 15th day of pregnancy (Rustia & Shubik, 1974) developed mainly neurinomas and neurosarcomas and also astrocytomas, ganglioneuromas and neurofibromas. Nakamura *et al.* (1989) induced multiple peripheral nervous system tumours in 75% of the progeny by transplacental administration of a single intraperitoneal injection of 100 mg/kg of ENU to pregnant female hamsters on the 16th day (the last day) of gestation. According to these authors, the histological, immunohistochemical and ultrastructural findings of tumours were similar to those of human neurofibroma and their plexiform growth pattern and the tumour distribution resembled those of human von Recklinghausen neurofibromatosis. Cardesa and Mohr (unpublished data) have obtained PNS neurinomas and neurofibromas in the progeny after a single intraperitoneal injection of 30 mg/kg of ENU to pregnant female hamsters on the 13th and 15th days. Only a limited number of plexiform neurofibromas were observed, which may be mainly attributed to the lower dose of ENU used in this study.

Rustia and Cardesa (1975) reported on three ganglioneuromas, which originated from ganglia of the sympathetic chain of hamsters after exposure to precursors of ENU during prenatal life in one case, and during their postnatal adult life in two cases. One of the tumours arose from the coeliac ganglion and the other two from thoracic ganglia. In the same publication, Rustia and Cardesa collected from the literature three other examples which developed after exposure to methylcholanthrene, diethylstilbestrol and urethane. Beniashvili (1990) has reported the induction of ganglioneuromas, ganglioneuroblastomas and neuroblastomas both by daily administration to hamsters of methylnitrosourea (10 mg/kg) and in offspring after the mothers were given a single intravenous injection of ENU (60 mg/kg) during pregnancy.

Dibutylnitrosourea injected subcutaneously into suckling hamsters induced neurosarcomas in various regions (Matsuyama & Suzuki, 1971). Subcutaneous injection of nitrosohexamethylenimine into adult hamsters produced four

subcutaneous neurosarcomas (Althoff *et al.*, 1973). Nitrosodiethylamine induced olfactory esthesioneuroepitheliomas (Herrold, 1964; Montesano & Saffiotti, 1968; Stenback, 1973) when administered subcutaneously, as did nitrosodimethylamine (Herrold, 1967).

Dimethylbenz[*a*]anthracene (DMBA) was injected intravenously (500 mg/kg) into pregnant hamsters (10th or 11th day of pregnancy), which were killed one hour after injection; embryonic brain fragments were intracerebrally injected into hamsters of various ages. Gangliogliomas and astrocytomas were then observed (Hosobuchi & Ishii, 1967). In the same set of experiments, the inoculation of fragments of embryonic hamster brain without treatment resulted in the induction of hamartomas and also of teratomas when the inoculum was contaminated with muscle, skin and other non-neural tissues.

COMPARATIVE ASPECTS

The resemblance of the neoplasms of the nervous system of the hamster to the corresponding human tumours is striking (Berman, 1967; Yohn, 1972; Rubinstein, 1982). This seems reasonable since the morphological substrate of the nervous system is very similar in all mammals (Zülch & Mennel, 1973). Neurogenic tumours account for a large number of the neoplasms seen in infancy and childhood (Rubinstein, 1972a). This clinical observation supports the validity of the hamster as a model for neurocarcinogenesis since the intracerebral injection of viruses into newborn animals and the transplacental exposure of fetuses to resorptive chemical carcinogens both lead to the development of neurogenic tumours in short periods of time.

Medulloblastomas in man are tumours that appear in early life and are generally localized in the cerebellum (Rubinstein, 1972a). In hamsters, medulloblastomas were reported 4–8 weeks after i.c. injection of human and simian adenovirus

(Ogawa *et al.*, 1969; Rapp *et al.*, 1969). Merkow *et al.* (1968) frequently observed that undifferentiated tumours caused by simian adenovirus 20 were morphologically indistinguishable from medulloblastomas and involved the vermis of the cerebellum by compression. The histological similarity of these tumours to their counterpart in man was pointed out by Rapp *et al.* (1969). In man, tumours with similar characteristics to the cerebellar medulloblastoma have been observed in the cerebrum and have been called 'primitive neuroectodermal tumours' (Hart & Earle, 1973) or 'extracerebellar medulloblastoma' (Cruz-Sanchez *et al.*, 1991). The human tumours that appear in early life have poor differentiation similar to those induced in hamsters by adenovirus 12 inoculation (Ogawa, 1989b), which have limited differentiation and histological features of cerebellar medulloblastoma. In the case of medulloblastoma exclusively found in the cerebellum, the original concept by Bailey and Cushing (1926) of the bipotential differentiation of medulloblastomas has received support (Herman & Rubinstein, 1984; Cruz-Sanchez *et al.*, 1989), as has its hypothesized origin from both the cerebellar external granular layer and the median germinal layer (Rubinstein, 1972b, 1985). Nagashima *et al.* (1984) found a lack of differentiation of JC virus-induced medulloblastomas to either glial or neuronal elements in immunocytochemical studies using the glial marker GFAP and the neuronal marker NSE. Takakura *et al.* (1987) found neither GFAP nor NSE in the original tumour cells. However, two years after *in vitro* propagation, 50% of tumour cells became positive for GFAP. The authors mention no neuronal differentiation in the *in vitro* growth. The JC virus-induced medulloblastomas in the hamster arose in the internal granular layer of the vermis or of the cerebellar hemispheres. It was originally hypothesized by ZuRhein and Varakis (1979) that this phenotypic

expression of malignant transformation follows viral infection of the undifferentiated cells of the outer granular layer which migrate downwards after having undergone mitoses. Subsequent investigators have supported this hypothesis and elucidated its mechanism (Nagashima *et al.*, 1984, 1986; Matsuda *et al.*, 1987; Ressetar *et al.*, 1990).

Sarcomas of the CNS in man are most frequently found in infants and children, and are uncommon in adults (Rubinstein, 1972a). In hamsters, meningeal sarcomas and intracerebral sarcomas develop in 5–10 weeks after i.c. injection of various viruses into newborns. The morphological resemblance of the sarcomas induced by polyomavirus to the rare leptomeningeal sarcomas of the human brain was reported by Rabson and Kirschstein (1960).

Choroid plexus papillomas, both benign and malignant, are rare intracranial tumours in man, found particularly during the first decade of life (Russell & Rubinstein, 1989). In hamsters, morphologically similar neoplasms have been induced within 4–8 weeks of i.c. injection of the Bryan strain of Rous sarcoma virus (Rabotti *et al.*, 1965) and 12–18 weeks after injecting SV40 (Duffell *et al.*, 1964). The induction of malignant forms was reported by Levenbook *et al.* (1968) and Shein (1970).

Ependymomas in man are evenly distributed through all age groups with the exception of those tumours of the 4th ventricle, which occur preferentially in the first decade of life (Fokes & Earle, 1969). Interestingly, in hamsters, the induction of ependymomas by SV40 (Eddy, 1962) and an avian adenovirus (CELO) (Mancini *et al.*, 1962) shows a longer latency period of 6–32 weeks than that seen in the induction of medulloblastomas, sarcomas and choroid plexus papillomas, which are typical tumours of infancy and childhood in man. In experiments with JC virus, induction of ependymomas was seen after late fetal, neonatal or three-days postnatal inoculation. Histologically, ependymo-mas in hamsters are frequently of the papillary variety, a tumour type rarely observed in man.

Gangliogliomas in hamsters, as in-duced by Hosobuchi and Ishii (1967), appeared after a latency period of 4–13 weeks, and showed a close morphological similarity to their human counterpart. In humans, a hamartomatous pathogenesis of gangliogliomas, which are seen in children and young adults, has been postulated (Rubinstein, 1972a). It is interesting that gangliogliomas and hamartomas in hamsters were induced in the same set of experiments.

In man, astrocytomas may arise at any age. In infancy and childhood, they are preferentially located in the midline, mainly in the brain stem and cerebellum. Hemispheric astrocytomas may occur in children, but are more frequently seen in adult humans (Rubinstein, 1972a). In hamsters, such astrocytomas appear early in life, 4–8 weeks after i.c. injection of Rous sarcoma virus to newborns (Rabotti & Raine, 1964). However, this tumour distribution pattern rather resembles that of the hemispheric astrocytomas of adult man. On the other hand, transplacentally induced gliomas appeared later, after a latency period of 35–80 weeks in the offspring of pregnant hamsters to which ENU had been administered (Ivankovic & Druckrey, 1968). Astrocytomas induced by the Mill Hill strain of Rous sarcoma virus and transplanted into cheek pouch of the hamster are histologically similar to the protoplasmic variant of human astro-cytoma. Subcutaneous transplants of the same tumour resemble the pilocytic astro-cytoma of adult man (Davies & Chesterman, unpublished data).

Glioblastoma multiforme, which has a preferentially hemispheric localization in humans and occurs in adult life, has been induced in hamsters after injection of polyoma-transformed cloned astrocytes (Shein, 1970). These results are in accordance with the currently dominant hypothesis on the histogenesis of glio-blastomas, which postulates that these tumours arise by neoplastic alteration and subsequent differentiation of mature astrocytes (Russel & Rubinstein, 1989). The development in hamster brains of glioblastoma multiforme within 24 weeks of inoculation with human papovavirus (JC), isolated from a patient with pro-gressive multifocal leukoencephalopathy (PML), was reported by Walker *et al.* (1973). PML is a degenerative disease of the human brain in which the scattered giant astrocytes usually present in the lesion cannot be distinguished from the malignant astrocytes of glioblastoma multiforme (ZuRhein, 1969).

Neurinomas and neurofibromas and their malignant forms in man are most frequently clinically apparent during the fourth, fifth and sixth decades of life and are 2–3 times more common in women than in men (Chason, 1971). In hamsters, these tumours are transplacentally induced in the offspring 35–80 weeks after administration of ENU or ethylurea and sodium nitrite to pregnant mothers (Ivankovic & Druckrey, 1968; Mennel & Zülch, 1972; Rustia & Shubik, 1974). As in humans, they show a significantly higher incidence in the female progeny (Rustia & Shubik, 1974). Grossly, trigeminal neurinomas of the hamster (Ivankovic & Druckrey, 1968) are com-parable to the classical acoustic neurinomas of man and particularly to the less frequent neurinomas of the Gasserian ganglion and trigeminal root reported by Schisano and Olivecrona (1960). Microscopically, the similarity of these hamster tumours to the human counterpart has been well docu-mented by Levenbook and Strizhachenko (1971) and Mennel and Zülch (1972), who showed that Antoni type A and B structures, as well as Verocay bodies, were present in the hamster tumours. Wagner–Meissner-like tactile corpuscles were also reported by Matsuyama and Suzuki (1971).

Prenatal and postnatal exposure to the powerful resorptive carcinogen ENU, a well established environmental carcinogen (Gichner & Veleminsky, 1967), provides an interesting model for neurocarcinogenesis in the hamster, which in turn may be useful in future attempts of extrapolation to human neurooncology. The induction in hamsters of neurogenic tumours of peripheral nervous system with a significantly higher incidence in the female progeny (50%) (Rustia & Shubik, 1974) establishes an experimental link with the sex-dependent neurogenic tumours frequently seen in man (Zülch & Mennel, 1973).

The plexiform structures in neurofibromas induced in hamsters (Rustia & Shubik, 1974; Nakamura *et al.*, 1989) show striking similarities with the plexiform neurofibromas induced in the rat (Cardesa *et al.*, 1989, 1990). The presence of the plexiform pattern in human peripheral nerve tumours is considered to be distinctive of neurofibromatosis (Harkin & Reed 1969; Asbury & Johnson, 1978). In hamsters and in rats, plexiform neurofibromas frequently develop together with neurofibrosarcomas. In man, severe cases of neurofibromatosis are also associated with neurofibrosarcomas (Riccardi & Eichner, 1986).

REFERENCES

Altavilla, G., Carra, L., Alberti, S., Corallini, A., Cavazzini, L., Fabris, G., Aleotti, A. & Barbanti-Brodano, G. (1983) BK virus-induced tumours in hamsters: a morphological, histochemical and ultrastructural study. *Oncology*, 40, 427–441

Althoff, J., Cardesa, A., Pour, P. & Mohr, U. (1973) Carcinogenic effect of *N*-nitrosohexamethylenimine in Syrian golden hamsters. *J. Natl Cancer Inst.*, 50, 323–329

Asbury A.K. & Johnson, P.C. (1978) Pathology of peripheral nerve. In: Bennington, J.L, ed., *Major Problems in Pathology*, Vol. 9. Philadelphia, Saunders, pp. 206–245

Bailey, P. & Cushing, H. (1926) *A Classification of the Tumours of the Glioma Group on a Histogenetic Basis With a Correlated Study of Prognosis*, Philadelphia, Lippincott

Beniashvili, D.Sh. (1990) Morphology of experimental tumours of the sympathetic nervous system. *Exp. Pathol.*, 39, 89–94

Berman, L.D. (1967) Comparative morphologic study of the virus-induced solid tumors of Syrian hamsters. *J. Natl Cancer Inst.*, 39, 847–901

Bucciarelli, R., Rabotti, G.F. & Dalton, J.A. (1967) Ultrastructure of gliomas induced in hamsters with Rous sarcoma virus. *J. Natl Cancer Inst.*, 38, 865–889

Bullon-Ramirez, A. (1962) *Anatomia Patológica de los Tumores del Sistema Nervioso*, Madrid, Editorial Paz Montalvo

Burger, P.C., Bigner, D.D. & Self, D.J. (1973) Morphologic observations of brain tumours in PD4 hamsters induced by four strains of avian sarcoma virus. *Acta Neuropathol.*, 26, 1–21

Cardesa, A., Rustia, M. & Mohr, U. (1982). Tumours of the nervous system. In: Turusov, V.S., ed., *Pathology of Tumours in Laboratory Animals*, Vol. III, *Tumours of the Hamster* (IARC Scientific Publications No. 34), Lyon, IARC, pp. 413–436

Cardesa, A., Ribalta, T., von Schilling, B., Palacín, A. & Mohr, U. (1989) Experimental model of tumours associated with neurofibromatosis. *Cancer*, 63, 1737–1749

Cardesa, A., Ribalta, T., Vogeley, K.T., Reifenberger, G., Wechsler, W. & Turusov, V.S. (1990). Tumours of the peripheral nervous system. In: Turusov, V.S. & Mohr, U., eds, *Pathology of Tumors in Laboratory Animals*, Vol. I, *Tumours of the Rat*, Second edition (IARC Scientific Publications No. 99), Lyon, IARC, pp. 699–724

Chason, J.L. (1971) Pathology of nervous system and skeletal muscle. In: Anderson, W.A.D., ed., *Pathology*, St. Louis, CV Mosby, pp. 1781–1862

Cheville, N.F. (1966) Studies on connective tissue tumors in the hamster produced by bovine papilloma virus. *Cancer Res.*, 26, 2334–2339

Corallini, A., Altavilla, G., Cecchetti, M.G., Fabris, G., Grossi, M.P., Balboni, P.G., Lanza, G. & Barbanti-Brodano, G. (1978) Ependymomas, malignant tumours of pancreatic islets, and osteosarcomas induced in hamsters by BK virus, a human papovavirus. *J. Natl Cancer Inst.*, 61, 875–883

Corallini, A., Altavilla, G., Carra, L., Grossi, M.P., Federspil, G., Caputo, A., Negrini, M. & Barbanti-Brodano, G. (1982) Oncogenicity of BK virus for immunosuppressed hamsters. *Arch. Virol.*, 73, 243–253

Costa, J., Yee, C., Tralka, T.S. & Rabson, A.S. (1976) Brief communication: Hamster ependymomas produced by intracerebral inoculation of a human papovavirus (MMV). *J. Natl Cancer Inst.*, 56, 863–864

Cruz-Sanchez, F.F., Rossi, M.L., Hughes, J.T., Esiri, M.M. & Coakham, H.B. (1989) Medulloblastoma: an immunohistological study of 50 cases. *Acta Neuropathol.*, 79, 205–210

Cruz-Sanchez, F.F., Rossi, M.L., Hughes, J.T. & Moss, T. (1991) Differentiation in embryonal neuroepithelial tumors. *Cancer*, 67, 965–976

De Estable, R.F., Rabson, A.S. & Kirschstein, R.L. (1965) Viral growth and viral oncogenesis in brains of newborn hamsters inoculated with polyoma virus. *J. Natl Cancer Inst.*, 34, 673–677

Della Porta, G. (1961) Induction of intestinal, mammary, and ovarian tumors in hamsters with oral administration of 20-methylcholanthrene. *Cancer Res.*, 21, 575–579

De Micco, C., Hassoun, J., Meyer, G. & Toga, M. (1986) Role of the blood-brain barrier in the establishment of the immune respose against polyoma virus-induced cerebral tumours in hamsters. *J. Neuroimmunol.*, 11, 301–310

Duffell, D., Hinz, R. & Nelson, E. (1964) Neoplasms in hamsters induced by simian virus 40: light and electron microscopic observation. *Am. J. Pathol.*, 45, 59–73

Eddy, B.E. (1962) Tumors produced in hamsters by SV40. *Fed. Proc.*, 21, 930–935

Ernst, H., Walter, G.F., Dasenbrock, C., Dungworth, D.L. & Mohr, U. (1991). Giant cell glioblastoma in a Syrian hamster. *Vet. Pathol.*, 28, 538–540

Fenner, F. (1976) Classification and nomenclature of viruses. *Intervirology*, 7, 1–116

Fokes, E.C. & Earle, K.M. (1969) Ependymomas: clinical and pathological aspects. *J. Neurosurg.*, 30, 585–594

Fortner, J.G. (1958a) An experimental prototype of human colon tumors. *Arch. Surg.*, 77, 627–633

Fortner, J.G. (1958b) Etiologic implications for spontaneous carcinogenesis in the Syrian hamster. In: *Proceedings of the 7th International Cancer Congress,* pp. 254–255

Fortner, J.G. & Gale, A.W. (1958) A spectrum of transplantable hamster tumors. *Proc. Am. Ass. Cancer Res.*, 2, 297–298

Garcia, H., Baroni, C. & Rappaport, H. (1961) Transplantable tumors of the Syrian golden hamster (Mesocricetus auratus). *J. Natl Cancer Inst.*, 27, 1323–1329

Gerber, P. & Kirschstein, R.L. (1962) SV40-induced ependymomas in newborn hamsters. I. Virus-tumor relationships. *Virology*, 18, 582–588

Gichner, T. & Veleminsky, J. (1967). The mutagenic activity of 1-alkylnitrosoureas and 1-alkyl-3-nitrosoguanidines. *Mutat. Res.*, 4, 207–212

Girardi, A.J., Sweet, B.H., Slotnick, V.B. & Hilleman, M.R. (1962) Development of tumours in hamsters inoculated in the neonatal period with vacuolating virus SV40. *Proc. Soc. Exp. Biol. (N.Y.)*, 109, 649–660

Greenlee, J.E., Narayan, O., Johnson, R.T. & Herndon, R.M. (1977) Induction of brain tumours in hamsters with BK virus, a human papovavirus. *Lab. Invest.*, 36, 636–641

Harkin, J.C. & Reed, R.J. (1969) Tumors of the peripheral nervous system. In: *Atlas of Tumor Pathology,* Washington, DC, Armed Forces Institute of Pathology, Second series, Fascicle 3

Hart, M.N & Earle, K.M (1973) Primitive neuroectodermal tumors of the brain in children. *Cancer*, 32, 890–897

Harvey, J.J. & East, J. (1971) The murine sarcoma virus (MSV). *Int. Rev. Exp. Pathol.*, 10, 265–360

Herman, M.M. & Rubinstein, L.J (1984). Divergent glial and neuronal differentiation in a cerebellar meduloblastoma in an organ culture system: *in vitro* occurrence of synaptic ribbons. *Acta Neuropathol.*, 65, 10–24

Herrold, K.M. (1964) Induction of olfactory neuroepithelial tumours in Syrian hamsters by diethylnitrosamine. *Cancer*, 17, 114–121

Herrold, K.M. (1967) Histogenesis of malignant liver tumours induced by dimethylnitrosamine. An experimental study in Syrian hamsters. *J. Natl Cancer Inst.*, 39, 1099–1111

Hosobuchi, Y. & Ishii, S. (1967) A new approach to hydrocarbon-induced brain tumors. *Arch. Neurol.*, 16, 664–675

Ivankovic, S. & Druckrey, H. (1968) Transplazentare Erzeugung maligner Tumoren des Nervensystems, I. Aethyl-nitroso-Harnstoff (ANH) an BD IX-Ratten. *Z. Krebsforsch.*, 71, 320–360

Kirkman, H. (1962) A preliminary report concerning tumors observed in Syrian hamsters. *Stanford Med. Bull.*, 20, 163–166

Kirschstein, R.L. & Gerber, P. (1962) Ependymomas produced after intracerebral inoculation of SV 40 into new-born hamsters. *Nature*, 195, 299–300

Lasneret, J., Chuat, J.C., Levy, J.P. & Boiron, M. (1965) Etude des tumeurs provoquées chez le hamster par le virus de la papillomatose bovine. *Pathol. Biol. Semaine Hop.*, 13, 1174–1179

Levenbook, I.S. & Strizhachenko, N.M. (1971) Morphology of tumors induced in hamster soft tissues by bovine adenovirus type 3. *Int. J. Cancer*, 8, 531–540

Levenbook, I.S., Chigirinsky, A.E., Tsetlin, E.M., Dodonova, N.N. & Altstein, A.D. (1968) Morphology of tumors induced in hamsters by simian adenoviruses. *Int. J. Cancer*, 3, 712–719

Luginbühl, H. (1962) Geschwuelste des Zentralnervensystems bei Tieren. *Acta Neuropathol.*, Suppl. I, 9–18

Luginbühl, H., Frankhauser, K.R. & McGrath, J.T. (1968) Spontaneous neoplasmas of the nervous system in animals. *Prog. Neurol. Surg.*, 2, 85–184

Mancini, L.O., Jates, V.J., Jasty, V. & Anderson, J. (1969) Ependymomas induced in hamsters inoculated with an avian adenovirus (CELO). *Nature*, 222, 190–191

Matsuda, M., Yasui, K., Nagashima, K. & Mori, W. (1987) Origin of medulloblastoma experimentally induced by human polyomavirus. *J. Natl Cancer Inst.*, 79, 585–591

Matsuyama, M. & Suzuki, H. (1971) Induction of neurosarcoma by injections of N-nitrosobutylurea in Syrian golden hamsters. *Experientia*, 27, 1459–1460

Mennel, H.D. & Zülch, K.J. (1972) Zur Morphologie transplacentar erzeugter neurogener Tumoren beim Goldhamster. *Acta Neuropathol.*, 21, 194–203

Merkow, L., Slifkin, M., Pardo, M. & Rapoza, N.P. (1968) Studies on the pathogenesis of simian adenovirus-induced tumors. III. The histopathology and ultrastructure of intracranial neoplasms induced by SV20. *J. Natl Cancer Inst.*, 41, 1051–1070

Mizobuchi, K., Motoi, M. & Ogawa, K. (1984) Undifferentiated neuroectodermal tumours induced by human adenovirus type 31 in Syrian hamsters. *Acta Pathol. Jpn.*, 34, 1313–1326

Montesano, R. & Saffiotti, U. (1968) Carcinogenic response of the respiratory tract of Syrian golden hamsters to different doses of diethylnitrosamine. *Cancer Res.*, 28, 2197–2210

Motoi, M. & Ogawa, K. (1985) Choroid plexus papilloma and giant cell glioblastoma induced in hamsters with bovine adenovirus type 3. *Acta Neuropathol.*, 66, 218–222

Mukai, N. (1976) Human adenovirus-induced embryonic neuronal tumor phenotype in rodents. *Prog. Neuropathol.*, 3, 89–128

Nagashima, K., Yasui, K., Kimura, J., Washizu, M., Yamaguchi, K. & Mori, W. (1984) Induction of brain tumours by newly isolated JC virus (Tokyo-1 strain). *Am. J. Pathol.*, 116, 455–463

Nagashima, K., Matsuda, M., Ikeda, K., Kimura-Kuroda, J., Yasui, K. & Mori, W. (1986) Induction of brain tumors experimentally by the JC virus. *Prog. Neuropathol.*, 6, 145–163

Nakamura, T., Hara, M. & Kasuga, T. (1989) Transplacental induction of peripheral nervous tumour in the Syrian golden hamster by N-nitroso-N-ethylurea. A new animal model for von Recklinghausen's neurofibromatosis. *Am J. Pathol.*, 135, 251–259

Nevin, S. (1938) Gliomatosis cerebri. *Brain*, 61, 170–191

Ogawa, K. (1989a) Embryonal neuroepithelial tumours induced by human adenovirus type 12 in rodents. 1. Tumour induction in the peripheral nervous system. *Acta Neuropathol.*, 77, 244–253

Ogawa, K. (1989b) Embryonal neuroepithelial tumours induced by human adenovirus type 12 in rodents. 2. Tumour induction in the central nervous system. *Acta Neuropathol.*, 78, 232–244

Ogawa, K., Hamayo, K., Jujii, Y., Matsuura, K. & Endo, T. (1969) Tumor induction by adenovirus type 12 and its target cell in the central nervous system. *Gann*, 60, 383–392

Ohashi, T., ZuRhein, G.M., Varakis, J.N., Padgett, B.L. & Walker, D.L. (1978) Experimental (JC virus-induced) intraocular and extraocular orbital tumours in the Syrian hamster. *J. Neuropathol. Exp. Neurol.*, 37, 667

Padgett, B.L., Walker, D.L., ZuRhein, G.M. & Varakis, J.N. (1977) Differential neuro-oncogenicity of strains of JC virus, a human polyoma virus, in newborn Syrian hamsters. *Cancer Res.*, 37, 718–720

Pour, P., Althoff, J. & Cardesa, A. (1973) Granular cells in tumors and in non-tumorous tissue. *Arch. Pathol.*, 95, 135–138

Pour, P., Cardesa, A., Althoff, J. & Mohr, U. (1974) Tumorigenesis in the nasal olfactory region of Syrian golden hamsters as a result of di-N-propylnitrosamine and related compounds. *Cancer Res.*, 34, 16–26

Pour, P., Mohr, U., Althoff, J., Cardesa, A. & Kmoch, N. (1976). Spontaneous tumours and common diseases in two colonies of Syrian hamsters. IV. Vascular and lymphatic systems and lesions of other sites. *J. Natl Cancer Inst.*, 56, 963–974

Quay, W.B., Ma Y.H., Varakis, J.N., ZuRhein, G.M., Padgett, B.L. & Walker, D.L. (1977) Modification of hydroxyindole-O-methyltransferase activity in experimental pineocytomas of hamsters induced by a human papovavirus (JC). *J. Natl Cancer Inst.*, 58, 123–127

Rabotti, G.F. & Raine, W.A. (1964) Brain tumors induced in hamsters inoculated intracerebrally at birth with Rous sarcoma virus. *Nature*, 204, 898–899

Rabotti, G.F., Raine, W.A. & Sellers, R.L. (1965) Brain tumors (gliomas) induced in hamsters by Bryan's strain of Rous sarcoma virus. *Science*, 147, 504–506

Rabson, A.S. & Kirschstein, R.L. (1960) Intracranial sarcomas produced by polyoma virus in Syrian hamsters. *Arch. Pathol.*, 69, 633–671

Rapp, F., Pauluzzi, S., Waltz, T.A., Burdine, J.A., Matsen, F.A. & Levy, B. (1969) Induction of brain tumors in newborn hamsters by simian adenovirus SA7. *Cancer Res.*, 29, 1173–1178

Ressetar, H.G., Walker, D.L., Webster, H. de F., Braun, D.G. & Stoner, G.L. (1990) Immunolabeling of JC virus large T-antigen in neonatal hamster brain before tumor formation. *Lab. Invest.*, 62, 287–296

Riccardi, V.M & Eichner J.E., eds (1986). *Neurofibromatosis*, Baltimore, Johns Hopkins University Press, pp. 162–168

Robl, M.G., Gordon, D.E., Lee, K.P. & Olson, C. (1972) Intracranial fibroblastic neoplasms in the hamster from bovine papilloma virus. *Cancer Res.*, 32, 2221–2225

Romanul, F.C.A., Roizman, B. & Luttrell, C.N. (1961) Studies of polyoma virus. Pathology and distribution of tumors produced in Syrian golden hamsters following intracranial or subcutaneous inoculation. *Bull. Johns Hopkins Hosp.*, 108, 1–15

Rubinstein, L.J. (1972a) Tumors of the central nervous system. In: *Atlas of Tumor Pathology*, Washington, DC, Armed Forces Institute of Pathology, second series, fascicle 6

Rubinstein, L.J. (1972b). Cytogenesis and differentiation of primitive central neuro-epithelial tumors. *J. Neuropathol. Exp. Neurol.*, 31, 7–26

Rubinstein, L.J. (1982) Tumors of the central nervous system. In: *Atlas of Tumor Pathology*, Washington DC, Armed Forces Institute of Pathology, second series, fascicle 6, supplement

Rubinstein, L.J. (1985). Embryonal central neuroepithelial tumors and their differentiating potential. *J. Neurosurg.*, 62, 795–805

Russel, D.S. & Rubinstein, L.J. (1989) *Pathology of Tumors of the Nervous System*, 5th ed., London, Edward Arnold

Rustia, M. (1974). Multiple carcinogenic effects of the ethylnitrosourea precursors ethylurea and sodium nitrite in hamsters. *Cancer Res.*, 34, 3232–3244

Rustia, M. & Shubik, P. (1974) Prenatal induction of neurogenic tumors in hamsters by precursors ethylurea and sodium nitrite. *J. Natl Cancer Inst.*, 52, 605–608

Rustia, M. & Cardesa, A. (1975) Ganglioneuromas in hamsters. *Acta Neuropathol.*, 32, 325–331

Schisano, G. & Olivecrona, H. (1960) Neurinomas of the gasserian ganglion and trigeminal root. *J. Neurosurg.*, 17, 306–322

Shein, H.M. (1968) Neoplastic transformation of hamster astrocytes in vitro by simian virus 40 and polyoma virus. *Science*, 159, 1476–1477

Shein, H.M. (1970) Neoplastic transformation of hamster astrocytes and choroid plexus cells in culture by polyoma virus. *J. Neuropathol Exp. Neurol.*, 29, 70–88

Schmidt, R.E., Eason, R.L., Hubbard, G.B., Young, J.T. & Eisenbrandt, D.L. (1983) *Pathology of Aging Syrian Hamsters*, Boca Raton, FL, CRC Press

Solleveld, H.A., Bigner, D.D., Averill, D.R., Jr, Bigner, S.H., Boorman, G.A., Burger, P.C., Gillespie, Y., Hubbard, G.B., Laerum, O.D., McComb, O.D., McGrath, J.T., Morgan, K.T., Peters, A., Rubinstein, L.J., Schoenberg, B.S., Schold, S.C., Swenberg, J.A., Thompson, M.B., Vandevelde, M. & Vinores, S.A. (1986) Brain tumors in man and animals: report of a workshop. *Environ. Health Perspect.*, 68, 155–173

Stenback, F. (1973) Glandular tumors of the nasal cavity induced by diethylnitrosamine in Syrian golden hamsters. *J. Natl Cancer Inst.*, 50, 895–901

Takakura, K., Inoya, H., Nagashima, K., Ikeda, K., Tomonaga, M. & Kondo, K. (1987) Viral neurooncogenesis., *Prog. Exp. Tumor Res.*, 30, 10–20

Uchida, S., Watanabe, S., Aizawa, T., Kato, K., Furuno, A. & Muto, T. (1976) Induction of papillary ependymomas and insulinomas in the Syrian golden hamster by BK virus, a human papovavirus. *Gann*, 67, 857–865

Uchida, S., Watanabe, S., Aizawa, T., Furuno, A. & Muto, T. (1979) Polyoncogenicity and insulinoma-inducing ability of BK virus, a human papovavirus, in Syrian golden hamsters. *J. Natl Cancer Inst.*, 63, 119–126

Varakis, J.N. & ZuRhein, G.M. (1976) Experimental pineocytoma of the Syrian hamster induced by a human papovavirus (JC). A light and electron microscopic study. *Acta Neuropathol.*, 35, 243–264

Varakis, J.N., ZuRhein, G.M., Padgett, B.L. & Walker, D.L. (1978) Induction of peripheral neuroblastomas in Syrian hamsters after injection as neonates with JC virus, a human polyoma virus. *Cancer Res.*, 38, 1718–1722

Walker, D.L., Padgett, B.L., Z§uRhein, G.M. & Albert, A.E. & Marsh, R.F. (1973) Human papovavirus (JC): induction of brain tumors in hamsters. *Science*, 181, 674–676

Walsh, J.W., Zimmer, S.G., Oeltgen, J. Markesbery, W.R. (1986) Invasiveness in primary intracranial tumours: part 1. An experimental model using cloned SV40 virus-produced hamster brain tumours. *Neurosurg.*, 19, 185–200

Yohn, D.S. (1972) Oncogenic viruses: expectations and applications in neuropathology. *Progr. Exp. Tumor Res.*, 17, 74–92

Zülch, K.J. & Mennel, H.D. (1973) Recent results in new models of transplacental carcinogenesis in rats. In: Tomatis, L. & Mohr, U. eds, *Transplacental Carcinogenesis* (IARC Scientific Publications No. 4), Lyon, IARC, pp. 29–44

ZuRhein, G.M. (1969) Association of papovavirions with a human demyelinating disease (progressive multifocal leukoencephalopathy). *Progr. Med. Virol.*, 11, 185–247

ZuRhein, G.M. (1983) Studies of JC virus-induced nervous system tumors in the Syrian hamster: a review. *Prog. Clin. Biol. Res.*, 105, 205–221

ZuRhein, G.M. (1987) Human viruses in experimental neuro-oncogenesis. *Cancer Campaign*, 10, 19–46

ZuRhein, G.M. & Varakis, J. (1975) Morphology of brain tumors induced in Syrian hamsters after inoculation with JC virus, a new human papovavirus. In: Korney, S., Tariska, S. & Gosztonyi, G., eds, *Proceedings, VIIth International Congress of Neuropathology (Budapest, 1974)*, Vol. I, Budapest, Akademial Kiado, Amsterdam, Excerpta Medica, pp. 479–481

ZuRhein, G.M. & Varakis, J.N. (1979) Perinatal induction of medulloblastomas in Syrian golden hamsters by a human polyoma virus (JC). In: Rice, J.M., ed., *Perinatal Carcinogenesis* (National Cancer Institute Monographs No. 51), Washington, DC, US Government Printing Office, pp. 205–208

ZuRhein, G.M., Albert, A.E., Padgett, B.L., Walker, D.L. & Marsh, R.F. (1974) Pathology of brain tumours induced in Syrian hamsters after inoculation with a papovavirus (JC) from human brain tissue. *J. Neuropathol. Exp. Neurol.*, 33, 173

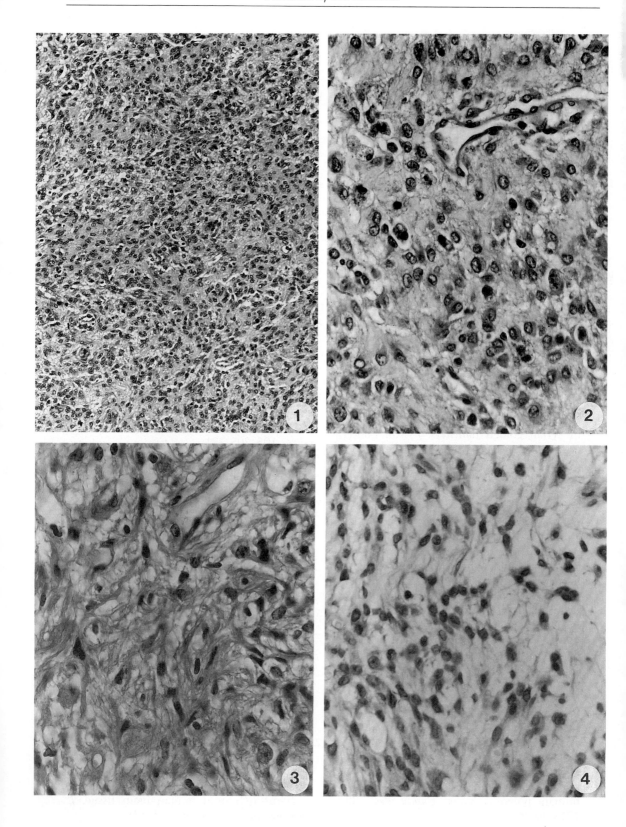

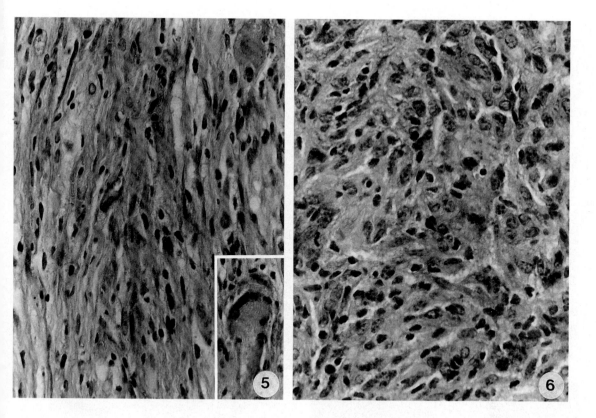

Figure 1. Astrocytoma originating in the pons. The neoplasm consists of uniform, rich astrocytic cellularity and moderate amounts of fibrillary matrix. Produced transplacentally by ethylurea and sodium nitrite. H & E; × 150. By courtesy of Dr M. Rustia.

Figure 2. Astrocytoma originating in the pons. Note the disposition of astrocytes in the proximity of blood vessel. Produced transplacentally by ethylurea and sodium nitrite. H & E; × 375. By courtesy of Dr M. Rustia.

Figure 3. Cerebral astrocytoma. The astrocytes exhibit a characteristic stellate shape, and contain abundant amounts of gliofibrillar material. Induced by the Mill Hill strain of the Rous sarcoma virus. H & E; × 450. By courtesy of Dr B.M.A. Davies and Dr F.C. Chesterman.

Figure 4. Astrocytoma. The astrocytes have a stellate shape and are arranged in a loose texture that corresponds to the pattern of growth of a protoplasmic astrocytoma. Cheek-pouch transplantation of a cerebral astrocytoma, induced by the Mill Hill strain of the Rous sarcoma virus. H & E; × 450. By courtesy of Dr B.M.A. Davies and Dr F.C. Chesterman.

Figure 5. Astrocytoma. The astrocytes have a compact texture and exhibit markedly elongated shape, corresponding to the pattern of growth of the pilocytic astrocytoma. Occasionally giant cells (inset) are seen within the tumour. Subcutaneous transplantation of a cerebral astrocytoma, induced by the Mill Hill strain of the Rous sarcoma virus. H & E; × 450. By courtesy of Dr B.M.A. Davies and Dr F.C. Chesterman.

Figure 6. Cerebral astrocytoma. The neoplasm shows an irregular arrangement of astrocytes with atypical nuclei and frequent mitoses. Induced by the Mill Hill strain of the Rous sarcoma virus. H & E; × 450. By courtesy of Dr B.M.A. Davies and Dr F.C. Chesterman.

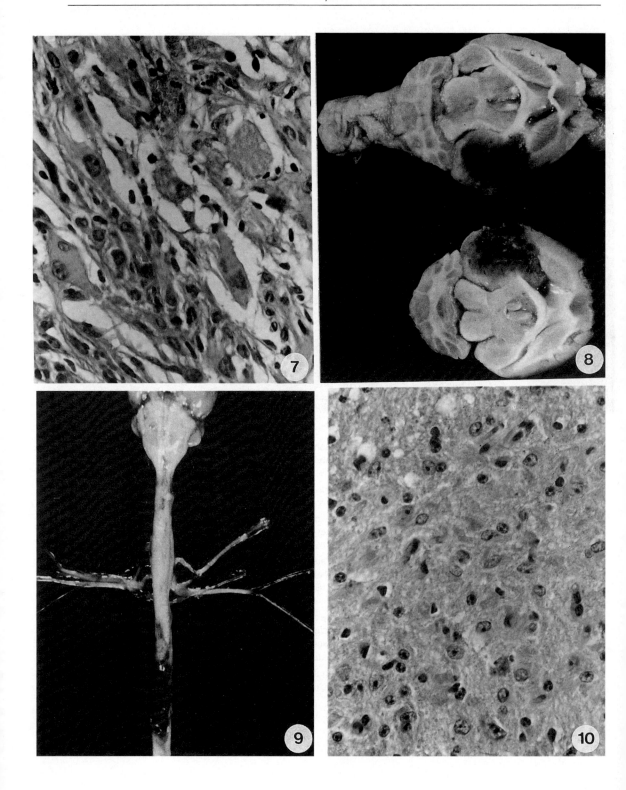

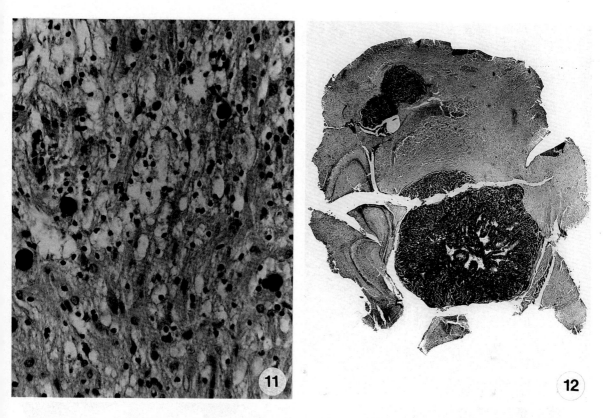

Figure 7. Cerebral astrocytoma (grade III). The neoplasm shows obvious pleomorphism and atypia, being composed of multinucleated astrocytes. Induced by the Mill Hill strain of the Rous sarcoma virus. H & E; × 450. By courtesy of Dr B.M.A. Davies and Dr F.C. Chesterman.

Figure 8. Mixed glioma originating in the region of the Ammon's horn. Induced prenatally by ENU. By courtesy of Professor H. Druckrey. By courtesy of Professor H. Druckrey.

Figure 10. Mixed glioma. The astrocytes are characterized by large nuclei with one prominent centrally located nucleolus. The oligodendroglia cells have small nuclei with marginal condensation of the chromatin. This area was observed in a cerebral astrocytoma induced by the Mill Hill strain of the Rous sarcoma virus. H & E; × 450. By courtesy of Dr B.M.A. Davies and Dr F.C. Chesterman.

Figure 11. Mixed glioma. Notice the predominance of oligodendrocytes with small hyperchromatic nuclei surrounded by a clear perinuclear halo. The characteristic feature in this case is the presence of the calcopherites. This area was observed in a cerebral astrocytoma induced by the Mill Hill strain of the Rous sarcoma virus. H & E; × 300. By courtesy of Dr B.M.A. Davies and Dr F.C. Chesterman.

Figure 12. Cerebral ependymoma involving the ventricular system. Induced by intracerebral injection of SV40 into newborn hamsters. H & E; × 8. From Eddy (1962) by courtesy of Dr B.E. Eddy.

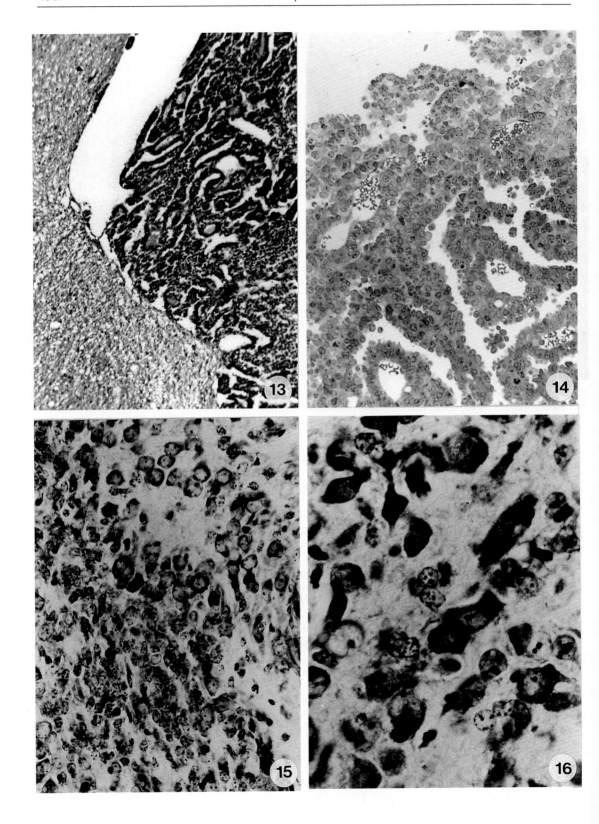

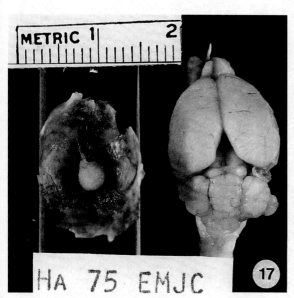

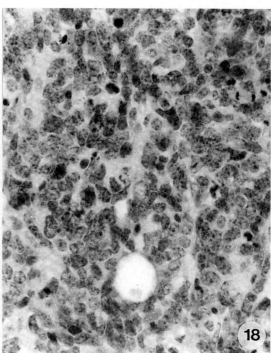

Figure 13. Papillary ependymoma arising from floor of 4th ventricle and projecting into its lumen. H & E; × 120

Figure 14. Portion from the surface of a choroid plexus papilloma. The cuboidal cells are supported by a delicate vascular stroma. Rare mitoses are present. Thick Epon section stained with toluidine blue; × 250

Figure 15. Ganglioglioma. Ganglion cells haphazardly intermixed with glia cells. H & E; × 340. From Hosobuchi & Ishii (1967), by courtesy of Dr Y. Hosobuchi.

Figure 16. Ganglioglioma. Note atypical ganglion cells. Klüver luxol blue stain; × 400. From Hosobuchi & Ishii (1967), by courtesy of Dr Y. Hosobuchi.

Figure 17. At top, pinealocytoma projecting from inner aspect of hamster calvarium in posterior midline. At bottom, dorsal aspect of brain where the encapsulated tumour had been easily dislodged from the area above the midbrain.

Figure 18. Pinealocytoma showing lobular pattern, scattered mitoses and a circular space. The tumour cell nuclei appear stippled. H & E; × 450

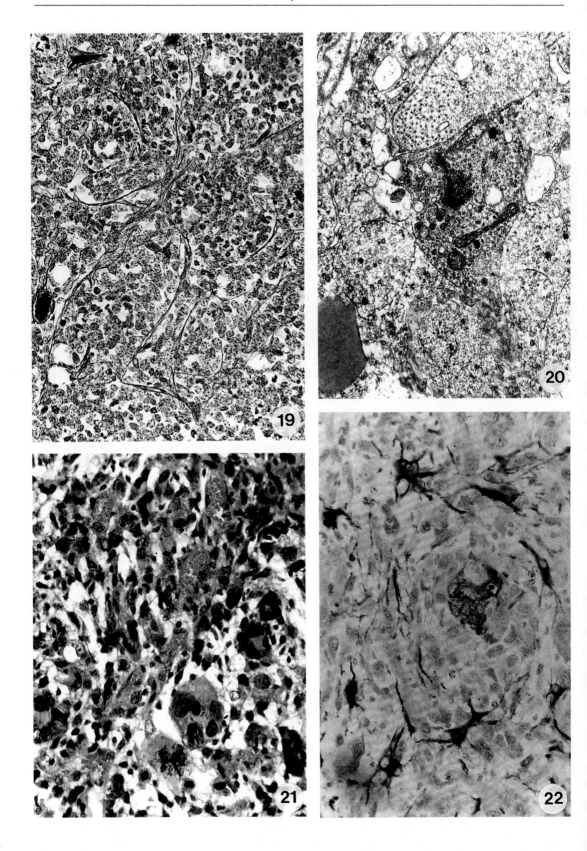

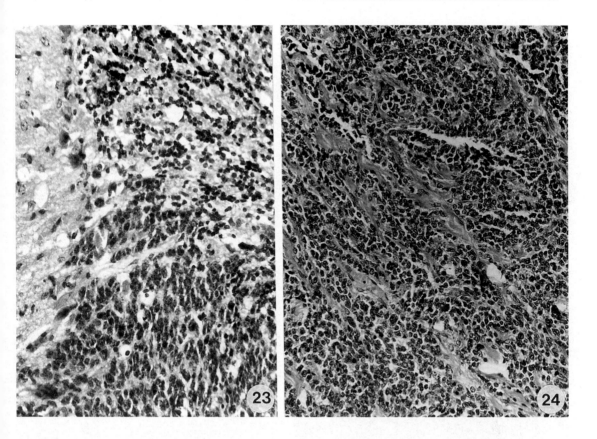

Figure 19. Reticular connective tissue stroma outlining the tumour lobules of pinealocytoma. Gomori silver stain; × 250

Figure 20. Electron micrograph of pinealocytoma: numerous cell processes contain dense-core and empty vesicles, microtubules and mitochondria. The process in the centre contains an aggregate of vesicle-crowned lamellae an organelle characteristic for pineocytes. × 20 500

Figure 21. Richly vascularized anaplastic astrocytic tumour (glioblastoma multiforme) with multi-nucleated giant cells and a atypical mitosis. H & E; × 350

Figure 22. Section of same brain tumour as in Figure 21, but stained for glial fibrillary acidic protein (GFAP) by the peroxidase-anti-peroxidase technique. Note especially the reaction product in the anaplastic giant cell in the centre. × 350

Figure 23. Cerebellar cortex with medulloblastoma arising from internal granular layer. H & E; × 250

Figure 24. Medulloblastoma. Nests of closely packed undifferentiated cells are separated by bundles of intervening hyaline material. Induced by simian adenovirus 7. H & E; × 180. By courtesy of Dr B. Levy and Dr F. Rapp.

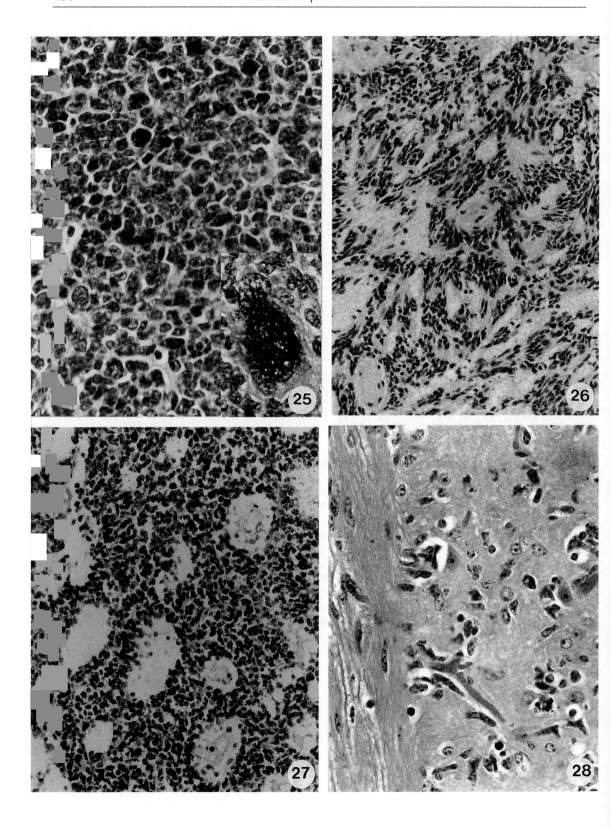

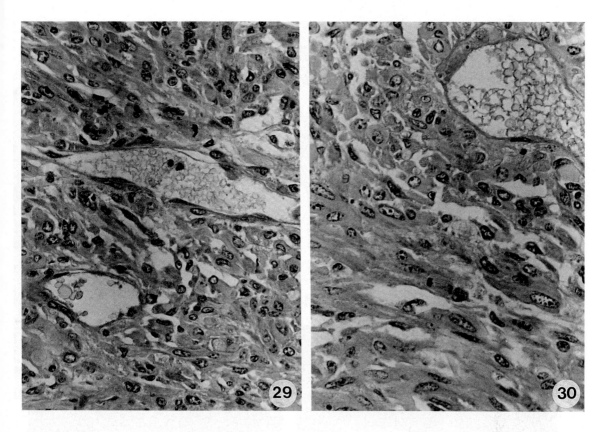

Figure 25. Medulloblastoma. Pleomorphic and anaplastic cells with small amount of cytoplasm. Notice the giant cell at low right-hand corner. Induced by simian adenovirus 7. H & E; × 450. By courtesy of Dr B. Levy and Dr. F. Rapp.

Figure 26. Medulloblastoma. Area of the tumour showing palisade arrangement of carrot-shaped cells and abundant intercellular fibrillary material. Induced by simian adenovirus 7. H & E; × 180. By courtesy of Dr B. Levy and F. Rapp.

Figure 27. Medulloblastoma. Area of tumour showing pseudo-rosette formations. Induced by simian adenovirus 7. H & E; × 150. By courtesy of Dr B. Levy and Dr F. Rapp.

Figure 28. Gliomatosis of spinal cord: tumour cells with hyperchromatic, oval, or angulated, or elongate nuclei are collected around neurons and blood vessels, or are scattered singly. H & E; × 450.

Figure 29. Intracerebral sarcoma. The tumour is formed by large spindle-shaped cells disposed around capillary blood vessels. Induced by murine sarcoma virus. H & E; × 450. By courtesy of Dr J.J. Harvey and Dr F.C. Chesterman.

Figure 30. Intracerebral sarcoma. Fusiform fibroblasts with frequent mitoses surround the blood vessels. Induced by murine sarcoma virus. H & E; × 450. By courtesy of Dr J.J. Harvey and Dr F.C. Chesterman

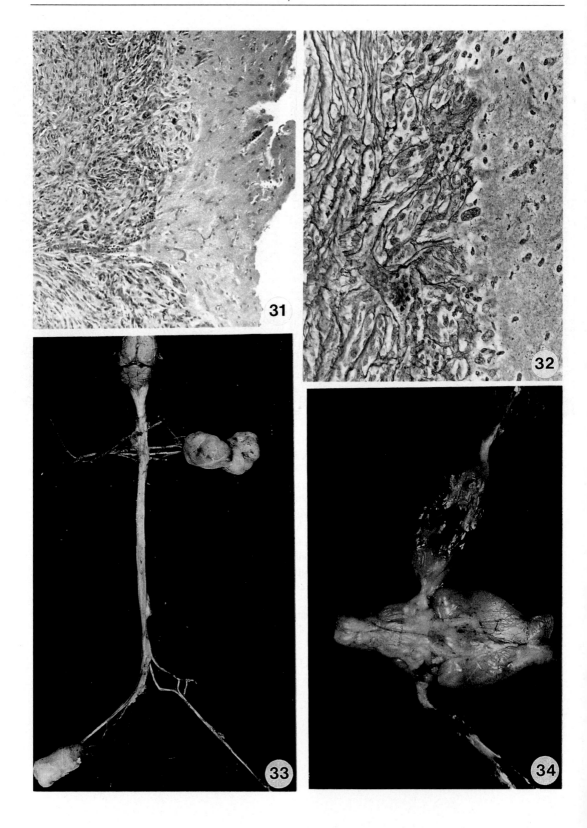

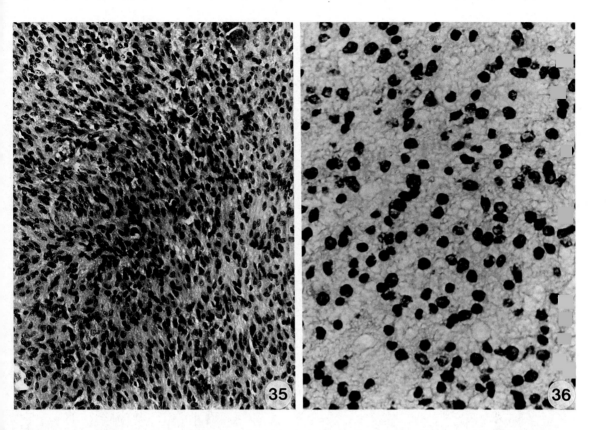

Figure 31. Fibrosarcoma of the meninges with focal extension into the subjacent cerebral cortex; 120

Figure 32. Reticulum framework in fibrosarcoma of the meninges. Gomori silver stain; × 250

Figure 33. Neurinomas originating in the right brachial as well as in the left lumbosacral plexus of the offspring, after a single intravenous injection of ENU at a dose of 60 mg/kg to the mother during late pregnancy. By courtesy of Dr D.Sh. Beniashvili.

Figure 34. Malignant neurinoma originating in the trigeminal (V) nerve, involving the gasserian ganglion. Induced prenatally by ENU. By courtesy of Professor H. Druckrey.

Figure 35. Neurinoma originating in the trigeminal (V) nerve, involving the gasserian ganglion. Well-differentiated Schwann cells are replacing the entire architecture of the ganglion. Induced transplacentally by ethylurea and sodium nitrite. H & E; × 170. By courtesy of Dr M. Rustia.

Figure 36. Neurinoma originating in the lumbosacral plexus. Note the moderate cellularity of Schwann cells, which are disposed between loose intercellular substance and exhibit round nuclei with homogeneous chromatin. Induced transplacentally by ethylurea and sodium nitrite. H & E; × 430. By courtesy of Dr M. Rustia.

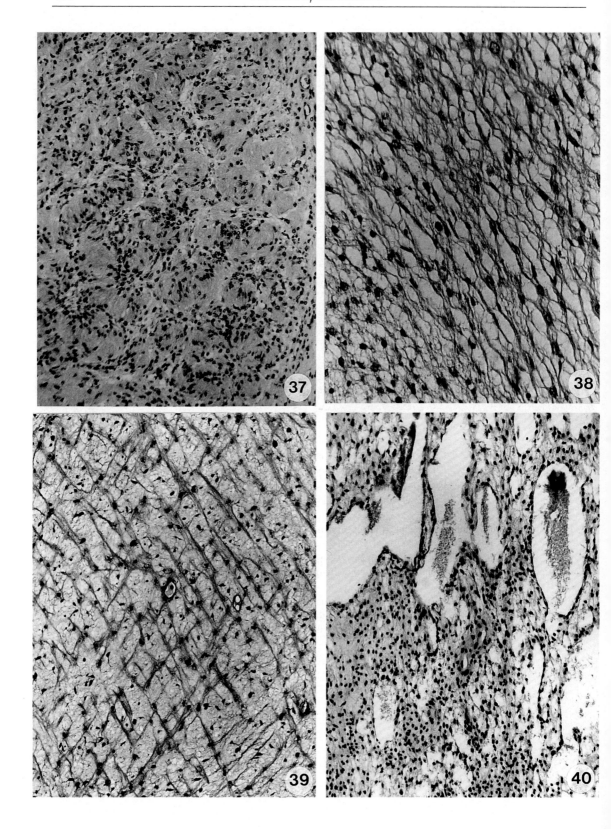

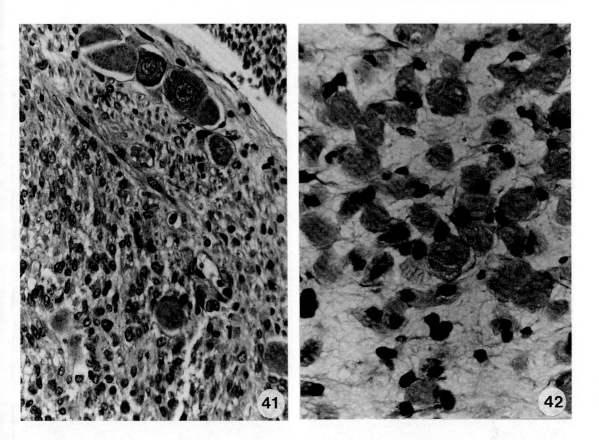

Figure 37. Neurinoma originating in the retroperitoneum. Note the presence of Schwann cells arranged in rhythmical structures of Antoni type A and the formation of Verocay bodies. Induced by ethylurea and sodium nitrite in adult hamster. H & E; × 110. By courtesy of Dr M. Rustia.

Figure 38. Neurinoma of reticular pattern originating from the hypoglossal (XII) nerve in the tongue. The cellular arrangement corresponds to Antoni type B. Note that the spindle-shaped Schwann cells form optically clear spaces containing amorphous material. Induced transplacentally by ethylurea and sodium nitrite. H & E; × 285. By courtesy of Dr M. Rustia.

Figure 39. Neurinoma originating in the mediastinum. The cellular arrangement corresponds to Antoni type B. Note rhomboid-like structures formed by the cytoplasmic elongations of Schwann cells. Induced transplacentally by ethylurea and sodium nitrite. H & E; × 170. By courtesy of Dr M. Rustia.

Figure 40. Neurinoma originating in the retroperitoneum. The neoplasm shows wide areas of cystic degeneration, containing amorphous, mucopolysaccharide-rich substance. Induced transplacentally by ethylurea and sodium nitrite. H. & E; × 145. By courtesy of Dr M. Rustia.

Figure 41. Neurinoma originating in the trigeminal (V) nerve, involving the gasserian ganglion. Note the displacement of the ganglionar elements by the proliferation of neoplastic Schwann cells. Induced transplacentally by ethylurea and sodium nitrite. H & E; × 300. By courtesy of Dr M. Rustia.

Figure 42. Lamellar structures in a conglomerate of Schwann cells, resembling tactoid-like formations. These structures can be found in both neurofibromas and neurinomas. In the present case they originated in the infra-orbital branch of the trigeminal (V) nerve. Induced transplacentally by ethylurea and sodium nitrite. H & E; × 430. By courtesy of Dr M. Rustia.

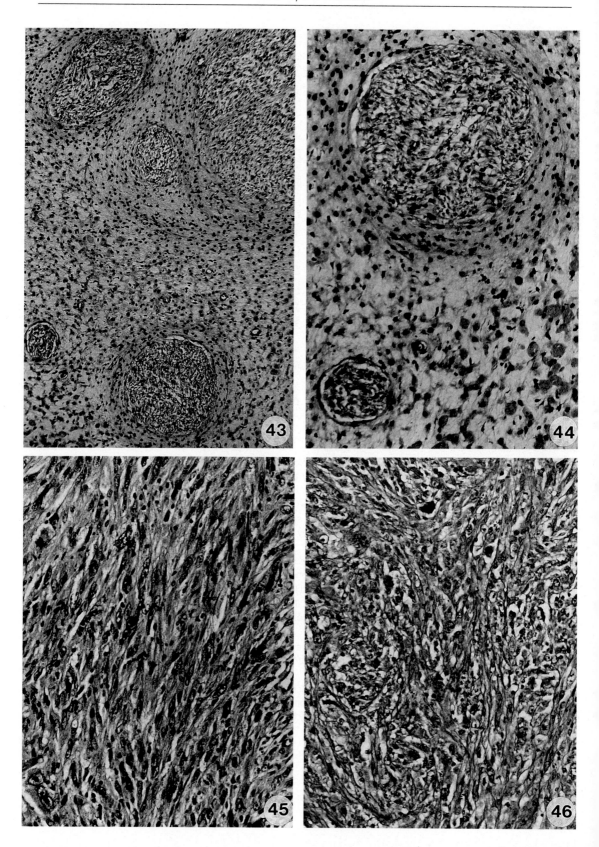

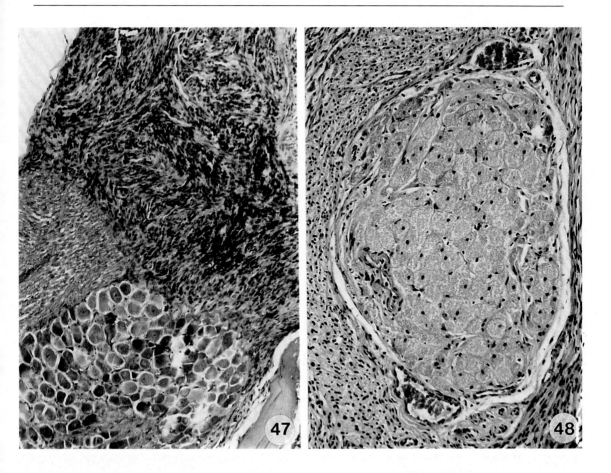

Figure 43. Plexiform neurofibroma originating in the suborbital branch of the trigeminal (V) nerve. Nerve trunks of various sizes are entrapped within the tumoral architecture, surrounded by the proliferation of Schwann cells. Induced transplacentally by ethylurea and sodium nitrite. H & E; × 75. By courtesy of Dr M. Rustia.

Figure 44. Plexiform neurofibroma originating in the suborbital branch of the trigeminal (V) nerve. Two nerve trunks are surrounded by the proliferation of Schwann cells with a tendency to form lamellar structures. Induced transplacentally by ethylurea and sodium nitrite. H & E; × 145. By courtesy of Dr M. Rustia.

Figure 45. Neurosarcoma originating in the retroperitoneum. The neoplasm is composed of bundles of spindle-shaped Schwann cells exhibiting a marked degree of anaplasia. Induced transplacentally by ethylurea and sodium nitrite. H. & E; × 170. By courtesy of Dr M. Rustia.

Figure 46. Neurosarcoma originating in the retroperitoneum. Note the delicate reticulum fibrils that extend in parallel rows among the spindle-shaped anaplastic Schwann cells. Induced transplacentally by ethylurea and sodium nitrite. Gomori's stain; × 170. By courtesy of Dr M. Rustia.

Figure 47. Malignant schwannoma with hypercellular intersecting cell bundles arising from peripheral nerve in vicinity of spinal ganglion. H & E; × 120

Figure 48. Spontaneous granular cell tumour originating in the uterine wall of a white hamster. Notice the circumscribed nodule of granular cells with excentric nuclei surrounded by smooth muscle fibres. H & E; × 115

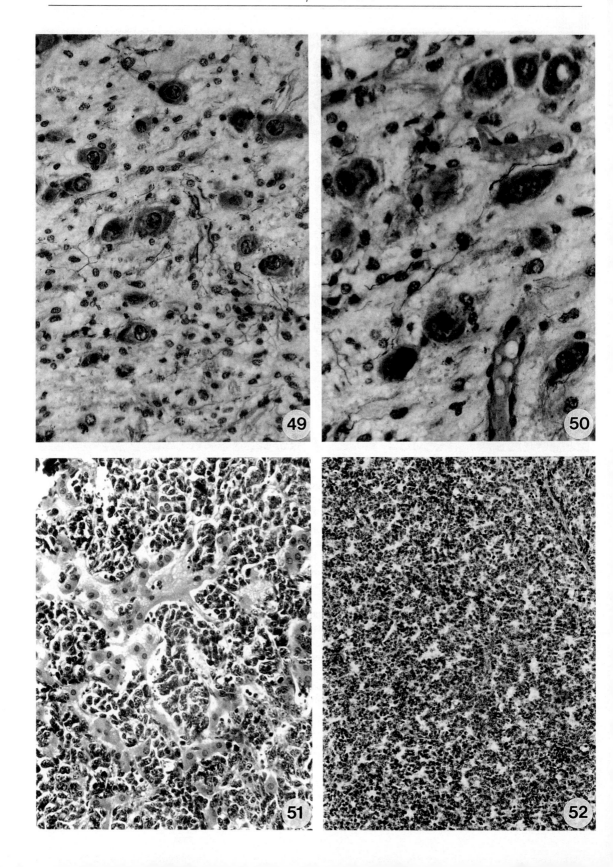

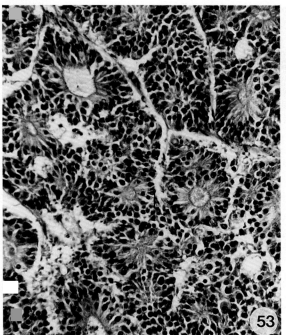

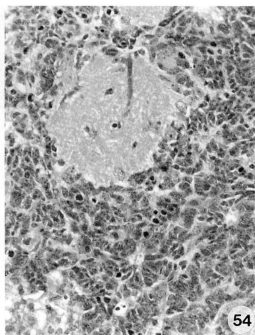

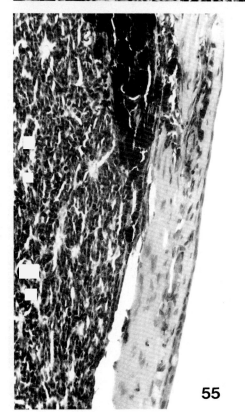

Figure 49. Ganglioneuroma originating from the thoracic segment of the sympathetic trunk. Ganglion cells appear irregularly distributed between Schwann cells. Notice the presence of neurofibrils. Induced by ethylurea and sodium nitrite in adult hamster. Bodian's stain; × 285

Figure 50. Ganglioneuroma originating from the thoracic segment of the sympathetic trunk. The ganglion cells show a tendency to form clusters. Induced by ethylurea and sodium nitrite in adult hamster. Bodian's stain; × 430

Figure 51. Neuroblastoma of the adrenal gland. Massive infiltration of the cortical tissue. H & E; × 250

Figure 52. Portion of a large intra-abdominal neuroblastoma exhibiting Homer–Wright rosettes. H & E; × 120

Figure 53. Esthesioneuroepithelioma originating in the olfactory region. The tumour is composed of columnar cells arranged around empty spaces, forming the so-called rosettes. H & E; × 190

Figure 54. Esthesioneuroblastoma with mitoses and Homer–Wright rosettes. Olfactory glomeruli on top. H & E; × 250

Figure 55. Retinoblastoma with several Homer–Wright rosettes. The tumour tissue appears compressed due to the marked increase in intraocular pressure. Sclera along right and pigmented choroidal cells on top. H & E; × 250

IARC Scientific Publications

No. 1
Liver Cancer
1971; 176 pages; ISBN 0 19 723000 8

No. 2
Oncogenesis and Herpesviruses
Edited by P.M. Biggs, G. de Thé and
L.N. Payne
1972; 515 pages; ISBN 0 19 723001 6

No. 3
N-Nitroso Compounds: Analysis and
Formation
Edited by P. Bogovski, R. Preussman
and E.A. Walker
1972; 140 pages; ISBN 0 19 723002 4

No. 4
Transplacental Carcinogenesis
Edited by L. Tomatis and U. Mohr
1973; 181 pages; ISBN 0 19 723003 2

No. 5/6
Pathology of Tumours in Laboratory
Animals. Volume 1: Tumours of the Rat
Edited by V.S. Turusov
1973/1976; 533 pages;
ISBN 92 832 1410 2

No. 7
Host Environment Interactions in the
Etiology of Cancer in Man
Edited by R. Doll and I. Vodopija
1973; 464 pages; ISBN 0 19 723006 7

No. 8
Biological Effects of Asbestos
Edited by P. Bogovski, J.C. Gilson,
V. Timbrell and J.C. Wagner
1973; 346 pages; ISBN 0 19 723007 5

No. 9
N-Nitroso Compounds in the
Environment
Edited by P. Bogovski and E.A. Walker
1974; 243 pages; ISBN 0 19 723008 3

No. 10
Chemical Carcinogenesis Essays
Edited by R. Montesano and L. Tomatis
1974; 230 pages; ISBN 0 19 723009 1

No. 11
Oncogenesis and Herpes-viruses II
Edited by G. de Thé, M.A. Epstein
and H. zur Hausen
1975; Two volumes, 511 pages; and
403 pages; ISBN 0 19 723010 5

No. 12
Screening Tests in Chemical
Carcinogenesis
Edited by R. Montesano, H. Bartsch
and L. Tomatis
1976; 666 pages; ISBN 0 19 723051 2

No. 13
Environmental Pollution and
Carcinogenic Risks
Edited by C. Rosenfeld and W. Davis
1975; 441 pages; ISBN 0 19 723012 1

No. 14
Environmental N-Nitroso Compounds.
Analysis and Formation
Edited by E.A. Walker, P. Bogovski and
L. Griciute
1976; 512 pages; ISBN 0 19 723013 X

No. 15
Cancer Incidence in Five Continents,
Volume III
Edited by J.A.H. Waterhouse, C. Muir,
P. Correa and J. Powell
1976; 584 pages; ISBN 0 19 723014 8

No. 16
Air Pollution and Cancer in Man
Edited by U. Mohr, D. Schmähl and
L. Tomatis
1977; 328 pages; ISBN 0 19 723015 6

No. 17*
Directory of On-Going Research in
Cancer Epidemiology 1977
Edited by C.S. Muir and G. Wagner
1977; 599 pages; ISBN 92 832 1117 0

No. 18
Environmental Carcinogens. Selected
Methods of Analysis. Volume 1: Analy-
sis of Volatile Nitrosamines in Food
Editor-in-Chief: H. Egan
1978; 212 pages; ISBN 0 19 723017 2

No. 19
Environmental Aspects of N-Nitroso
Compounds
Edited by E.A. Walker, M. Castegnaro,
L. Griciute and R.E. Lyle
1978; 561 pages; ISBN 0 19 723018 0

No. 20
Nasopharyngeal Carcinoma:
Etiology and Control
Edited by G. de Thé and Y. Ito
1978; 606 pages; ISBN 0 19 723019 9

No. 21
Cancer Registration and its Techniques
Edited by R. MacLennan, C. Muir,
R. Steinitz and A. Winkler
1978; 235 pages; ISBN 0 19 723020 2

No. 22
Environmental Carcinogens: Selected
Methods of Analysis. Volume 2:
Methods for the Measurement of Vinyl
Chloride in Poly(vinyl chloride), Air,
Water and Foodstuffs
Editor-in-Chief: H. Egan
1978; 142 pages; ISBN 0 19 723021 0

No. 23
Pathology of Tumours in Laboratory
Animals.
Volume II: Tumours of the Mouse
Editor-in-Chief: V.S. Turusov
1979; 669 pages; ISBN 0 19 723022 9

No. 24
Oncogenesis and Herpesviruses III
Edited by G. de-Thé, W. Henle and
F. Rapp
1978; Part I: 580 pages;
Part II: 512 pages; ISBN 0 19 723023 7

No. 25
Carcinogenic Risk: Strategies for
Intervention
Edited by W. Davis and C. Rosenfeld
1979; 280 pages; ISBN 0 19 723025 3

No. 26*
Directory of On-going Research in
Cancer Epidemiology 1978
Edited by C.S. Muir and G. Wagner
1978; 550 pages; ISBN 0 19 723026 1

No. 27
Molecular and Cellular Aspects of
Carcinogen Screening Tests
Edited by R. Montesano, H. Bartsch
and L. Tomatis
1980; 372 pages; ISBN 0 19 723027 X

No. 28*
Directory of On-going Research in
Cancer Epidemiology 1979
Edited by C.S. Muir and G. Wagner
1979; 672 pages; ISBN 92 832 1128 6

No. 29
Environmental Carcinogens. Selected
Methods of Analysis. Volume 3:
Analysis of Polycyclic Aromatic Hydro-
carbons in Environmental Samples
Editor-in-Chief: H. Egan
1979; 240 pages; ISBN 0 19 723028 8

No. 30
Biological Effects of Mineral Fibres
Editor-in-Chief: J.C. Wagner
1980; Two volumes, 494 pages & 513
pages; ISBN 0 19 723030 X

No. 31
N-Nitroso Compounds: Analysis,
Formation and Occurrence
Edited by E.A. Walker, L. Griciute,
M. Castegnaro and M. Börzsönyi
1980; 835 pages; ISBN 0 19 723031 8

No. 32
Statistical Methods in Cancer Research.
Volume 1: The Analysis of Case-
control Studies
By N.E. Breslow and N.E. Day
1980; 338 pages; ISBN 92 832 0132 9

*(out of print)

No. 33*
Handling Chemical Carcinogens in the
Laboratory
Edited by R. Montesano, H. Bartsch,
E. Boyland, G. Della Porta, L. Fishbein,
R.A. Griesemer, A.B. Swan and
L. Tomatis
1979; 32 pages; ISBN 0 19 723033 4

No. 34
Pathology of Tumours in Laboratory
Animals.
Volume III: Tumours of the Hamster
Editor-in-Chief: V.S. Turusov
1982; 461 pages; ISBN 0 19 723034 2

No. 35*
Directory of On-going Research in
Cancer Epidemiology 1980
Edited by C.S. Muir and G. Wagner
1980; 660 pages; ISBN 0 19 723035 0

No. 36
Cancer Mortality by Occupation and
Social Class 1851–1971
Edited by W.P.D. Logan
1982; 253 pages; ISBN 0 19 723036 9

No. 37
Laboratory Decontamination and
Destruction of Aflatoxins B1, B2, G1,
G2 in Laboratory Wastes
Edited by M. Castegnaro, D.C. Hunt,
E.B. Sansone, P.L. Schuller, M.G.
Siriwardana, G.M. Telling, H.P. van
Egmond and E.A. Walker
1980; 56 pages; ISBN 0 19 723037 7

No. 38*
Directory of On-going Research in
Cancer Epidemiology 1981
Edited by C.S. Muir and G. Wagner
1981; 696 pages; ISBN 0 19 723038 5

No. 39
Host Factors in Human Carcinogenesis
Edited by H. Bartsch and B. Armstrong
1982; 583 pages; ISBN 0 19 723039 3

No. 40
Environmental Carcinogens: Selected
Methods of Analysis. Volume 4: Some
Aromatic Amines and Azo Dyes in the
General and Industrial Environment
Edited by L. Fishbein, M. Castegnaro,
I.K. O'Neill and H. Bartsch
1981; 347 pages; ISBN 0 19 723040 7

No. 41
N-Nitroso Compounds:
Occurrence and Biological Effects
Edited by H. Bartsch, I.K. O'Neill,
M. Castegnaro and M. Okada
982; 755 pages; ISBN 0 19 723041 5

No. 42
Cancer Incidence in Five Continents
Volume IV

Edited by J. Waterhouse, C. Muir,
K. Shanmugaratnam and J. Powell
1982; 811 pages; ISBN 0 19 723042 3

No. 43
Laboratory Decontamination and
Destruction of Carcinogens in Laboratory Wastes: Some N-Nitrosamines
Edited by M. Castegnaro, G. Eisenbrand, G. Ellen, L. Keefer, D. Klein,
E.B. Sansone, D. Spincer, G. Telling
and K. Webb
1982; 73 pages; ISBN 0 19 723043 1

No. 44
Environmental Carcinogens: Selected
Methods of Analysis.
Volume 5: Some Mycotoxins
Edited by L. Stoloff, M. Castegnaro,
P. Scott, I.K. O'Neill and H. Bartsch
1983; 455 pages; ISBN 0 19 723044 X

No. 45
Environmental Carcinogens: Selected
Methods of Analysis.
Volume 6: N-Nitroso Compounds
Edited by R. Preussmann, I.K. O'Neill,
G. Eisenbrand, B. Spiegelhalder
and H. Bartsch 1983;
508 pages; ISBN 0 19 723045 8

No. 46*
Directory of On-going Research in
Cancer Epidemiology 1982
Edited by C.S. Muir and G. Wagner
1982; 722 pages; ISBN 0 19 723046 6

No. 47
Cancer Incidence in Singapore
1968–1977
Edited by K. Shanmugaratnam,
H.P. Lee and N.E. Day
1983; 171 pages; ISBN 0 19 723047 4

No. 48
Cancer Incidence in the USSR (2nd
Revised Edition)
Edited by N.P. Napalkov, G.F.
Tserkovny, V.M. Merabishvili,
D.M. Parkin, M. Smans and C.S. Muir
1983; 75 pages; ISBN 0 19 723048 2

No. 49
Laboratory Decontamination and
Destruction of Carcinogens in
Laboratory Wastes: Some Polycyclic
Aromatic Hydrocarbons
Edited by M. Castegnaro, G. Grimmer,
O. Hutzinger, W. Karcher, H. Kunte,
M. Lafontaine, H.C. Van der Plas,
E.B. Sansone and S.P. Tucker
1983; 87 pages; ISBN 0 19 723049 0

No. 50*
Directory of On-going Research in
Cancer Epidemiology 1983
Edited by C.S. Muir and G. Wagner
1983; 731 pages; ISBN 0 19 723050 4

No. 51
Modulators of Experimental
Carcinogenesis
Edited by V. Turusov and R. Montesano
1983; 307 pages; ISBN 0 19 723060 1

No. 52
Second Cancers in Relation to Radia-
tion Treatment for Cervical Cancer:
Results of a Cancer Registry
Collaboration.
Edited by N.E. Day and J.C. Boice, Jr
1984; 207 pages; ISBN 0 19 723052 0

No. 53
Nickel in the Human Environment
Editor-in-Chief: F.W. Sunderman, Jr
1984; 529 pages; ISBN 0 19 723059 8

No. 54
Laboratory Decontamination and
Destruction of Carcinogens in
Laboratory Wastes: Some Hydrazines
Edited by M. Castegnaro, G. Ellen,
M. Lafontaine, H.C. van der Plas,
E.B. Sansone and S.P. Tucker
1983; 87 pages; ISBN 0 19 723053

No. 55
Laboratory Decontamination and
Destruction of Carcinogens in
Laboratory Wastes: Some
N-Nitrosamides
Edited by M. Castegnaro, M. Bernard,
L.W. van Broekhoven, D. Fine,
R. Massey, E.B. Sansone, P.L.R.
Smith, B. Spiegelhalder, A. Stacchini,
G. Telling and J.J. Vallon
1984; 66 pages; ISBN 0 19 723054 7

No. 56
Models, Mechanisms and Etiology of
Tumour Promotion
Edited by M. Börzsönyi, N.E. Day,
K. Lapis and H. Yamasaki
1984; 532 pages; ISBN 0 19 723058 X

No. 57
N-Nitroso Compounds: Occurrence,
Biological Effects and Relevance to
Human Cancer
Edited by I.K. O'Neill, R.C. von Borstel,
C.T. Miller, J. Long and H. Bartsch
1984; 1013 pages; ISBN 0 19 723055 5

No 58
Age-related Factors in Carcinogenesis
Edited by A. Likhachev, V. Anisimov
and R. Montesano
1985; 288 pages; ISBN 92 832 1158 8

No. 59
Monitoring Human Exposure to
Carcinogenic and Mutagenic Agents
Edited by A. Berlin, M. Draper,
K. Hemminki and H. Vainio
1984; 457 pages; ISBN 0 19 723056 3

*(out of print)

No. 60
Burkitt's Lymphoma: A Human Cancer
Model
Edited by G. Lenoir, G. O'Conor and
C.L.M. Olweny
1985; 484 pages; ISBN 0 19 723057 1

No. 61
Laboratory Decontamination and Des-
truction of Carcinogens in Laboratory
Wastes: Some Haloethers
Edited by M. Castegnaro, M. Alvarez,
M. Iovu, E.B. Sansone, G.M. Telling
and D.T. Williams
1985; 55 pages; ISBN 0 19 723061 X

No. 62*
Directory of On-going Research in
Cancer Epidemiology 1984
Edited by C.S. Muir and G. Wagner
1984; 717 pages; ISBN 0 19 723062 8

No. 63
Virus-associated Cancers in Africa
Edited by A.O. Williams, G.T. O'Conor,
G.B. de Thé and C.A. Johnson
1984; 773 pages; ISBN: 0 19 723063 6

No. 64
Laboratory Decontamination and Des-
truction of Carcinogens in Laboratory
Wastes: Some Aromatic Amines and
4-Nitrobiphenyl
Edited by M. Castegnaro, J. Barek,
J. Dennis, G. Ellen, M. Klibanov,
M. Lafontaine, R. Mitchum, P. van
Roosmalen, E.B. Sansone,
L.A. Sternson and M. Vahl
1985; 84 pages; ISBN: 92 832 1164 2

No. 65
Interpretation of Negative
Epidemiological Evidence for
Carcinogenicity
Edited by N.J. Wald and R. Doll
1985; 232 pages; ISBN 92 832 1165 0

No. 66
The Role of the Registry in Cancer
Control
Edited by D.M. Parkin, G. Wagner and
C.S. Muir
1985; 152 pages; ISBN 92 832 0166 3

No. 67
Transformation Assay of Established
Cell Lines: Mechanisms and
Application
Edited by T. Kakunaga and H. Yamasaki
1985; 225 pages; ISBN 92 832 1167 7

No. 68
Environmental Carcinogens: Selected
Methods of Analysis.
Volume 7: Some Volatile Halogenated
Hydrocarbons
Edited by L. Fishbein and I.K. O'Neill
1985; 479 pages; ISBN 92 832 1168 5

No. 69*
Directory of On-going Research in
Cancer Epidemiology 1985
Edited by C.S. Muir and G. Wagner
1985; 745 pages; ISBN 92 823 1169 3

No. 70
The Role of Cyclic Nucleic Acid Adducts
in Carcinogenesis and Mutagenesis
Edited by B. Singer and H. Bartsch
1986; 467 pages; ISBN 92 832 1170 7

No. 71
Environmental Carcinogens: Selected
Methods of Analysis. Volume 8: Some
Metals: As, Be, Cd, Cr, Ni, Pb, Se, Zn
Edited by I.K. O'Neill, P. Schuller and
L. Fishbein
1986; 485 pages; ISBN 92 832 1171 5

No. 72
Atlas of Cancer in Scotland, 1975–1980:
Incidence and Epidemiological
Perspective
Edited by I. Kemp, P. Boyle, M. Smans
and C.S. Muir
1985; 285 pages; ISBN 92 832 1172 3

No. 73
Laboratory Decontamination and
Destruction of Carcinogens in
Laboratory Wastes:Some Anti-
neoplastic Agents
Edited by M. Castegnaro, J. Adams,
M.A. Armour, J. Barek, J. Benvenuto,
C. Confalonieri, U. Goff, G. Telling
1985; 163 pages; ISBN 92 832 1173 1

No. 74
Tobacco: A Major International Health
Hazard
Edited by D. Zaridze and R. Peto
1986; 324 pages; ISBN 92 832 1174 X

No. 75
Cancer Occurrence in Developing
Countries
Edited by D.M. Parkin
1986; 339 pages; ISBN 92 832 1175 8

No. 76
Screening for Cancer of the Uterine
Cervix
Edited by M. Hakama, A.B. Miller and
N.E. Day
1986; 315 pages; ISBN 92 832 1176 6

No. 77
Hexachlorobenzene: Proceedings of
an International Symposium
Edited by C.R. Morris and J.R.P. Cabral
1986; 668 pages; ISBN 92 832 1177 4

No. 78
Carcinogenicity of Alkylating Cytostatic
Drugs
Edited by D. Schmähl and J.M. Kaldor
1986; 337 pages; ISBN 92 832 1178 2

No. 79
Statistical Methods in Cancer
Research Volume III: The Design and
Analysis of Long-term Animal
Experiments
By J.J. Gart, D. Krewski, P.N. Lee,
R.E. Tarone and J. Wahrendorf
1986; 213 pages; ISBN 92 832 1179 0

No. 80*
Directory of On-going Research in
Cancer Epidemiology 1986
Edited by C.S. Muir and G. Wagner
1986; 805 pages; ISBN 92 832 1180 4

No. 81
Environmental Carcinogens:
Methods of Analysis and Exposure
Measurement. Volume 9: Passive
Smoking
Edited by I.K. O'Neill, K.D. Brunnemann,
B. Dodet and D. Hoffmann
1987; 383 pages; ISBN 92 832 1181 2

No. 82
Statistical Methods in Cancer
Research. Volume II: The Design and
Analysis of Cohort Studies
By N.E. Breslow and N.E. Day
1987; 404 pages; ISBN 92 832 0182 5

No. 83
Long-term and Short-term Assays for
Carcinogens: A Critical Appraisal
Edited by R. Montesano, H. Bartsch,
H. Vainio, J. Wilbourn and H. Yamasaki
1986; 575 pages; ISBN 92 832 1183 9

No. 84
The Relevance of N-Nitroso Compounds to Human Cancer: Exposure
and Mechanisms
Edited by H. Bartsch, I.K. O'Neill and
R. Schulte-Hermann
1987; 671 pages; ISBN 92 832 1184 7

No. 85
Environmental Carcinogens: Methods
of Analysis and Exposure Measurement. Volume 10: Benzene and
Alkylated Benzenes
Edited by L. Fishbein and I.K. O'Neill
1988; 327 pages; ISBN 92 832 1185 5

No. 86*
Directory of On-going Research in
Cancer Epidemiology 1987
Edited by D.M. Parkin and
J. Wahrendorf
1987; 685 pages; ISBN: 92 832 1186 3

No. 87*
International Incidence of Childhood
Cancer
Edited by D.M. Parkin, C.A. Stiller,
C.A. Bieber, G.J. Draper. B. Terracini
and J.L. Young
1988; 401 pages; ISBN 92 832 1187 1

*(out of print)

No. 88
Cancer Incidence in Five Continents,
Volume V
Edited by C. Muir, J. Waterhouse,
T. Mack, J. Powell and S. Whelan
1987; 1004 pages; ISBN 92 832 1188 X

No. 89*
Methods for Detecting DNA Damaging
Agents in Humans: Applications in
Cancer Epidemiology and Prevention
Edited by H. Bartsch, K. Hemminki and
I.K. O'Neill
1988; 518 pages; ISBN 92 832 1189 8

No. 90
Non-occupational Exposure to Mineral
Fibres
Edited by J. Bignon, J. Peto and
R. Saracci
1989; 500 pages; ISBN 92 832 1190 1

No. 91
Trends in Cancer Incidence in
Singapore 1968–1982
Edited by H.P. Lee, N.E. Day and
K. Shanmugaratnam
1988; 160 pages; ISBN 92 832 1191 X

No. 92
Cell Differentiation, Genes and Cancer
Edited by T. Kakunaga, T. Sugimura,
L. Tomatis and H. Yamasaki
1988; 204 pages; ISBN 92 832 1192 8

No. 93*
Directory of On-going Research in
Cancer Epidemiology 1988
Edited by M. Coleman and J. Wahrendorf
1988; 662 pages; ISBN 92 832 1193 6

No. 94
Human Papillomavirus and Cervical
Cancer
Edited by N. Muñoz, F.X. Bosch and
O.M. Jensen
1989; 154 pages; ISBN 92 832 1194 4

No. 95
Cancer Registration: Principles and
Methods
Edited by O.M. Jensen, D.M. Parkin,
R. MacLennan, C.S. Muir and R. Skeet
1991; 296 pages; ISBN 92 832 1195 2

No. 96
Perinatal and Multigeneration
Carcinogenesis
Edited by N.P. Napalkov, J.M. Rice,
L. Tomatis and H. Yamasaki
1989; 436 pages; ISBN 92 832 1196 0

No. 97
Occupational Exposure to Silica and
Cancer Risk
Edited by L. Simonato, A.C. Fletcher,
R. Saracci and T. Thomas
1990; 124 pages; ISBN 92 832 1197 9

No. 98
Cancer Incidence in Jewish Migrants
to Israel, 1961-1981
Edited by R. Steinitz, D.M. Parkin,
J.L. Young, C.A. Bieber and L. Katz
1989; 320 pages; ISBN 92 832 1198 7

No. 99
Pathology of Tumours in Laboratory
Animals, Second Edition, Volume 1,
Tumours of the Rat
Edited by V.S. Turusov and U. Mohr
1990; 740 pages; ISBN 92 832 1199 5

No. 100
Cancer: Causes, Occurrence and
Control
Editor-in-Chief: L. Tomatis
1990; 352 pages; ISBN 92 832 0110 8

No. 101
Directory of On-going Research in
Cancer Epidemiology 1989/90
Edited by M. Coleman and
J. Wahrendorf
1989; 828 pages; ISBN 92 832 2101 X

No. 102
Patterns of Cancer in Five Continents
Edited by S.L. Whelan, D.M. Parkin
and E. Masuyer
1990; 160 pages; ISBN 92 832 2102 8

No. 103
Evaluating Effectiveness of Primary
Prevention of Cancer
Edited by M. Hakama, V. Beral,
J.W. Cullen and D.M. Parkin
1990; 206 pages; ISBN 92 832 2103 6

No. 104
Complex Mixtures and Cancer Risk
Edited by H. Vainio, M. Sorsa and
A.J. McMichael
1990; 441 pages; ISBN 92 832 2104 4

No. 105
Relevance to Human Cancer of
N-Nitroso Compounds, Tobacco
Smoke and Mycotoxins
Edited by I.K. O'Neill, J. Chen and
H. Bartsch
1991; 614 pages; ISBN 92 832 2105 2

No. 106
Atlas of Cancer Incidence in the
Former German Democratic Republic
Edited by W.H. Mehnert, M. Smans,
C.S. Muir, M. Möhner and D. Schön
1992; 384 pages; ISBN 92 832 2106 0

No. 107
Atlas of Cancer Mortality in the
European Economic Community
Edited by M. Smans, C. Muir and
P. Boyle
1992; 213 pages +44 coloured maps;
ISBN 92 832 2107 9

No. 108
Environmental Carcinogens:
Methods of Analysis and Exposure
Measurement. Volume 11:
Polychlorinated Dioxins and
Dibenzofurans
Edited by C. Rappe, H.R. Buser,
B. Dodet and I.K. O'Neill
1991; 400 pages; ISBN 92 832 2108 7

No. 109
Environmental Carcinogens:
Methods of Analysis and Exposure
Measurement. Volume 12:
Indoor Air
Edited by B. Seifert, H. van de Wiel,
B. Dodet and I.K. O'Neill
1993; 385 pages; ISBN 92 832 2109 5

No. 110
Directory of On-going Research in
Cancer Epidemiology 1991
Edited by M.P. Coleman and
J. Wahrendorf
1991; 753 pages; ISBN 92 832 2110 9

No. 111
Pathology of Tumours in Laboratory
Animals, Second Edition. Volume 2:
Tumours of the Mouse
Edited by V. Turusov and U. Mohr
1994; 800 pages; ISBN 92 832 2111 1

No. 112
Autopsy in Epidemiology and Medical
Research
Edited by E. Riboli and M. Delendi
1991; 288 pages; ISBN 92 832 2112 5

No. 113
Laboratory Decontamination
and Destruction of Carcinogens
in Laboratory Wastes: Some
Mycotoxins
Edited by M. Castegnaro, J. Barek,
J.M. Frémy, M. Lafontaine, M. Miraglia,
E.B. Sansone and G.M. Telling
1991; 63 pages; ISBN 92 832 2113 3

No. 114
Laboratory Decontamination
and Destruction of Carcinogens
in Laboratory Wastes: Some Polycyclic
Heterocyclic Hydrocarbons
Edited by M. Castegnaro, J. Barek,
J. Jacob, U. Kirso, M. Lafontaine,
E.B. Sansone, G.M. Telling and
T. Vu Duc
1991; 50 pages; ISBN 92 832 2114 1

No. 115
Mycotoxins, Endemic Nephropathy and
Urinary Tract Tumours
Edited by M. Castegnaro, R. Plestina,
G. Dirheimer, I.N. Chernozemsky and
H. Bartsch
1991; 340 pages; ISBN 92 832 2115 X

*(out of print)

No. 116
Mechanisms of Carcinogenesis in Risk
Identification
Edited by H. Vainio, P. Magee,
D. McGregor and A.J. McMichael
1992; 615 pages; ISBN 92 832 2116 8

No. 117
Directory of On-going Research in
Cancer Epidemiology 1992
Edited by M. Coleman, E. Demaret and
J. Wahrendorf
1992; 773 pages; ISBN 92 832 2117 6

No. 118
Cadmium in the Human Environment:
Toxicity and Carcinogenicity
Edited by G.F. Nordberg, R.F.M. Herber
and L. Alessio
1992; 470 pages; ISBN 92 832 2118 4

No. 119
The Epidemiology of Cervical Cancer
and Human Papillomavirus
Edited by N. Muñoz, F.X. Bosch,
K.V. Shah and A. Meheus
1992; 288 pages; ISBN 92 832 2119 2

No. 120
Cancer Incidence in Five Continents,
Vol. VI
Edited by D.M. Parkin, C.S. Muir,
S.L. Whelan, Y.T. Gao, J. Ferlay
and J. Powell
1992; 1020 pages; ISBN 92 832 2120 6

No. 121
Time Trends in Cancer Incidence and
Mortality
By M. Coleman, J. Estève P. Damiecki,
A. Arslan and H. Renard
1993; 820 pages; ISBN 92 832 2121 4

No. 122
International Classification of Rodent
Tumours. Part I. The Rat
Editor-in-Chief: U. Mohr
1992-1996; 10 fascicles of 60–100
pages; ISBN 92 832 2122 2

No. 123
Cancer in Italian Migrant
Populations
Edited by M. Geddes, D.M. Parkin,
M. Khlat, D. Balzi and E. Buiatti
1993; 292 pages; ISBN 92 832 2123 0

No. 124
Postlabelling Methods for the Detection
of DNA Damage
Edited by D.H. Phillips, M. Castegnaro
and H. Bartsch 1993; 392 pages;
ISBN 92 832 2124 9

No. 125
DNA Adducts: Identification and
Biological Significance
Edited by K. Hemminki, A. Dipple,
D.E.G. Shuker, F.F. Kadlubar,
D. Segerbäck and H. Bartsch
1994; 478 pages; ISBN 92 832 2125 7

No. 126
Pathology of Tumours in Laboratory
Animals, Second Edition. Volume 3:
Tumours of the Hamster
Edited by V.S. Turusov and U. Mohr
1966; 465 pages; ISBN 92 836 2126 5

No. 127
Butadiene and Styrene: Assessment of
Health Hazards
Edited by M. Sorsa, K. Peltonen, H.
Vainio and K. Hemminki
1993; 412 pages; ISBN 92 832 2127 3

No. 128
Statistical Methods in Cancer Research.
Volume IV. Descriptive Epidemiology
By J. Estève, E. Benhamou and
L. Raymond
1994; 302 pages; ISBN 92 832 2128 1

No. 129
Occupational Cancer in Developing
. Countries
Edited by N. Pearce, E. Matos,
H. Vainio, P. Boffetta and M. Kogevinas
1994; 191 pages; ISBN 92 832 2129 X

No. 130
Directory of On-going Research in
Cancer Epidemiology 1994
Edited by R. Sankaranarayanan,
J. Wahrendorf and E. Démaret
1994; 800 pages; ISBN 92 832 2130 3

No. 132
Survival of Cancer Patients in Europe:
The EUROCARE Study
Edited by F. Berrino, M. Sant,
A. Verdecchia, R. Capocaccia,
T. Hakulinen and J. Estève
1995; 463 pages; ISBN 92 832 2132 X

No. 134
Atlas of Cancer Mortality in Central
Europe
W. Zatonski, J. Estève, M. Smans,
J. Tyczynski and P. Boyle
1996; 175 pages + 40 coloured maps
ISBN 92 832 2134 6

No. 136
Chemoprevention in Cancer Control
Edited by M. Hakama, V. Beral,
E. Buiatti, J. Faivre and D.M. Parkin
1996; 160 pages; ISBN 93 832 2136 2

No. 137
Directory of On-Going Research in
Cancer Epidemiology 1996
Edited by R. Sankaranarayanan, J.
Wahrendorf and E. Démaret
1996; 810 pages; ISBN 93 832 2137 0

IARC Monographs on the Evaluation of Carcinogenic Risks to Humans

Volume 1*
Some Inorganic Substances,
Chlorinated Hydrocarbons, Aromatic
Amines, N-Nitroso Compounds, and
Natural Products
1972; 184 pages; ISBN 92 832 1201 0

Volume 2*
Some Inorganic and Organometallic
Compounds
1973; 181 pages; ISBN 92 832 1202 9

Volume 3*
Certain Polycyclic Aromatic
Hydrocarbons and Heterocyclic
Compounds
1973; 271 pages; ISBN 92 832 1203 7

Volume 4
Some Aromatic Amines, Hydrazine
and Related Substances, N-Nitroso
Compounds and Miscellaneous
Alkylating Agents
1974; 286 pages; ISBN 92 832 1204 5

Volume 5*
Some Organochlorine Pesticides
1974; 241 pages; ISBN 92 832 1205 3

Volume 6*
Sex Hormones
1974; 243 pages; ISBN 92 832 1206 1

Volume 7*
Some Anti-Thyroid and Related
Substances, Nitrofurans and Industrial
Chemicals
1974; 326 pages; ISBN 92 832 1207 X

Volume 8
Some Aromatic Azo Compounds
1975; 357 pages; ISBN 92 832 1208 8

Volume 9
Some Aziridines, N-, S- and O-Mustards
and Selenium
1975; 268 pages; ISBN 92 832 1209 6

Volume 10*
Some Naturally Occurring
Substances
1976; 353 pages; ISBN 92 832 1210 X

Volume 11*
Cadmium, Nickel, Some Epoxides,
Miscellaneous Industrial Chemicals
and General Considerations on Volatile
Anaesthetics
1976; 306 pages; ISBN 92 832 1211 8

Volume 12
Some Carbamates, Thiocarbamates
and Carbazides
1976; 282 pages; ISBN 92 832 1212 6

Volume 13
Some Miscellaneous Pharmaceutical
Substances
1977; 255 pages; ISBN 92 832 1213 4

Volume 14*
Asbestos
1977; 106 pages; ISBN 92 832 1214 2

Volume 15*
Some Fumigants, the Herbicides
2,4-D and 2,4,5-T, Chlorinated
Dibenzodioxins and Miscellaneous
Industrial Chemicals
1977; 354 pages; ISBN 92 832 1215 0

Volume 16
Some Aromatic Amines and Related
Nitro Compounds – Hair Dyes,
Colouring Agents and Miscellaneous
Industrial Chemicals
1978; 400 pages; ISBN 92 832 1216 9

Volume 17
Some N-Nitroso Compounds
1978; 365 pages; ISBN 92 832 1217 7

Volume 18
Polychlorinated Biphenyls and
Polybrominated Biphenyls
1978; 140 pages; ISBN 92 832 1218 5

Volume 19*
Some Monomers, Plastics and
Synthetic Elastomers, and Acrolein
1979; 513 pages; ISBN 92 832 1219 3

Volume 20*
Some Halogenated Hydrocarbons
1979; 609 pages; ISBN 92 832 1220 7

Volume 21
Sex Hormones (II)
1979; 583 pages; ISBN 92 832 1521 4

Volume 22
Some Non-Nutritive Sweetening Agents
1980; 208 pages; ISBN 92 832 1522 2

Volume 23*
Some Metals and Metallic Compounds
1980; 438 pages; ISBN 92 832 1523 0

Volume 24
Some Pharmaceutical Drugs
1980; 337 pages; ISBN 92 832 1524 9

Volume 25
Wood, Leather and Some Associated
Industries.
1981; 412 pages; ISBN 92 832 1525 7

Volume 26
Some Antineoplastic and Immuno-

suppressive Agents.
1981; 411 pages; ISBN 92 832 1526 5

Volume 27
Some Aromatic Amines, Anthraqui-
nones and Nitroso Compounds, and
Inorganic Fluorides Used in Drinking
Water and Dental Preparations
1982; 341 pages; ISBN 92 832 1527 3

Volume 28
The Rubber Industry
1982; 486 pages; ISBN 92 832 1528 1

Volume 29
Some Industrial Chemicals and Dyestuffs
1982; 416 pages; ISBN 92 832 1529 X

Volume 30
Miscellaneous Pesticides
1983; 424 pages; ISBN 92 832 1530 3

Volume 31
Some Food Additives, Feed Additives
and Naturally Occurring Substances
1983; 314 pages; ISBN 92 832 1531 1

Volume 32
Polynuclear Aromatic Compounds,
Part 1: Chemical, Environmental and
Experimental Data.
1983; 477 pages; ISBN 92 832 1532 X

Volume 33*
Polynuclear Aromatic Compounds,
Part 2: Carbon Blacks, Mineral Oils
and Some Nitroarenes
1984; 245 pages; ISBN 92 832 1533 8

Volume 34
Polynuclear Aromatic Compounds,
Part 3: Industrial Exposures in
Aluminium Production, Coal
Gasification, Coke Production, and
Iron and Steel Founding
1984; 219 pages; ISBN 92 832 1534 6

Volume 35
Polynuclear Aromatic Compounds:
Part 4: Bitumens, Coal-Tars and Derived Products, Shale-Oils and Soots
1985; 271 pages; ISBN 92 832 1535 4

Volume 36
Allyl Compounds, Aldehydes, Epoxides
and Peroxides
1985; 369 pages; ISBN 92 832 1536 2

Volume 37
Tobacco Habits Other than Smoking;
Betel-Quid and Areca-Nut Chewing;
and Some Related Nitrosamines
1985; 291 pages; ISBN 92 832 1537 0

*(out of print)

Volume 38
Tobacco Smoking
1986; 421 pages; ISBN 92 832 1538 9

Volume 39
Some Chemicals Used in Plastics and
Elastomers
1986; 403 pages; ISBN 92 832 1239 8

Volume 40
Some Naturally Occurring and
Synthetic Food Components, Furo-
coumarins and Ultraviolet Radiation
1986; 444 pages; ISBN 92 832 1240 1

Volume 41
Some Halogenated Hydrocarbons
and Pesticide Exposures
1986; 434 pages; ISBN 92 832 1241 X

Volume 42
Silica and Some Silicates
1987; 289 pages; ISBN 92 832 1242 8

Volume 43
Man-Made Mineral Fibres and Radon
1988; 300 pages; ISBN 92 832 1243 6

Volume 44
Alcohol Drinking.
1988; 416 pages; ISBN 92 832 1244 4

Volume 45
Occupational Exposures in Petroleum
Refining; Crude Oil and Major Petroleum Fuels.
1989; 322 pages; ISBN 92 832 1245 2

Volume 46
Diesel and Gasoline Engine Exhausts
and Some Nitroarenes
1989; 458 pages; ISBN 92 832 1246 0

Volume 47
Some Organic Solvents, Resin
Monomers and Related Compounds,
Pigments and Occupational Exposures
in Paint Manufacture and Painting
1989; 535 pages; ISBN 92 832 1247 9

Volume 48
Some Flame Retardants and Textile
Chemicals, and Exposures in the
Textile Manufacturing Industry
1990; 345 pages; ISBN: 92 832 1248 7

Volume 49
Chromium, Nickel and Welding
1990; 677 pages; ISBN: 92 832 1249 5

Volume 50
Some Pharmaceutical Drugs
1990; 415 pages; ISBN 92 832 1259 9

Volume 51
Coffee, Tea, Mate, Methylxanthines
and Methylglyoxal
1991; 513 pages; ISBN: 92 832 1251 7

Volume 52
Chlorinated Drinking-Water; Chlori-
nation By-products; Some other Halogenated Compounds; Cobalt and
Cobalt Compounds
1991; 544 pages; ISBN: 92 832 1252 5

Volume 53
Occupational Exposures in Insecticide
Application, and Some Pesticides
1991; 612 pages; ISBN 92 832 1253 3

Volume 54
Occupational Exposures to Mists and
Vapours from Strong Inorganic Acids;
and other Industrial Chemicals
1992; 336 pages; ISBN 92 832 1254 1

Volume 55
Solar and Ultraviolet Radiation
1992; 316 pages; ISBN 92 832 1255 X

Volume 56
Some Naturally Occurring Substances:
Food Items and Constituents, Heterocyclic Aromatic Amines and Mycotoxins
1993; 600 pages; ISBN 92 832 1256 8

Volume 57
Occupational Exposures of Hair-
dressers and Barbers and Personal
Use of Hair Colourants; Some Hair
Dyes, Cosmetic Colourants, Industrial
Dyestuffs and Aromatic Amines
1993; 428 pages; ISBN 92 832 1257 6

Volume 58
Beryllium, Cadmium, Mercury and
Exposures in the Glass Manufacturing
Industry
1994; 444 pages; ISBN 92 832 1258 4

Volume 59
Hepatitis Viruses
1994; 286 pages; ISBN 92 832 1259 2

Volume 60
Some Industrial Chemicals
1994; 560 pages; ISBN 92 832 1260 6

Volume 61
Schistosomes, Liver Flukes and
Helicobacter pylori
1994; 270 pages; ISBN 92 832 1261 4

Volume 62
Wood Dusts and Formaldehyde
1995; 405 pages; ISBN 92 832 1262 2

Volume 63
Dry cleaning, Some chlorinated
Solvents and Other Industrial
Chemicals
1995; 551 pages; ISBN 92 832 1263 0

Volume 64
Human Papillomaviruses
1995; 409 pages; ISBN 92 832 1264 9

Volume 65
Printing Processes, Printing Inks,
Carbon Blacks and Some Nitro
Compounds
1996; 578 pages; ISBN 92 832 1265 7

Supplements to Monographs

Supplement No. 1*
Chemicals and Industrial Processes
Associated with Cancer in Humans
(IARC Monographs, Volumes 1 to 20)
1979; 71 pages; ISBN 92 832 1402 1

Supplement No. 2
Long-Term and Short-Term Screening
Assays for Carcinogens:
A Critical Appraisal
1980; 426 pages; ISBN 92 832 1404 8

Supplement No. 3*
Cross Index of Synonyms and Trade
Names in Volumes 1 to 26
1982; 199 pages; ISBN 92 832 1405 6

Supplement No. 4*
Chemicals, Industrial Processes and
Industries Associated with Cancer in
Humans (IARC Monographs,
Volumes 1 to 29)
1982; 292 pages; ISBN 92 832 1407 2

Supplement No. 5*
Cross Index of Synonyms and Trade
Names in Volumes 1 to 36
1985; 259 pages; ISBN 92 832 1408 0

Supplement No. 6
Genetic and Related Effects: An
Updating of Selected IARC
Monographs from Volumes 1 to 42
1987; 729 pages; ISBN 92 832 1409 9

Supplement No. 7
Overall Evaluations of Carcinogenicity:
An Updating of IARC Monographs
Volumes 1 to 42
1987; 440 pages; ISBN 92 832 1411 0

Supplement No. 8
Cross Index of Synonyms and Trade
Names in Volumes 1 to 46
1989; 346 pages; ISBN 92 832 1417 X

*(out of print)

IARC Technical Reports

No. 1
Cancer in Costa Rica
Edited by R. Sierra, R. Barrantes,
G. Muñoz Leiva, D.M. Parkin, C.A.
Bieber and N. Muñoz Calero
1988; 124 pages; ISBN 92 832 1412 9

No. 2*
SEARCH: A Computer Package to
Assist the Statistical Analysis of
Case-Control Studies
Edited by G.J. Macfarlane, P. Boyle
and P. Maisonneuve
1991; 80 pages; ISBN 92 832 1413 7

No. 3
Cancer Registration in the European
Economic Community
Edited by M.P. Coleman and E.
Démaret
1988; 188 pages; ISBN 92 832 1414 5

No. 4
Diet, Hormones and Cancer: Methodo-
logical Issues for Prospective Studies
Edited by E. Riboli and R. Saracci
1988; 156 pages; ISBN 92 832 1415 3

No. 5
Cancer in the Philippines
Edited by A.V. Laudico, D. Esteban and
D.M. Parkin
1989; 186 pages; ISBN 92 832 1416 1

No. 6
La genèse du Centre international de
recherche sur le cancer
By R. Sohier and A.G.B. Sutherland
1990, 102 pages; ISBN 92 832 1418 8

No. 7
Epidémiologie du cancer dans les
pays de langue latine
1990, 292 pages; ISBN 92 832 1419 6

No. 8
Comparative Study of Anti-smoking
Legislation in Countries of the
European Economic Community
By A. J. Sasco, P. Dalla-Vorgia and
P. Van der Elst
1992; 82 pages; ISBN: 92 832 1421 8
Also available in French
(ISBN 92 832 2402 7)

No. 9
Epidémiologie du cancer dans les
pays de langue latine
1991; 346 pages; ISBN 92 832 1423 4

No. 10
Manual for Cancer Registry Personnel
Edited by D. Esteban, S. Whelan,
A. Laudico and D.M. Parkin
1995; 400 pages; ISBN 92 832 1424 2

No. 11
Nitroso Compounds: Biological
Mechanisms, Exposures and Cancer
Etiology
Edited by I. O'Neill and H. Bartsch
1992; 150 pages; ISBN 92 832 1425 X

No. 12
Epidémiologie du cancer dans les
pays de langue latine
1992; 375 pages; ISBN 92 832 1426 9

No. 13
Health, Solar UV Radiation and
Environmental Change
By A. Kricker, B.K. Armstrong, M.E.
Jones and R.C. Burton
1993; 213 pages; ISBN 92 832 1427 7

No. 14
Epidémiologie du cancer dans les
pays de langue latine
1993; 400 pages; ISBN 92 832 1428 5

No. 15
Cancer in the African Population of
Bulawayo, Zimbabwe, 1963–1977
By M.E.G. Skinner, D.M. Parkin,
A.P. Vizcaino and A. Ndhlovu
1993; 120 pages; ISBN 92 832 1429 3

No. 16
Cancer in Thailand 1984–1991
By V. Vatanasapt, N. Martin, H. Sriplung,
K. Chindavijak, S. Sontipong,
S. Sriamporn, D.M. Parkin and J. Ferlay
1993; 164 pages; ISBN 92 832 1430 7

No. 18
Intervention Trials for Cancer
Prevention
By E. Buiatti
1994; 52 pages; ISBN 92 832 1432 3

No. 19
Comparability and Quality Control in
Cancer Registration
By D.M. Parkin, V.W. Chen, J. Ferlay,
J. Galceran, H.H. Storm and
S.L. Whelan
1994; 110 pages; plus diskette;
ISBN 92 832 1433 1
Also available in French
(ISBN 92 832 2403 5)
and Spanish
(ISBN 92 832 0402 6)

No. 20
Epidémiologie du cancer dans les
pays de langue latine
1994; 346 pages; ISBN 92 832 1434 X

No. 21
ICD Conversion Programs for Cancer
By J Ferlay
1994; 24 pages plus diskette;
ISBN 92 832 1435 8

No. 22
Cancer in Tianjin
By Q.S. Wang, P. Boffetta, M. Kogevinas
and D.M. Parkin
1994; 96 pages; ISBN 92 832 1433 1

No. 23
An Evaluation Programme for Cancer
Preventive Agents
By Bernard W. Stewart
1995; 40 pages; ISBN 92 832 1438 2

No. 24
Peroxisome Proliferation and its
Role in Carcinogenesis. Views and
expert opinions of an IARC Working
Group
1995; 85 pages; ISBN 92 832 1439 0

No. 25
Combined Analysis of Cancer Mortality
in Nuclear Workers in Canada, the
United Kingdom and the United States
of America
By E. Cardis, E.S. Gilbert, L. Carpen-
ter, G. Howe, I. Kato, J. Fix, L. Salmon,
G. Cowper, B.K. Armstrong, V. Beral,
A. Douglas, S.A. Fry, J. Kaldor,C. Lavé,
P.G. Smith, G. Voelz and L. Wiggs
1995; 160 pages; ISBN 92 832 1440 4

*(out of print)

Directories of Agents being Tested for Carcinogenicity

No. 14
Edited by M.-J. Ghess, J.D. Wilbourn and H. Vainio
1990; 369 pages; ISBN 92 832 1314 9

No. 15
Edited by M.-J. Ghess, J.D. Wilbourn and H. Vainio
1992; 317 pages; ISBN 92 832 1315 7

No. 16
Edited by M.-J. Ghess, J.D. Wilbourn and H. Vainio
1994; 294 pages; ISBN 92 832 1316 5

No. 17
Edited by A. Meneghel and J.D. Wilbourn
1996; 360 pages; ISBN 92 832 1317 3

Non-serial publications

Alcool et Cancer
By A. Tuyns
1978; 48 pages; ISBN 92 832 2401 9

Cancer Morbidity and Causes of Death among Danish Brewery Workers
By O.M. Jensen
1980; 143 pages; ISBN 92 832 1403 X

Directory of Computer Systems Used in Cancer Registries
By H.R. Menck and D.M. Parkin
1986; 236 pages

Facts and Figures of Cancer in the European Community
By J. Estève, A. Kricker, J. Ferlay and D.M. Parkin
1993; 52 pages; ISBN 92 832 1437 4

IARC Monographs and Technical Reports are available from the World Health Organization Distribution and Sales, CH-1211 Geneva 27 (Fax: +41 22 791 4857) and from WHO Sales Agents worldwide.

IARC Scientific Publications are available from Oxford University Press, Walton Street, Oxford, UK OX2 6DP (Fax: +44 1865 267782).

All IARC Publications are also available directly from IARCPress, 150 Cours Albert Thomas, F-69372 Lyon cedex 08, France (Fax: +33 72 73 83 02; E-mail: press@iarc.fr).